Genes, Hearing, and Deafness
From Molecular Biology to Clinical Practice

Edited by

Alessandro Martini
Audiology and ENT Clinical Institute
University of Ferrara
Ferrara Italy

Dafydd Stephens
School of Medicine
Cardiff University
Cardiff Wales

Andrew P Read
Department of Medical Genetics
St Mary's Hospital
Manchester UK

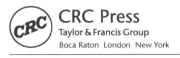

CRC Press
Taylor & Francis Group
Boca Raton London New York

CRC Press is an imprint of the
Taylor & Francis Group, an **informa** business

CRC Press
Taylor & Francis Group
6000 Broken Sound Parkway NW, Suite 300
Boca Raton, FL 33487-2742

First issued in paperback 2019

© 2007 by Taylor & Francis Group, LLC
CRC Press is an imprint of Taylor & Francis Group, an Informa business

No claim to original U.S. Government works

ISBN-13: 978-0-415-38359-2 (hbk)
ISBN-13: 978-0-367-38899-7 (pbk)

A CIP record for this book is available from the British Library.
Library of Congress Cataloging-in-Publication Data

Composition by Egerton + Techset.

Visit the Taylor & Francis Web site at
http://www.taylorandfrancis.com

and the CRC Press Web site at
http://www.crcpress.com

Contents

List of contributors   v

Preface   ix

PART I: GENETICS AND HEARING IMPAIRMENT

1   Understanding the genotype: basic concepts   3
Andrew P Read

2   Understanding the phenotype: basic concepts in audiology   19
Silvano Prosser, Alessandro Martini

3   Newly emerging concepts in syndromology relevant to audiology   39
and otolaryngology practice
William Reardon

4   Deafblindness   55
Claes Möller

5   Nonsyndromic hearing loss: cracking the cochlear code   63
Rikkert L Snoeckx, Guy Van Camp

6   Age-related hearing impairment: ensemble playing of environmental and genetic factors   79
Lut Van Laer, Guy Van Camp

7   Noise-related hearing impairment   91
Ilmari Pyykkö, Esko Toppila, Jing Zou, Howard T Jacobs, Erna Kentala

8   Otosclerosis: a genetic update   111
Frank Declau, Paul Van De Heyning

9   Mitochondrial DNA, hearing impairment, and ageing   121
Kia Minkkinen, Howard T Jacobs

PART II: CURRENT MANAGEMENT

10   Psychosocial aspects of genetic hearing impairment   145
Dafydd Stephens

11   Attitudes of deaf people and their families towards issues surrounding genetics   163
Anna Middleton

12   Genetics of communication disorders   173
Elisabetta Genovese, Rosalia Galizia, Rosamaria Santarelli, Edoardo Arslan

13   Audiometric profiles associated with genetic nonsyndromal hearing   185
impairment: a review and phenotype analysis
Patrick L M Huygen, Robert Jan Pauw, Cor W R J Cremers

14   Early detection and assessment of genetic childhood hearing impairment   205
Agnete Parving

15   What genetic testing can offer   213
      Paolo Gasparini, Andrew P Read

16   Pharmacotherapy of the inner ear   219
      Ilmari Pyykkö, Esko Toppila, Jing Zou, Erna Kentala

17   Diagnosis and management strategies in congenital middle and external ear anomalies   239
      Frank Declau, Paul Van De Heyning

18   Cochlear implantation in genetic deafness   253
      Richard Ramsden, Shakeel Saeed, Rhini Aggarwal

19   Auditory neuropathy caused by the otoferlin gene mutation   263
      Constantino Morera, Laura Cavallé, Diego Collado, Felipe Moreno

PART III: THE FUTURE

20   Innovative therapeutical strategies to prevent deafness and to treat tinnitus   271
      Jian Wang, Matthieu Guitton, Jérôme Ruel, Rémy Pujol, Jean-Luc Puel

21   Stem cells in the inner ear: advancing towards a new therapy for hearing impairment   279
      Marcelo N Rivolta

22   Tissue transplantation into the inner ear   289
      Mats Ulfendahl

23   Gene therapy of the inner ear   299
      M Pfister, A K Lalwani

24   Mechanisms for hair cell protection and regeneration in the mammalian organ of Corti   305
      Sara Euteneuer, Allen F Ryan

Index   313

Contributors

Rhini Aggarwal
Department of Otolaryngology
Manchester Royal Infirmary
Manchester UK

Edoardo Arslan
Department of Audiology and Phoniatrics
University of Padova
Padova Italy

Laura Cavallé
Department of Otorhinolaryngology
University Hospital La Fe
Valencia Spain

Diego Collado
Department of Otorhinolaryngology
University Hospital La Fe
Valencia Spain

Cor W R J Cremers
Department of Otolaryngology
Radboud University Medical Center
Nijmegen The Netherlands

Frank Declau
Department of Otorhinolaryngology,
    Head and Neck Surgery and
    Communication Disorders
University of Antwerp
Antwerp Belgium

Sara Euteneuer
Department of Surgery/Otolaryngology
University of California San Diego (UCSD)
    School of Medicine
La Jolla CA USA

Department of Otorhinolaryngology
St. Elisabeth-Hospital
Ruhr-University Boschum School of Medicine
Bochum Germany

Rosalia Galizia
Department of Audiology and Phoniatrics
University of Padova
Padova Italy

Paolo Gasparini
Medical Genetics
Department of Reproductive Sciences and Development
University of Trieste
Trieste Italy

Elisabetta Genovese
Department of Audiology and Phoniatrics
University of Padova
Padova Italy

Matthieu Guitton
INSERM, U583
Laboratoire de Physiopathólogie et Thérapie des Déficits
Sensoriels et Moteurs
Montpellier France

Patrick L M Huygen
Department of Otolaryngology
Radboud University Medical Center
Nijmegen The Netherlands

Howard T Jacobs
Institute of Medical Technology
University of Tampere
Tampere Finland

Erna Kentala
Department of Otolaryngology
University of Helsinki
Helsinki Finland

A K Lalwani
Department of Otolaryngology and
    Head and Neck Surgery
University of Tübingen
Tübingen Germany

Alessandro Martini
Audiology and ENT Clinical Institute
University of Ferrara
Ferrara Italy

Anna Middleton
Institute of Medical Genetics
School of Medicine
Cardiff University
Cardiff Wales

Kia Minkkinen
Institute of Medical Technology
University of Tampere
Tampere Finland

Claes Möller
Department of Audiology
The Swedish Institute of Disability Research
Örelro University Hospital
Örelro Sweden

Felipe Moreno
Institute of Molecular Genetics
Hospital Ramon y Cajal
Madrid Spain

Constantino Morera
Department of Otorhinolaryngology
University Hospital La Fe
Valencia Spain

Agnete Parving
Department of Audiology
HS Bispebjerg Hospital
Copenhagen Denmark

Robert Jan Pauw
Department of Otolaryngology
Radboud University Medical Center
Nijmegen The Netherlands

Markus Pfister
Department of Otolaryngology and
Head and Neck Surgery
University of Tübingen
Tübingen Germany

Silvano Prosser
Audiology Unit and ENT Clinical Institute
University of Ferrara
Ferrara Italy

Jean-Luc Puel
INSERM, U583
Laboratoire de Physiopathólogie et
    Thérapie des Déficits Sensoriels
    et Moteurs
UMR-S583
Université Montpellier
Montpellier France

Rémy Pujol
INSERM, U583
Laboratoire de Physiopathólogie et Thérapie des Déficits
Sensoriels et Moteurs
UMR-S583
Université Montpellier
Montpellier France

Ilmari Pyykkö
Department of Otolaryngology
University of Tampere
Tampere Finland

Richard Ramsden
Department of Otolaryngology
Manchester Royal Infirmary
Manchester UK

Andrew P Read
Department of Medical Genetics
St Mary's Hospital
Manchester UK

William Reardon
Our Lady's Hospital for Sick Children
Dublin Ireland

Marcelo N Rivolta
Centre for Stem Cell Biology
Department of Biomedical Sciences
University of Sheffield
Sheffield UK

Jérôme Ruel
INSERM, U583
Laboratoire de Physiopathólogie et
    Thérapie des Déficits Sensoriels et Moteurs
Montpellier France

Allen F Ryan
Department of Surgery/Otolaryngology
    and Neuroscience
University of California San Diego (UCSD)
    School of Medicine
La Jolla CA USA

Shakeel Saeed
Department of Otolaryngology
Manchester Royal Infirmary
Manchester UK

Rosamaria Santarelli
Department of Audiology and Phoniatrics
University of Padova
Padova Italy

Rikkert L Snoeckx
Department of Medical Genetics
University of Antwerp
Antwerp Belgium

Dafydd Stephens
School of Medicine
Cardiff University
Cardiff Wales

Esko Toppila
Institute of Occupational Health
Helsinki Finland

Mats Ulfendahl
Center for Hearing and
*   Communication Research*
Karolinska Institutet
Stockholm Sweden

Guy Van Camp
Department of Medical Genetics
University of Antwerp
Antwerp Belgium

Paul Van De Heyning
Department of Otorhinolaryngology, Head and
*   Neck Surgery and Communication Disorders*
University of Antwerp
Antwerp Belgium

Lut Van Laer
Department of Medical Genetics
University of Antwerp
Antwerp Belgium

Jian Wang
INSERM, U583
Laboratoire de Physiopathólogie et hérapie des Déficits
Sensoriels et Moteurs
Montpellier France

Jing Zou
Department of Otolaryngology
University of Tampere
Tampere Finland

Preface

Frequently, hearing impairment has been considered to require no more than the provision of a hearing aid, with little understanding of the need for thorough aetiological investigation to ensure prevention and remediation where possible and structured rehabilitation programmes, if the distressing personal and social consequences of hearing impairment are to be avoided.

It is worth pointing out that one in every 1,000 new-born babies suffers from congenital severe or profound hearing impairment. Furthermore, epidemiological studies demonstrate that the percentage of the population who have a hearing impairment that exceeds 45 dB HL and 65 dB HL are about 1.3% and 0.3% between the ages of 30 and 50 years, and 7.4% and 2.3% between the ages of 60 and 70 years, respectively (Davis, 1989). Hearing loss has for some time, been considered a permanent effect and consequence of factors such as infections, ototoxicity, trauma and ageing. In recent years, molecular biology and molecular genetics have made a key contribution to the understanding of the normal and defective inner ear, not only in congenital profound hearing impairment but also in late onset/progressive hearing impairment.

The HEAR and GENDEAF projects

In September 1994, when a Preparatory Workshop for the Constitution of a European study group on genetic deafness was held in Milan, only four loci of non-syndromal hearing impairment and only three genes responsible for syndromal hearing impairment had been discovered, whereas at the time of writing, some 45 genes which can cause non-syndromal hearing impairment have been identifies and over 110 loci found.

The importance of establishing common terminology and definitions and co-ordinating the multi-disciplinary approach was the core aim of HEAR project-European Concerted Action HEAR (Hereditary Deafness: Epidemiology and Clinical Research 1996–1999). The idea was to deal with the problem of combining clinical in-depth family and phenotype studies with basic molecular genetics and gene mapping methods in a more standardized way, with the aim of establishing a stable international collaboration. The initiative also wanted to create a bank of updated information on these disorders that would be useful not only to experts but to the entire scientific community in identifying sources of information and specialized centres to which specific cases may be referred. This project stimulated a considerable amount of work in this field leading to developments in molecular genetics and the mapping of human loci associated with hearing disorders. The numerous and scattered loci mapped reflect a heterogeneous set of genes and mechanisms responsible for human hearing and suggest a complicated interaction between these genes (Lalwani and Castelein, 1999).

GENDEAF European Union Thematic Network Project 2001–2005 has helped to further open and widen the analysis of genotype/phenotype correlations, the effects of deafness on the family and the psychosocial aspects (also involving patient associations).

This book is aimed as a follow up of these two projects. It endeavours to provide a broad and up to date overview of genetic hearing impairment for audiologists, otolaryngologists, paediatricians and clinical geneticists to improve the quality of care for the large group of patients with suspected genetic hearing impairment. It does not set out to be a comprehensive description of syndromes such as the excellent and complete text of Toriello, Reardon, and Gorlin (2004), but to provide an easily read sourcebook for those students and clinicians with an interest in this field.

The book is divided into three parts:

The first part reports the important elements of current knowledge of the various situations in which genes have an influence on inner ear dysfunction. Chapters 1 and 2 provide the reader with an appropriate background, presenting an introduction to auditory function, basic genetics and genetic techniques significant to this field. Chapter 3 does not list the various syndromes, but intends to discuss and help clinicians to interpret the signs in order to better understand how molecular genetics can be informative. Chapter 4 tackles the complex genetic aspect of deaf/blindness. Chapter 5 analyses the role of the various genes as a causative of non-syndromal hearing loss. Chapters 6 to 9 analyse the responsibility of genetic factors in certain complex situations such as ageing, noise exposure, ototoxic drugs and otosclerosis.

Part II discusses current approaches to and management of hearing impairment in different ways. Thus Chapters 10 and 11 review the psychosocial impact of genetic hearing impairment and how culturally Deaf people react to genetic interventions. Chapter 12 looks at the related area of genetic factors in speech and language while Chapters 13 to 15 provide guidance on the identification of specific genotypes from phenotypic information, steps which should be taken in this respect in deaf children and how geneticists approach such a challenge. Developments in the pharmacological approach to hearing impairment and tinnitus are covered in Chapters 16 and 20, while Chapters 17 to 19 discuss the medical and surgical management of specific genetic disorders affecting the outer/middle ear, the cochlea and the cochlear nerve respectively.

Finally, the third part delves into our future and is an update of various lines of research covering a range of therapeutic strategies. These include the use of stem cells, tissue transplantation into the inner ear, gene therapy and finishes with an overview of the important process of apoptosis and how it can be prevented.

The contributing experts are all authoritative in their fields and have been asked to present up to date, concise and brief reviews of their particular subject matter; the reader should find this book follows the rapid pace of change in medical science.

Alessandro Martini
Dafydd Stephens
Andrew P Read
Editors

Part I
Genetics and hearing impairment

1 Understanding the genotype: basic concepts

Andrew P Read

Introduction

This chapter is for readers who feel threatened by genetics, who are apt to see genetics as a malignant growth, taking over familiar areas of medicine and rendering them strange and incomprehensible. It is a survival kit but also an entry ticket to this most intellectually exciting area of biomedical science. Genetics is not taking over medicine; it is burrowing under it and rearranging the foundations. Genetics is relevant to hearing and deafness at two levels. In everyday clinical practice, effective diagnosis and management of patients require some familiarity with common patterns of inheritance and with the availability, use, and limitations of genetic tests. More fundamentally, to understand the causes and pathology of hearing impairments, we need to understand the molecular pathology of the genes that program cells in the inner ear. What follows is a review of the concepts and vocabulary of genetics as it applies to both these levels. Italicised words are defined in the Glossary at the end of this chapter. For readers who would like more detail, references are given below to the relevant sections of Strachan & Read Human Molecular Genetics; the text of the second edition ("S&R2") is freely available on the NCBI Bookshelf website (1).

Genes, DNA, and chromosomes

These are the three most basic elements in genetics. "Genes," like elephants, are easier to recognize than to define. Unlike elephants, genes are recognised in two fundamentally different ways:

- As determinants of characters that segregate in pedigrees according to Mendel's laws
- As functional units of DNA

Genes recognised in the first way are rather formal, abstract entities. In retrospect, their connection to physical objects began early, with the recognition of chromosomes and crystallised with Avery's 1943 demonstration that the genetic substance of bacteria was DNA. However, it was not until the 1970s that physical investigation of genes acquired any clinical relevance. Developments in molecular genetics in no way make formal mendelian genetics obsolete. The ability to recognize mendelian pedigree patterns and calculate genetic risks remains an essential clinical skill, while understanding the relation between the DNA sequence and an observable character is a central intellectual challenge of genetics.

DNA is the molecule that carries genetic information. For understanding most of genetics, it is sufficient to view DNA as a long chain of four types of unit called A, G, C, and T. Organic chemists define the structure of A, G, C, and T as nucleotides (nts), each composed of a base (adenine, guanine, cytosine, or thymine) linked to a sugar, deoxyribose, and a phosphate. Watson and Crick in 1953 showed how DNA consists of two polynucleotide chains wrapped round one another in a double helix. The two strands fit together like the two halves of a zip, with A on one chain always next to T on the other, and G always opposite C. As Watson and Crick famously remarked, "it has not escaped our notice that the specific pairing we have postulated immediately suggests a possible copying mechanism for the genetic material." Note, however, that in itself the Watson-Crick structure sheds no light on how the sequence of nucleotides along a DNA chain might control the characteristics of an organism—understanding of that process only began to dawn in the 1960s. Chapter 1 of S&R2 provides rather more detail on DNA structure and function.

Geneticists use some conventions and shortcuts in describing DNA that can confuse the unwary.

- The terms base, nucleotide, and base pair (bp) are normally used interchangeably to describe the A, G, C, and T units of a DNA chain, although strictly they mean different things. A double helix with 100 units in each chain is 100 bases, 100 nt, or 100 bp long (not 200).

- Looking at the detailed chemical structure shows that DNA chains are not symmetrical. The two ends are different and so the sequence AGTC is not the same as the sequence CTGA. The ends are labelled 5′ ("5 prime") and 3′, and it is a universal convention that sequences are always written in the 5′→3′ direction. It is just as wrong and unnatural to write a sequence in the 3′→5′ direction as it is to write an English word from right to left. This may seem a trivial and pedantic point, but its importance comes from the fact that the two chains in a Watson–Crick double helix run in opposite directions (the structure is described as antiparallel). Thus the strand complementary to AGTC is not TCAG but (5′→3′) GACT.

- Geneticists are no happier than anybody else about the way this makes a sequence and its complement look very different, and they get round it by a convention that makes the relation between the sequence of a gene, a messenger RNA (mRNA), and (via a table of the genetic code) a protein all immediately obvious. So for most purposes you can forget about 5′ and 3′, but the convention needs mentioning because otherwise readers with enquiring minds will run up against seemingly baffling inconsistencies. (see section 3.2 for the detail.)

"Chromosomes" (Fig. 1.1) are seen in cells when they divide. These visible chromosomes represent the DNA packaged into a set of compact bundles so that it can be divided up between the daughter cells. The 46 human chromosomes (23 pairs) each contain between 45 and 280 million base pairs (Mb) of DNA in the form of a single immensely long double helix. Before a cell divides, it replicates all its DNA. When the chromosomes become visible, each consists of two identical sister chromatids, each containing a complete copy of the DNA of that chromosome. Cell division separates the two chromatids, sending one into each daughter cell, and in their normal state each chromosome consists of a single chromatid but with the DNA somewhat decondensed and fluffed out so that it is not visible under the microscope. Even in this state, the DNA is still quite highly structured. It exists as chromatin, a complex of DNA, and various proteins, particularly histones. Chapter 2 of S&R2 describes and illustrates the structure and function of chromosomes.

Back in the 1880s, biologists recognised that there were two types of cell division. The usual form is mitosis. This precisely divides the replicated genetic material between the two daughter cells so that each is genetically identical. All the normal cells of a person are derived by repeated mitosis from the original fertilised egg. That is why you can use a blood, skin, or any other sample to study somebody's DNA; it is the same in every cell (more or less). Gametes (sperm and egg) are formed by a special process, meiosis, which has two purposes. It halves the number of chromosomes so that a 23-chromosome sperm fertilizes a 23-chromosome egg to produce a 46-chromosome zygote. It also shuffles genes so that every sperm or egg that a person produces contains a novel combination of the genes he or she inherited from his or her mother and father. Mendelian pedigree patterns are a consequence of the events of meiosis. Linkage analysis, which maps a gene to a specific chromosomal region, also depends on features of meiosis, as detailed below.

Note the disparity between chromosomes and DNA. The smallest chromosome abnormality visible under the microscope involves around 5 Mb of DNA. Molecular genetic techniques are most efficient when dealing with no more than 1000 bp (1 kb) of DNA. New techniques that fill the gap between these two scales ("molecular cytogenetics") have been important recent drivers of genetic discovery.

Patterns of inheritance

Humans have around 25,000 genes and every human genetic character must depend on the action of very many genes, together with environmental factors. However, for some variable characters, presence or absence of the character depends, in most people and in most circumstances, on variation in a single gene. These are the mendelian or single-gene characters that are by far the easiest genetic characters to analyse. When following the segregation of alternative forms of a gene (alleles)

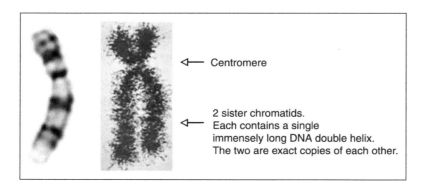

Figure 1.1 The structure of a chromosome as seen in a cell dividing by mitosis. (*Left image*) chromosome 9 as seen in a conventional cytogenetic preparation. The two sister chromatids are tightly pressed together. The banding pattern (G-banding) is produced by partial digestion with trypsin before staining with Giemsa stain. It helps the cytogeneticist to recognize chromosome abnormalities. (*Right image*) chromosome 9 as seen under the electron microscope. Threads of chromatin of diameter 30 nm can be seen, which form loops attached to a central protein scaffold (not visible). DNA is highly packaged even within the 30 nm thread. Overall, chromosome 9 is about 10 μm long and contains about 5 cm of DNA.

←— Centromere

←— 2 sister chromatids.
Each contains a single immensely long DNA double helix.
The two are exact copies of each other.

through a pedigree, the alleles are conventionally designated by upper and lower case forms of the same letter, e.g., "A" and "a."

The art of human pedigree interpretation is to make a judgment of the most likely mode of inheritance. The two main questions are the following questions:

▧ Is the character dominant or recessive?
▧ Is the gene autosomal, X-linked, or mitochondrial?

An initial hypothesis is formed by asking the following questions:

▧ Does each affected person have an affected parent? If so, the condition is probably dominant; if not, either it is recessive or something more complex is going on.
▧ Are there any sex effects? If not (affects both sexes, can be transmitted from father to son, from father to daughter, from mother to son, or from mother to daughter), the character is probably autosomal. If yes, it may be X-linked. Y-linked pedigrees are possible in theory but are unlikely in human diseases. Characters that are transmitted only by the mother, but affect both sexes, may be mitochondrial.

The pedigree is then tested for consistency with the initial hypothesis by writing in presumed genotypes. If this process requires special coincidences (an unrelated person marrying in, who happens to carry the same disease allele; a new mutation), alternative hypotheses are tested. The most likely interpretation is the one that requires the fewest coincidences. It is important to stress that for most pedigrees these interpretations are provisional because families are too small to be sure. Sometimes past experience tells us that a particular condition is always inherited in a particular way, but this is often not the case and particularly not with nonsyndromic hearing impairment.

Pedigree description of autosomal dominant inheritance. Both males and females can be affected. The disorder is transmitted from generation to generation and can be transmitted in all possible ways—female to female, female to male, male to female, or male to male. With human autosomal dominant diseases, affected people are almost always heterozygotes; when married to an unaffected person each offspring has a 50:50 chance of inheriting the mutant allele. In small families, the mode of inheritance can be difficult to determine, but transmission of a rare condition across three generations is good evidence for dominant inheritance. Many dominant conditions are variable (even within families) and may skip generations (nonpenetrance, see below).

Pedigree description of autosomal recessive inheritance. Both males and females can be affected. Both parents are usually unaffected heterozygous carriers, and the risk for any given child is 1 in 4. Recessive inheritance is likely when unaffected parents have more than one affected child, especially if the parents are consanguineous. In most cases, there is only one affected individual in the family, making the pedigree pattern hard to identify, but in large multiply inbred kindreds,

affected individuals may be seen in several branches of the family.

Pedigree description of X-linked inheritance. Many X-linked diseases are seen only or almost only in males; where females are affected, they may be more mildly or more variably affected. The X chromosome is transmitted to a male from his mother and never from his father, so male-to-male transmission rules out X-linked inheritance. The line of inheritance in a pedigree must go exclusively through females (or affected males). All daughters of an affected male are carriers.

Having the wrong number of chromosomes is usually fatal; yet males and females manage to be healthy despite having different numbers of X chromosomes. This is because of a special mechanism, X inactivation or Lyonisation (named after its discoverer, Mary Lyon). In each early embryo, each cell somehow counts the number of X chromosomes it contains. If there are two, each cell picks one at random and permanently inactivates it. The chromosome is still there, but the genes on it are permanently switched off. If there are more than two X chromosomes, all except one are inactivated. Thus every cell, male or female, has only one active X chromosome.

X inactivation happens only once in the early embryo, but the decision as to which X to inactivate is remembered. As the few cells of the early XX embryo divide and divide, whichever X was inactivated in the mother cell is inactivated in both daughter cells. Thus, an adult woman is a mosaic of clones, some derived from cells that inactivated her father's X and others that inactivated her mother's X. If the woman is a heterozygous carrier of an X-linked disease, some of her cells will be using just the good X and others just the bad X. Depending on the nature of the disease, this may be evident as a patchy phenotype, as in some skin conditions, or there may just be an averaging effect, as in hemophilia. Either way, the distinction between dominant and recessive is not as obvious in X-linked as in autosomal conditions. For males, of course, there is no question of dominance or recessiveness because here are no heterozygotes.

Pedigree description of mitochondrial inheritance. The mitochondria in cells have their own little piece of DNA, probably a leftover from their origin as endosymbiotic bacteria. It is tiny compared to the nuclear genome (16.5 kb and 37 genes, compared to 3.2 million kb and around 24,000 genes; see S&R2 section 7.1.1), but mutations in the mitochondrial DNA are important causes of hearing loss (and other problems). A person's mitochondria come exclusively from the egg; the sperm contributes none. Thus, mitochondrial conditions are passed on only by the mother (matrilineal inheritance). An affected mother transmits the condition to her children of either sex. The resulting pedigrees can look very like autosomal dominant pedigrees unless they are large enough for the exclusively maternal transmission to be obvious.

Cells contain many mitochondria, and it often happens that these are a mixture of normal and mutant versions (heteroplasmy). Heteroplasmy, unlike nuclear genetic mosaicism (see below), can be passed from mother to child, because the egg

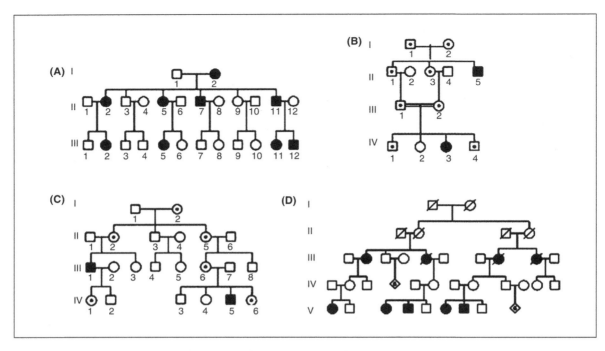

Figure 1.2 Autosomal dominant (A), autosomal recessive (B), X-linked (C), and mitochondrial (D) pedigree patterns. Squares represent males; circles, females. Blacked-in symbols are individuals affected by the condition. Dots in a symbol indicate a phenotypically normal carrier. An unshaded diamond-shaped symbol containing a number, e.g., 6 means 6 unaffected offspring, sexes not specified. Consanguineous marriages can be highlighted by a double marriage line. Generations are numbered in Roman and individuals are numbered across each generation in Arabic numerals. These are ideal pedigrees; those encountered in the clinic are rarely so clear-cut.

contains many mitochondria. Mitochondrial mutations show a particularly poor correlation between genotype and phenotype—for example, the A3243G mutation has been identified as the cause of nonsyndromal hearing loss in some people but diabetes in others (2).

Figure 1.2 shows ideal pedigrees for the main modes of inheritance. Note the conventions used in drawing pedigrees.

Several factors commonly complicate pedigree interpretation:

- *Nonpenetrance.* This describes the situation where a person carries a gene that would normally cause them to have a condition but does not show the condition. Evidence for this can come from the pedigree (an unaffected person who has an affected parent and an affected child) or from DNA testing. The cause is straightforward: a rare lucky combination of other genes or environmental factors may occasionally rescue the person from the condition. Penetrance can be age related, as in late onset hearing loss. Mitochondrial conditions are especially likely to show reduced penetrance. Nonpenetrance is a serious pitfall in genetic counselling.
- *New mutations.* For dominant or X-linked conditions that seriously diminish reproductive prospects, many new cases are caused by fresh mutations. This is not normally the case for recessive conditions.
- *Mosaicism.* A person carrying a new mutation may have a mixture of mutant and nonmutant cells if the mutation happened in one cell of the early embryo. This can directly

affect their phenotype and can also produce an unusual pedigree pattern if their gonads contain some mix of normal and mutant cells. Such germinal mosaicism explains why occasionally a phenotypically normal person with no family history produces two or more offspring affected by a dominant condition.

- *Phenocopies.* People who clinically have the condition, but for a nongenetic reason. Obviously, this is a major problem in interpreting pedigrees of hearing loss.
- *Deaf–deaf marriages.* These can make it impossible to work out who inherited what from whom.

Genes as functional units of DNA

Overview

Back in the 1940s, Beadle and Tatum recognised that the primary function of a gene is to direct the synthesis of a protein. In modern terms, the sequence of A, G, C, and T nucleotides in the DNA is used to specify the sequence of amino acids in the polypeptide chain of a protein. In essence, the process consists of two steps:

1. An RNA copy is made of the gene sequence (transcription).
2. The nucleotide sequence in the RNA is used to specify the sequence in which amino acids are assembled into a protein, via the genetic code (translation).

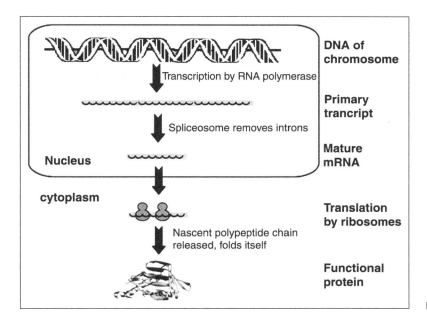

Figure 1.3 Essentials of gene expression.

In slightly more detail (Fig. 1.3):

1. A decision is made to transcribe a particular small segment of the continuous DNA strand.
2. An RNA copy of the whole gene sequence (the primary transcript) is made by the enzyme RNA polymerase.
3. The primary transcript is processed, mainly by cutting out introns (see below) and splicing together exons, to produce the mature mRNA.

4. The mRNA moves out from the nucleus to the cytoplasm, where a complicated machinery comprising ribosomes and transfer RNAs (tRNAs) translates it. In the genetic code, (Fig. 1.4) three consecutive nts form a codon, coding for one amino acid. Since there are 64 possible codons to encode only 20 amino acids, most amino acids are encoded by more than one codon. When the ribosome encounters any one of three stop codons (UGA, UAA, or UAG), it detaches from the mRNA and releases the newly synthesised polypeptide chain.

Transcription

Transcription starts when a large multiprotein complex including RNA polymerase is assembled at a particular point on the DNA. DNA sequences (promoters) that are able to bind the complex mark the genes, which are quite thinly scattered along either strand of the double helix. The DNA-binding proteins of the complex (transcription factors) include some that are universal and others that are present only in specific cells or tissues, or in response to specific signals. Other proteins stabilize or destabilize the complex purely through protein–protein interactions (co-activators and co-repressors). This specific and variable activation or repression of transcription is the major way in which cells establish their identity (muscle cells, neurons, and lymphocytes all contain the same genes, but activate them differentially) and control their activity. Not surprisingly, mutations in the genes encoding transcription factors are a major cause of genetic disease, including hereditary deafness.

	2nd base in codon				
	U	**C**	**A**	**G**	
U	Phe	Ser	Tyr	Cys	U
	Phe	Ser	Tyr	Cys	C
	Leu	Ser	STOP	STOP	A
	Leu	Ser	STOP	Trp	G
C	Leu	Pro	His	Arg	U
	Leu	Pro	His	Arg	C
	Leu	Pro	Gln	Arg	A
	Leu	Pro	Gln	Arg	G
A	Ile	Thr	Asn	Ser	U
	Ile	Thr	Asn	Ser	C
	Ile	Thr	Lys	Arg	A
	Met	Thr	Lys	Arg	G
G	Val	Ala	Asp	Gly	U
	Val	Ala	Asp	Gly	C
	Val	Ala	Glu	Gly	A
	Val	Ala	Glu	Gly	G

(1st base in codon / 3rd base in codon)

Figure 1.4 The genetic code. This code is almost universal in all living organisms, although the small protein synthesis apparatus within mitochondria uses a slightly modified version.

The primary transcript is an RNA molecule corresponding precisely to the DNA sequence of the gene. RNA is chemically virtually identical to DNA, with small differences:

- RNA has ribose where DNA has deoxyribose
- RNA has uracil (U) wherever the corresponding DNA has thymine.

These small differences allow the cell to target different enzymes to RNA and DNA so that they perform different functions in the cell. DNA is the central archive of genetic information; RNA molecules have quite a variety of different roles (Table 1.1). RNA is single stranded simply because cells do not contain enzymes to synthesise a complementary strand. Splicing, ribosomes, and transfer RNA are described below.

If the DNA sequence at some point reads AGTC, the RNA transcribed from this strand would read GACU, writing the sequences, as always, in the $5' \rightarrow 3'$ direction. This is where the convention mentioned above is brought in to make life simpler. Rather than give the sequence of the DNA strand that was used as a template in transcription, we give the sequence of the opposite strand (the "sense strand"). This is GACT, and so, immediately relates to the RNA sequence. Gene sequences are always written in this way.

Processing the primary transcript: exons and introns

In 1977, a wholly unexpected and baffling feature of our genes was discovered. At that time, the broad outlines of transcription and translation had been identified through work on the bacterium *Escherichia coli*. But in 1977, researchers discovered that in humans and chickens, the coding sequence of a gene was split into several noncontiguous segments (exons) separated by noncoding introns. This exon–intron organisation turned out to be typical of the great majority of genes in all eukaryotes (organisms higher than bacteria). There is no seeming logic in the number or size of introns. Over the whole human genome, the average number is eight, but for different genes, it varies from 0 to over 100. Their size also varies enormously, from a dozen nts up to over 100 kb. Exons also vary in size from a few nucleotides up to several kb, though the distribution is more clustered around 100 to 150 bp. Introns are usually bigger than exons—the average in humans is 1300 bp—and so the majority of most genes consists of noncoding sequence. Table 1.2 shows some typical examples. Arguably, this exon–intron organisation allows novel proteins to evolve by shuffling exons that encode functional modules; but it is fair to say that nobody predicted that our genes would be organised in this way, and it still remains one of the most remarkable aspects of the human genome.

Overall, the average human gene is 27 kb long, has nine exons averaging 145 bp, and the introns average 3365 bp—but as the table shows, the range is very wide. Note that the "size in genome" figure refers to the transcribed sequence (exons + introns) and does not include the promoter or other regulatory sequences.

Within the cell nucleus, the primary transcript is processed by physically cutting out the introns that are degraded and splicing together the exons. This is done by a complex machine, the spliceosome, which consists of numerous proteins plus some small RNA molecules. Spliceosomes recognize introns in the primary transcript through details of the nucleotide sequence. Introns nearly always start with GU and end with AG. In themselves those signals would not be sufficient—most GU or AG dinucleotides do not function as splice sites. Splice sites are recognised when the invariant GU or AG is embedded in a broader consensus sequence.

For many genes—at least 40% of all human genes, probably the majority—primary transcripts can be spliced in more than one way, so that several isoforms are produced. There may also be alternative start points for transcription. Thus, a single gene often encodes more than one protein. Much of this alternative

Table 1.1 A partial list of the types of RNA in a cell

RNA species	Typical size	Role in cell
Messenger RNA (>100,000 types)	500–15,000 nt	Mediators of gene expression
Ribosomal RNA (2 species)	4700, 1900 nt	Structural and functional components of the ribosome
Transfer RNA (ca. 50 species)	Ca. 80 nt	Each ferries a specific amino acid to the ribosome and base pairs with the appropriate codon in the mRNA
Small nuclear and nucleolar RNAs (many types)	Typically ca. 100 nt	Control mRNA splicing and other RNA processing
Micro-RNA (several hundred types)	20–22 nt	A recently discovered class believed to be important regulators of gene expression

Abbreviation: nt, nucleotide.

Table 1.2 Structures of some human genes

Gene	Size in genome (kb)	No. of exons	Average exon size (bp)	Average intron size (bp)	Exons as % of primary transcript
Interferon A6 (IFNA6)	0.57	1	570	—	100
Insulin (INS)	1.4	3	154	483	32
Class 1 HLA (HLA-A)	2.7	7	160	269	41
Collagen VII (COL7A1)	51	118	78	358	18
Phenylalanine hydroxylase (PAH)	78	13	206	6264	3.4
Cystic fibrosis (CFTR)	189	27	227	7022	3.2
Dystrophin (DMD)	2090	79	178	26615	0.7

splicing is functional and may be controlled according to the needs of the cell, though in some cases it may just reflect inefficiencies in the machinery. Figure 1.5 shows a typical human gene, with large introns and several alternative splice isoforms.

Mutations that alter splice signals are a major cause of malfunction of genes. Researchers have found it difficult to predict when a sequence change near an intron–exon boundary will affect splicing, and probably this class of mutations often goes unrecognised when it does not alter the invariable GU...AG signal. The only sure way to identify splicing patterns is to study mRNA extracted from appropriate cells.

To complete processing of the primary transcript, a specific nonstandard nt (the "cap") is added to the 5′ end and a string of around 200 A nts is added to the 3′ end [the poly(A) tail]. The mature mRNA is now ready to move to the cytoplasm to be translated.

Translation

In the cytoplasm, ribosomes engage the 5′ end of mRNA molecules. Ribosomes are huge multimolecular complexes comprising two large RNA molecules (ribosomal RNA) and around 100 proteins. The ribosomes physically slide along the mRNA until they encounter a start signal. This is the codon AUG embedded in a consensus ("Kozak") sequence. At this signal, they start assembling amino acids into a polypeptide chain, moving along the mRNA and incorporating the appropriate amino acid in response to each triplet codon, according to the genetic code (Fig. 1.4). Amino acids are brought to the ribosome by yet another class of small RNA molecule, tRNAs. Ultimately, which amino acid is incorporated in response to which codon depends on which tRNA carries that amino acid, which in turn is determined by the specificity of the enzymes that join amino acids onto tRNA molecules. There is no evident logic in the code. It is a sort of frozen accident; it could

perfectly well have been different, but once arrived at, any mutation that changed it in an organism would cause such chaos as to be lethal.

Translation continues until a stop codon (UAG, UAA, or UGA) is encountered, at which point the ribosomes detach from the mRNA and release the newly synthesised polypeptide chain. This may then undergo a whole series of specific enzyme-catalysed modifications—cleaving off parts, attaching sugars or other residues—before being transported to the location inside or outside the cell where it is required.

Note that only part of the mature mRNA carries the code for protein. Although the introns have all been removed within the nucleus, the remaining exonic sequence includes the two untranslated ends of the mRNA—the 5′ untranslated sequence (5′UT) between the cap and the start codon, and the 3′UT between the stop codon and the poly(A) tail. Both these untranslated sequences are important for correct control of translation and mRNA stability, so changes in them can have consequences for gene function. However, we understand very little of the detail; so, it is usually impossible to predict whether a mutation in either of these sequences will be pathogenic.

Overview of the human genome

Our genome (one copy of chromosome 1, one copy of chromosome 2, etc.) comprises about 3.2×10^9 bp of DNA. There are about 24,000 protein-coding genes on current estimates; this figure is provisional because there is no sure-fire way of recognising genes. Genes are scattered quite thinly and apparently randomly along the chromosomes, with no evident reason why a gene is in one place rather than another. Figure 1.6 shows an example. This figure also illustrates one of the main computer programs (genome browsers) used to make sense of the raw human-genome sequence in the public databases.

About 1.5% of our genome codes for protein. So what does the other 98.5% do?

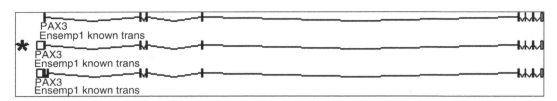

Figure 1.5 A typical human gene. The diagram shows a 100 kb section of chromosome 2 containing the *PAX3* gene, which encodes three isoforms. The horizontal lines represent the primary transcripts. Vertical bars represent exons; the lines linking each set of exons represent the introns. Solid bars are coding sequence; open bars are the 5′ and 3′ untranslated sequences. The transcript marked by an asterisk has eight exons that in total make up 3% of the primary transcript. *Source*: From Ref. 3.

■ The transcribed gene sequences, as explained above, include the 5′ and 3′ untranslated sequences and also all the introns. Genes, including their introns, account for about 20% of our genome.

■ Gene expression is regulated by nontranscribed sequences. Most obviously, this includes the promoter, which lies immediately upstream of the gene, but other regulatory elements ("enhancers" and "locus control regions") may be situated anything up to 1Mb either side of the transcribed sequence. These poorly understood elements bind activating or repressing proteins, and the DNA may loop round so that physically it lies close to the promoter of the gene it regulates. Alternatively, the regulatory proteins may trigger chemical modification of the histone proteins in chromatin, causing a structural change in the chromatin. Chromatin configuration ("open" vs. "closed") is a key determinant of gene activity. Much current interest attaches to identifying and investigating noncoding sequences that are highly conserved in evolution (i.e., are little changed between humans, mice, and, maybe, other organisms), on the assumption that evolutionary conservation implies an important function. Such conserved noncoding sequences make up around 3% of our genome.

■ Exploring our DNA reveals many nonfunctional copies of active genes. These pseudogenes are believed to have arisen through accidental duplication of a gene. Once there are two copies, there is no pressure of natural selection to prevent mutated versions of one copy being transmitted to the offspring.

■ As well as the 24,000 protein-coding genes, we have other genes whose product is a functional RNA. These include all the classes of non-mRNA shown in Table 1.1. The computer programs that are used to identify genes in the raw genome sequence are very poor at identifying genes that do not encode proteins; so, we have little idea how many such genes we have. A large fraction of our genome is at least occasionally transcribed, but it is not known how much of this is functional and how much is just mistakes by the transcription machinery. Micro-RNAs (miRNAs), in particular, are a very hot topic in research. Some workers believe miRNAs will turn out to control much of the way our genome functions.

■ Some DNA sequences control chromosome structure and function. These include centromeres, telomeres (the ends of chromosomes, which are marked by special structures), and scaffold attachment regions that bind the DNA in large (20–100kb) loops to the central protein core of the chromosome.

Some 50% of our DNA consists of repetitive sequences. That is, the same sequence is present several times in the genome. A small proportion of this represents genes that are present in many copies, particularly the genes that encode the various functional RNA molecules shown in Table 1.1. The rest fall into two categories:

■ *Tandem repeats*: The same sequence is repeated a few to several thousand times one after another at a particular location in the DNA. Tandem repeats are important for the structure of centromeres and telomeres; other tandem

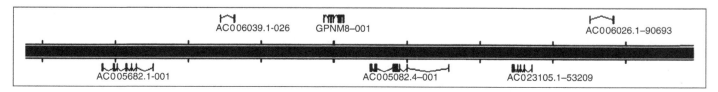

Figure 1.6 Genes in a 0.5 Mb stretch of the short arm of human chromosome 7. The chromosome is shown as a thick black line. Genes are shown as exons (*vertical lines*) linked together to show how they are spliced. Note the small proportion of the total sequence that is occupied by exons. Genes shown above the line are transcribed from left to right, using the upper DNA strand as the sense strand; those below the line use the lower strand and so are transcribed in the opposite direction (remember that the two strands of the double helix are antiparallel). *Source*: From Ref. 3.

repeats are thought to arise from mistakes in DNA replication ("stuttering") and are not functional but are important research tools for gene mapping (microsatellites, see below).

- *Interspersed repeats*: The same sequence is present at many different locations in the genome. The great majority of all repetitive DNA, and about 45% of the entire human genome, is made up of families of repeats that have, or had in the past, the ability to replicate themselves within the genome, almost like viruses. Scientists argue about whether these "transposon-derived repeats" are useless "junk DNA" or whether they have some beneficial function. Studying these repeats reveals much about the evolution of mammalian genomes. We have about 1,200,000 copies of one family, the 280bp Alu sequence, and about 600,000 copies (mostly incomplete) of the 6.5kb LINE1 sequence.

One cannot fail to be struck by the contrast between, on the one hand, our anatomy and physiology, where we constantly encounter marvels of natural engineering, elegant functional adaptation, and beautiful fitness for purpose, and, on the other hand, our genome, which seems disorganised and chaotic. Maybe there is some deep organising principle of genomes that we do not understand, but more probably, it is because natural selection has no interest in a tidy genome, just as long as it works.

Mapping and identifying genes

Two ways of identifying genes

At the start of this chapter, I described the two ways genes are recognised, as functional units of DNA or as determinants of mendelian characters. These two views underlie the two broad strategies for identifying genes.

Genes as functional DNA units are identified by careful study of the genome sequence ("annotating the sequence"). Computer programs scan the sequence for open reading frames—stretches of the DNA that can be read as protein code without hitting a stop codon. Figure 1.7 shows a hypothetical example.

This sort of analysis is fairly straightforward in bacteria, but in higher organisms, the open reading frames are fragmented by introns. Programs must try to identify fragments of coding sequence flanked by plausible splice sites and thinly scattered through much longer regions of noncoding DNA. As mentioned above, even this route is not available for genes that encode functional RNAs rather than proteins. As a result, gene predictions are uncertain and provisional until supported by laboratory identification of the predicted mRNA.

In the laboratory, for technical reasons, it is convenient to study mRNA in the form of synthetic DNA copies [complementary DNA (cDNA)]. Because cDNAs represent only a small fraction of our genome (maybe 2%) but contain all the protein-coding information, much human genome research has focused on cDNAs. Databases compiled by industrial-scale sequencing of small segments of cDNAs (expressed sequence tags) prepared from different tissues are important resources for identifying genes and for seeing which genes are expressed in a given tissue.

Genes as determinants of mendelian characters cannot be picked out in this way. No amount of analysis of the DNA sequence databases, or sequencing of cDNAs, could produce anything labeled "Late-onset hearing loss" or "Pendred syndrome." Genes defined in this way can only be found by studying families where the condition is segregating.

Genetic mapping

The principle of genetic mapping of a mendelian character is to find a chromosomal segment whose segregation in a family or series of families exactly parallels the segregation of the character being investigated. Figure 1.8 shows the principle.

Chromosomal segments are followed through pedigrees by using genetic markers. A genetic marker can be any character that is variable in a population and is inherited in a mendelian fashion. In practice, DNA polymorphisms are invariably used. Two types of common DNA variants are the main tools for current genetic mapping:

- *Single nucleotide polymorphisms (SNPs)*: The history of our species has endowed us with a rather counterintuitive pattern of variability in our DNA. Most nucleotides are the same in all of us, with occasional rare variants, but about 1 nucleotide in every 300 is polymorphic, with two alternatives being reasonably common in populations worldwide. Around 10 million SNPs have been identified. Almost all are in the 98% of our DNA that does not code for protein, and they have no phenotypic effect.
- *Microsatellites*: These are a subgroup of the tandem repetitive DNA in which the repeating unit is a two-, three-, or four-nt sequence. Often, the number of units in the repeated block varies from person to person. For example, everybody might have a run of CACACACA... at a particular location on chromosome 3, but in some people there might be 10 CA units, in others 11, 12, 13, etc.

```
5′  CCTATGGCATGGTCTCGCTAAACATTCCACATCGTGCATAGCGGC  3′
3′  GGATACCGTACCAGAGCGATTTGTAAGGTGTAGCACGTATCGCCG  5′
```

Figure 1.7 Looking for an open reading frame. Both strands of the DNA are shown. Any ATG triplet (reading 5′→3′ as always) could mark the start of an open reading frame (AUG in a mRNA). But each of the underlined ATGs leads quickly to a stop codon, TGA, TAA, or TAG when the sequence is read 5′→3′ in triplets. Only the double-underlined ATG starts an open reading frame, suggesting it might mark the translation start of a gene. A real gene should have an open reading frame of 100 amino acids or more.

Either type of marker can be easily scored by standard laboratory methods (see S&R2 section 17.1.3 for details).

The protocol for mapping a mendelian condition consists, in principle, of the following:

1. The starting point is a large family, or more often a collection of families, in which the condition of interest is segregating. DNA samples must be obtained from all family members, and the diagnoses carefully confirmed by an experienced clinician.
2. All the DNA samples are typed for a genetic marker.
3. The results are checked to see whether segregation of the marker follows segregation of the condition. The test statistic is the lod score, calculated by computer. This is the logarithm of the odds of linkage versus no linkage. A lod score of 3.0 corresponds to the conventional $p < 0.05$ threshold. (See S&R2 section 11.3 for an explanation of lod scores.)
4. Assuming the lod score falls short of 3.0, try another marker and keep trying marker after marker until you find evidence of linkage. In a typical family collection, about 300 microsatellites or 1000 SNPs would be required to test every chromosomal segment.
5. When convincing linkage is found, the chromosomal location of the relevant DNA polymorphism (which can be looked up in public databases) identifies the approximate location of the disease gene. If the marker tracks nearly but not quite always with the disease, other markers from nearby on the chromosome can be used to define the minimal chromosomal segment that tracks completely with the disease. This defines the candidate region that must contain the disease gene.

Positional cloning

Once a candidate region has been defined by genetic mapping, we need to find which gene within that region is mutated to cause the condition. In years past, this endeavour, called positional cloning, was a massive undertaking that often involved years of intensive toil by small armies of postdoctoral scientists. Now that we have the human genome sequence, it is very much easier. We can search the public databases to draw up a list of the genes within the candidate region. Hopefully, the list will be not more than a few dozen. These are then prioritised for investigation based on any available knowledge about their function, domain of expression, etc. A gene causing nonsyndromal hearing loss should be expressed in the inner ear, and ideally it should encode an ion channel, motor protein, or gap junction protein, since these are the commonest genes involved in hearing loss. A gene causing syndromal hearing loss should be expressed during the development of the ear and the other organs involved, and ideally, it should encode a transcription factor.

Given a candidate gene, its sequence is then examined in a panel of unrelated individuals who have the condition being investigated. The correct gene is one that is mutated in those people but not in unaffected controls. The techniques used to do this are the same as those used in genetic testing (see below).

How genes go wrong

The mechanics of mutations

As we have seen, the route from genotype (the DNA sequence) to phenotype (an observable character) is long and complex.

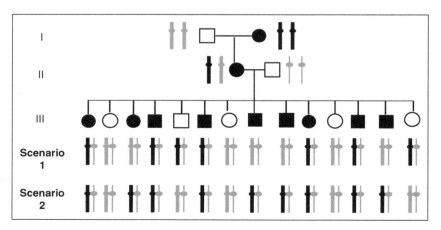

Figure 1.8 The principle of genetic mapping. The diagram shows two possible ways a specific chromosome might segregate in a family in which hearing loss is being transmitted as an autosomal dominant trait. The mother in generation II (II-1) inherited her hearing loss from her father. The chromosome that she inherited from her father is shown in bold. In Scenario 1, there is no relation between whether an offspring in generation III inherits hearing loss and whether they inherit the marked chromosome. This suggests that the gene responsible for the hearing loss is not on that particular chromosome but on one of the other 22 that II-1 received from her father. In Scenario 2, inheritance of the bold chromosome exactly parallels inheritance of hearing loss. If this happens sufficiently often, it would suggest that the hearing-loss gene is carried on that chromosome. This is the principle of linkage analysis. However, in real life, pairs of chromosomes swap segments during each meiosis, so what we have to follow through the pedigree is a chromosomal segment rather than a whole chromosome.

Inevitably, it can go wrong in many different ways. Table 1.3 lists the main things that can go wrong.

Frameshifts are best explained by an example. Consider a string of letters that is to be read as a series of three-letter words:

- The big bad boy hit the cat. . . .

If we add or delete one letter, from then on the whole message is corrupted:

- The bix gba dbo yhi tth eca t
- The bib adb oyh itt hec at. . . . .

When the ribosomes translate an mRNA, the reading frame is fixed by the AUG start codon, and there is no further check. So just as in the above examples, it can be thrown out by insertions or deletions. Frameshifts result not only from insertion or from deletion of any number of nucleotides that is not a multiple of three but also from splicing mutations or exon deletions

that remove a nonintegral number of codons. Since 5% (3/64) of random codons are stop codons, when ribosomes read an mRNA out of frame, it is usually not long before they encounter a stop codon. Unexpectedly, premature stop codons (whether due to frameshifts or nonsense mutations) usually do not result in production of a truncated protein. Instead, in most cases, the mRNA is broken down and the result is no product. This "nonsense mediated decay" probably functions to protect the cell against deleterious effects of partially functional proteins.

A major distinction is between mutations that totally abolish gene expression or totally wreck the product and those that lead to an abnormal degree of expression or to a recognizable but abnormal product. As indicated in the table, this is not always easy to predict just by looking at the sequence change and may need to be checked experimentally. Many missense mutations have no effect on the function of the gene product, but this is virtually impossible to predict—as genetic diagnostic laboratories have learned to their cost.

Table 1.3 How genes go wrong

Type of change	Likely effect	Whether function should be totally abolished
Delete all of the gene	Total absence of product	Yes
Delete one or more exons	Variable	Generally yes, but missing exon(s) may not be necessary for gene function or may be used in only one splice isoform
Mutation in promoter	May change level of expression of the gene	Generally no, but hard to predict
Missense mutation in coding sequence	Replace one amino acid with another	Not unless that amino acid is vital to the function
Synonymous change in coding sequence	Replaces one codon for an amino acid with another for the same amino acid	Usually no effect, but sometimes the change may affect splicing
Nonsense mutation	Mutate an amino acid codon to a stop codon	Usually yes
Frameshift mutation	Insert or delete 1, 2, or any number of nts that is not a multiple of 3, so as to change the reading frame	Usually yes
Change invariant GT … AG splice signal	Exon may be skipped, or intronic material retained in the mature mRNA	Usually yes, but it may just alter balance of splice isoforms
Mutations in 5′UT or 3′UT	Might affect stability of mRNA	Unlikely, but hard to predict
Mutations in introns	None, unless they affect splicing	Usually no, but effects on splicing are hard to predict

Abbreviations: bp, base pair; nt, nucleotide.
Source: From Ref. 3.

The effects of mutations

In attempting to think through the likely effect of a mutation, the first question to ask is whether it causes a loss of function or a gain of function.

- *Loss of function* results from complete gene deletions, most frameshift, nonsense, and splice site mutations, and from some missense mutations. All mutations that cause complete loss of function of a gene would be expected to have the same phenotypic effect. What this effect is depends on how vital the function is and the other allele. Assuming the other allele functions normally, cells of a heterozygous person have 50% of the normal amount of the gene product. For many genes, this is sufficient for normal function; the person is normal and the condition is recessive. The common frameshifting mutation in *connexin 26*, 35delG, is an example. In some cases 50% is not sufficient ("haploinsufficiency"), a heterozygote will be affected and the condition is dominant. Loss of function mutations in the *PAX3* gene causing Type 1 Waardenburg syndrome are an example of haploinsufficiency. Mutations causing a partial loss of function might be expected to have similar but milder effects, though much depends on the details.
- *Gain of function* does not usually mean gain of an entirely novel function—this happens in tumours when chromosomal rearrangements may combine exons of two genes, but it is almost unknown among inherited mutations. Rather, it means a gene being expressed inappropriately—at the wrong level, in the wrong cell, in response to the wrong signal, etc. Alternatively, it can mean that the product of the mutated gene is toxic or interferes with the working of the cell. For example, some missense mutations in connexin 26 cause dominant hearing loss because the abnormal protein causes gap junctions between cells to behave abnormally. This is called a dominant negative effect. Gain-of-function mutations are likely to produce dominant effects because the gain of function is present even in a heterozygous person. Since the effect depends on the presence of the gene product, these are normally missense mutations.

Genotype–phenotype correlations are the Holy Grail of clinical molecular genetics. We would like to be able to see a change in the DNA sequence and predict what effect that would have on the person carrying it. Very seldom is that possible. Although we know many genes that, when mutated, can cause hearing loss, it is unrealistic to expect that a given mutation will always cause a specific degree of loss, a specific audiogram configuration, or a specific age of onset in every mutation carrier. Even mendelian conditions do not really depend on just a single gene, and the innumerable genetic and environmental differences between people are likely to have some effect on the phenotype. Thus, although it is always sensible to look for genotype–phenotype correlations, we should not hold exaggerated hopes of what we might find.

Genetic testing

The central problem in genetic testing is to see the one particular piece of DNA of interest against a background of the 6×10^9 bp of irrelevant DNA in every cell. There are two general solutions to this:

- Selectively amplify the sequence of interest to such an extent that the sample consists largely of copies of that sequence.
- Pick out the sequence of interest by hybridising it to a matching sequence that is labeled, e.g., with a fluorescent dye.

In the past, selective amplification was achieved by cloning the sequence into a bacterium, but nowadays the polymerase chain reaction (PCR) is universally used. For details of this technique see S&R2 section 6.1; for present purposes, it suffices to know that PCR allows the investigator to amplify any chosen sequence of up to a few kilobases to any desired degree in a few hours. All that is necessary is to know a few details of the actual nucleotide sequence that is to be amplified and to order some specific reagents (PCR primers) from one of the firms that custom-produce these. Almost all genetic testing involves PCR, although some companies make kits based on alternative methods, mainly to avoid the royalty payments required of users of the patented PCR process. The big limitation of PCR is that it can only be used to amplify sequences of, at most, a few kilobases. It is not possible to PCR-amplify a whole gene (average size 27 kb), still less a whole chromosome (average size 100 Mb).

Hybridisation depends on the fact that the two strands of the DNA double helix can be separated ("denatured") by brief boiling, and when the resulting single-stranded DNA solution is cooled, each Watson strand will try to find a matching Crick strand. If a dye-labeled single strand corresponding to the sequence of interest (a "probe") is added, some of the test DNA will stick to the probe and can be isolated, followed, or characterised by using the label. Hybridisation was important in the now largely obsolete technique of Southern blotting, and it has regained importance as the principle behind microarrays ("gene chips").

Various applications of PCR and/or hybridisation make it relatively straightforward to check any predetermined short stretch of a person's DNA—but the key word is "short." In general, each exon of a gene must be the subject of a separate test, and when DNA is sequenced, a maximum of around 500 to 700 bp can be sequenced in a single test. Details of how these methods work are given in S&R2 sections 6.3 and 17.1, but the key point to appreciate is that our ability to answer questions about a person's DNA depends crucially on the precision with which the question is posed.

Consider three possible questions:

1. Does this patient have any genetic cause for her hearing loss?

2. Does this patient have any mutation in her *connexin 26* genes that could explain her hearing loss?

3. Does this patient have the 35delG mutation in her *connexin 26* genes?

Question 1 is unanswerable in any diagnostic setting—it might well be too challenging even for a PhD project. Question 3, on the other hand, can be answered cheaply and in an afternoon. Question 2 lies somewhere in between. To answer it, it would be necessary to examine the entire gene. For *connexin 26*, this is fairly simple because it is a small gene with only two exons. The same question in Type 1 Usher syndrome is a very different proposition. Several different genes can cause Type 1 Usher syndrome, and they are large—MYO7A for example has 50 exons. Most diagnostic laboratories would not be willing to devote so much effort to a single case, and even if they were willing, the cost would be high. Gene chips and/or developments in laboratory automation may, in the near future, make such problems much more tractable—but it remains true that the key to successful genetic testing is to pose a precise question.

DNA technology is developing very fast. Sequencing and genotyping become cheaper every year and new technologies allow both to be done on scales that were unthinkable a few years ago. Some companies claim to be developing methods that would allow a person's entire genome to be sequenced in a few days for a few thousand dollars. Optimists and pessimists alike dream of the day when everybody's complete genome sequence will be stored in vast databases; they differ only in their reaction to this prospect. Among all this heady talk, it is important to remember that DNA analysis can reveal only those things about us that are genetically determined.

References

1. Strachan T, Read AP. Human Molecular Genetics. 2nd ed. Oxford: Bios Scientific Publishers, 1999 on the NCBI Bookshelf: http://www.ncbi.nlm.nih.gov/entrez/query.fcgi?db = Books (accessed 31st May 2005).
2. Mitomap www.mitomap.org (accessed 31st May 2005).
3. Ensembl genome browser www.ensembl.org/Homo_sapiens/ (accessed 23rd February 2005).

Glossary

Allele: One or several possible forms of a particular gene, which may or may not be pathological.

Autosome: Any chromosome other than the X or Y sex chromosomes.

Autosomal Dominant: The pedigree pattern seen when an allele at an autosomal locus causes a dominant character.

Autosomal Recessive: The pedigree pattern seen when an allele at an autosomal locus causes a recessive character.

Base: The heterocyclic rings of atoms that form part of nucleotides. Chemically, adenine and guanine are purines, cytosine, thymine, and uracil are pyrimidines.

Base Pair: The A-T and G-C pairs in the DNA double helix. They are held together by hydrogen bonds.

Carrier: An unaffected person with one pathogenic and one normal allele at a locus. Best restricted to heterozygotes for recessive conditions, but the word is sometimes applied to unaffected people with a gene for an incompletely penetrant or late-onset dominant condition.

cDNA: A DNA copy of a mRNA, made in the laboratory. DNA is more stable than RNA and can be cloned, sequenced, and manipulated in ways that RNA cannot.

Chromatin: A nonspecific term for the DNA-protein complex in which the DNA of eukaryotic cells is packaged. Heterochromatin is a highly condensed genetically inert form of chromatin, characteristic of the centromeres of chromosomes; the alternative is euchromatin.

Coactivator: A protein that helps to assemble the various protein components needed to initiate transcription by binding to several components of the complex.

Corepressor: A protein that works in the same way as a co-activator, but to opposite effect.

Codon: The trio of nucleotides in a gene or mRNA that encodes one amino acid. Codons in the mRNA base pair with anticodons in the tRNA.

Consanguineous: Parents are consanguineous if they are blood relatives. Since ultimately everybody is related, a practical working definition is that the parents are second cousins or closer relatives. Second cousins are children of first cousins; first cousins are children of sibs.

Dominant: A character that is manifest in a heterozygote.

Dominant Negative Effect: An inhibitory effect, seen in a heterozygote when a mutant protein prevents the normal version from functioning by sequestering it in nonfunctional dimers or multimers.

Eukaryote: Any organism higher than bacteria. Characterised by cells with a membrane-bound nucleus, internal organelles, DNA in the form of chromatin and genes with introns.

Exon: The parts of the DNA or primary transcript of a gene that are retained in the mature mRNA.

Expressed Sequence Tag (EST): A partial sequence, typically around 300 nt, of a cDNA—incomplete but sufficient to recognise it uniquely.

Genetic Marker: Any character used to follow a segment of a chromosome through a pedigree. SNPs and microsatellites are the genetic markers of choice.

Genotype: The genetic constitution of a person. One can talk of the genotype at a single locus, or the overall genotype. Cf. Phenotype.

Germinal Mosaicism: Mosaicism affecting the gonads, so that a person can produce sperm or eggs representing each genotype present in the mosaic.

Haploinsufficiency: The situation where a 50% level of function of a locus is not sufficient to produce a fully normal phenotype. It causes loss-of-function mutations to produce dominant conditions.

Haplotype: A series of alleles at linked loci on the same physical chromosome.

Heterozygous: Having two different alleles at a locus.

Homozygous: Having two identical alleles at a locus.

Hybridisation: The process where two single strands of DNA or RNA that have complementary sequences stick together to form a double helix.

Intron: The parts of a primary transcript of a gene that are removed and degraded during splicing. It is sometimes called intervening sequences (IVS).

Isoforms: Different forms of the protein product or mature mRNA of a single gene produced by alternative splicing of exons or the use of alternative start sites—a normal feature of gene expression.

Locus: The position that a gene occupies on a chromosome. Since people have a pair of each autosome, a person has two alleles (identical or different) at each autosomal locus.

Locus Heterogeneity: Locus heterogeneity is seen when indistinguishable mendelian disorders can be caused by mutations at more than one locus. This is a common finding in genetics, e.g., Usher syndrome Type 1 can be caused by mutations at loci on the long arm of chromosome 14 (14q31), the long arm of chromosome 11 (11q13) or the short arm of chromosome 11 (11p13).

Lod Score: The statistical outcome of linkage analysis. It is the logarithm of the odds of linkage versus no linkage. A lod score above +3 gives significant evidence for linkage, and a score below −2 gives significant evidence against linkage.

Lyonisation: An alternative name for X inactivation, a phenomenon discovered by Mary Lyon.

Marker: See Genetic marker.

Meiosis: The specialised cell division that produces sperm and eggs. It consists of two successive cell divisions that ensure each gamete contains 23 chromosomes with a novel combination of genes.

Mendelian: A character or pedigree pattern that follows Mendel's laws because it is determined at a single chromosomal location. Characters determined by combinations of many genes are called multifactorial, complex, or nonmendelian.

Microsatellite: A small run of tandem repeats of a very simple DNA sequence, usually 1 to 4 bp, for example $(CA)_n$.

Microarray: A postage-stamp size wafer of silicon or glass carrying a large arrayed set of single-stranded oligonucleotides corresponding to parts of the sequence of one or more genes. When fluorescently labelled PCR-amplified genomic DNA or cDNA is hybridised to the array, the pattern of hybridisation can be used to read off the sequence, to check which genes are expressed in a tissue, or to genotype a sample for a large number of SNPs in parallel.

Mitosis: The normal process of cell division by which each daughter cell receives an exact and complete copy of all the DNAA in the mother cell.

Mosaic: An individual who has two or more genetically different cell lines derived from a single zygote (because of a fresh mutation or chromosomal mishap).

Nonpenetrance: It describes the situation when a person carrying a gene for a dominant character does not manifest the character. This is because of the effects of other genes or of environmental factors.

Nucleotide: The units out of which DNA and RNA chains are constructed. It consists of a base linked to a sugar (deoxyribose in DNA, ribose in RNA) linked to a phosphate group. A nucleoside is the same but without the phosphate.

Obligate Carrier: A person who is necessarily a carrier by virtue of the pedigree structure. For autosomal recessive conditions, this normally means the parents of an affected person, for X-linked recessive conditions, a woman who has affected or carrier offspring and also affected brothers or maternal uncles. A woman who has only affected offspring is not an obligate carrier of an X-linked condition, because new mutations are frequent in X-linked (but not autosomal recessive) pedigrees.

Open Reading Frame: A stretch of genomic DNA that could be translated into protein without encountering a stop codon.

Penetrance: The probability that a phenotype will be seen with a given genotype.

Phenocopy: An individual who has the same phenotype as a genetic condition under study, but for a nongenetic reason, e.g., somebody with nongenetic deafness in a family where genetic deafness is segregating. Phenocopies can be a major problem in genetic mapping.

Phenotype: The observed characteristics of a person (including the result of clinical examination). Compare with Genotype.

Poly(A) Tail: The string of around 200 consecutive A nucleotides that is added on to the 3′ end of most mRNAs. It is important for the stability of mRNA.

Polymerase Chain Reaction (PCR): A method for selectively copying a defined short (no more than a few kilobases) segment of a large or complex DNA molecule. The basis of most genetic testing.

Primary Transcript: The initial result of transcribing a gene: an RNA molecule corresponding to the complete gene sequence, introns as well as exons.

Probe: A labelled piece of DNA that is used in a hybridisation assay to identify complementary fragments. Depending on the application, probes may be pieces of cloned natural DNA around 1 kb long, or much shorter (20–30 nt) pieces of synthetic DNA.

Promoter: The DNA sequence immediately upstream of a gene that binds RNA polymerase and transcription factors, so that the gene can be transcribed.

Pseudogene: A nonfunctional copy of a working gene. Pseudogenes are quite common in our genome and represent the failed results of abortive evolutionary experiments.

Recessive: A character that is manifest only in the homozygous state and not in heterozygotes.

Sibs (Siblings): Brothers and sisters, regardless of sex. A sibship is a set of sibs.

SNP (Single Nucleotide Polymorphism): The main class of genetic marker used for very high-throughput genotyping. About 1 nucleotide in every 300 is polymorphic. Most SNPs have no phenotypic effect, but some may contribute to susceptibility to common complex diseases.

Southern Blotting: A method of studying DNA based on separating fragments by size and hybridising them to a labelled probe. It is largely superseded by PCR, which entails much less work but still used for some special applications. It is named after its inventor; Northern blotting and Western blotting are similar techniques used on RNA and proteins, respectively—the names are jokes.

Transcription Factor: A protein that binds the promoters of genes so as to activate transcription. Basal transcription factors are involved in transcription of all genes; tissue-specific transcription factors cause different cells to express different subsets of their genes.

X–Inactivation: The mysterious process by which every human cell has only a single working X chromosome, regardless of how many X chromosomes are present.

X-Linked Inheritance: X-linked inheritance is seen when a condition is caused by an allele located on the X chromosome.

2 Understanding the phenotype: basic concepts in audiology

Silvano Prosser, Alessandro Martini

Introduction

Knowledge in audiology, as in many other medical fields, advances discontinuously, paralleling developments in technology applied to scientific research. After the eras of psychoacoustics, tympanic measurements, electrophysiological responses, and otoacoustic emissions, it is apparent today that molecular biochemistry will play an important role in the exploration of auditory function. From a clinical point of view, it will transform the classification of hearing impairment and the possibilities for new therapeutic approaches.

Studies in molecular genetics are accumulating an impressive quantity of knowledge on the aetiopathology of hearing loss, as the mapping and cloning of genes reveal their functions in the inner ear, its structural organisation, and its homeostasis. Currently, several hundred chromosomal loci have been identified and associated with syndromal and nonsyndromal hearing impairments. This number has been estimated to represent about half of the genetic changes resulting in hearing impairments. Thus, genetic factors have to be considered in diagnostic audiology much more frequently than in the past. At present, clinical audiology has to meet two requirements. First, there is the need for deeper knowledge of the pathophysiological changes that gene mutations induce in the auditory system; second, there is a need for new audiological diagnostic tools sensitive enough to elucidate these changes. This could help to better define the phenotype and narrow, to within a reasonable range, the set of genetic investigations necessary.

Pure-tone hearing–threshold measurements

The principal audiometric test entails measuring the auditory thresholds for pure tones. Results indicate the minimum sound pressure levels (dB SPL) that evoke the minimal auditory sensation within the frequency range between 125 and 8000 Hz. International standards define the SPL threshold values for normal hearing, and, after normalisation, relate them to 0 dB hearing loss (HL). Threshold increments up to 25 dB HL, although irrelevant for medicolegal purposes, may be valuable for diagnostic purposes. Two separate measures of the hearing threshold, respectively air-conducted (through an earphone or an insert) or bone-conducted (a vibrator on the forehead or the mastoid process) stimuli, permit the distinction between two main kinds of hearing losses: conductive and sensorineural. The first show a normal bone-conducted and an elevated air-conducted hearing threshold. The second show equal values of the two thresholds. There are also mixed hearing losses, which have elements of both conductive and sensorineural losses. When a marked difference exists between the hearing thresholds of the two ears, noise masking is needed for the better ear, in order to ensure that a sensation evoked in the better ear does not interfere with the sensation elicited in the worse ear.

A diagnosis of conductive hearing loss made by pure-tone audiometry indicates a dysfunction of the external or middle ear, but its origin cannot be pinpointed without otoscopic examination and admittance measurement. A diagnosis of sensorineural hearing loss indicates dysfunction in either the cochlea or the auditory pathway: other investigations are needed to confirm the site of the lesions. Clinical pure-tone audiometry, such as the psychoacoustical tests described below, is based on a stimulus-response behavioural model, which requires active cooperation and attentive attitude by the subject being tested. Simulators, individuals with low levels of vigilance and reduced attention may give unreliable results, i.e., a hearing threshold poorer than the actual threshold or one excessively variable at retest. Three- to five-year-old children can reliably perform pure-tone audiometry. Younger children can be examined by special conditioning procedures.

Table 2.1 Relevant terms and definitions

Hearing threshold level

It means the threshold value averaged over frequencies
0.5, 1, 2, and 4 kHz in the better ear

Hearing threshold levels (0.5–4 kHz)	Frequency ranges
Mild: over 20 and <40	Low: up to and equal to 500 Hz
Moderate: over 40 and <70 dB	Mid: over 500 up to and equal to 2000 Hz
Severe: over 70 and <95 dB	High: over 2000 up to and equal to 8000 Hz
Profound: equal to and over 95 dB	Extended high: over 8000 Hz

Types of hearing impairment

Unilateral: one ear has either >20 dB pure-tone average or one frequency exceeding 50 dB, with the other ear better than or equal to 20 dB

Asymmetrical: >10 dB difference between the ears in at least two frequencies, with the pure-tone average in the better ear worse than 20 dB

Progressive: a deterioration of >15 dB in the pure-tone average within a 10-year period. Results in those aged over 50 years should be treated with some caution. In all cases the time-scale and patient age should be specified

Conductive: related to disease or deformity of the outer/middle ears. Audiometrically, there are normal bone-conduction thresholds (<20 dB) and an air-bone gap >15 dB averaged over 0.5-1-2 kHz

Mixed: related to combined involvement of the outer/middle ears and inner ear/cochlear nerve. Audiometrically >20 dB HL in the bone-conduction threshold together with >15 dB air-bone gap averaged over 0.5-1-2 kHz

Sensorineural: related to disease/deformity of the inner ear/cochlear nerve with an air-bone gap <15 dB averaged over 0.5-1-2 kHz

Sensory: a subdivision of sensorineural related to disease or deformity in the cochlea

Neural: a subdivision of sensorineural related to a disease or deformity in the cochlear nerve

A relative contraindication to pure-tone audiometry may be the presence of occluding wax in the ear canal, since this may be responsible for a conductive loss of 20 to 30 dB HL. By examining patients suspected of having noise-induced hearing loss, an unexposed interval of 16 hours is needed to avoid false results due to "temporary threshold shift" phenomena.

Commonly, the hearing threshold is measured at frequencies separated by octave intervals, from 0.125 to 8 kHz. The addition of intermediate frequencies (1.5, 3, 6, 10, and 12 kHz) may improve the overall threshold estimate. Indeed, as the threshold values of contiguous frequencies are correlated, the more the frequencies recorded, the less the probability of the errors associated with a single-frequency threshold measurement. The measurement error for air-conduction testing is usually estimated within ± 5 dB, and it is about twice that figure for bone-conduction testing. These errors mainly originate from the transducers' incorrect positioning as well as subject-related factors.

The accuracy of the pure-tone hearing threshold is crucial in defining any progression of the hearing impairment (1). Some genetic hearing impairments show this characteristic. Hence, the first pure-tone threshold has to be measured with high precision, since it will then be the reference for successive threshold comparisons.

Table 2.1 gives relevant terms and definitions, derived from Stephens (2), on the basis of recommendations of the HEAR European project.

Relationship between pure–tone hearing thresholds and auditory damage

External and middle ear

A variety of genetic syndromes can affect the anatomy of these structures. By altering the sound transmission to the cochlea, they present as a conductive hearing impairment. Such anomalies range from simple stenosis of the external meatus to total lack of the tympano-ossicular complex, with intermediate conditions including an atretic external canal, an absence of the tympanic bone, and a lack or fusion of the ossicles, stapes fixation, and atretic Eustachian tube. [See Van de Heyning (3) for an otosurgical classification.] Even in young children, the consequences of these anomalies can be measured by means of auditory-evoked potentials presented by air and bone conduction. Two extreme pathological pictures may be taken as a reference to predict the pure-tone threshold: (*i*) Simple atresia of the external meatus causes a 30 to 35 dB conductive hearing impairment due to the attenuation of the sounds directed to the tympanic membrane. (*ii*) A complete lack of the tympanic function causes a 60 to 70 dB conductive hearing loss, essentially due to the attenuation of the acoustical energy directed to the cochlea. Between these two extremes, the hearing loss may vary in respect to the anatomical structures involved and their consequence on auditory function (Fig. 2.1).

Inner ear

Inner ear lesions resulting in a sensorineural hearing loss show a moderate relationship with the pure-tone threshold. An elevated threshold at high frequencies indicates damage to the basal portion of the cochlea. An elevated threshold for low frequencies suggests damage of the apical portion. Schuknecht's (4) studies on the comparison of audiograms to cochlear histology ("cochleograms") corroborates such a relationship. A further distinction involves the degree of hearing loss. Based on the role of outer and inner hair cells, we can assume that a total loss of outer cells causes a hearing impairment of 55 and 65 dB for low- and high-frequency ranges, respectively. A complete loss of inner hair cells should cause a profound hearing impairment (95 dB HL to total hearing loss). In practice, the lesions usually involve both the outer and the inner hair cells, with the proportions depending on the causative factor. Apart from these observations, other conditions have to be considered, in which the audiogram–histology relationship may break down.

One of these is that the cochlea may appear anatomically normal in its microscopic structure, but the biochemical–metabolic processes responsible for its function and homeostasis are altered. In addition, there are several other cochlear sites of damage than those examined in the traditional cochlear histological studies, locations that molecular genetics has demonstrated. These include the gap-junction system, the ionic-transport channels, the synaptic organisation, as well as some components of extracellular matrix (5,6). Such alterations may affect auditory function in different ways, independently of the anatomical loss of hair cells. A second exception to the audiogram–cochlear damage correspondence is represented by the possible existence of cochlear dead regions. A dead region is a section of the cochlear partition where inner hair cells are totally lacking. This condition is not reflected in the audiogram, since frequencies that should be processed by the dead zone are made audible by contiguous zones when the stimulus intensity is high enough to generate a mechanical pattern spreading towards them (off-frequency listening). Finally, another limitation of pure-tone measurements is that the typical "auditory residue" observable at low frequencies in profound hearing loss is difficult to attribute unquestionably to an auditory rather than a tactile sensation (Fig. 2.2) (7).

Cochlear nerve

Pure-tone thresholds are relatively resistant to lesions involving the cochlear nerve. Schuknecht et al. (8) demonstrated in animal studies that only a lesion involving over 75% of the nerve fibres causes effects evident in the pure-tone threshold. In humans, the vestibular Schwannomas represent the most common clinical cause of cochlear nerve lesions. Among patients with this pathology, about 80% show a hearing impairment, although the amount of hearing loss correlates only poorly with the tumour size. For those cases with a high-frequency hearing loss, a mechanism was suggested in which the most external nerve fibres coming from the basal cochlea would be the most vulnerable to compression by the tumour. There are, however, many exceptions to this picture. In fact, the hearing may be variously compromised in relation to the complex effects resulting from tumour growth: for instance, demyelinisation (9), neural ischaemia, indirect cochlear damage due to a reduced blood supply from the compressed labyrinthine artery, and retrograde degeneration (10).

Automated procedures for self-recording hearing thresholds

Modern audiometers often incorporate automated modalities to record the hearing threshold. The most popular, based on an adaptive procedure, is known as Békésy audiometry. This technique requires the subject to control the stimulus intensity according to his responses. Pure tones are either continuous or interrupted (2.5/sec) at continuously changing frequencies or at the discrete frequencies of the classical audiometry, whereas intensity changes in steps of 2.5 or 5 dB.

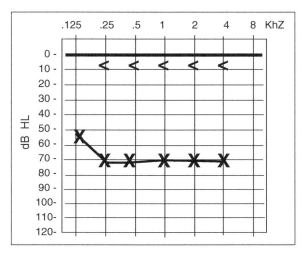

Figure 2.1 An example of conductive hearing loss (normal bone-conduction threshold) due to a severe malformation of external-middle ear.

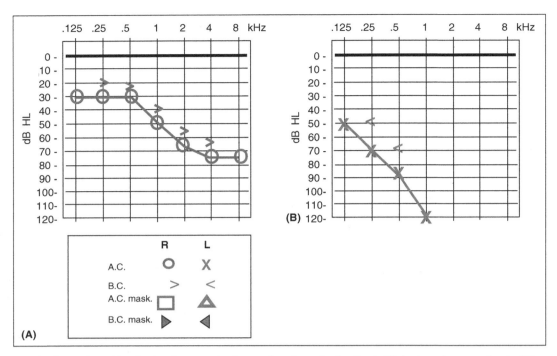

Figure 2.2 (A) An example of sensorineural hearing loss (bone-conduction equal to air-conduction threshold) due to an inner ear disorder. This common threshold configuration may approximately suggest the type and distribution of the lesion within the cochlea: at the basal end (high frequencies), probable involvement of both outer and inner hair cells; at the apex (low frequencies), probable involvement of half of the population of outer hair cells. (B) This threshold profile is common in profound hearing loss and could indicate residual function in hair cells at the apex. However, the thresholds recorded in response to low frequency and very intense tones could be due to vibrotactile perception.

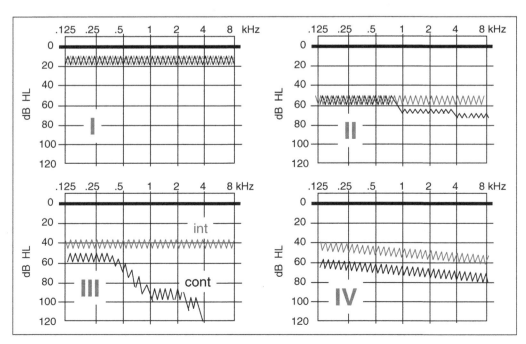

Figure 2.3 Classification of Békésy audiometry tracings. Type I (overlapping of thresholds for continuous and interrupted stimuli) is observable in normal hearing and conductive hearing loss. Type II (small excursions with a continuous stimulus) is observable in cochlear lesions. Type III (progressively diverging thresholds) can be found in eighth nerve disorders. Type IV can be observed in cochlear and retrocochlear lesions. Type V, not shown here, display a threshold change in interrupted tones worse than that for continuous tones; it is associated with nonorganic hearing loss.

The subject's task consists of pressing a button when he perceives the signal and releasing it when he hears nothing. Accordingly, the intensity decreases and increases by the preset steps and rates. Finally, the instrument produces graphic tracings of the up–down intensity excursions around the threshold. A reliable test takes from 30 seconds to 2 minutes for each frequency.

In addition to the threshold estimate, Békésy audiometry has proved to be sensitive to different kinds of hearing impairment. Its diagnostic potential is based on the comparison of hearing threshold tracings in response to continuous and interrupted tones. Four patterns have been identified (Fig. 2.3): type I, usually found in normal hearing and conductive loss; type II, mainly found in sensorineural loss with recruitment; type III, suggesting a retrocochlear involvement; and type IV, observable either in cochlear or in eight-nerve lesions. An additional type V has often been observed in nonorganic hearing loss (11). Today, more reliable diagnostic tools exist for identifying the lesion site of a hearing loss. Békésy audiometry, however, may be recommended in selected cases when more precision is needed in estimating the hearing threshold. Indeed, threshold values obtained with automated audiometry are more sensitive, on average, than those obtained with classical audiometry, and twice as stable at retest (12). The best estimates in either terms of absolute sensitivity or the test–retest variability have been obtained by an interrupted stimulus of 500 ms duration, 50% on–off and with 4 to 5 dBs attenuation rate (13).

An alternative automated technique is based on methods of frequency scanning (Audioscan). This may explore the auditory threshold with a resolution of up to 64 points/octave. Different from the Békésy technique, the pure-tone stimuli are delivered at a fixed intensity. The subject's task is to press a button when he perceives the stimulus. At the end of the frequency scan, the intensity increases by a predetermined step, and the scan restarts. The intensity levels perceived by the subject are stored, and finally the instrument provides a profile of the pure-tone threshold. The threshold is estimated with a precision comparable to that of Békésy audiometry, with measurement errors typically ranging between 3.5 and 4.5 dB. Since many frequencies can be tested other than those recordable by classical audiometry, the threshold profile often exhibits characteristic "notches," indicating some frequency-related discontinuities of the hearing acuity. These notches may be described in terms of frequency range, depth, and intensity level (14), and they define the so-called "threshold fine structure." The exact meaning of the notches is still controversial: Perhaps they represent some interference between the cochlear mechanical input and output, in a similar way to the fine structure of otoacoustic emissions. Although it has been empirically determined that the notch amplitude should be at least 15 dB to be considered pathological (15), it is still unclear whether and when the threshold fine structure could reflect a fully healthy ear rather than the early signs of auditory damage (16). The presence of notches in the threshold fine structure has been assumed to be the marker of a carrier condition for certain

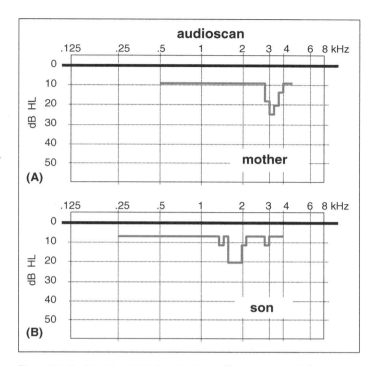

Figure 2.4 Auditory thresholds from Audioscan (frequency scanning), where notches are apparent at 3 to 4 kHz, and 1.5 to 2 kHz. The two audiograms have been obtained from a mother and son, both healthy carriers (on classical audiometry) of a genetic hearing loss. *Source*: From Ref. 15.

genetic mutations responsible for hearing impairment (17,18). However, these observations have not been confirmed at least in the context of other categories of genetic hearing impairment, including some nonsyndromal, recessive forms (19).

Compared with Békésy audiometry, the Audioscan technique is apparently more sensitive in detecting threshold notches that could identify carriers of genetic mutations (Fig. 2.4). However, it has been also remarked that the prevalence of notches in a normal control population is around 15% to 20% (20).

Estimating a progressive hearing impairment

The causative factors of hearing impairment often result in a progressive deterioration over time. A typical example consists of noise-induced hearing loss (NIHL). In addition, there are several genetic conditions, mostly nonsyndromal dominant, where the progressive worsening of the hearing may represent a phenotypical feature. Knowing that a certain genetic hearing impairment will progress with age to a predictable degree could facilitate the planning of therapy or rehabilitation. However, three significant factors make the evaluation of a worsening hearing loss problematic, especially when conducted over a long time span. The first concerns test modality: Instruments and examiners may introduce errors into the threshold

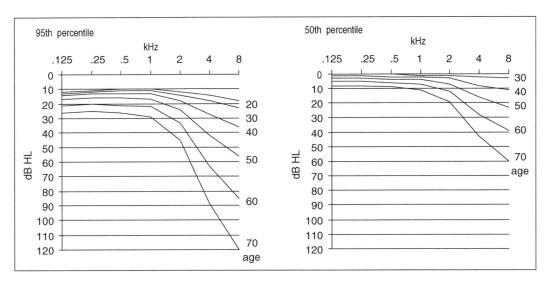

Figure 2.5 Reference auditory thresholds for different ages, according to ISO 7029 (1984) (22) and based on an "otologically normal" male population. Data are displayed for the 50th and 95th percentiles, respectively. Due to the wide range of variability, the estimate of any age effect in an individual patient is quite approximate. A criterion for selecting the candidates with a genetic diagnosis could be a hearing threshold exceeding the 95th percentile (24).

estimates, of the order of at least 5 dB. The other two factors are subject dependent and consist of the effects of age and the intrasubject, test–retest variability of the responses. The impact of these two factors is difficult to predict for any individual because every subject reacts to age and retest conditions in particular ways. Nevertheless, since we have to account for these factors, it is feasible to rely on the mean age-related threshold data and the test–retest variability as derived from wide population samples. The subtraction of these, more general, effects enables us to broadly estimate the specific effects such as those related to noise exposure or to genetic factors. Indeed, these estimates when applied to a single case study incorporate a variable degree of uncertainty, depending on the statistical properties of the reference sample data (21). ISO 1999 (22) and ISO 7029 (23) provide data used to calculate the age-related hearing loss for a reference population. In fact, the age-related hearing loss can be predicted even if within a wide confidence interval, for instance, 50 dB between 10th and 90th percentile for 60-year-old subjects (Fig. 2.5). For this reason, considerable criticism has been made of the utility of correcting the threshold values for age. Today this problem is further complicated due to the uncertain definition of "presbyacusis." In fact, it is likely that many cases formerly defined as "presbyacusis" and included in the reference population are actually cases of genetic hearing impairments. Although gene mutations responsible for age-related hearing loss have been demonstrated only in animals, epidemiological data (25,26) show that half the variance associated with "presbyacusis" may be attributed to genetic factors.

In contrast to the age effect, intrasubject variability of threshold measurements is easily predictable. Robinson et al. (27) provided useful data for test–retest variability: Two

audiograms recorded separately in time may differ by 1.4 dB on an average, with a standard deviation of 5.7 dB and a maximum difference of 18.5 dB.

Figure 2.6 shows an example of how the progression of hearing loss may be apparent. The data are derived from a group of patients belonging to families with nonsyndromal hearing impairment (28). They show remarkable differences in the

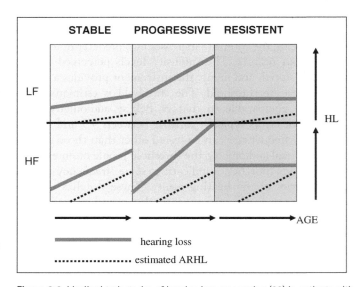

Figure 2.6 Idealised trajectories of hearing loss progression (28) in patients with hereditary nonsyndromal hearing impairment. Compared to the age-related hearing loss (*dotted lines*) the hearing impairment may be "stable" (hearing deterioration due to age only), "progressive" (deterioration due to age plus a genetic factor), and "resistant" (no age effect). Also, mixed figures exist, with different progression at low and high frequencies. *Abbreviations*: ARHL, age related hearing loss; HF, high frequencies; HL, hearing loss; LF, low frequencies.

progression of the hearing loss over time, from very rapid progression to a stable hearing loss, with other forms showing a different rate of progression for low and high frequencies.

More accurate data analyses such as those reported by Huygen et al. (29) are helpful in defining certain genetic hearing impairments (DFNA2,5,6/14,9,10,15,20/26,21) with precise temporal progression of hearing loss and the threshold profile. Although these data are representative of a small number of families, they are relevant since they could throw light on the pathophysiological mechanisms underlying some genetic mutations.

Audiometric classification and threshold profile

Although only a broad relationship exists between cochlear pathology and pure-tone audiogram, it is popular to classify the audiograms according to their shapes. Indeed, certain audiometric profiles may lead to a diagnostic hypothesis. For the diagnosis of genetic hearing impairments, an audiometric classification could be helpful to recognise specific phenotypes, and then, to isolate the corresponding genotypes. Table 2.2 shows the definitions as proposed by the European Working Group on genetic hearing impairments (2), which allows for the audiometric classification shown in Figure 2.7.

As underlined by Hinchcliffe (30), classifying the audiograms is a pattern recognition exercise, which may have mathematical (31,32) or matrices-based solutions. The latter approach, three frequency bands x four threshold levels, was implemented by Sorri et al. (33). Among the conclusions from a study of the classification of audiograms in genetic hearing impairment (34), it was noted that the particular difficulty was in ascertaining a clear phenotype–genotype relationship. For this reason, it was also proposed that additional classificatory data such as progression or age correction be included in an attempt to improve our understanding of the phenotype–genotype relationship.

It appears today that the pure-tone threshold profile is of little value for the diagnosis of genetic hearing impairments.

Observations on temporal changes of hearing thresholds have demonstrated that apparently typical profiles, for instance a U-shaped profile, can substantially change to a downward-sloping pattern involving the high frequencies (Fig. 2.8) (29).

On genotype–phenotype relationships

For many cases, genetic hearing impairment is recognised to be due to a definite gene mutation. For other forms, mainly syndromal, such a relationship is less clear. Indeed, different phenotypes may be the expression of different mutations on the same gene, a condition defined as allelic mutation by geneticists. For example, different mutations of the same COL11A1 gene on chromosome 1p21 can cause two distinct syndromes: Marshall syndrome and Stickler syndrome type 2, both characterised by different progressive hearing losses, skeletal abnormalities, myopia, and craniofacial dysmorphism (35). Also, types 1 and 3 of Waardenburg syndrome (dystopia canthorum in type 1, musculoskeletal anomalies in type 3) and the hearing-and-craniofacial syndrome are caused by allelic mutations of the PAX3 gene (transcription factor) on chromosome 2q35 (36,37). In addition, there are other combinations of gene mutations contributing to complicate the genotype–phenotype relationship: Mutations on multiple genes may be expressed as a similar phenotype, a condition defined as genetic heterogeneity by geneticists. In fact, heterogeneity hides the clinical features that could allow grouping the members of a family with a single locus mutation. A typical example consists of Usher syndrome type I in which the phenotype is a congenital profound hearing loss, retinitis pigmentosa, and vestibular areflexia. This syndrome is, however, recognised to be associated with at least seven different genes (type Ia: USH1A, Ib: MYO7A: Ic: USH1C, Id: CDH23; Ie: USH1E; If: PCDH15; and Ig: USH1G), which result in the same clinical picture.

Another confounding factor in the genotype–phenotype relationship stems from the possibility that the mutation effects can attain clinical relevance at different ages. Thus, the first symptom could precede the appearance of the second symptom,

Table 2.2 Audiometric profiles: classification criteria

Low frequency ascending	>15 dB from the poorer low-frequency thresholds to the higher frequencies
Midfrequency U-shaped	>15 dB difference between the poorest thresholds in the midfrequencies, and those at higher and lower frequencies
High frequencies gently sloping	15–29 dB difference between the mean of 0.5 and 1 kHz and the mean of 4 and 8 kHz
High frequencies steeply sloping	>30 dB difference between the mean of 0.5 and 1 kHz and the mean of 4 and 8 kHz
Flat	<15 dB difference between the mean 0.25/0.5 kHz thresholds, the mean of 1 and 2 kHz, and the mean of 4 and 8 kHz

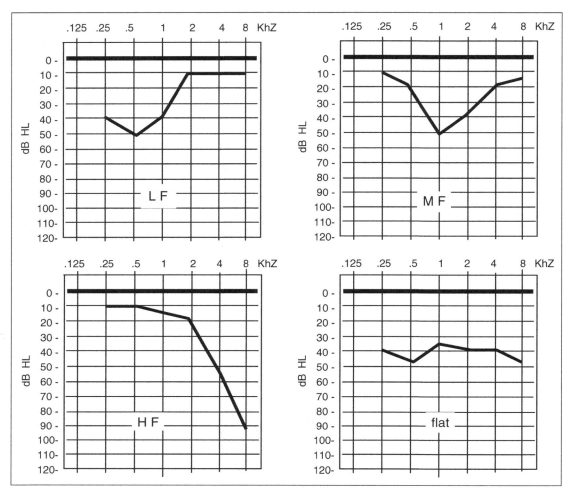

Figure 2.7 Typical pure-tone hearing profiles, as defined by the European working group HEAR (2). *Abbreviations*: HF, high frequencies; LF, low frequencies; MF, middle frequencies.

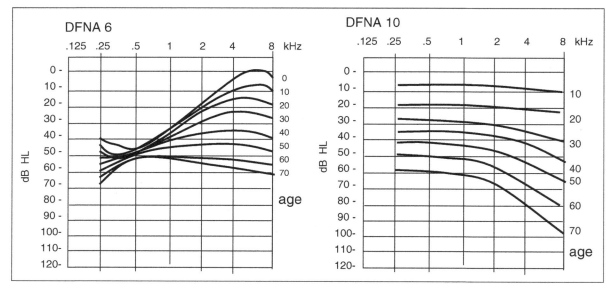

Figure 2.8 Examples of hearing loss progression as modelled by averaging the data of several families. Evaluating hearing loss in relation to age-related typical audiogram may allow a better definition of phenotypes associated with certain gene mutations. *Source*: From Ref. 29.

crucial for classifying the condition, by many years. For example, in Usher syndrome types I and II, hearing loss is congenital, but retinitis pigmentosa, the crucial symptom, may be delayed until adolescence.

Finally, distinguishing between syndromal and nonsyndromal hearing impairments may be clinically difficult. A reason may be that an apparently isolated hearing loss can be concomitant with other anomalies that are not easily recognizable. A second reason can be that an allelic mutation, although involving the same gene, can express either as a nonsyndromal or as a syndromal hearing impairment. An example is given by the mutation of the gene *SLC26A4*, responsible for either Pendred syndrome or the recessive form DFNB4 (38). Even autosomal-dominant (DFNA) and -recessive (DFNB) forms can be caused by mutations on the same gene. For example, mutations on the same gene *MYO7A* are associated with either a dominant (DFNA11) or a recessive (DFNB37) form (39). In addition, mutations of the gene *GJB2(Cx26)* may be expressed as DFNA3 (dominant) and as DFNB1 (recessive) (40).

Topodiagnosis of hearing loss

Classical audiometry comprises a group of tests aimed at distinguishing between two phenomena: "loudness recruitment," associated with lesions in the cochlea and "pathological adaptation," associated with lesions of the cochlear nerve. To enhance the diagnostic sensitivity by cross-checking the results, these tests are often arranged in the form of a diagnostic battery. At present, they are rarely used because other diagnostic tools [auditory brain stem response (ABR), admittance, and otoacoustic emissions (OAE)] are available to provide more reliable data (41).

"Recruitment" is a loudness distortion caused by an abnormality or a loss of the cochlear outer hair cells. The effect of such a condition is that within the audibility range, equal increments of stimulus intensity are perceived louder when compared to normally hearing subjects. For instance, while a level variation of 1 dB evokes the minimal sensation in the normal subject, variations of 0.25 to 0.5 dB are sufficient to evoke the same sensation in a subject with a cochlear hearing loss. The impairment of the active cochlear mechanism, residing in outer hair cells, accounts for both threshold elevation and loudness recruitment (42).

In contrast, "pathological adaptation" is typically due to a functional reduction of the cochlear nerve fibres, normally around 30,000 in number. In such a condition, the nerve trunk cannot sustain a constant sensation over time. For instance, the sensation of a pure tone at an intensity near the threshold quickly disappears after a few seconds, to be restored after an appropriate stimulus increment (43).

Table 2.3 summarises the tests that are still regarded as having a clinical value. This selection is determined by the hearing-threshold characteristics such as right–left symmetry, degree of hearing loss, and threshold profile.

Traditionally, the clinical goal of these test batteries was the early identification of potentially life-threatening retrocochlear lesions such as, for example, vestibular schwannoma. This often led to the interpretation of the tests results dichotomously, on the basis of a separation between cochlear and retrocochlear lesions. Although clinically useful, this separation may not reflect a parallel separation in the pathophysiological mechanisms. In fact, damage firstly located within the cochlea can progressively

Table 2.3 Topodiagnostic audiometric tests

	Stimuli	Task	Positive results
Recruitment test			
Short increment sensitivity index	Pure tones 20 dB SL + 1 dB	Detection of increments (Δi)	>75%
Alternate binaural loudness balance	Pure tones binaurally alternated from 0 dB SL, with 10–20 dB successive increments	Loudness binaural balance	Binaural balance of loudness within ±10 dB HL
Luescher	Pure tones, 40 dB SL, amplitude modulated between 0.25 and 2 dB	Detection of modulation	<1 dB
Pathological adaptation test			
Carhart–Rosemberg	Pure tones (0.5–1–2 kHz) + 5 dB SL, successive 5 dB increments, 1 min duration	Detection	Total intensity increment >35 dB/1 min
Supra threshold adaptation test	Pure tones (0.5–1–2 kHz) 100 dB HL, 1 min duration	Detection after 1' stimulation	Absence of auditory sensation

involve the spiral ganglion neurons, and conversely, degenerative phenomena of cochlear nerve fibres can involve the cochlear epithelium in a retrograde way. In practice, common examples of concomitant cochlear and neural dysfunction, often yielding ambiguous results to recruitment and adaptation tests, are represented by cases of NIHL, "presbyacusis," and, although rarely, vestibular schwannoma.

Identifying cochlear dead regions

A number of histopathological observations (4,44) showed that some cases of sensorineural hearing loss are characterised by a complete lack of inner hair cells in a limited area of the cochlear partition. Since neural activation strictly depends upon the inner hair cells, their absence prevents any mechano-electrical transduction from taking place in the region involved ("cochlear dead region"). However, as briefly mentioned earlier, pure-tone audiometry may be insensitive to dead regions. In fact, the cochlear mechanical pattern induced by a sinusoidal stimulus at the frequency corresponding to a dead zone can activate the neural fibres originating from the boundary regions, where a sufficient number of inner hair cells may provide the transduction. For instance, if the dead zone comprises the 3 to 4 kHz cochlear region, the corresponding neurons are not activated. However, 3 to 4 kHz stimuli of high intensity can stimulate the 1- to 2-kHz, more apical, region where inner hair cells are available for transduction. This phenomenon is defined as downward spread of excitation. Thus, the pure-tone threshold does not indicate the true condition of the cochlea, since a moderate hearing loss is apparent where, in fact, a cochlear dead zone actually exists. Based on these arguments, Moore et al. (45,46) proposed a clinical test [threshold equalising noise: TEN test (TEN test)] specifically designed to identify cochlear dead regions in patients with sensorineural hearing impairment. This test, easily performed, is based on the repeated recording of pure-tone thresholds under different levels of broadband noise masking. A dead zone is revealed at the frequencies where the pure-tone threshold increases more than 10 dB, despite the fact that masking is at a level below the unmasked threshold of those frequencies (Fig. 2.9). Although the clinical results are, so far, somewhat controversial (47) with regard to congenital hearing impairments (48) and the implications on hearing aid benefit (49), this test represents a significant attempt to improve the definition of cochlear damage through a simple behavioural test.

Middle-ear admittance and stapedial reflexometry

The dynamic measurements of tympanic admittance are of remarkable value for the diagnosis of middle-ear pathology. In

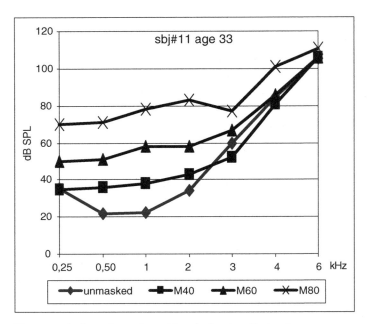

Figure 2.9 Audiometric test for cochlear dead regions. The hearing threshold (dB SPL) increases at the frequencies affected by masking, whereas the threshold at the frequencies above the level of masking remains unchanged. This happens, for the case shown, with masking of 30 and 50 dB SPL (M40, M60). With masking of 70 dB SPL (M80), the threshold above 3 kHz increases more than 10 dB, although for these frequencies, the level of masking is below the threshold. This figure suggests the presence of a cochlear dead region with boundaries at 3 to 4 kHz. *Source:* Author's data.

particular, reactive components of admittance are sensitive to the physical condition of the tympanic membrane, the ossicular chain, the contents of the middle ear, and the Eustachian tube function. The changes of admittance as a function of different air pressure applied to external ear canal are recorded as "tympanograms." Based on their morphology, tympanograms can be grouped into different classes, each reflecting a particular functional condition of the tympano-ossicular complex (50–52). Figure 2.10 shows a simple classification.

The measurement of admittance changes following the stapedial-muscle contraction, represents another important source of information relative to the functioning of middle–inner ear, cochlear nerve, and brain stem structures (53). Stapedial-reflex measures investigate a wide spectrum of functions due to the long neural arc linking the input (acoustical stimulus) to output (stapes-muscle contraction) (Fig. 2.11). Stapedial contraction is bilateral with high-intensity stimuli (over 85 dB HL), irrespective of the stimulated ear. The cochleostapedial arc is multisynaptic (54), with a short arc for the reflex ipsilateral to the stimulated ear, and a longer arc, crossing the brain stem, for the contralateral contraction. The complex of superior olivary nuclei constitutes the bridge between the cochlear nuclei and the facial motor nuclei, where motor fibres depart to innervate the muscles. Due to the complexity of the cochleostapedial arc, there are many pathological conditions that can alter the reflex. In addition to those

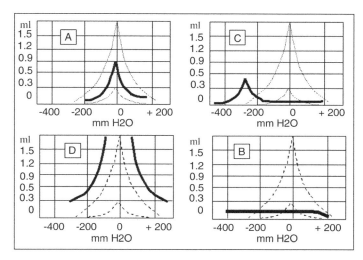

Figure 2.10 Simple classification of the principal tympanograms. Normally (**A**), the maximal admittance (compliance) coincides with a condition of equal air pressure between the external ear and the middle ear cavity (0 mm H$_2$O horizontal axis). (**B**) indicates low admittance values, irrespective of the air pressure changes: this figure is common in otitis media with effusion. In (**C**) the maximal admittance peaks at a negative air pressure, indicating a middle-ear pressure lower than external pressure (defective Eustachian tube). (**D**) reflects admittance values exceeding the instrument's capacity: usually this picture is associated with a discontinuity of the ossicular chain or a healed perforation.

involving the auditory periphery of the stimulated ear, (middle ear, inner ear, and cochlear nerve), there are also brain stem lesions, and those involving the nonstimulated ear (middle ear and stapedial muscle) and its facial nerve. To test the stapedial reflex, pure-tone stimuli and broadband noise are used. The difference between an elevated pure-tone threshold and the stapedial-reflex threshold is a valid diagnostic index. When it is less than 55 dB, it indicates a compressed auditory dynamic range, a feature reflecting cochlear damage (55); otherwise, retrocochlear involvement may be suspected. Pathological cochlear nerve adaptation in the stimulated ear is revealed by a

decay of the stapedial contraction for acoustical stimuli delivered for 10 seconds (56).

Another reflex variant consists of two peaks of admittance variations occurring at the start and at the end of the stimuli (the on–off effect). This finding may suggest an early otosclerotic focus affecting the stapes mobility at the oval window (57). Stapedial-reflex measures can also be used to indirectly estimate the hearing threshold (58). As a first approximation, the presence of a stapedial reflex elicited by an 85 dB stimulus can exclude a severe-to-profound hearing loss. Other predictions may be drawn from the difference of the stapedial threshold elicited by broadband noise and by pure tones. In normally hearing subjects, the noise threshold is 10 dB more sensitive than that for pure tones. In cochlear damage, this difference tends to disappear, whereas in severe-to-profound hearing losses, the probability of evoking a stapedial reflex, even at the highest stimulus intensity, decreases progressively. Table 2.4 summarises some conditions of the stapedial reflex and their possible associations with hearing impairments.

Otoacoustic emissions

Otoacoustic emissions are acoustical waveforms of small amplitude emitted by the cochlea in response to transient stimuli [transient-evoked otoacoustic emissions (TEOAEs)] or pairs of sinusoidal stimuli [distortion product otoacoustic emissions (DPOAEs)]. These responses are regarded as the ideal tools in the development of systems for universal neonatal screening. In fact, they may be rapidly recorded (3–5 minutes per subject) even by trained assistants. Independent of the kind of stimulus, otoacoustic emissions are the expression of the integrity of the outer hair cell system (59–61).

TEAOEs are evoked by transient stimuli of about 80 dB SPL. They represent small amounts of acoustical energy transmitted backward from the cochlea through the middle ear.

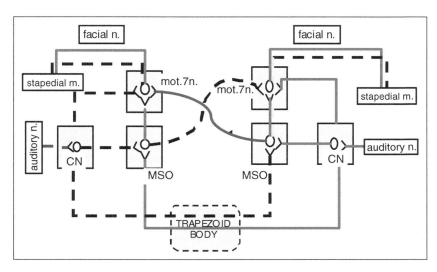

Figure 2.11 Schematic view of the cochleostapedial arc. Continuous and dashed lines are for the right and left arcs, respectively. The complex pathway accounts for the sensitivity of the reflex to a wide spectrum of disorders. *Abbreviations:* CN, cochlear nucleus; MSO, media superior olivary complex.

Table 2.4 Acoustic reflex prediction test

Acoustic reflex threshold difference (white noise–pure tones)	Acoustic reflex white noise	Hearing loss
>20	Anywhere	Normal hearing
15–19	≤80	Normal hearing
15–19	>80	Normal-mild hearing loss
10–14	Anywhere	Mild-moderate
<10	≤90	Severe
<10	>90	Profound

DPOAEs are evoked by stimuli consisting of two pure tones, with the frequencies having a ratio of 1.22 (for example, $f1 = 1000\,Hz$ and $f2 = 1220\,Hz$). In response to this complex stimulus, the cochlea generates and backwardly reflects a series of partials, the most intense of which is at the frequency corresponding to $2f1–f2$. By the use of f2 frequencies equal in value to those used in the classical audiometry, the amplitude of the DPOAE may be reported as a "DP-gram" (Fig. 2.12).

The efficiency of otoacoustic emissions as a screening tool is due to their presence/absence, which has proved to be capable of separating the babies with a hearing threshold better than 35 dB HL (present OAEs) from those with a hearing threshold worse than 45 dB HL (absent OAEs). This characteristic is then used as a criterion for identifying the "fail" cases, for which a hearing loss may be suspected, and in which a diagnostic investigation is needed.

In addition to their use for the screening for congenital hearing impairment, OAEs are also employed as a topodiagnostic test to detect early cochlear damage and, more importantly, to demonstrate the function of the normal outer hair cells in the context of auditory neuropathy. If cochlear damage is present, the amplitude and occurrence of OAEs decrease with the amount of hearing loss. It is thought that their changes could indicate outer hair-cell dysfunction before it is seen as an elevation of the hearing threshold. This latter condition occurs when at least 30% of outer hair cells are not functional.

In addition, the response pattern in OAEs has proved to be very stable also in time, and this feature may provide reliable longitudinal monitoring of cochlear function in subjects at a risk of sensorineural loss.

Auditory-evoked potentials

Among the range of neural electrical potentials recordable in response to auditory stimulation, those originating from the auditory periphery are widely employed in clinical settings, particularly with infants because they can provide reliable and objective measures of auditory sensitivity.

Electrocochleography

The first potential recordable by surface electrodes in response to transient stimuli is due to the activation of the more distal portion of the cochlear nerve. The same neural activity, also defined as the global action potential (AP) of the cochlear nerve, can be recorded in the "near field" through a transtympanic electrode, a technique called electrocochleography (ECochG) (62,63).

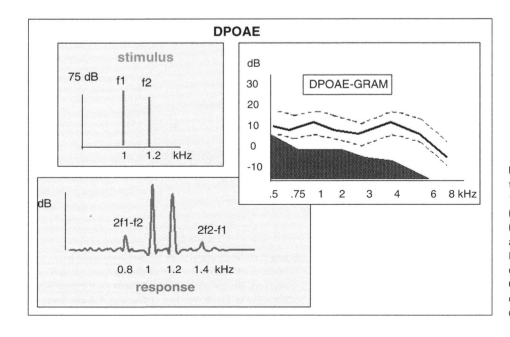

Figure 2.12 (*Stimulus*) DPOAEs are evoked by a two-tone complex (f1, f2) with a frequency ratio of 1.22 and an intensity of 55 to 70 dB SPL. (*Response*) In response to this stimulus, a partial (2f1-f2) or distortion product is reflected backward and acoustically recorded in the external ear. The DPOAE amplitude may be plotted in the function of the f2 frequency, as DP-gram (*insert*). Otoacoustic emissions are reliable indicators of outer hair-cells integrity. *Abbreviation*: DPOAE, distortion product otoacoustic emissions.

In addition to the AP, ECochG also records two receptor potentials, the cochlear microphonic and the summating potentials. The electrophysiological threshold of the AP is highly correlated to the psychoacoustical threshold (Fig. 2.13). For this reason, ECochG is retained as the most precise tool for objectively measuring the hearing threshold and the auditory peripheral function in children. Since, in clinical ECochG, the AP is evoked by transient stimuli, a limitation of the threshold estimates is that the AP threshold is directly comparable to the behavioural threshold only at frequencies between 1 and 4 kHz. Measurements of the AP including latency and amplitude changes, as a function of the stimulus intensity, provide information about the nature of the hearing loss (64), whether sensorineural or conductive. In addition, its morphology may be broadly indicative of the threshold profile. The AP is not detectable in those with hearing thresholds below 90 dB HL.

Transtympanic ECochG is considered a second-choice diagnostic tool, at least for children, since it requires a general anaesthesia.

Auditory brain stem response

The portion of the auditory pathway between the cochlear nerve and the subthalamic region (65) gives rise to a succession of six to seven potentials recordable by surface electrodes, in response to transient acoustical stimuli. The electrical sources of the first three components of ABR have been identified as the cochlear nerve (I, II) and cochlear nucleus, superior olive, and trapezoid body nuclei (III). The other components (IV, V, and VI) also show multiple origins, mainly from structures contralateral to the stimulated ear (lateral lemniscus, inferior colliculus, and medial geniculate body). Due to the multiple electrical sources contributing to each potential, the correlation between an altered potential and the anatomical site of lesion is quite low. On the other hand, the regular succession of the ABR components depends on synchrony of discharge of the neural units, which are activated in succession following the cochlear mechanical response to impulsive stimulation. Hence, the presence or absence of the components, their latency, the interwave latency differences, and the interaural latencies are reliable indicators of cochlear nerve and brain stem auditory pathway function (66,67).

Among the ABR components, wave V can be detected at a stimulus intensity near the behavioural threshold. The ABR wave V threshold evoked by transients correlates significantly with the behavioural threshold at 1 to 4 kHz, with an error of about ±15 dB (Fig. 2.14). As the ABR is easily recordable during spontaneous sleep or under slight sedation, it is considered to be a first-choice technique for examining the hearing of small children. These may be those identified as a "fail" by a neonatal screening but also includes all the other children up to two to three years of age requiring an objective measurement of their auditory sensitivity. Response parameters of the ABR in children younger than two years have to rely on appropriate normative data since the latencies of the ABR components are prolonged at birth, and then progressively "mature," reaching the adult values approximately at the age of two years (68).

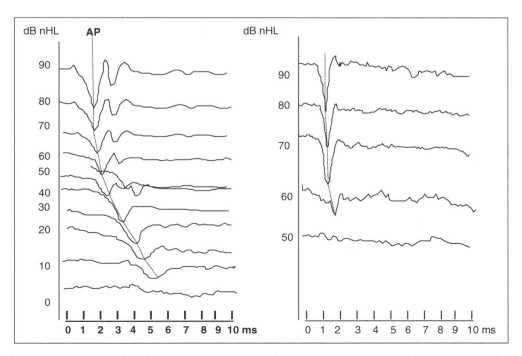

Figure 2.13 Electrocochleographic recording of the global AP of the cochlear nerve. (*Left*) normal hearing, AP well defined at 10 dB nHL. (*Right*) hearing loss, AP defined up to 60 dB nHL, with latencies relatively stable. This feature may suggest the presence of loudness recruitment. *Abbreviation*: AP, action potential.

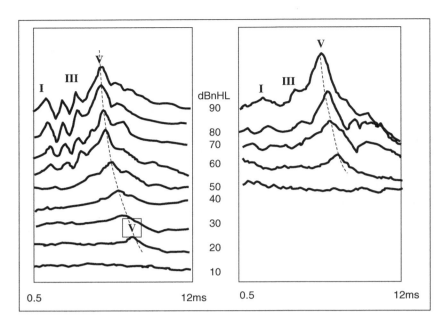

Figure 2.14 (*Left*) Auditory brain stem response (ABR) from a normally hearing subject. Wave V is defined down to 20 dB nHL. This component allows for threshold estimates at frequencies of 2 to 4 kHz. (*Right*) ABR in a case of conductive hearing loss; wave V defined to 60 dB nHL, increased latency, normal I to V interval.

A common finding in the children is an elevation of wave V threshold due to otitis media with effusion. Those with conductive hearing loss show an increase in the latency of all the ABR components, with a I–V interval in the normal range. Those with cochlear sensorineural hearing loss, in addition to an elevation in wave V threshold, show components that, at high stimulus intensity, are normal in latency. This picture can suggest the presence of loudness recruitment. Those in whom any component cannot be evoked by the maximal stimulus intensity are strongly suspected of having a profound hearing loss.

ABR in children presenting with a language disorder enables us to distinguish whether it is secondary to a defect of the auditory periphery or to more central dysfunction at the level of the brain stem (Fig. 2.15). In a small group of the latter, imaging techniques may also document organic lesions within the central nervous system. Conversely, in the majority, only a variety of ABR abnormalities can be demonstrated, ranging from a prolonged I–V interval to a complete abolition of the evoked response. The first is generally interpreted as a consequence of a delay in maturation of the brain stem auditory pathway. The most marked alterations may suggest severe disorganisation of neural discharge synchrony. It is still unclear whether this reflects dysfunction affecting the whole brain stem auditory pathway or the consequence of more limited damage,

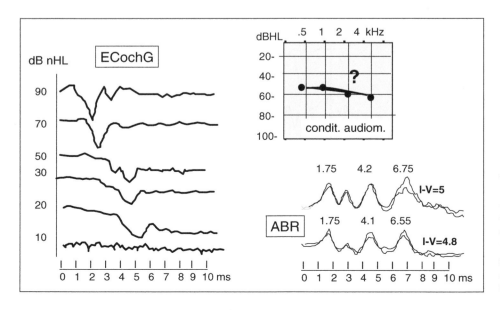

Figure 2.15 ECochG and ABR in a four-year-old child with a severe language disorder and uncertain results to conditioned response audiometry (*peep show*). The 20 dB nHL action-potential threshold excludes a damage in the auditory periphery. Conversely, ABR shows a prolonged I to V interval (normal values up to 4.4 msec), and this may suggest a delay in maturation of the brain stem auditory pathway. *Abbreviations*: ABR, auditory brain stem response; ECochG, electrocochleography.

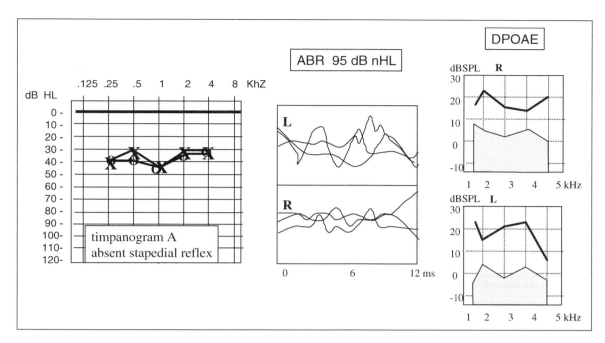

Figure 2.16 In some cases, ABR result is undefined, despite a normal or slightly enhanced hearing threshold. When this finding is associated with normal OAEs, the clinical figure is defined as "auditory neuropathy." In the case shown, a five-year-old child had abnormal language development and presented with a marked lexical reduction and defective connected language. *Abbreviations*: ABR, auditory brain stem response; DPOAE, distortion product otoacoustic emission; L, left ear; R, right ear.

involving the inner hair cell—first auditory neuron complex (69). This latter condition has been hypothesised as explaining the clinical finding broadly defined as "auditory neuropathy" (70). The typical picture of this clinical entity, with an aetiology still undefined, consists of a normal or slightly impaired pure-tone threshold, indefinable ABR components, normal OAEs (Fig. 2.16), and poor speech recognition.

Auditory steady state response

Auditory steady state response (ASSRs) are recorded in response to an ongoing sinusoidal stimulus (carrier), periodically modulated in amplitude [amplitude modulation (AM)] or frequency at a rate of about 100/sec. Unlike transient responses such as the ABR, which show typical variations measurable in the time-domain (i.e., latency), ASSRs are potentials with frequency components remaining constant in amplitude and phase for the duration of the sustained stimulus.

The ASSR recording technique is the same as for the ABR, but the signal analysis is different. ASSRs are analysed in the frequency domain through spectral analysis techniques. Their electrical amplitude is usually much lower than the electroencephalogram (EEG) baseline amplitude. Hence, the response is detected by specific statistical algorithms that operate simultaneously with the acquisition of the bioelectrical signal.

The cochlea reacts to an AM sinusoidal stimulus by activating the hair cells in the region corresponding to the carrier frequency. Although the resultant neural activation arises from a restricted area of the basilar membrane (the carrier is frequency specific), it also takes the same periodicity of the modulation frequency (Fig. 2.17). Thus, the neural response to the modulation frequency primarily originates at the level of the first auditory afferent neuron, while the cochlear nuclei and other brain stem nuclei preserve this information (71).

The clinical interest in ASSRs lies in the possibility of testing the auditory sensitivity to low frequencies, even in children under slight sedation, because vigilance and sedation have little influence on these potentials. The ASSR electrophysiological thresholds are less sensitive than behavioural thresholds to pure tones (Fig. 2.18). In adults, the difference is between 10 and 20 dB (73,74), whereas in children, this difference is more difficult to evaluate. Subjects with sensorineural hearing loss show a closer accord of the two thresholds, and this effect is probably associated with loudness recruitment. The use of acoustical stimuli simultaneously modulated in amplitude and frequency can probably improve ASSR detection in children (75,76).

Speech audiometry

Speech audiometry was initially aimed at obtaining audiometric measurements more relevant to communication difficulties than pure-tone audiometry. Speech material has also proved to be particularly sensitive to lesions involving the auditory central nervous system (77,78). Its clinical sensitivity could be further enhanced by manipulating the primary speech signal,

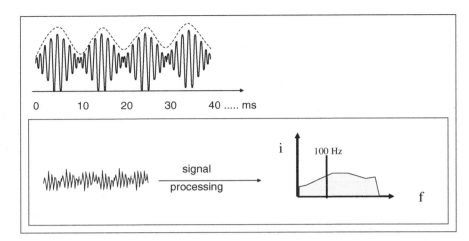

Figure 2.17 Steady-state responses are evoked by ongoing pure tones modulated in amplitude or frequency (*upper*, 1 kHz carrier frequency amplitude modulated at 100 Hz). The neural response to modulation is physically smaller than EEG amplitude. A specific signal analysis recognises the modulation frequency within the bioelectrical signal. (*Lower* insert, spectral analysis indicates the 100 Hz component emerging from EEG noise.) *Abbreviation*: EEG, electroencephalogram.

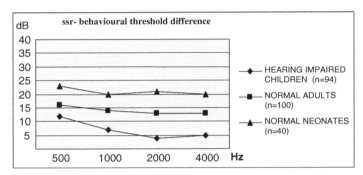

Figure 2.18 Difference between SSR and behavioural thresholds in children and adults. For comparison, the SSR thresholds in normal neonates are also shown. *Abbreviation*: SSR, steady state responses. *Source*: From Ref. 72.

for instance by changes in the frequency, temporal, and linguistic domains, or indirectly, by delivering the speech signal under physical (noise masking) or informative masking (competition).

The clinical use of speech audiometry for the site-of-lesion diagnosis of auditory disorders is limited today. Imaging techniques are more reliable for exploration of the central nervous system. Conversely, speech audiometry is mainly used to evaluate the results following any rehabilitative intervention such as ear surgery, hearing aids, and implantable devices. Speech audiometry, indeed, may provide functional estimates of the single-subject auditory performance, by comparing the pre- and posttreatment results.

Performance scores and hearing impairment

The traditional techniques of speech audiometry are based on the administration of stimulus material consisting of 10 to 20 speech items (words and sentences) arranged in lists. The speech items within a list are balanced for lexical occurrence and phonetic distribution and are acoustically calibrated. Each list is delivered at a fixed level of intensity, according to the psychoacoustical method of "constant stimuli," through headphones or loudspeakers in the free field. The subject's task

consists of repeating each item, and the percentages of correct responses relative to each list are plotted as a function of the intensity. This is defined as the "intelligibility function." The correct response rate or intelligibility is influenced by numerous variables other than those represented by the hearing acuity. Some are cognitive factors concerning the individual; others concern the test techniques. Among these is the score variability depending on the number of items within each list (Fig. 2.19). Because this may consistently affect the intermediate portion of the intelligibility function, i.e., around the 50% [speech reception threshold (SRT)], it may lead to uncertain results when two intelligibility functions are compared as, for example, in order to evaluate a pre/post-treatment effect. For scores of 50% and 95%, the variability given by two standard deviations corresponds to 32% and 13.8%, respectively, with 10 items per list (79).

The SRT may be also measured by adaptive procedures (80). These enable us to obtain the intensity levels corresponding to a fixed percentage of intelligibility, e.g., 25%, 50%, and 75%. The most common adaptive procedure is the simple up–down technique, in which the speech items are serially presented with an intensity that changes according to the subject's responses. Following a correct response, the intensity is decreased; following an incorrect response, intensity is increased. Intensity steps are usually between 2 and 5 dB. After 8 to 12 reversals, the test is over, and the SRT is calculated in dB as the mean of the median values between each reversal. In normally hearing subjects, in conductive and cochlear hearing loss (Fig. 2.20), the SRT correlates within ±5 dB with the average pure-tone threshold (0.5-1-2 kHz). However, in cochlear losses, the shape of the intelligibility function may be influenced by the perceptual distortions of intensity, frequency, and time, since they can adversely affect phoneme discrimination (42,81). Patients with retrocochlear hearing impairment or defective neural transduction often present with difficulty of speech recognition, particularly for high-intensity signals. Patients with lesions within the brain stem or involving the parietotemporal cortex may show performance on speech tests remarkably worse than those predicted from pure-tone thresholds.

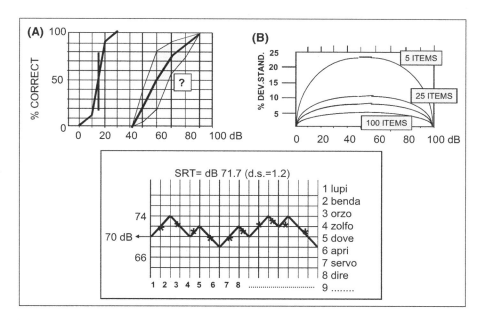

Figure 2.19 In speech audiometry, the scores of correct responses are affected by an intrinsic variability, depending on the number of items within the list. The speech audiogram (A) shows two intelligibility functions, one from a normal subject and one from a patient with a hearing impairment. For the latter, the range of variability (±2 SD) is shown, as expected for a 10-items list, (B) shows the standard deviation as a function of the number of items. The lower insert depicts the format used for adaptive procedures. Each stimulus consists of a different word, and intensity changes according to whether the responses are correct or incorrect. For this simple up–down procedure, the speech reception threshold (50% correct responses) is given by averaging the median intensities between the peaks and the troughs.

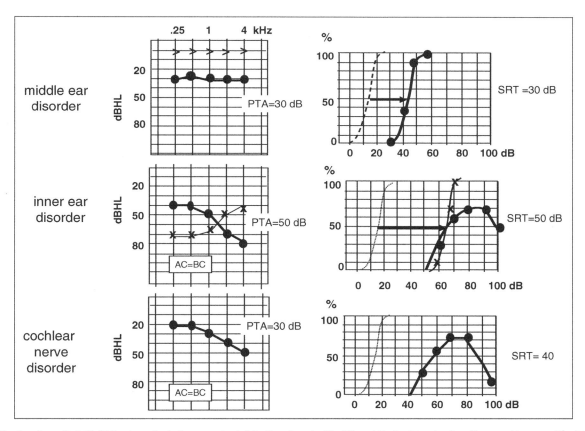

Figure 2.20 The function of intelligibility also reflects the perceptual distortions found with different kinds of hearing loss. Compared to normal (*pointed function*), in middle ear disorders, the SRT is shifted by the same amount as the pure-tone hearing threshold (PTA, 0.5-1-2 kHz). In inner ear disorders, the maximum intelligibility may be less than 100% due to perceptual disorders typical of cochleopathies. In retrocochlear disorders (cochlear nerve and brain stem), the SRT is shifted by an amount greater than that predicted from the PTA. In addition, a progressive reduction of intelligibility with intensity is sometimes observable ("roll-over effect"). *Abbreviations*: PTA, pure tone average; SRT, speech reception threshold.

Such results may be sensitised by the use of special speech materials in which redundancy is decreased by changing the acoustical properties of the speech signal or by adding other competing signals.

Although speech audiometry has been excluded from the test battery originally recommended in individuals with a suspected genetic hearing impairment (82), it has recently provided useful results in the characterisation of some forms of dominant nonsyndromal hearing impairments.

For example, the progressive forms, DFNA2 and DFNA5, show a deterioration in the rate of speech recognition that occurs relatively slowly over time. On the other hand, DFNA9 and DFNA10, with a later onset, show a more rapid deterioration, with an intelligibility reduction estimated at 1.8% per year (83–85). Such findings could indicate that, in DFNA2 and DFNA5, the cochlear damage is relatively stable, whereas in DFNA9 and DFNA10, in which speech test scores are similar to those of "presbyacusis," the damage tends to involve structures other than the outer hair cells (86,87).

References

1. Pennings RJE, Huygen PLM, VanCamp G, et al. A review of progressive phenotypes in nonsyndromic autosomal dominant hearing impairment. Audiol Med 2003; 1:47–55.
2. Stephens D. Audiological terms. In: Martini A, Mazzoli M, Stephens D, Read A, eds. Definitions, Protocols & Guidelines in Genetic Hearing Impairment. London: Whurr, 2001:9–16.
3. Van de Heyning P, Claes J, Brokx J, et al. Surgical management of hearing impairment in audiological medicine. In: Luxon L, Furman F, Martini A, Stephens D, eds. Textbook of Audiological Medicine. London: Martin Dunitz, 2003:603–640.
4. Schuknecht HF. Further observations on the pathology of presbyacusis. Arch Otolaryngol 1964; 80:369–382.
5. Raphael Y, Altshuler RA. Structure and innervation of the cochlea. Brain Res Bull 2003; 60:397–422.
6. Cryns K, VanCamp G. Deafness genes and their diagnostic applications. Audiol Neuro otol 2004; 9:2–22.
7. Boothroyd A, Cawkwell S. Vibrotactile thresholds in pure tone audiometry. Acta Otolaryngol 1979; 69:381–387.
8. Schuknecht HF, Woellner R. An experimental and clinical study of deafness for lesions of the cochlear nerve. J Laryngol Otol 1955; 69:75–97.
9. Lehnhardt E. Neuro-axonal recruitment: a result of selective compression. J Laryngol Otol 1990; 104:185–190.
10. Spoendlin H. Retrograde degeneration of the cochlear nerve. Acta Otolaryngol 1975; 79:266–275.
11. Jerger J, Herer G. An unexpected dividend in Bekesy audiometry. J Speech Hear Disord 1961; 26:390–391.
12. Erlandsson B, Hakansson H, Ivarsson A, et al. Comparison of the hearing threshold measured by manual pure-tone and by self-recording (Bekesy) audiometry. Audiology 1979; 18:414–429.
13. McCommons RB, Hodge DC. Comparison of continuous and pulsed tone for determining Bekesy threshold measurements. J Acoust Soc Am 1969; 45:1499–1503.
14. Laroche C, Hetu R. A study of the reliability of automatic audiometry by the frequency scanning method (Audioscan). Audiology 1997; 36:1–18.
15. Stephens D, Meredith R, Sirimanna, et al. Application of the Audioscan in the detection of carriers of genetic hearing loss. Audiology 1995; 34:91–97.
16. Mauermann M, Long GR, Kollmeier B. Fine structure of hearing threshold and loudness perception. J Acoust Soc Am 2004; 116:1066–1080.
17. Parving A. Reliability of Bekesy threshold tracing in identification of carriers of genes for an X-linked disease with deafness. Acta Otolaryngol 1978; 85:40–44.
18. Meredith R, Stephens D, Sirimanna T, et al. Audiometric detection of carriers of Usher's type II. J Audiol Med 1992; 1: 11–19.
19. Cohen M, Francis M, Luxon L, et al. Dips on Bekesy or Audioscan fail to identify carriers of autosomal recessive non-syndromic hearing loss. Acta Otolaryngol 1996; 116:5121–527.
20. Stephens D, Francis M. The detection of carriers of genetic hearing loss. In: Martini A, Read A, Stephens D, eds. Genetics and hearing impairment. London: Whurr, 1996:100–108.
21. Dobie RA. The relative contributions of occupational noise and aging in individual cases of hearing loss. Ear Hear 1992; 13: 19–27.
22. International Standard Organization. ISO 1999. Acoustics-determination of occupational noise exposure and estimation of noise-induced hearing impairment. Geneva, ISO 1990.
23. International Standard Organization. ISO 7029. Acoustics-threshold of hearing by air conduction as a function of age and sex for otologically normal persons. Geneva, ISO 1984.
24. Wuyts FL, Van de Heyning PH, Decalu F. Audiometric criteria for linkage analysis in genetic hearing impairment. In: Stephens D, Read A, Martini A, eds. Developments in Genetic Hearing Impairment. London: Whurr, 1998:54–55.
25. Karlsson KK, Harris JR, Svartengren M. Description and primary results from an audiometric study of male twins. Ear Hear 1997; 18:114–120.
26. Gates GA, Couropmitree NN, Myers RH. Genetic associations in age-related hearing thresholds. Arch Otolaryngol Head Neck Surg 1999; 125:275–280.
27. Robinson DW. Long-term repeatability of the pure-tone hearing threshold and its relation to noise exposure. Br J Audiol 1991; 25:219–235.
28. Martini A, Prosser S, Mazzoli M, et al. Contribution of age related factors to the progression of nonsyndromic hereditary hearing impairment. J Audiol Med 1996; 5:141–156.
29. Huygen PLM, Pennings RJE, Cremers CWR. Characterizing and distinguishing progressive phenotypes in nonsyndromic autosomal dominant hearing impairment. Audiol Med 2003; 1:37–46.
30. Hinchcliffe R. The threshold of hearing. In: Luxon L, Furman F, Martini A, Stephens D, eds. Handbook of Audiological Medicine. London: Martin Dunitz, 2003:213–247.

31. Job A, Delplace F, Anvers P, et al. Analyze automatique d'audiogramme visant à la surveillance épidémiologique di cohortes exposée aux bruits impulsifs. Rev Epidem Santè Pub 1993; 41:407–520.

32. Ozdamar X, Eilers RE, Miskiel E, et al. Classification of audiograms by sequential testing using a dynamic Bayesian procedure. J Acoust Soc Am 1990; 88:2171–2179.

33. Sorri M, Muhli A, Maeki-Torkko E, et al. Unambiguous system for describing audiogram configurations. J Audiol Med 2000; 9: 160–169.

34. Martini S, Milani M, Rosignoli M, et al. Audiometric patterns of genetic non-syndromal sensorineural hearing loss. Audiology 1997; 36:228–236.

35. Griffith AJ, Sprunger LK, Sirko-Osada DA, et al. Marshall syndrome associated with a slicing defect at the COL11A1 locus. Am J Hum Genet 1998; 62:816–823.

36. Asher JH, Sommer A, Morell R, et al. Missense mutation in the parallel domain of PAX3 causes craniofacial-deafness-hand syndrome. Hum Mut 1996; 7:30–35.

37. Friedman B, Friedman JM, Shulz M, et al. Recent advances in the understanding of syndromic forms of hearing loss. Ear Hear 2003; 24:289–302.

38. Li XC, Everett LA, Lawani AK, et al. A mutation in PDS causes non-syndromic recessive deafness. Nat Gen 1998; 18:215–217.

39. Hasson T, Heintzelman MB, Santos-Sacchi J, et al. Expressions in the cochlea and retina of myosin VIIa, the gene product defective in Usher syndrome type Ib. Proc Natl Acad Sci 1995; 92:9815–9819.

40. Chang EH, VanCamp G, Smith RJH. The role of connexins in human disease. Ear Hear 2003; 24:314–323.

41. Hall JW. Classic site-of-lesion tests. In: Rintelmann WF, ed. Hearing assessment. 2nd ed. Needham Heights, MD: Allyn & Bacon, 1991:669–679.

42. Glasberg BR, Moore BCJ. Psychoacoustic abilities of subjects with unilateral and bilateral cochlear impairments and their ability to understand speech. Scand Audiol 1989; suppl 32:1–25.

43. Rosenberg P. Abnormal auditory adaptation. Archs Otolaryngol 1971; 89:89–97.

44. Borg E, Canlon B, Engstroem B. Noise induced hearing loss. Literature review and experiments in rabbits. Scand Audiol 1995; 24(suppl 40):1–147.

45. Moore BCJ, Huss M, Vickers DA, et al. A test for the diagnosis of dead regions in the cochlea. Br J Audiol 2000; 34:205–224.

46. Moore BCJ. Dead regions in the cochlea: diagnosis, perceptual consequences and implication for the fitting of hearing aids. Trends Amplif 2001; 5:1–34.

47. Summers V, Molis MR, Musch H, et al. Identifying dead regions in the cochlea: psycophysical tuning curves and tone detection in threshold equalizing noise. Ear Hear 2003; 24:133–142.

48. Moore BCJ, Killen T, Munro KJ. Application of TEN test to hearing-impaired teenagers with severe-to-profound hearing loss. Int J Audiol 2003; 42:465–474.

49. Vickers DA, Moore BCJ, Baer T. Effects of low-pass filtering on the intelligibility if speech in quiet for people with and without dead regions at high frequencies. J Acoust Soc Am 2001; 110:1164–1175.

50. Jerger J, Jerger S, Mauldin L. Studies in impedance audiometry. I. Normal and sensorineural ears. Arch Otolaryngol 1972; 96:513–523.

51. Jerger J, Anthony L, Jerger S, Mauldin L III. Studies in impedance audiometry. III. Middle ear disorders. Arch Otolaryngol 1974; 99:165–171.

52. Liden G, Bjorkman G, Nyman H. Tympanometry and acoustic impedance. Acta Otolaryngol 1977; 83:140–145.

53. Hayes D, Jerger J. Pattern of acoustic reflex and auditory brainstem response abnormality. Acta Otolaryngol 1981; 92:199–202.

54. Borg E. On the neural organization of the acoustic middle ear reflex: a physiological and anatomical study. Brain Res 1973; 49:101–123.

55. Metz O. Threshold of reflex contraction of muscles of middle ear and recruitment of loudness. Arch Otolaryngol 1952; 55:536–543.

56. Anderson H, Barr B, Wedenberg E. Early diagnosis of the eight nerve tumors by acoustic reflex tests. Acta Otolaryngol 1970; suppl 263:232–237.

57. Bel J, Causse P, Michaux R, et al. Mechanical explanation of the on-off effect (diphasic impedance change) in otospongiosis. Audiology 1976; 15:128–140.

58. Hall JW. Predicting hearing level from the acoustic reflex: a comparison of three methods. Arch Otolaryngol 1978; 104:601–606.

59. Gorga M, Neely S, Bergman B, et al. Otoacoustic emissions from normal-hearing and hearing-impaired subjects: distortion product responses. J Acoust Soc Am 1993; 93:2050–2060.

60. Prieve BA, Gorga M, Schmidt A, et al. Analysis of transient-evoked otoacoustic emissions in normal-hearing and hearing-impaired ears. J Acoust Soc Am 1993; 93:3308–3319.

61. Prieve BA, Fitzgerald TS, Schulte LE, et al. Basic characteristics of distortion product otoacoustic emissions in infants and children. J Acoust Soc Am 1997; 102:2871–2879.

62. Eggermont JJ. Basic principles for electrocochleography. Acta Oto laryngol 1974; 316 (suppl):7–16.

63. Arslan E, Prosser S, Conti G, Michelini S. Electrocochleography and brainstem potentials in the diagnosis of the deaf child. Int J Pediatr Otorhinolaryngol 1982; 5:251–259.

64. Yoshie N. Diagnostic significance of electrocochleogram in clinical audiometry. Audiology 1973; 12:504–539.

65. Moeller AR. Neural generators of the brainstem auditory evoked potentials. Sem Hear 1998; 19:11–27.

66. Starr A, Achor J. Auditory brainstem responses in neurological disease. Arch Neurol 1975; 32:761–768.

67. Starr A, Hamilton A. Correlation between confirmed sites of neurological lesions and abnormalities of far-field auditory brainstem responses. Electroencephal Clin Neurophysiol 1976; 41:596–608.

68. Salamy R. Maturation of auditory brainstem response from birth through early childhood. J Clin Neurophysiol 1984; 1:293–329.

69. Kraus N, Ozdamar O, Stein L, et al. Absent auditory brain stem response: peripheral hearing loss or brain stem dysfunction? Laryngoscope 1984; 94:400–406.

70. Starr A, Picton TW, Sininger Y, et al. Auditory neuropathy. Brain 1996; 119:741–753.

71. Langner G, Schreiner CE. Periodicity coding in the inferior colliculus of the cat. I. Neuronal mechanisms. J Neurophysiol 1988; 60:1799–1822.

72. Perez-Abalo MC, Savio G, Toores A, et al. Steady state responses to multiple amplitude-modulated tones: an optimized method to test frequency-specific thresholds in hearing impaired children and normal hearing subjects. Ear Hear 2001; 22:200–211.

73. Rance G, Rickards FW, Cohen LT, et al. The automated prediction of hearing thresholds in sleeping subjects using auditory steady-state evoked potentials. Ear Hear 1995; 16:499–507.

74. Herdmann AT, Stapells DR. Thresholds determined using the monotic and dichotic multiple auditory steady state response technique in normal hearing subjects. Scand Audiol 2001; 30:41–49.

75. John MS, Brown DK, Muir PJ, et al. Recording auditory steady-sate responses in young infants. Ear Hear 2004; 25: 539–553.

76. Lins OG, Picton TW. Auditory steady state responses to multiple simultaneous stimuli. Electroencephal Clin Neurophysiol 1995; 96:420–432.

77. Bocca E, Calearo C. Central hearing processes. In: Jerger J, ed. Modern developments in audiology. New York: Academic Press, 1963:337–370.

78. Jerger J, Jerger SW. Clinical validity of central auditory tests. Scand Audiol 1975; 4:147–163.

79. Lyregaard P. Towards a theory of speech audiometry tests. In: Martin M, ed. Speech Audiometry. London: Taylor & Francis, 1987: 33–67.

80. Levitt H. Adaptive testing in audiology. Scand Audiol 1978; 6(suppl):241–291.

81. Festen JM. Contribution of comodulation masking release and temporal resolution to the speech–reception threshold masked by interfering noise. J Acoust Soc Am 1993; 94: 1725–1736.

82. Stephens D. Audiometric investigation of probands. In: Martini A, Mazzoli M, Stephens D, Read A, eds. Definitions, Protocols & Guidelines in Genetic Hearing Impairment. London: Whurr, 2001:29–31.

83. De Leeheener EMR, Huygen PLM, Wayne S, et al. The DFNA 10 phenotype. Ann Otol Rhinol Laryngol 2001; 110:861–866.

84. De Leeheener EMR, Huyhen PLM, Coucke PJ, et al. Longitudinal and cross-sectional phenotype analysis in a new, large Dutch DFNA 2/KCNQ4 family. Ann Otol Rhinol Laryngol 2002; 111: 267–274.

85. De Leenheer EMR, vanZuijlen DA, Van Laer L, et al. Further delineation of the DFNA5 phenotype. Results of speech recognition tests. Ann Otol Rhinol Laryngol 2002; 111:639–641.

86. Bom SJH, De Leeheener EMR, Leamrie FX, et al. Speech recognition scores related to age and degree of hearing impairment in DFNA2/KCNQ4 and DFNA9/COCH. Arch Otolaryngol 2001; 127:1045–1048.

87. Ketharpal U. DFNA9 is a progressive audiovestibular dysfunction with a microfibrillar deposit in the inner ear. Laryngoscope 2000; 110:1379–1384.

3 Newly emerging concepts in syndromology relevant to audiology and otolaryngology practice

William Reardon

Clinical basics—the descriptive language of dysmorphology

Dysmorphologists recognise four essential categories of birth defect. Firstly "deformations," which means that the birth defect results from abnormal mechanical forces acting to distort an otherwise normal structure. These often occur quite late in gestation after normal initial formation of organs, but the growth and subsequent development of these organs or structures are hampered by the mechanical force. An example of one such birth defect might be a club foot (talipes), but it needs to be borne in mind that talipes is not always the result of a deformation and can result from other categories of birth defect.

Secondly, "disruptions," are structural defects caused by actual destruction of previously normal tissue. This type of birth defect could be consequent on haemorrhage or poor blood flow during development to a particular region of the developing fetus. Disruptional abnormalities generally affect several different tissue types within a well-demarcated anatomical region.

Thirdly, "dysplasias," being abnormal cellular organisation or function within a specific tissue type throughout the body, resulting in clinically apparent structural changes. A good example of a dysplasia is a skeletal dysplasia, resulting in

"dwarfing," where the patient's short stature is caused by a major gene mutation causing a dysplasia of the cartilage, with the result that the bones do not elongate.

The fourth type of birth defect is "malformation." This term is reserved for abnormalities caused by failure of the embryonic process; in other words, the particular tissue or organ is arrested, delayed or misdirected, causing permanent abnormalities of the structure. This was a structure, which never pursued normal development. Many malformations are the result of genetic mutations and can result in a malformation syndrome affecting several different body systems and causing a range of different clinical signs of birth defects in the individual patient.

In contrast to deformations and disruptions, malformations suggest an error occurring early in gestation, either in tissue differentiation or during the development of individual organ systems. Likewise it should be inferred that since both deformations and disruptions usually affect structures, which have undergone normal initial development, the presence of a birth defect thus classified does not signify an intrinsic abnormality of the tissues involved. Furthermore, it follows that there is rarely a cause for concern about mental retardation or other hidden future medical problems if the birth defect in a child is determined to be a disruption or a deformation—unless there has been structural damage to the brain as part of the birth defect.

The relationship of birth defects to one another

Four distinct relationships are recognised and these will be outlined.

Single system defects

Malformations comprising a local region of a single organ system of the body account for the majority of birth defects. Representative examples include cleft lip, congenital heart disease, and congenital dislocation of the hip.

Associations

Clinical signs, which occur together in a nonrandom fashion and result in a recognisable "pattern," but whose single underlying cause remains unknown are said to represent an association. A good example is a fairly common condition seen in newborn babies and recognised by the pattern of birth defects. The condition is VATER association, comprising vertebral abnormalities, anal atresia, tracheo-oesophageal fistula, renal abnormalities and limb defects. The cause(s) of this condition is not known. Chromosome and other genetic studies are invariably normal in the affected patient. What is recognised is that a child with tracheo-oesophageal fistula, who will present with inability to swallow on day 1 or 2 of life, needs to have careful examination for these other clinical features, which are sometimes associated. So, it acts as a prompt to the astute clinician to look for some of the more cryptic birth defects such as the vertebral abnormalities, which might otherwise be overlooked but have serious long-term sequelae.

Sequences

Some patterns of multiple birth defects result from a cascade of seemingly unrelated events but which actually follow from a single developmental event/defect. Consequently, this primary abnormality interferes with normal embryological and fetal development to result in the birth of a child who appears to have separate and distinct abnormalities, possibly involving widely separated body areas and organ systems. For instance, in Potter sequence, the primary abnormality is absent kidneys. The failure to produce urine results in a greatly reduced volume of amniotic fluid around the baby, which in turn leads to mechanical constraint on the baby with deformations such as limb bowing, joint contractures, and compressed facial features, known as Potter's facies. These deformations are elements of the sequence of events, which follow from the primary defect, which is the absent kidneys.

Syndromes

A particular set of congenital anomalies repeatedly occurring in a generally consistent pattern is known as a "syndrome." In contrast to an association, a syndrome suggests that the link between the various anomalies is fairly consistent from patient to patient. Often a syndrome is differentiated from an association by the identification of the underlying cause, which explains the seemingly disparate clinical elements of the syndrome. Consequently, it will be understood that a syndrome may be caused by a chromosomal problem (Down syndrome), a biochemical defect (Smith–Lemli–Opitz syndrome), a Mendelian genetic defect (Treacher Collins syndrome), or an environmental agent (fetal alcohol syndrome).

Since this particular term, syndrome, is at the heart of this discussion, a few points of elaboration may be in order. Birth defect syndromes are usually recognised from the report of a single or a few individual cases which bear a resemblance to one another. With the publication of further cases, this emerging new syndrome is expanded by the inclusion of other birth defects not observed in the original reports. Likewise, these follow-on publications tend to throw light on the natural history of the condition, clarify the prognosis, and, with luck, establish a causation or identify a new investigation, which is diagnostic. This is a period of natural tension between aspiring authors, anxious to publish their cases and expand the clinical documentation of the new syndrome, and journal editors and referees, who have a duty to keep the literature free of impurities but also an obligation to publish genuine cases, which do add to the sum total of knowledge in relation to the newly emerging/emerged condition. However, in the absence of hard objective laboratory investigations, cases that are wrongly attributed can and sometimes do get published, resulting in confusion in the emerging literature. One can then understand why it is that for newly emerging, individually rare, conditions, based on relatively few cases, the clinical basis of the diagnosis may remain "soft" for a considerable period. It is worth quoting directly from Aase (1), "even after considerable refinement, however, diagnoses based on clinical observations show a great range of latitude and there may be no "gold standard" against which a particular patient can be compared. ...there is inherent variability in the manifestations of most dysmorphic disorders, both in type and in severity of structural abnormalities... Syndrome diagnosis still relies heavily on the ability of the clinician to detect and to correctly interpret physical and developmental findings and to recognise patterns in them."

The impact of gene identification and the altered environment of clinical practice

This chapter addressed a decade ago might have had a strong emphasis on the need for careful phenotypic examination of patients with a view to gathering together adequate pedigrees to pursue linkage and aspire to gene identification. For many well-defined syndromes, these goals have now been attained and current molecular strategies are increasingly turning toward non-Mendelian conditions, often characterised as associations. There is an increasing reliance on molecular cytogenetics to investigate patients whose clinical conditions, occurring sporadically within their families, have previously been unexplained. Much of this work stems from observations of Flint and others in the mid-1990s that up to 7% of unexplained mental retardation could be caused by subtelomere deletions of chromosomes in patients whose gross chromosomal examination was normal (2,3). As a result of this new focus of research into previously undiagnosable cases, new syndromes are emerging, many of them of relevance to the audiological physician and his/her surgical counterpart.

Meanwhile, rare or poorly defined syndromes continue to be subject to ongoing research studies with a view to identifying causative mutations underlying those conditions and easing diagnostic controversies in cases on the margins of those diagnoses. In parallel with these active research developments, clinicians have worked to apply many of the lessons learned from syndromes and conditions for which diagnostic genetic tests have now become available to enhance clinical management of patients and families with these conditions. It would be impossible in this contribution to allude to all of the advances relevant to syndromology of audiological medicine and otolaryngology practice, so the author proposes to focus on specific examples, which demonstrate the principles above outlined.

Identifying a genetic basis for a sporadically occurring condition—CHARGE association becomes a syndrome

CHARGE association was first described in 1979 by Hall in 17 children with multiple congenital anomalies, who were ascertained because of choanal atresia (4). Low-set, small, and malformed ears were identified among several of these cases, and associated clinical observations encompassing congenital heart defects, ocular colobomas, deafness, hypogenitalism, facial palsy, and developmental delay were noted as inconsistent findings across the patient cohort. Writing in the same year, Hittner et al. (5) reported 10 children, ascertained for colobomatous microphthalmia, with essentially the same constellation of clinical malformations. The term CHARGE was first proposed by Pagon et al. (6) to reflect the major clinical clues to this diagnosis, such as coloboma, heart defect, atresia choanae, retarded growth, or ear anomalies/deafness. As recognised by Graham (7), the characteristic asymmetry of the clinical findings and the frequent absence of either choanal atresia or coloboma made diagnosis difficult in many cases, and several patients looked like they "might" have CHARGE association, but, without a diagnostic test, the clinical designation of such cases remained dubious. Experienced clinical geneticists often seized upon the ear morphology, the typically cup-shaped ear, as a clue to diagnosis in these marginal cases (Fig. 3.1).

An important clinical landmark was reached in 2001 when Amiel et al. (8) reported absence or hypoplasia of the semicircular canals on temporal bone computed tomography

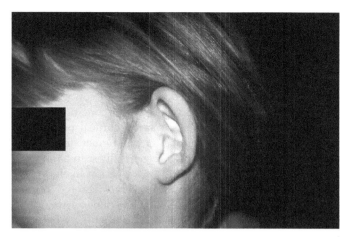

Figure 3.1 Cupped, prominent ear, in a patient with CHARGE syndrome. *Abbreviation*: CHARGE, coloboma, heart defect, atresia choanae, retarded growth, ear anomalies/deafness.

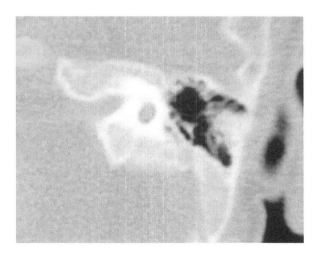

Figure 3.2 CHARGE syndrome—axial computed tomography of the petrous bone at the level of the internal auditory meatus at the expected level of the horizontal semicircular canal, which is absent. The crus of the posterior semicircular canal should also be seen at this level indicating complete absence of the semicircular canals (with thanks to Dr. E. Phelan). *Abbreviation*: CHARGE, coloboma, heart defect, atresia choanae, retarded growth, ear anomalies/deafness.

scanning as a core feature of CHARGE association (Fig. 3.2). Likewise, a large-scale clinical study by the same group, of clinical characteristics of patients with CHARGE association, unsurprisingly showed many other clinical features occurring as uncommon but probably integral features of the syndrome (9). In addition to reporting semicircular canal hypoplasia on temporal bone scans in 12 of 12 cases, these authors also drew attention to asymmetric crying facies, esophageal and laryngeal anomalies, renal malformations, and facial clefts among patients with CHARGE association.

Despite these important clinical increments in recognising the totality of the spectrum of associated anomalies, the cause of the condition remained unidentified. A teratogenic aetiology had been proposed but no specific agent had been identified common to women who had had such children (7). A few instances of parent-to-child transmission had been recorded (7), suggesting, in this subpopulation of CHARGE cases at least, a genetic, autosomal-dominant basis. Other evidence for a genetic basis was drawn from observation of concordance of the condition in monozygotic twins and discordance in dizygotic twins (7). Although it was routine clinical practice for clinical geneticists to undertake chromosomal analysis in CHARGE association cases, this was generally seen as an exercise in hope rather than a realistic investigation likely to give an abnormality. Most such cases resolutely showed normal chromosomal analysis. Hurst et al. (10) had drawn attention to a de novo chromosomal rearrangement, a seemingly balanced whole arm chromosomal rearrangement between chromosomes 6 and 8 in a child with typical clinical features of CHARGE, but there being no further evidence to substantiate this as an important finding, it was equally likely that it was a red herring and not of aetiological significance.

All of this changed however when Vissers et al. (11) used the comparative genome hybridisation approach to screen CHARGE patients for submicroscopic copy number changes with a view to identifying microdeletions or duplications in patients with CHARGE association. They identified a CHARGE case with 8q12 clones deleted in a region of approximately 5 Mb. Recognising the possible value of Hurst's report and obtaining DNA from her case, these researchers then hybridised genomic DNA from Hurst's patient onto the chromosome 8 BAC array and identified two submicroscopic deletions overlapping with the earlier 5Mb 8q12 critical region. Proceeding from these important initial data, no deletions were identified in 17 other cases of CHARGE. Nine genes were identified within this critical region and sequencing of these genes identified mutations within a specific locus, CHD7, in 10 of the 17 patients with CHARGE association not related to 8q12 submicroscopic deletions. The CHD genes are a family of genes encoding chromodomain helicase DNA-binding proteins, a family of proteins thought to have pivotal roles in early embryonic development by affecting chromatin structure and gene expression. The findings of Vissers et al. (11) clearly establish that haploinsufficiency of the CHD7 gene results in CHARGE features. Interestingly, and as might have been predicted, the individual with the microdeletion has relatively severe mental retardation in association with the core clinical features of CHARGE—presumably this represents the haploinsufficiency of genes adjacent to CHD7, whose specific absence accounts for the typical CHARGE features.

What of the seven individuals for whom neither deletions nor mutations were identified within this locus? It is already known that CHARGE can be associated with chromosome 22q11.2 deletion syndrome-like phenotype, a cytogenetic deletion syndrome more readily associated with clinical stigmata of Di George sequence, velocardiofacial syndrome, and Cayler syndrome (12). Consequently the emerging data confirm that

CHARGE is a genetically heterogeneous condition, most cases being caused by haploinsufficiency of CHD7, but some other cases may possibly represent an extended chromosome 22q11.2 microdeletion syndrome and other cases an as yet unidentified genetic causation. However, it is now fair to recognise that most cases of CHARGE do share an underlying genetic basis, irrespective of variability in clinical signs and that the condition might correctly be termed a syndrome under the distinction outlined above.

Improved cytogenetics identifies new syndromes with specific audiological and ENT relevance. Clinical and cytogenetic interaction can result in recognition of abnormal chromosomes

One of the questions most posed to geneticists relates to the origins of "new" syndromes. Of course the conditions referred to as new are not new. They have always existed but have not been previously recognised as distinct clinical entities. New syndromes emerge through the medical literature all the time. In the past, these have frequently comprised clinical reports of instructive families or individuals, but a particular trend of the last few years has been the identification of syndromes with specific chromosomal abnormalities which are deemed to be clinically recognisable. Consequently, seeing a patient in whom one is reminded of one of these new cytogenetic syndromes, the clinician has a definite idea of what investigations he/she might request of their laboratory in seeking to establish the underlying diagnosis in that particular patient.

Deletions of chromosome 1p36 represent a good instance of special relevance to clinicians dealing with deafness in the context of developmental delay. Shapira et al. presented clinical details of 14 patients with deletion of chromosome 1p36 and identified that the condition was much more common than previously recognised by the then prevailing cytogenetic techniques. Exploiting fluorescent in-situ hybridisation (FISH) and other advances in cytogenetic technology facilitated the identification of the syndrome in cases where this had not previously been possible. Moreover, the clinical phenotype described was strongly suggestive of a pattern of malformations, which should be clinically recognisable. Thus the clinician, by redirecting the attention of cytogeneticists toward this area of the karyotype, might assist in identification of the underlying chromosomal abnormality and thus solve the diagnostic issue for the patient (13). In fact it is clear from reading this paper that the clinicians were able to make the diagnosis clinically once they had become accustomed to the phenotype from the first few cytogenetically positive cases. Following that breakthrough paper, there were several other reports of this syndrome being recognised by clinicians elsewhere; these are well summarised by Slavotinek et al. in a major review article (14).

The clinical profile of affected individuals, which has been crystallised from these reported experiences is one of motor delay and hypotonia (90% +), moderate to severe mental retardation (90% +), pointed chin (80%), seizures (70% +), clinodactyly and/or short fifth finger (60% +), ear asymmetry (55% +), low-set ears (55% +), hearing deficits (55% +), and other variable features, including congenital heart disease and cleft lip, and/or palate. Some have commented on a horizontality of the eyebrows, which they find clinically valuable in alerting them to this syndromic diagnosis but that is inconstant, as any examination of published photographs shows. If present, it is a valuable clue. However, for this author at least, the clue is often the shape of the chin, which is pointed and often rather prominent (Fig. 3.3).

While the low-set ears and ear asymmetry may be noted in audiology or ENT clinics, the main concern will often relate to hearing abnormalities. These have been characterised as high frequency bilateral sensorineural hearing loss in 8 of 18 cases in one report, a further two cases having conductive loss characterised as severe degree (15). It is valuable to know that experienced dysmorphologists will often recognise children with this syndrome clinically, despite a normal karyotype report, and discussion with cytogeneticist colleagues will often lead to reevaluation of the original chromosome report and the identification of the underlying deletion.

A further example of this clinical–cytogenetic interaction proving valuable in identification of an underlying causative chromosomal abnormality occurs in relation to chromosome 4qter deletion. The existence of a syndrome

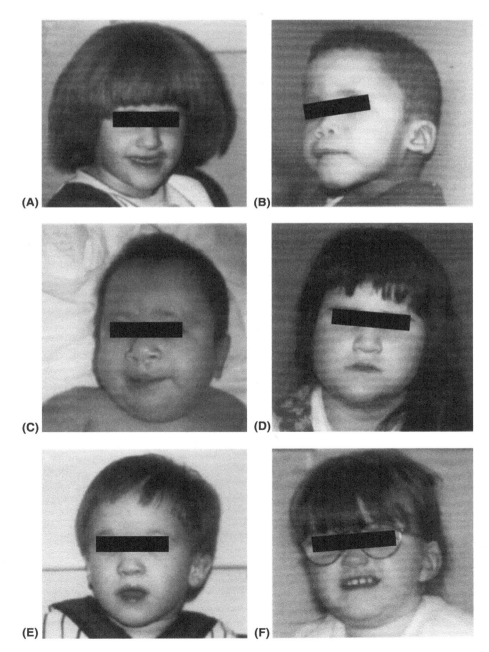

Figure 3.3 Facial characteristics seen in six children with chromosome 1p36 deletion. Note especially the horizontality of the eyebrows, which is a good clinical sign but not universal. The pointed chin, cases B, D, and E especially, is another good clinical clue. (Kindly reproduced from Ref. 14 by permission of the BMJ Publishing Group.)

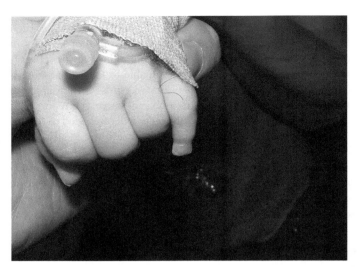

Figure 3.4 Tail of a nail sign in chromosome 4q–syndrome.

The patient was the youngest of three sisters born to unrelated parents. At the age of one, she presented with an acute respiratory arrest. Laryngotracheobronchoscopy showed multiple haemorrhagic regions in the trachea and main bronchi, consistent with acute respiratory arrest. No obstructive or other cause for this was identified. Routine investigations including basic chromosomes were normal. A genetics referral led to some new points being established—specifically there was no facial dysmorphism, but the developmental history was suggestive of slight parental concern in that milestones were not being achieved at the same rate as had occurred in the older siblings. Specifically, as she got older, it became clear that speech was delayed. The only clinical sign was an abnormal fifth fingernail unilaterally (Fig. 3.4), which prompted the clinical geneticists to ask for cytogenetic reevaluation with specific reference to chromosome 4q. A tiny deletion was shown on extended banding review of the chromosomes (Fig. 3.5).

Subsequently this child developed severe palatal insufficiency, with little evidence of gag reflex on video fluoroscopy (Fig. 3.6), which led to gastrostomy and direct feeding. Following fundoplication, airway function improved greatly and eventually it was possible to reinstigate oral feeding. Oropharyngeal hypotonia and palatal dysfunction are a well-established feature of the 4q–syndrome, frequently leading to the need for tracheostomy and gastrostomy. Several such cases are described. Considering the numbers of children who have these surgical procedures, it ought to be worth clinically examining the nails for tail of the nail sign and reviewing the chromosomes for evidence of 4q-abnormality, which can be familial and asymptomatic in some individuals.

comprising developmental delay, hypertelorism, often cleft palate and palatal dysfunction, low-set ears, poor growth, and abnormal fifth finger nails has been known for many years (16). Indeed, this latter sign has been recognised by Flannery as the main clue to the diagnosis and led him to coin the term "tail of a nail" syndrome for the condition (17). However, the deletion can be subtle cytogenetically, and, the patient's clinical condition being mild, be missed. Such a case arose in this author's own practice recently.

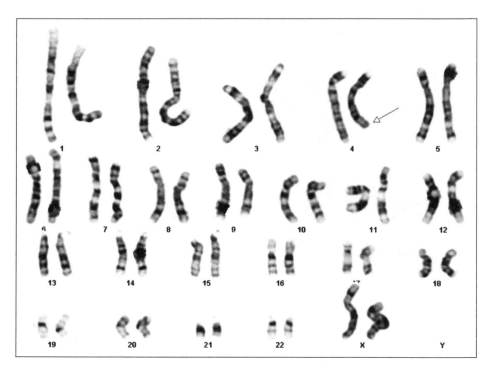

Figure 3.5 The karyotype of the patient with "tail of a nail" sign is shown. Note specifically the arrowed deletion of chromosome 4qter. (With thanks to Mr. A. Dunlop.)

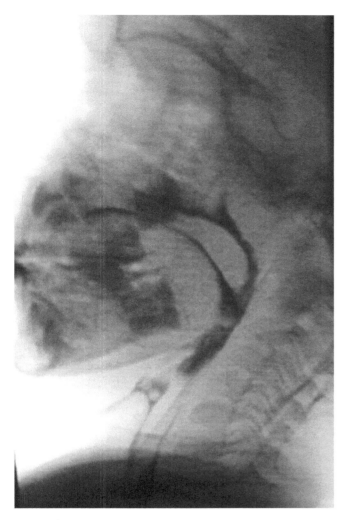

Figure 3.6 Swallowing study of 4q–showing the aspiration from the pharynx into the trachea, which is often seen in children with this chromosomal abnormality and can lead to life-threatening consequences.

New clinical signs and associations are crystallised which are relevant to audiological physicians and surgeons

It is difficult to conceive that the practice of medicine can, after all the generations of our antecedents, still throw up new clinical signs. Perhaps it is not so much the clinical sign itself, which is new, as the recognition of that sign as a marker for a specific genetic disease or syndrome. A case in point with particular relevance to the clinical examination of ears has come to light over the last few years and now bears the eponym Mowat–Wilson syndrome, after the pair of principal observers, Drs. David Mowat and Meredith Wilson.

In 1998, Mowat et al. published a series of six children bearing a distinctive facial phenotype, in association with mental retardation, microcephaly, short stature, and, in four of the six, neonatal Hirschsprung's disease (18). Severe constipation was present in all

six. Having established a deletion of chromosome 2q22–23 in one of these patients, the authors then proceeded to review the literature of clinical data from published cases with visible deletions in this region of chromosome 2q and felt there were strong facial resemblances between the features on the six cases under report and the case previously identified by Lurie et al. (19). Mowat et al. observed that following the recognition of the phenotype in the first two cases in their series, the next three cases were recognised within a six-month period. This phenomenon exemplifies the important learning process, which dysmorphologists often comment upon and call "getting your eye in"—essentially a learning period during which one recognises the phenotype and, having so done, recognises the pattern in future consultations with other patients. This learning stage is an important process in the emergence of any new dysmorphic syndrome. It also follows that if the original authors identified five patients within a few months that the syndrome must be a relatively common problem and these cases were unlikely to be unique cases.

Subsequent events have shown that such is indeed the correct conclusion—a review by the original authors in 2003 recorded 45 cases from several continents (20). In the interim period between the publication of the original observations and the review, the genetic basis of the syndrome had been established as involving the ZFHX1B gene on chromosome 2q22-q23. Some patients, as in the case reported by Lurie et al. (19) and the original observation by Mowat et al. (18), had large deletions encompassing this locus and surrounding regions, occasionally resulting in cytogenetic deletions visible down the microscope. Most patients however had intragenic mutations of ZFHX1B and the clue to undertaking this confirmatory test in these individuals lay in the phenotype.

Reflecting on the fundamental facial features, Mowat et al. (20) drew attention to a prominent chin, hypertelorism, deep-set eyes, a broad nasal bridge, saddle nose, prominent rounded nasal tip, posteriorly rotated ears, and large uplifted ear lobes. Commenting on the configuration of the ear lobes, which they described "as like orecchiette pasta or red blood corpuscles in shape, is a consistent and easily recognised feature." (Figs. 3.7 and 3.8).

The point that needs to be established is that a new syndrome has emerged, which is identifiable on the basis of clinical features and that the recognition of those clinical features is the key to directing investigation toward the ZFHX1B gene for mutation analysis. Perhaps the clinical sign itself is not new—indeed it is likely that this condition has always existed, but the relevance of the clinical signs and their specific causal association with ZFHX1B have only recently emerged.

A similar phenomenon is beginning to emerge in relation to some cases of choanal atresia. Most cases of this malformation arise as isolated clinical findings and many patients are never investigated beyond a brief consideration of whether the choanal atresia may represent a presentation of CHARGE syndrome. Most cases arise as new events in the family and, if taken, the family history is unremarkable. One aspect of history, which is frequently not sought, is the history of the pregnancy,

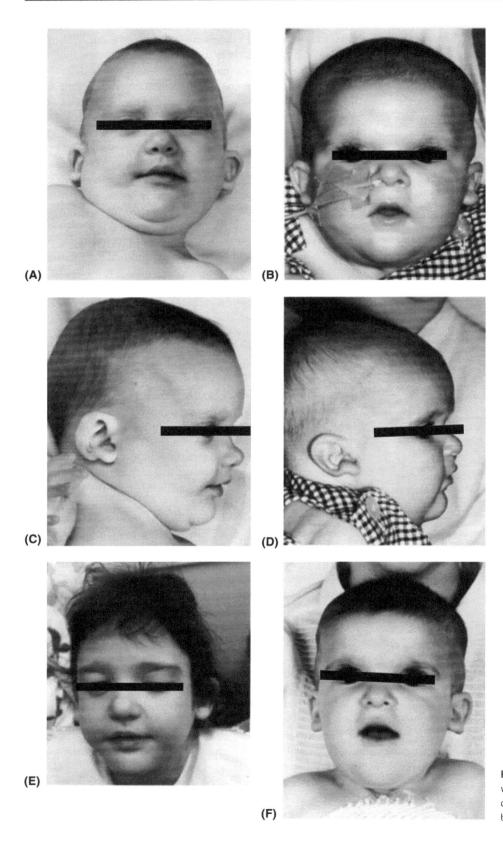

Figure 3.7 The facial appearance of two children with Mowat–Wilson syndrome in infancy and childhood is shown. (Kindly reproduced from Ref. 20 by permission of the BMJ Publishing Group.)

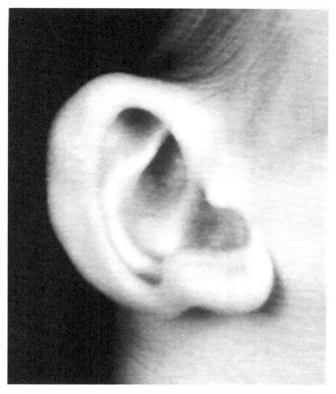

Figure 3.8 The characteristic ear appearance in Mowat–Wilson syndrome is shown. (Kindly reproduced from Ref. 20 by permission of the BMJ Publishig Group.)

and, in particular, a history of maternal medication. In fact, a trickle of cases since Greenberg first observed choanal atresia in the offspring of a woman exposed to carbimazole in pregnancy (21) have supported a likely causal effect for choanal

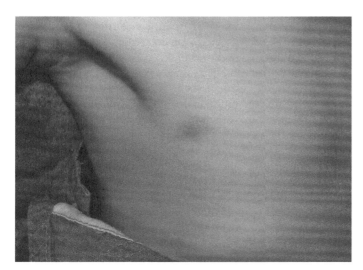

Figure 3.9 Nipple hypoplasia in carbimazole exposure is demonstrated. Some children have had complete absence of nipple formation in association with choanal atresia in this teratogenic syndrome.

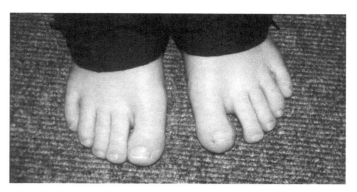

Figure 3.10 Broad halluces seen in association with deafness in a case of Keipert syndrome. *Source*: From Ref. 24.

atresia in several cases of carbimazole exposure (22,23), which may be associated with oesophageal atresia, nipple aplasia or hypoplasia, and dysmorphic facial features in some instances (Fig. 3.9).

As with the ear abnormalities in 2q deletion syndrome, choanal atresia related to the ingestion of carbimazole during pregnancy has long existed but the association has been overlooked by failure to take the history of the pregnancy. The lesson is that for cases of isolated choanal atresia, it is worth taking a detailed history of the pregnancy and looking carefully at the nipples of the baby.

Often the diagnostic significance of a specific clinical sign can be obscured by lack of reports or failure to observe the sign in cases with the condition. It certainly seems that this observation is true in respect of Keipert syndrome, in which condition deafness is associated with broad thumbs and halluces (Fig. 3.10). Only a handful of reports have recognised this rare diagnosis, but the author is aware of at least three further cases, which have been brought to his attention following a report of a classical case (24). Apart from the broad thumbs, there was general reduction in the terminal phalanges on radiology with a large thumb epiphysis (Fig. 3.11). It is likely that there are many other cases of this syndrome currently unrecognised for want of clinical examination.

Molecular genetics of known syndromes informs clinical classification and explains some previous contradictions

Antley–Bixler syndrome

Antley–Bixler syndrome is a condition derived from the eponymous 1975 report of a patient with craniosynostosis, radiohumeral synostosis and femoral bowing (25). Over 30 subsequent cases have been described, sometimes as single events, often as sibships. In common with other children with severe craniosynostosis, many of these children have significant audiological problems, complicating a clinical profile, which already encompasses craniofacial, dental, orthopaedic and endocrine

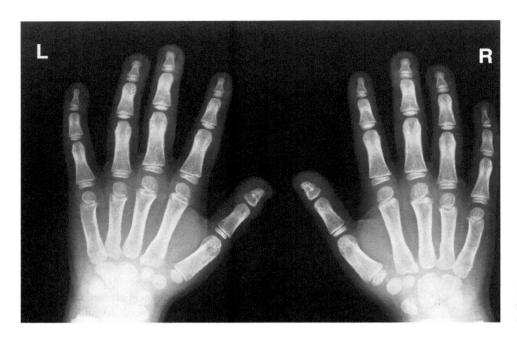

Figure 3.11 Short terminal phalanges in Keipert syndrome. Note also the abnormally large epiphysis in the thumbs. *Source*: From Ref. 24.

elements. Genital abnormality is an inconstant element of the condition. However, the syndrome is very difficult to distinguish from two other clinical disorders: Pfeiffer syndrome with large joint synostosis, in which the genital malformations are absent, and fluconazole embryopathy. In the latter condition, mothers taking fluconazole have given birth to children with a clinical picture, which closely resembles Antley–Bixler syndrome and may be indistinguishable (26). The observation of clitoromegaly in a single case of Antley–Bixler syndrome led one group of authors to pursue this line of enquiry further. They observed abnormalities of steroid biogenesis in 7 out of 16 patients with a clinical presentation consistent with Antley–Bixler syndrome, finding mutations of the *FGFR2* (*fibroblast growth factor receptor 2*) gene in a further seven cases. This led to the authors postulating that there were different forms of Antley–Bixler syndrome—those associated with steroid biogenesis abnormalities and those whose clinical phenotype might reflect *FGFR* mutation only (27). This suggestion has been developed further and mutations in cytochrome P450 oxidoreductase identified in children with disordered steroidogenesis, ambiguous genitalia, and Antley–Bixler syndrome, this condition segregating as an autosomal recessive disorder in contrast with the new dominant mutation of *FGFR2*, which gives a similar phenotype, but for the absence of genital ambiguity (28). Not only has the molecular genetics resolved the differences between the overlapping clinical phenotypes but it has also given an understandable reason for the genital ambiguity in some families, which was not apparent in the *FGFR2*-related forms. Finally the fluconazole embryopathy phenotype can be readily understood in the context of considering the mode of action of that antifungal agent. Fluconazole acts through the cytochrome P450 enzyme C-14 α demethylase, principally inhibiting the demethylation of lanosterol, the predominant sterol of the fungal cell wall. Although one of the therapeutic advantages of fluconazole is the improved specificity it shows for the fungal cytochrome P450 enzyme complex, the embryopathy is likely to reflect relative adrenal insufficiency in infants who develop features of the embryopathy in mothers exposed to fluconazole during pregnancy. The identification of mutations in the *POR* gene consolidates this likely mechanism of action as the basis of the fluconazole embryopathy and the phenotypic overlap with *FGFR2* mutation and *POR* mutation. Thus clinical observations, in this instance the identification of ambiguous genitalia in a single case, which can initially seem rather disparate, can be crucial to the ultimate understanding of the pathological spectrum in all its variations and the apparent contradictions can be elided.

Pendred syndrome
There are several other good examples of this in conditions, which are considered more "mainstream" with respect to deafness syndromology. If we look at Pendred syndrome, the classical diagnostic triad of deafness, goitre, and a positive perchlorate discharge test have been shown to be relatively poor identifiers of affected individuals. The substitution of radiological malformation in the form of Mondini malformation or dilatation of the vestibular aqueduct greatly enhances diagnosis and identification of affected individuals (29,30). Indeed, in clinical practice, the use of the perchlorate discharge test has largely been supplanted. Likewise the identification of mutations in the *PDS* gene on chromosome 7q has greatly added to the investigative tools available in recognising this syndrome in all its manifestations (31). Over 100 mutations of the gene are now known, though a small number are much more prevalent than others, some of which have only been observed on a single occasion. The deployment of these new forms of investigation has facilitated the resolution of diagnostic conundrums posed by particular interesting cases and families. For instance,

Gill et al. presented a case in which the proband had been dead for 35 years (32). The patient had been congenitally deaf and hypothyroid, the deafness having been assumed to be secondary to the hypothyroidism. Temporal bone sections had been stored and on review, 35 years later, a grossly dilated vestibular aqueduct was identified. An affected younger sibling was identified and investigated, revealing typical clinical and radiological findings of Pendred syndrome. The developmental delay in the index case was clearly attributable to the congenital hypothyroidism, a very rare complication in the profile of Pendred syndrome.

Likewise there have been perplexing families reported, whose clinical conditions have been resolvable by molecular approaches. The best example of such is the Brazilian family recorded by Billerbeck et al. (33). Goitre associated with deafness and a positive perchlorate discharge test was observed in at least two affected individuals in the highly consanguineous pedigree under consideration. To complicate matters, the family emanated from a region of endemic goitre. The likely diagnosis of Pendred syndrome was offset by the observation of positive perchlorate test in the absence of hearing loss in other individuals in the pedigree, while others were recorded with deafness alone or goitre as a sole finding. The identification of mutations in the PDS gene facilitated the wider exploration of the underlying pathology in this confusing pedigree. It transpired that the index case, satisfying all typical diagnostic parameters for Pendred syndrome, did harbour a homozygous deletion in exon 3 of the gene, resulting in a frameshift and premature stop. An additional two individuals in the pedigree also shared this genotype, and thus had Pendred syndrome. However, several deaf individuals in the pedigree were not homozygous for the PDS mutation, suggesting a likely alternative autosomal recessive cause for deafness in these patients. Moreover six individuals in the family with goitre did not have PDS gene mutations and the likely cause for the goitre in these was the endemic iodine deficiency (34). Accordingly the clinical classification of this family has been established as comprising three distinct conditions—Pendred syndrome, goitre related to endemic iodine deficiency, and nonsyndromic deafness. Similar phenomena have been observed and formally established in another confusing family (35).

Waardenburg syndrome
Waardenburg syndrome and the various subtypes of this condition provide one of the most elegant examples of how good clinical observation, careful family studies, and integration of molecular data can powerfully combine to enhance understanding of clinical observations, which, initially at least, seemed to be at variance with received wisdom, ultimately resulting in the recognition of new disease processes. It is worth briefly reviewing the progress, which has been made relating to this group of disorders.

The original observation of deafness with heterochromia irides, white forelock, and white skin patches dates from 1951 (36). Some 20 years later, it was the observations of Arias that

the dystopia canthorum segregated with deafness in some families but not in others, which led to the separation of type I (with dystopia) from type II (37). Subsequent reports were less amenable to classification: the observation by Shah et al. in 1981 of infants with Hirschsprung disease and white forelock, seemingly inherited in autosomal recessive manner (38) and the report from Klein in 1983 of a patient with features of Waardenburg syndrome type I associated with severe arm hypoplasia and arthrogryposis of the wrists and hands (39).

Aided by careful attention to phenotype and, in particular, to dystopia canthorum, linkage studies on Waardenburg syndrome type I (WSI) led to identification of mutations in the PAX3 gene on chromosome 2 (40,41). Subsequent studies have established that almost all cases conforming to the WSI phenotype have mutations at this locus and there is no substantial evidence for genetic heterogeneity. However, deafness is a variable feature of the syndrome among WSI individuals, with Read and Newton citing a prevalence of 52% in their experience (42). This seems not to be related to the nature of the mutation and the exact cause of this variation in penetrance remains unclear. However, identification of mutations in PAX3 has considerably aided our understanding of clinically confusing situations outlined above. Klein–Waardenburg syndrome, also known as WSIII, has proven to be another phenotype of PAX3 mutation. In some instances, this is due to a contiguous gene deletion involving the PAX3 locus and adjacent regions of chromosome 2q35, but in others, intragenic mutations of PAX3 have been found, either in the homozygous or in the heterozygous state. A good example is the family reported by Woolnik et al. in which parents with WSI shared a mutation for PAX3, the offspring being homozygous for the mutation, Y90H, and having the WSIII phenotype (43). In mice, homozygosity of PAX3 mutations results in severe neural tube defects and lethality. Likewise a phenotype of exencephaly and severe contracture and webbing of the limbs in human kind has been speculated to be consistent with a severe PAX3 mutation in homozygous form (44). Indeed screening patients with neural tube defects for PAX3 mutation led to the identification of one patient with a myelomeningocele who, on close examination, was shown to have mild features of WSI, which were also seen to segregate with the mutation in several family members (45). Less predictable was the finding that craniofacial-deafness-hand syndrome is allelic to WSI, being caused by an exon 2 missense mutation in affected members of this unique family. The phenotype comprises autosomal-dominant deafness, with hypoplasia of the nasal bones, telecanthus, nasolacrimal duct absence/obstruction, ulnar deviation of the hands, and flexion contractures of the ulnar digits (46). Notably there are no features of pigmentary disturbance in this pedigree. The mutation in this family is a missense mutation, resulting in substitution of asparagine by lysine (N47K). However, alternative mutation of this asparagine residue to histidine in another family results in a more typical clinical outcome of WSIII in affected individuals. However, unlike the PAX3 mutations seen in homozygous form in some WSIII patients, this N47H mutation causes WSIII in heterozygous form (47). More commonly however, the WSIII phenotype is seen as a consequence of compound heterozygosity for *PAX3* mutation. The likely explanation for these seemingly contradictory observations lies in the effects of the mutation on the function of the *PAX3* mutant protein. Indeed, there is evidence for this from the work of DeStefano et al. (48) who studied the relationship between mutation type and clinical sequelae in 271 WS individuals, representing 42 unique *PAX3* mutations. Deletions of the homeodomain were most significantly correlated with significant clinical findings and were seen especially to correlate strongly with white forelock.

In parallel with these emerging insights into the clinical phenotypes attributable to genetic mutation at the *PAX3* locus, there has been considerable advance on the understanding of the genetic basis of WSII and related disorders. Mutations in the *MITF* gene on chromosome 3p have been established in several families conforming to the clinical definition of WSII. Other clinically interesting phenomena associated with mutation at this locus have also been observed. Deafness is more common as a clinical finding of WSII than is the case in WSI, being observed in approximately 80% of cases (42). However, the absence of pigmentary abnormalities in many patients, or the presence of such features in only very subtle form, does lead to difficulty in discrimination between WSII and patient with nonsyndromic deafness. Indeed Read has confirmed this clinical observation at molecular level with his observation that 10% of cases with a clinical diagnosis of WSII in fact have mutations at the *Connexin 26* locus and do not have WSII at all (49). As often happens, once the molecular genetics of a syndrome become established, conditions, which had been considered to represent clinically distinct syndromes have been recognised as allelic forms, due to the identification of a mutation at the same locus. Tietz syndrome is a case in point. The syndrome dates from the 1963 report of Tietz of a family in which deafness segregated as a dominant trait over six generations but always in association with albinism. The irides were blue, with albinoid fundi, the hair being blond, and the skin very fair. *MITF* mutation was shown as the basis of this syndrome of albinism and deafness (50). Foremost among the clinical observations, which underlay this syndrome was the cosegregation of albinism and deafness in affected individuals as autosomal-dominant traits. Albinism is more often and classically observed as an autosomal recessive trait in clinical genetics. However, families were also known in whom WSII and ocular albinism existed but in which the pattern of cosegregation was not as clear-cut. This was known as the Waardenburg syndrome type II with ocular albinism (WSII-OA) phenotype. Such pedigrees are rare, but Morrell et al. studied one such pedigree, establishing an intragenic deletion within the *MITF* locus. Individuals with the OA phenotype were shown to have homozygosity or heterozygosity for the R402Q mutation in the *tyrosinase* gene, which functionally reduces the catalytic activity of the tyrosinase enzyme, in addition to the *MITF* mutation (51). These observations led the authors to

propose that the WSII-OA phenotype is consequent on digenic interaction between *MITF* and tyrosinase, a gene regulated by *MITF*.

Not all cases of WSII phenotype have mutation of the *MITF* locus. Indeed, online mendelian inheritance in man (OMIM) currently lists four loci for WSII, respectively, termed WSIIA-D. However, only the *MITF* locus is confirmed and to date, this represents the sole locus for WSII at which mutations have been established, which result in the WSII phenotype. *MITF* is a key activator for tyrosinase, a major enzyme in melanogenesis and critical for melanocyte differentiation. *PAX3* transactivates the *MITF* promoter and is assisted in doing so by another gene *SOX10*. Not surprisingly, this latter is also an important gene in WS phenotypes and specifically in the WS4 clinical spectrum.

The term WS4 relates, as outlined above, to the observations of Hirschsprung disease in association with other phenotypic characteristics of WS. In a study of a large Mennonite family, many of whose members had Hirschsprung disease, sometimes associated with low-grade features of WS (white forelock in 7.6% of cases), Puffenberger et al. identified a causative mutation in the *endothelin receptor B gene (EDNRB)* on chromosome 13 (52). This was an interesting mutation, which showed dosage sensitivity. Homozygotes have a 74% chance of showing Hirschsprung disease against a 21% chance in heterozygotes. This was a seminal finding, leading not only to the identification of a genetic basis for many cases of nonsyndromic Hirschsprung disease, but also to mutation of the *EDNRB* locus in families conforming to the Waardenburg-Shah phenotype (WS4) (53) as well as the recognition of an allelic condition, albinism, black lock, cell migration disorder of the neurocytes of the gut, and deafness (ABCD) syndrome (54). The latter refers to a child with deafness, albinism, a black lock in the right temporo-occipital region, and spots of retinal depigmentation, in whom severe intestinal innervation defects were established. These clinical findings were causally attributed to homozygosity for a C to T transition in the *EDNRB* gene resulting in a stop codon with no production of normal protein possible.

Prompted by these observations and encouraged by the knowledge that mutation of the *endothelin 3 gene* in mouse results in a phenotype similar to WS4, Edery et al. searched for and reported mutations of the *EDN3* gene in patients with Waardenburg-Shah syndrome (55). Subsequently mutations at this same locus have been found in other cases of WS4 but also in isolated cases of Hirschsprung disease and even in a patient with Hirschsprung disease associated with central hypoventilation syndrome. It is now known that *EDNRB* has a strictly defined role in governing migration of the precursor cells of the enteric nervous system into the colon. Binding sites for *SOX10* enhance the migration of these enteric nervous system cells. Not surprisingly, then, the *SOX10* gene, on chromosome 22q13, is also associated with WS phenotypes. Specifically several patients with WS4 phenotype have been described due to mutation at this locus. Moreover, a patient thought to have a separate condition, Yemenite deaf–blind hypopigmentation syndrome, was also reported with *SOX10* mutation (56). Likewise, *SOX10* mutations have been recorded in patients with pigmentary disturbance and deafness suggestive of WS but in whom rectal biopsy is normal. Nonetheless, the patients have persistent bowel symptoms suggestive of bowel obstruction. This establishes that aganglionosis is not the only mechanism associated with intestinal dysfunction in *SOX10* mutation (57). Other clinically important phenomena have been observed in the spectrum of *SOX10*-associated disease. Donnai presented details of an adult deaf female with raindrop pigmentation of the skin, in whom a *SOX10* mutation was established (58). A further set of patients was identified with WS4 features associated with a peripheral neuropathy and/or central hypomyelinating neuropathy associated with *SOX10* mutation (57,59). This neurological variant is now known as peripheral demyelinating neuropathy, central demyelinating leukodystrophy, Waardenburg syndrome, and Hirschsprung disease (PCWH), and recent work has established that this more severe phenotype occurs because truncated, mutant SOX10 proteins with potent dominant negative activity escape the nonsense medicated decay pathway (60).

To summarise, mutations at five distinct loci, *PAX3*, *MITF*, *EDNRB*, *EDN3*, and *SOX10*, have been described in association with Waardenburg syndrome phenotypes. However, careful attention to clinical examination and investigation in these patient groups has contributed enormously to an enhanced understanding of the molecular mechanisms, the mutational spectrum, and the embryological events, which underlie the differing presentations of Waardenburg syndrome.

Phenotypic studies of syndromes with an already established genetic basis enhances clinical data, patient management and drives further research

The cloning of a gene and the establishment of causative mutations at that locus for various phenotypes are sometimes seen as an end in itself. To researchers engaged on such research, this does represent a momentous milestone. However, to clinicians, families with the condition and those charged with delivery of medical services to such patients and families, the identification of mutations does not usually change patient care other than by facilitating identification of others in the kindred who themselves have inherited the mutation and might benefit from specific screening measures for covert disease. What the identification of mutations underlying a specific syndrome does allow is more detailed phenotypic studies of that condition and encourage the clinical "teasing out" of clinically overlapping conditions, so that it can become clearly established as to what particular pathology applies in an individual patient or family.

A good example of this is provided by the dilated vestibular aqueduct syndrome (Fig. 3.12). Dilatation of the vestibular aqueduct has been known since 1978. Several series of deaf patients with this radiological phenomenon had been published,

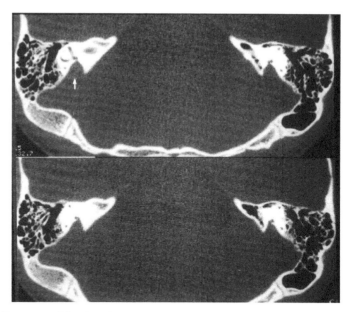

Figure 3.12 Dilatation of the vestibular aqueduct is shown in a typical case of Pendred syndrome. *Source*: From Ref. 29.

resulting in over 200 cases being identified and reported in radiological and ENT literatures. It appears that none of these patients had been recognised as having an underlying genetic syndrome and indeed it is never addressed in any of these publications as to whether any of the patients included in the various series were related. Phelps recognised that almost all cases of Pendred syndrome manifest dilatation of the vestibular aqueduct (30,61) and there has since been a mushrooming of interest in this radiological marker of deafness. This interest in investigating deaf patients more systematically and in seeking to identify the precise basis of the deafness has established that dilatation of the vestibular aqueduct is not confined to Pendred syndrome. Indeed, it is not at all surprising, considering the shared pathology of ion transporter defects seen in both conditions, that renal tubular acidosis and deafness, a distinct autosomal recessive condition, should share this characteristic with Pendred syndrome (62). There are now suggestions that there may be a genetically distinct autosomal recessive syndrome of dilatation of the vestibular aqueduct and deafness separate from Pendred syndrome and for which the locus remains to be established (63). Such claims, whether they will be validated in time or not, are only possible because of detailed phenotypic work, which has continued following the identification of the genetic basis of Pendred syndrome and the incorporation of such mutational studies into clinical practice. The best estimate currently available is that Pendred syndrome mutation accounts for about 86% of cases of vestibular aqueduct dilatation (29).

Likewise with respect to branchio-oto-renal (BOR) syndrome, the cloning and identification of mutation at the *EYA1* gene has shown that there are other clinically overlapping phenotypes, which are not due to mutation at this locus. Among families, comprising the majority, which do owe their clinical phenotype to *EYA1* mutation, there has been enhanced incorporation of genetic data into patient care and management. Chang et al. have furnished their data incorporating 40 families with 33 distinct mutations segregating and have identified the major features as deafness in 98.5%, preauricular pits in 83.6%, branchial anomalies in 68.5%, and renal anomalies in 38.2% (64). However, other phenotypes have also been associated with mutation at this locus, including cataract and anterior ocular defects (65), Otofaciocervical syndrome (66) and a contiguous gene deletion syndrome, which is clinically characterised by BOR syndrome but with additional clinical features of Duane eye retraction syndrome, hydrocephalus, and aplasia of the trapezius muscle (67). In addition to these allelic diseases emerging from BOR-related studies, there has also been clarification of those families whose clinical phenotype appears to suggest a likely diagnosis of BOR but for whom mutation at *EYA1* was not established and linkage data suggested that the disease phenotype was a function of mutation at another locus. A good example of this is provided by the large kindred forming the basis of the report of another BOR locus on chromosome 14q (68). This pedigree, comprising over 40 affected individuals, differs from the classical BOR syndrome profile in that only approximately 25% had branchial arch-related defects, the age of onset of deafness was much later and more variable than is generally seen in *EYA1*-related deafness, and no renal malformations or anomalies are reported in the clinical data furnished on the family. Purists might argue with the nosology of the syndrome as BOR3, but it is difficult to argue against this in light of the clinical finding of branchial defects in 25% of affected individuals. The mutational basis of this, to date unique, family remains unresolved at this time, but it is worth noting that other "nonsyndromic deafness" loci map to the same region on linkage (DFNA23 and DFNB35). The designation BOR2 has been given to another hitherto unique dominant pedigree mapping to chromosome 1q (69). Such a designation is certainly more contentious as the family had always been considered clinically distinct from BOR by the absence of cervical fistulae, renal anomalies, and the presence of lip pits. However, there is no doubt that this pedigree represents another form of autosomal-dominant deafness associated with preauricular sinuses.

BOR syndrome also represents an example of how learning that a member of a specific gene family can cause a particular phenotype extends the opportunities for establishing molecular pathology in clinically related situations. *EYA1* is one of four related human loci, and mutations at another of the genes in this family, *EYA4*, have been reported in deafness of autosomal-dominant nonsyndromic type (70).

References

1. Aase JM. Diagnostic Dysmorphology. Plenum Medical Book Company. New York, 1990.
2. Knight SJL, Flint J. Perfect endings: a review of subtelomeric probes and their use in clinical diagnosis. J Med Genet 2000; 37: 401–409.
3. Flint J, Knight S. The use of telomere probes to investigate submicroscopic rearrangements associated with mental retardation. Curr Opin Genet Dev 2003; 13:310–316.
4. Hall BD. Choanal atresia and associated multiple anomalies. J Pediatr 1979; 95:395–398.
5. Hittner HM, Hirsch NJ, Kreh GM, Rudolph AJ. Colobomatous microphthalmia, heart disease, hearing loss and mental retardation: a syndrome. J Pediatr Ophthalmol Strabismus 1979; 16: 122–128.
6. Pagon RA, Graham JM, Zonana J, Young SL. Congenital heart disease and choanal atresia with multiple anomalies. J Pediatr 1981; 99:223–227.
7. Graham JM Jr. A recognizable syndrome within CHARGE association: Hall-Hittner syndrome. Am J Med Genet 2001; 99: 120–123.
8. Amiel J, Attie-Bitach T, Cormier-Daire V, et al. Temporal bone anomaly proposed as a major criteria for diagnosis of CHARGE syndrome. Am J Med Genet 2001; 99:124–127.
9. Tellier AL, Cormier-Daire V, Abadie V, et al. CHARGE syndrome: report of 47 cases and review. Am J Med Genet 1998; 76: 402–409.
10. Hurst JA, Meinecke P, Baraitser M. Balanced t(6;8)(6p8p;6q8q) and the CHARGE association J Med Genet 1991; 28:54–55.
11. Vissers LELM, van Ravenswaaij CMA, Admiraal R, et al. Mutations in a new member of the chromodomain gene family cause CHARGE syndrome. Nat Genet 2004; 36:955–957.
12. de Lonlay-Debeney P, Cormier-Daire V, Amiel J, et al. Features of DiGeorge syndrome and CHARGE association in five patients. J Med Genet 1997; 34:986–989.
13. Shapira S, McCaskill C, Northrup H, et al. Chromosome 1p36 deletions: the clinical phenotype and molecular characterization of a common newly delineated syndrome. Am J Hum Genet 1997; 61:642–650.
14. Slavotinek A, Shaffer LG, Shapira SK. Monosomy 1p36. J Med Genet 1999; 36:657–663.
15. Heilstedt HA, Wu YQ, May K, et al. Bilateral high frequency hearing loss is commonly found in patients with the 1p36 deletion syndrome. Am J Hum Genet Suppl 1998; 63:A106.
16. Lin AE, Garver KL, Diggans G, et al. Interstitial and terminal deletions of the long arm of Chromosome 4: further delineation of phenotypes. Am J Med Genet 1988; 31:533–548.
17. Flannery DB. Tale of A Nail; Proceedings of the Greenwood Genetics Center. 1993; 12:90.
18. Mowat DR, Croaker GDH, Cass DT, et al. Hirschsprung Disease, microcephaly, mental retardation, and characteristic facial features: delineation of a new syndrome and identification of a locus at chromosome 2q22-q23. J Med Genet 1998; 35:617–623.
19. Lurie IW, Supovitz KR, Rosenblum-Vos LS, Wulfsberg EA. Phenotypic variability of del (2)(q22-q23): report of a case and review of the literature. Genet Couns 1994; 5:11–14.
20. Mowat DR, Wilson MJ, Goossens M. Mowat-Wilson syndrome. J Med Genet 2003; 40:305–310.
21. Greenberg F. Choanal atresia and athelia: methimazole teratogenicity or a new syndrome? Am J Med Genet 1987; 28:931–934.
22. Myers AK, Reardon W. Choanal atresia—a recurrent feature of Fetal Carbimazole syndrome. Clin Otolaryngol 2005; 30:375–377.

23. Lam WWK, Keng WT, Metcalfe K, et al. Fetal Carbimazole—characteristic facial features. 11th Manchester Birth Defects Conference. Manchester, 2004.

24. Reardon W, Hall CM. Broad thumbs and halluces with deafness: a patient with Keipert syndrome. Am J Med Genet 2003; 118A: 86–89.

25. Antley RM, Bixler D. Trapezoidocephaly, midfacial hypoplasia and cartilage abnormalities with multiple synostoses and skeletal fractures. Birth Defects 1975; XI:397–401.

26. Aleck KA, Bartley DL. Multiple malformation syndrome following Fluconazole use during pregnancy: report of an additional patient. Am J Med Genet 1997; 72:253–256.

27. Reardon W, Smith A, Honour JW, et al. Evidence for digenic inheritance in some cases of Antley-Bixler syndrome? J Med Genet 2000; 37:26–32.

28. Flück CE, Tajima T, Pandey AV, et al. Mutant P450 oxidoreductase causes disordered steroidogenesis with and without Antley-Bixler syndrome. Nat Genet 2004; 36:228–230.

29. Reardon WO, Mahoney CF, Trembath R, Jan H, Phelps PD. Enlarged vestibular aqueduct: a radiological marker of Pendred syndrome and mutation of the PDS gene. Quart J Med 2000; 93:99–104.

30. Phelps PD, Coffey RA, Trembath RC, et al. Radiological malformations of the ear in Pendred Syndrome. Clin Radiol 1998; 53:268–273.

31. Everett LA, Glaser B, Beck JC, et al. Pendred syndrome is caused by mutations in a putative sulphate transporter gene. Nat Genet 1997; 17:411–422.

32. Gill H, Michaels L, Phelps PD, Reardon W. Histopathological findings suggest the diagnosis in an atypical case of Pendred syndrome. Clin Otolaryngol 1999; 24:523–526.

33. Billerbeck AEC, Cavaviere H, Goldberg AC, Kalil J, Medeiros-Neto G. Clinical and genetic studies in Pendred syndrome. Thyroid 1994; 4:279–284.

34. Kopp P, Arseven OK, Sabacan L, et al. Phenocopies for deafness and goiter development in a large inbred Brazilian kindred with Pendred's syndrome associated with a novel mutation in the PDS gene. J Clin Endocrinol Metab 1999; 84:336–341.

35. Vaidya B, Coffey R, Coyle B, et al. Concurrence of Pendred syndrome, autoimmune thyroiditis and simple goiter in one family. J Clin Endocrinol Metab 1999; 84:2736–2738.

36. Waardenburg PJ. A new syndrome combining developmental anomalies of the eyelids, eyebrows, and nose root with pigmentary defects of the head hair and with congenital deafness. Am J Hum Genet 1951; 3:195–250.

37. Arias S. Genetic heterogeneity in the Waardenburg syndrome. Birth Defects Original Article Series 1971; 7:87–101.

38. Shah KN, Dalal SJ, Sheth PN, Joshi NC, Ambani LM. White forelock, pigmentary disorder of the irides and long segment Hirschsprung disease: possible variant of Waardenburg syndrome. J Pediatr 1981; 99:432–435.

39. Klein D. Historical background and evidence for dominant inheritance of the Klein-Waardenburg syndrome (type III). Am J Med Genet 1983; 14:231–239.

40. Tassabehji M, Read AP, Newton V, et al. Waardenburg syndrome patients have mutations in the human homologue of the Pax-3 paired box gene. Nature 1992; 355:635–636.

41. Baldwin CT, Hoth CF, Amos JA, da-Silva EO, Milunsky. An exonic mutation in the HuP2 paired domain gene causes Waardenburg's syndrome. Nature 1992; 355:637–638.

42. Read AP, Newton V. Waardenburg syndrome. In: Martini, Read, Stephens, eds. Genetics and Hearing Impairment. London Whurr, 1996.

43. Woolnik B, Tukel T, Uyguner O, et al. Homozygous and heterozygous inheritance of PAX3 mutations causes different types of Waardenburg syndrome. Am J Med Genet 2003; 122A:42–45.

44. Ayme S, Philip N. Possible homozygous Waardenburg syndrome in a fetus with exencephaly. J Med Genet 1995; 59:263–265.

45. Hol FA, Hamel BCJ, Geurds MPA, et al. A frameshift mutation in the gene for PAX3 in a girl with spina bifida and mild signs of Waardenburg syndrome. J Med Genet 1995; 32:52–56.

46. Sommer A, Bartholomew DW. Craniofacial-Deafness-Hand Syndrome Revisited. Am J Med Genet 2003; 123A:91–94.

47. Hoth CF, Milunsky A, Lipsky N, et al. Mutations in the paired domain of the human PAX3 gene cause Klein-Waardenburg syndrome (WS-III) as well as Waardenburg syndrome type I (WS-I). Am J Hum Genet 1993; 52:455–462.

48. DeStefano AL, Couples LA, Arnos KS, et al. Correlation between Waardenburg syndrome phenotype and genotype in a population of individuals with identified PAX3 mutations. Hum Genet 1998; 102:499–506.

49. Read AP. Genes Hearing and Deafness—from Molecular Biology to Clinical Practice. Caserta, Italy, 2005.

50. Amiel J, Watkin PM, Tassabehji M, Read AP, Winter RM. Mutation of the MITF gene in albinism-deafness syndrome (Tietz syndrome). Clin Dysmorph 1998; 7:17–20.

51. Morell R, Spritz RA, Ho L, et al. Apparent digenic inheritance of Waardenburg syndrome type 2 (WS2) and autosomal recessive ocular albinism (AROA). Hum Mol Genet 1997; 6:659–664.

52. Puffenberger EG, Hosoda K, Washington SS, et al. A missense mutation of the endothelin-B receptor gene in multigenic Hirschsprung's disease. Cell 1994; 79:1257–1266.

53. Syrris P, Carter ND, Patton MA. Novel missense mutation of the endothelin-B receptor gene in a family with Waardenburg-Hirschsprung disease. Am J Med Genet 1999; 87:69–71.

54. Verheij JBG, Kunze J, Osinga JC, van Essen AJ, Hofstra RMW. ABCD syndrome is caused by a homozygous mutation in the EDNRB gene. Am J Med Genet 2002; 108:223–225.

55. Edery P, Attie T, Amiel J, et al. Mutation of the endothelin-3 gene in the Waardenburg-Hirschsprung disease (Shah-Waardenburg syndrome). Nat Genet 1996; 12:442–444.

56. Bondurand N, Kuhlbrodt K, Pingault V, et al. A molecular analysis of the Yemenite deaf-blind hypopigmentation syndrome: SOX10 dysfunction causes different neurocristopathies. Hum Mol Genet 1999; 8:1785–1789.

57. Pingault V, Guiochon-Mantel A, Bondurand N, et al. Peripheral neuropathy with hypomyelination, chronic intestinal pseudo-obstruction and deafness: a developmental "neural-crest syndrome" related to a SOX10 mutation. Ann Neurol 2000; 48:671–676.

58. Donnai D. The Carter Lecture. British Society of Human Genetics. York, September 2004.

59. Inoue K, Tanabe Y, Lupski J. Myelin deficiencies in both the central and the peripheral nervous systems associated with a SOX10 mutation. Ann Neurol 1999; 46:313–318.

60. Inoue K, Khajavi M, Ohyama T, et al. Molecular mechanism for distinct neurological phenotypes conveyed by allelic truncating mutations. Nat Genet 2004; 36:361–369.

61. Phelps PD. Large vestibular aqueduct: large endolymphatic sac? J Laryngol Otol 1996; 110:1103–1104.

62. Berrettini S, Neri E, Forli F, et al. Large vestibular aqueduct in distal renal tubular acidosis. High-resolution MR in three cases. Acta Radiol 2001; 42:320–322.

63. Pryor SP, Madeo AC, Reynolds JC, et al. SLC26A4/PDS genotype-phenotype correlation in hearing loss with enlargement of the vestibular aqueduct (EVA): evidence that Pendred syndrome and non-syndromic EVA are distinct clinical and genetic entities J Med Genet 2005; 42:159–165.

64. Chang EH, Mebezes M, Meyer NC, et al. Branchio-Oto-Renal Syndrome: the mutation spectrum in EYA1 and its phenotypic consequences. Hum Mutat 2004; 23:582–589.

65. Azuma N, Hirakiyama A, Inoue T, Asaka A, Yamada M. Mutations of a human homologue of the Drosophila eyes absent gene (EYA1) detected in patients with congenital cataracts and ocular anterior segment anomalies. Hum Mol Genet 2000; 9:363–366.

66. Rickard S, Parker M, van't Hoff W, et al. Oto-facial-cervical (OFC) syndrome is a contiguous gene deletion syndrome involving EYA1: molecular analysis confirms allelism with BOR syndrome and further narrows the Duane syndrome critical region to 1 cM. Hum Genet 2001; 108:398–403.

67. Vincent C, Kalatzis V, Compain S, et al. A proposed new contiguous gene syndrome on 8q consists of branchio-oto-renal (BOR) syndrome, Duane syndrome, a dominant form of hydrocephalus and trapeze aplasia; implications for the mapping of the BOR gene. Hum Mol Genet 1994; 3:1859–1866.

68. Ruf RG, Berkman J, Wolf MTF, et al. A gene locus for branchio-otic syndrome maps to 14q21.3–24.3. J Med Genet 2003; 40:515–519.

69. Kumar S, Deffenbacher K, Marres HAM, Cremers CWRJ, Kimberling WJ. Genome-wide search and genetic localization of a second gene associated with autosomal dominant branchio-oto-renal syndrome: clinical and genetic implications. Am J Hum Genet 2000; 66:1715–1720.

70. Wayne S, Robertson NG, DeClau F, et al. Mutations in the transcriptional activator EYA4 cause late-onset deafness at the DFNA10 locus. Hum Mol Genet 2001; 10:195–200.

4 Deafblindness

Claes Möller

Introduction

Deafblindness comprises a number of heterogeneous hearing and vision disorders. These disorders can be caused by trauma, diseases, and different genetic syndromes. The two senses hearing and vision are the primary communication tools for humans; their action is complementary and they enhance each other. To be fast and reliable, communication between humans relies on vision and hearing. Since communication is derived from the Latin word "communicare," which means to do things together, it is obvious that a loss of these two senses can be catastrophic. For example, in noisy environments where it is difficult to hear, visual input such as body language and expressions can supplement our understanding. Likewise, when vision is poor, hearing plays a major role in the localisation of sounds and detection of danger etc.

The definition deafblindness comprises many different forms of impairments. A person with deafblindness can be profoundly deaf and completely blind, completely deaf with visual impairment, completely blind with hearing impairment, or have a hearing and vision dysfunction. As mentioned before, vision and hearing interact, thus deafblindness is 1 + 1 = 3.

A widely used definition is by the Northern European committee on disability who in 1980 stated as follows: A person is deafblind when he/she has a severe degree of combined visual and auditory impairment. Some deafblind people are totally deaf and blind, whereas others have residual hearing and residual vision.

Another categorisation of deafblindness is to discuss these disorders as either congenital or acquired deafblindness.

Congenital deafblindness

Congenital deafblindness is extremely rare: about 1 in 10,000 newborn babies is affected. Causes of congenital deafblindness include genetic syndromes, premature birth, infections, etc. Subjects with complete congenital deafblindness very often have other dysfunctions such as mental retardation, cerebral palsy, etc. Due to the lack of vision and hearing, the subject has to rely on sensory influx from smell, taste, and touch. This also gives a severe risk of sensory deprivation, which might enhance a mild mental retardation. Subjects with congenital deafblindness need an environment with extremely good professional communication skills. The communication training is lifelong and relies heavily on tactile sign language and input via the remaining senses—touches, smell, and taste. When working with persons with congenital deafblindness, the goals have so far been to open new channels for communication.

During the previous years, very promising achievements have been made through the advent of cochlear implants (CI). If a child with congenital deafblindness does not have severe brain damage, early cochlear implantation might result in hearing and even in speech. In other syndromes associated with additional brain damage, the goal of CI is simply to create sound awareness and basic recognition of sounds. Thus, in the future, CI will probably dramatically change communication skills for many persons with congenital deafblindness. Similar vision implants have not yet proved to be successful but ongoing research will probably result in similar achievements.

Today (2006), at least 20 different genetic syndromes are known to cause congenital deafblindness. In some of these, the genes have been identified and cloned. Because of the rarity of these genetic conditions and difficulties in assessment, congenital deafblindness can sometimes be missed and hidden due to other dysfunctions and, thus, attributed to other conditions.

Acquired deafblindness

As in congenital deafblindness, there are many causes of acquired deafblindness. The prevalence of acquired deafblindness is hard to estimate, in part depending on the definition. Usually only young and middle-aged people are included and most of the syndromes known today have clinical features present from childhood or young adulthood. It should be noted, however, that in old people, a severe hearing loss as well as a severe visual loss caused by conditions such as cataracts, macular degeneration, and age-related hearing loss will create a severe communication problem. Thus, age-related deafblindness is not caused by syndromes but will result in the same impairment, which if not compensated, will increase dementia and other disorders.

Today (2006), more than 50 hereditary syndromes are known to cause acquired deafblindness. Out of those, at present, in around 40 different syndromes, the gene has been localised and in quite a few, the gene has been identified. Many of these syndromes have proven to be heterogeneous with many different genes causing the same or similar phenotypes (1).

Some deafblind syndromes

The following syndromes are described in more detail below:

- Usher syndrome (US)
- Alström syndrome
- Norrie disease
- Mohr–Tranebjaerg syndrome
- Wolfram syndrome
- Refsum syndrome

Usher syndrome

The three clinical features of US are retinitis pigmentosa (RP), hearing loss/deafness, and vestibular dysfunction/areflexia. US is an autosomal recessive disorder. The prevalence of US differs in different countries but approximately 50% of all people affected with deafblindness have US (2). The disease was first described by Albrecht von Graefe in 1858 with the occurrence of RP and congenital deafness in three brothers. The next to describe the disease was Charles Usher in 1914. He described deafness and RP in several families in England. Another historic landmark was the recognition by Julia Bell in 1933 of the hearing loss variation in US (3).

Retinitis pigmentosa

RP is a description of several different disorders of the retina. The disease in the retina is degeneration. A hallmark for RP is "bones spicules," which are caused by release of pigment from the pigment epithelium, forming black spots in the retina. The degeneration starts in the rods, and the cones are affected later. This will give rise to different symptoms such as glare sensitivity, night blindness, and progressive reduction of the visual field. RP is present in many heterogeneous disorders, and it can be inherited in autosomal dominant, or recessive as well as sex-linked patterns. A large number of genes causing RP have been identified.

Classification

Classification of US can be made from the phenotype or the genotype. The clinical classification is at present based on three

Table 4.1 The genetic subtypes of Usher syndrome

Type	Chromosome	Gene
Usher IB	11q13.5	*MYO7A*
Usher IC	11p15.1	*USH1C*
Usher ID	10q22.1	*CDH23*
Usher IE	21q21	Unknown
Usher IF	10q21-22	*PCDH15*
Usher IG	17q24-25	*SANS*
Usher IIA	1q41	*Usherin*
Usher IIB	3p23-24.2	Unknown
Usher IIC	5q14.3-q21.3	*VLGR1*
Usher III	3q25	*Clarin*

clinical subtypes I, II, and III (4). Table 4.1 shows the current classification of US based on molecular genetic studies (5). (Note that Usher 1A (6) is no longer valid since the families were later found to have mutations in MYO7A.)

US type I

Hearing: The hearing loss is congenital, profound bilateral deafness. The audiogram might sometimes show a little residual hearing at low frequencies (corner audiogram). The profound deafness does not allow development of speech. The habilitation of children with type I US has dramatically changed during recent years with the introduction of CI. If implantation is made early in life (before two years of age), the results are excellent and will result in hearing and spoken language as well as benefiting sound localisation later in life when vision deteriorates.

Vision: The degeneration is progressive, bilateral, and symmetrical. The degeneration starts in the periphery. The initial symptoms are glare sensitivity, night blindness, and, later, constricted visual fields. The first visual symptoms can be observed in early childhood. The child is insecure in darkness, clumsy, etc. The fundus changes are seen rather late, thus the first reliable diagnostic tool is electroretinography (ERG). This can show changes as early as in the first or second year of life. The progress of RP in type I is slow and most persons will have central vision with approximately 5° visual field at the age of 50 to 60 years. The RP is often complicated by cataracts (80%).

Balance: Subjects with type I have bilateral vestibular areflexia (deaf in the vestibular-balance organs). This is a hallmark of type I and the clinical symptoms are late motor milestones, late walking age (>18 months), and clumsiness, especially in darkness. The bilateral vestibular areflexia, which will cause the late walking age, is the first obvious symptom of a possible US. This is easily assessed in small children by using video-Frenzel during rotation. Thus screening for vestibular deficiency in deaf and hearing-impaired children, and a finding of a bilateral vestibular areflexia, will in approximately 30% to 40% of these children result in a diagnosis of US (2).

So far, six different genetic loci have been identified for Type I US (Table 4.1).

- *Usher type Ib*: This common form of Usher type I has been linked to chromosome 11q13.5 and is caused by mutation of the *myosin VIIa (MYO7A)* gene. This protein is believed to act on the cytoplasmic actin filaments (7). A mouse model (shaker-1) has been found for Usher type Ib. The mouse is deaf and has vestibular areflexia but no RP (8). The gene is expressed in many organs. The MYO7A gene is large and at present (2005) more than 80 different mutations have been reported.

- *Usher type Ic*: The gene is linked to chromosome 11p14-p15.1 and was first described in the French Acadian population of Louisiana, U.S.A. (9). The gene product is named *Harmonin* and is suggested to play a role in transmission of nerve impulses. The exact function of *Harmonin* is not yet fully understood.

- *Usher type Id*: This condition is linked to chromosome 10q and is caused by mutations in the *Cadherin (CDH23)* gene (10). A mouse model for Usher type Id, called the Waltzer mouse, exists. In this mouse, the stereocilia and the kinocilium are disrupted (11).

- *Usher type Ie*: The locus has been linked to chromosome 21q21. The gene is not yet identified. Only one family from Morocco has been found (12).

- *Usher type If*: This form is linked to chromosome 10q21 and has been found in a few families. The protein is related to otocadherin and the gene is expressed both in the retina and in the inner ear. The gene has now been named *Protocadherin 15 (PCDH15)* and it seems to be necessary for development of the neurological system. A mouse model of Usher type If has been created, which is called the Ames Waltzer mouse (13).

- *Usher type Ig*: This form is linked to chromosome 17q24-25 and has been found in two different families. Mutations are found in the *SANS* gene, which is involved in a functional network together with *harmonin, cadherin 23*, and *myosin VIIa* (14). Thus, the genes of Usher type I seems to interact with each other and in the future new research will probably reveal a close interaction between these genes and maybe between genes causing type II and III condition as well. Today it is believed that Usher type Ib and Usher type Id are the most common genotypes.

US type II

Hearing: The first symptom in US type II is a congenital or extremely early–acquired sensorineural hearing loss. The hearing loss is bilateral, symmetrical, and moderate to severe. The audiogram is down sloping with a mild-to-moderate loss at lower frequencies and a severe-to-profound loss at higher frequencies. The hearing loss is in most cases stable but a mild progression can be seen from the fourth decade. The hearing benefits from bilateral hearing aid amplification as early as possible.

Vision: The visual problems are similar to those in Type I. The course of RP (progression of visual acuity loss and visual field loss) might be milder in Usher type II compared with Usher type I (15).

Balance: vestibular function is normal.

So far, three different genetic loci have been found with mutations (Table 4.1).

- *US type IIa*: This is the most common form. It has been linked to chromosome 1q and the mutation 2299delG is the single most common form of mutation (16). The mutations are found in a gene named *Usherin*, which codes for a novel protein in the extracellular matrix and in cell-surface receptors. *Usherin* is found in many organs. Its exact function is still unclear. US type IIa seems to account for more than 70% of all subjects with Usher type II (17). Genetic testing is available on a clinical basis.

- *US type IIb*: This form is linked to chromosome 3p23-24.2 and has been localised in one family. The gene is not known (18).

- *US type IIc*: Type IIc has been linked to chromosome 5q14 and has so far been reported in four families. The gene is named *VLGR1*; the protein is still unknown (19,20).

US type III

Hearing: Patients affected with type III have a congenital or early bilateral sensorineural hearing loss. It differs from type II in one important respect: The progression of hearing loss is rapid and results in acquired profound deafness at the age of 30 to 40 years (21).

Vision: The progression of RP can so far not be separated from the clinical picture found in type I and type II (21).

Balance: The vestibular function is, in most cases, normal during childhood but might progress similar to the hearing loss (21).

The prevalence of type III is low in the United States and in Europe except for Finland. In Finland, a founder effect is known and type III accounts for nearly 40% of all Finnish Usher affected (22). At present, one gene has been linked to chromosome 3q25. So far, nine mutations have been identified in US type III (23).

Prevalence of US

The prevalence of US in different parts of the world is not very well known. One large epidemiological prevalence study from Sweden has confirmed a prevalence rate of type I, 1.6/100,000, type II, 1.4/100,000, and type III, 0.3/100,000. These prevalence figures are likely to be underestimates due to the late age at which US is diagnosed. The prevalence of type I is significantly higher in the northern parts of Sweden, which indicates a founder effect (24). Very few other studies are representative for a larger geographic area.

New and ongoing studies (2005) have indicated that there are genotype–phenotype correlations with differences between different types. The current genotype and phenotype knowledge of US will probably in the near future produce new insights and thus hopefully new possibilities for treatment and eventually cure. Treatment modalities could be antioxidants, growth hormone factors, or gene or stem cell therapy.

Alström syndrome

Alström syndrome is a rare autosomal recessively inherited disorder, which affects many organs. Approximately 300 subjects are known today but many new cases are being added as the disorder is better characterised. The disease was first described in 1959 by the Swedish doctor Carl Henry Alström (25). It is characterised by multiple organ system involvements, with much heterogeneity. Features include RP, sensorineural hearing loss, cardiomyopathy, obesity, diabetes mellitus type 2, increased serum lipids, other endocrine disturbances, liver dysfunction, pulmonary symptoms, and different developmental and behaviour disturbances. The disorder has different clinical appearances during childhood and young adulthood (26):

- *Zero to two years*: The first symptom is RP with early retinal pigmentary degeneration. This is first demonstrated by light sensitivity and nystagmus. A severe deterioration of cone function and later a progressive deterioration of rod function are found. In Alström syndrome, the diagnosis of RP is usually made before the age of two years by electroretinography (ERG) and fundoscopy. During the first year of life, 50% of children suffer from a cardiomyopathy, which can be misinterpreted as pulmonary infection. The cardiomyopathy is severe and life threatening.
- *Two to four years*: The RP will progress with diminished darkness sensitivity and diminished vision fields. The child is clumsier than other children. Most children have a rapid growth, with childhood obesity in nearly all children. A rapid weight gain is usually observed even before two years of age. During these years, the child might have numerous upper airway infections as well as urinary infections.
- *Four to six years*: A continued rapid gain of weight and in many children elevated blood lipids. More than 50% develop diabetes type 2 during childhood. During these years, a progressive hearing loss is apparent but sometimes the diagnosis is missed due to all the other organ dysfunctions.
- *Six to twelve years*: visual function is rapidly deteriorating and during age of 12 to 15 years, most children will be blind. As this age, other dysfunctions such as liver, kidney, heart problems, etc. can develop.
- *Twelve to eighteen years*: Nearly all are blind, and besides RP, most have also developed cataract. The hearing disorder is in some cases progressive from moderate to severe and at older ages, profound bilateral deafness. The cardiomyopathy might reappear; thus, regular monitoring of cardiac functions is vital.

The heterogeneity in Alström syndrome is extensive. The author knows of five individuals who all are above 20 years of age. They are all blind, have a severe/profound progressive hearing loss; they all have diabetes, elevated lipids, and liver, kidney, and cardiac dysfunctions (unpublished observations). Very few persons with Alström syndrome are over 40 years of age. Developmental milestones are delayed in approximately 50%. These can be fine motor skills, language delay, and autistic-spectrum behaviour abnormalities (27).

One causative gene has so far been mapped to chromosome 2p (28). The gene is ALMS1. This gene probably interacts with genetic modifiers, which could explain the large heterogeneity. A mouse model has been created. The findings from the mouse model suggest that ALMS1 has a role in intracellular trafficking (29,30). Since Alström syndrome is a very complex disorder affecting many organs and with a large heterogeneity, it is likely that other genes are also involved in this disorder.

Norrie disease

This disorder was first described by Gordon Norrie in 1933. It was, however, Mette Warburg, in 1961, who reported seven cases of a hereditary degenerative disease found in seven generations in a Danish family, suggesting the name of the disorder. (31). Norrie disease belongs to the category of congenital deafblindness. The inheritance is X-linked. The symptoms of Norrie disease are variable and may include many organs.

Hearing: A progressive hearing loss with variable progression is found during early childhood. In most cases, profound deafness is found at the age of 30 years. The localisation of the hearing loss is in the cochlea (unpublished observations by the author).

Vision: A congenital severe vision loss or congenital blindness is often present. The vision loss is due to several abnormalities such as iris atrophy, retinopathy, pseudoglioma, and cataracts.

Usually severe mental retardation and microcephaly are found and other dysfunctions can include cryptorchidism and hypogonadism (32).

The gene (NDP) is located on chromosome Xp11.4 and has been cloned. Because of the small size of the Norrie gene, mutation detection in Norrie disease is particularly simple and fast (33). The protein product of the NDP gene is called norrin, and is a secreted protein.

Mohr–Tranebjaerg syndrome

The Mohr–Tranebjaerg syndrome is an X-linked recessive disorder. In 1960, Mohr and Mageroy described a family where four generations were affected with a progressive form of deafness. The family was Norwegian. Originally, it was reported as a nonsyndromic X-linked recessive deafness. Tranebjaerg et al. in 1992 and 1995 did a reinvestigation and discovered several visual dysfunctions in the family.

Vision: The visual loss is severe and includes myopia, decreased visual acuity, constricted visual fields, and abnormal electroretinograms. A severe retinal degeneration is found.

Hearing: The hearing loss is progressive and will eventually be profound. A combination of cochlear loss and auditory neuropathy might be found (unpublished observations by the author).

As well as the hearing and vision deficiencies described above, there are central nervous system disorders such as dystonia, spasticity, dysphagia, dysarthria, tremor, hyperreflexia, and mental deterioration. Behavioural and psychiatric abnormalities are also common. In addition to the Norwegian family, other families have been described. There seems to be a clinical heterogeneity; so far, the Norwegian family have had the most severe symptoms. In this family, mental deficiency and blindness as well as deafness were found in nearly all individuals (34).

Linkage analysis located the causative gene to Xq22, close to a gene found in X-linked Alport syndrome. In 1999, Wallace and Murdock found that the underlying defect is in the mitochondrial oxidative phosphorylation chain (35).

Wolfram syndrome

Wolfram syndrome was first described in 1938 by Wolfram and Wagener, who described a family with juvenile diabetes mellitus and optic atrophy (36). Wolfram syndrome is also named DIDMOAD (diabetes insipidus, diabetes mellitus, optic atrophy, and deafness). The syndrome is autosomal recessive. The disorder is heterogeneous and many studies are based on case reports and family studies.

Vision: Optic atrophy is the main feature of this disorder. The atrophy of the optic nerve can be visualised by fundoscopy and magnetic resonance imaging and imaging findings have revealed atrophy of the optic nerve, chiasma, and optic tracts.

Hearing: The pattern of hearing loss is unusual, with low-frequency loss. The severity is variable from mild to profound. It has been demonstrated that patients with nonsyndromic, low-frequency hearing loss also might have mutations in the Wolframin gene-1 (37).

Other neurological abnormalities that might be apparent include mental retardation. Imaging findings in Wolfram syndrome have revealed atrophy of the optic nerve, chiasma, and tracts as well as atrophy of the brain stem and cerebellum. The diabetes could be both diabetes insipidus and diabetes mellitus where the onset usually is early (juvenile).

Wolfram syndrome has so far been localised to two different genes (*WFS1* and 2). *WFS1* is localised to chromosome 4p. More than 120 mutations have been identified in *WFS1*; the most common mutation described is in exon 8 (38). The second type, *WFS2*, is also linked to chromosome 4p (39). Recent research has suggested that the Wolfram gene might be expressed in the canalicular reticulum, which is a special form of the endoplasmic reticulum in the inner ear. Thus, the Wolframin genes might play a role in inner ear homeostasis.

This might also explain the low-frequency hearing loss found, which shows similarities to Menière's syndrome.

Refsum disease

The disorder is named after Sigvard Refsum who in 1949 described the visual and neurological symptoms (40). The clinical findings of Refsum disease are RP, chronic polyneuropathy, cerebellar dysfunction, and hearing loss/deafness. Other symptoms described are ichthyosis and dysplasia of the skeleton. In 1963, Klenk and Kahlke discovered accumulation of fatty acids and phytanic acid. The probable cause is a diminished ability to degrade phytanic acid. The accumulation will cause degeneration in different organs (41). It has been suggested that a diet free of chlorophyll and other food that might contain phytol will reduce the amount of unresolved phytanic acid in the blood, and thus reduce the progression of symptoms or even make a clinical improvement. This has not yet been convincingly proven.

Vision: The vision loss is RP of a mild type with late onset blindness. In-depth studies of RP in Refsum disease have so far not been performed.

Hearing: The hearing loss is moderate to severe and down sloping; in many patients it is progressive. Recent findings have suggested that the localisation of the hearing loss is not in the inner ear but rather in the auditory nerve (auditory neuropathy) (42).

Refsum disease is a heterogeneous disorder. One gene has been localised to chromosome 10p (43); however, recent studies have shown that many patients with Refsum disease do not have mutations in this gene. The prevalence of Refsum syndrome is so far unknown but the resemblance between Refsum and US might result in false diagnosis in some patients with Refsum syndrome, which will result in wrong treatment and rehabilitation. Thus testing for Refsum syndrome should always be made if a patient with RP and sensorineural hearing loss has other clinical symptoms such as polyneuritis, ichthyosis, etc.

An early designation called "infantile Refsum disease" was used for a similar congenital, very severe deafblind disorder with high morbidity and early mortality. This disorder also has phytanic acid accumulation, but due to other causes. It is suggested that the designation "infantile Refsum" should be avoided (44).

Summary

"I went to the doctor and he told me that I would go deaf and blind. He does not know when, but it might be in the near future. Then the doctor abruptly left the room. No! Not my hearing, not my vision! It is not fair! How could God do this to me? Why wasn't I told until I was grown up? Somebody help me!!!"

The gradual loss of hearing and vision creates stress, anxiety, grief, and horror. Deafblindness should be described as a functional entity with the two major channels for communication being hampered. The rapid progress of gene identification and cloning might in the near future lead to better medical and, hopefully, genetic treatment. The new discoveries of antioxidants and growth-hormone factors along with the increasing understanding of the physiology of vision and hearing will result in new treatment modalities. These new insights into genetics combined with more advanced diagnostic tools for assessment of vision and hearing will make early and correct diagnosis in most cases possible. Early diagnosis and prognosis will give better habilitation, rehabilitation, and treatment. Another important outcome of the new genetic discoveries are the possibilities of information to patients and family concerning aetiology, which in many cases will reduce fear and misunderstanding that will foster more realistic expectations and allow better rehabilitation, and, hopefully, in the future, treatment.

References

1. Omim http//www.ncbi.nlm.nih.gov.
2. Kimberling WJ, Möller C. Clinical and molecular genetics of Usher syndrome. Am Acad Audiol 1995; 6:63–72.
3. Bell J. Retinitis pigmentosa and allied diseases. In: Pearson K, ed. Treasury of Human Inheritance. London: Cambridge University Press, 1933:1–29.
4. Smith RJ, Berlin CI, Hejtmancik JF, et al. Clinical diagnosis of the Usher syndromes. Am J Med Genet 1994; 50:32–38.
5. van Camp G, Smith RJ. Hereditary Hearing Loss Homepage, http://webhost.ua.ac.be/hhh.
6. Kaplan J, Gerger S, Bonneau D, et al. A gene for Usher syndrome type I (USH1A) maps to chromosome 14q. Genomics 1992; 14:979–987.
7. Kimberling WJ, Möller CG, Davenport S, et al. Linkage of Usher syndrome type I gene (USH1B) to the long arm of chromosome 11. Genomics 1992; 14:988–994.
8. Gibson R, Walsh J, Mburu P, et al. A type VII myosin encoded by the mouse deafness gene shaker-1. Nature 1995; 374:62–64.
9. Smith RJ, Lee EC, Kimberling WJ, et al. Localisation of two genes for Usher syndrome type I to chromosome 11. Genomics 1992; 14:995–1002.
10. Wayne S, Kaloustian V, Schloss M, et al. Localisation of the Usher syndrome type Id gene (USH1D) to chromosome 10. Hum Mol Genet 1996; 5:1689–1692.
11. Di Palma F, Holme RH, Bryda EC, et al. Mutations in CDH23, encoding a new type of cadherin, cause stereocilia disorganisation in waltzer, the mouse model for Usher syndrome type 1D. Nat Genet 2001; 27:103–107.
12. Chaib H, Kaplan J, Gerber S, et al. A newly identified locus for Usher syndrome type I, USH1E, maps to chromosome 21q21. Hum Mol Genet 1997; 6:27–31.
13. Ahmed ZM, Riazuddin S, Bernstein SL, et al. Mutations of the protocadherin gene PCDH15 cause Usher syndrome type 1F. Am J Hum Genet 2001; 69:25–34.
14. Weil D, El-Amraoui A, Masmoudi S, et al. Usher syndrome type I G (USH1G) is caused by mutations in the gene encoding SANS, a protein that associates with the USH1C protein, harmonin. Hum Mol Genet 2003; 12:463–471.
15. Sadeghi M, Eriksson K, Kimberling WJ, Sjöström A, Möller C. Long-term visual prognosis in Usher syndrome type I and II. Scand J Ophtalmol 2005. In Press.
16. Kimberling W, Weston M, Möller C, et al. Localisation of Usher syndrome type II to chromosome 1q. Genomics 1990; 7:245–249.
17. Weston M, Eudy J, Möller C, et al. Genomic structure and identification of novel mutations in usherin, the gene responsible for Usher syndrome type IIa. Am J Hum Genet 2000; 66:1199–1210.
18. Hmani M, Ghorbel A, Boulila-Elgaied A, et al. A novel locus for Usher syndrome type II, USH2B, maps to chromosome 3 at 3p23-24.2. Eur J Hum Genet 1999; 7:363–367.
19. Pieke-Dahl S, Möller CG, Astuto LM, Cremers CW, Gorin MB, Kimberling WJ. Genetic heterogeneity of Usher syndrome type II: localisation to chromosome 5q. J Med Genet 2004; 44:256–262.
20. Weston MD, Luijendijk MW, Humphrey KD, Möller C, Kimberling WJ. Mutations in the VLGR1 gene implicate G-protein signalling in the pathogenesis of Usher syndrome type II. Am J Hum Genet 2004; 74:357–366.
21. Sadeghi M, Cohn ES, Kimberling WJ, Tranebjaerg L, Möller C. Audiological and vestibular features in affected subjects with USH3: a genotype/phenotype correlation. Int J Audiology 2005. In Press.
22. Pakarinen L, Sankila EM, Tuppurainen K, Karjalainen S, Helena K. Usher syndrome type III (USH3): the clinical manifestations in 42 patients. Scand J Log phon 1995; 20:141–150.
23. Joensuu T, Blanco G, Pakarinen L, et al. Refined mapping of the Usher syndrome type III locus on chromosome 3, exclusion of candidate genes, and identification of the putative mouse homologous region. Genomics 1996; 38:255–263.
24. Sadeghi M, Kimberling WJ, Tranebjaerg L, Möller C. The prevalence of Usher syndrome in Sweden:a nation-wide epidemiological and clinical survey. Audiol Med 2004; 2:220–228.
25. Alström CH, Hallgren B, Nilsson LM, Åsander A. Retinal degeneration combined with obesity, diabetes mellitus and neurogenous deafness: a specific syndrome distinct from Laurence-Moon-Biedel syndrome. A clinical, endocrinological and genetic examination based on a large pedigree. Acta Psychiatr Neurol Scand 1959; 34(suppl 1229):1–35.
26. Hopkinson I, Marshall JD, Paisey RB, Carrey C, Macdermott. Alström's syndrome. Available at http://www.genetests.org. Accessed Aug 2005.
27. Marshall JD, Bronson R, Collin G, et al. New Alström syndrome phenotypes based on the evaluation of 182 cases. Arch Intern Med 2005; 165:675–683.
28. Collin GB, Marshall JD, Cardon LR, Neshina PM. Homozygosity mapping of Alström syndrome to chromosome 2p. Hum Mol Genet 1997; 6:213–219.
29. Collin GB, Marshall JD, Ikeda A, et al. Mutations in ALMS1 cause obesity, type 2 diabetes and neurosensory degeneration in Alström syndrome. Nat Genet 2002; 31:74–78.

30. Collin GB, Bronson R, Marshall J, et al. ALMS1-disruped mice recapitulate human Alström syndrome. Hum Mol Genet 2005; 15:2323–2333.

31. Warburg M. Norrie's disease: a new hereditary bilateral pseudotumor of the retina. Acta Ophthal 1961; 39:757–772.

32. Warburg M. Norrie disease, a congenital progressive oculo-acoustico-cerebral degeneration. Acta Ophthal 1966; 89(suppl): 1–147.

33. Berger W, Meindl A, van de Pol TJ, et al. Isolation of a candidate gene for Norrie disease by positional cloning. Nat Genet 1992; 1:199–203.

34. Tranebjaerg L, Schwartz C, Eriksen H, et al. A new X-linked recessive deafness syndrome, blindness, dystonia, fractures and mental deficiency is linked to Xq22. J Med Genet 1995; 32:257–263.

35. Wallace DC, Murdock DG. Mitochondria and dystonia: the movement disorder connection? Proc Nat Acad Sci 1999; 96:1817–1819.

36. Wolfram D, Wagener HP. Diabetes mellitus and simple optic atrophy among siblings: report of four cases. Mayo Clin Proc 1938; 13:715–718.

37. Gurtler N, Kim Y, Mhatre A, et al. Two families with non-syndromic low frequency hearing loss harbor novel mutations in Wolfram syndrome gene 1. J Mol Med 2005; 83:553–560.

38. Hardy C, Khanim F, Torres R, et al. Clinical and molecular genetic analysis of 19 Wolfram syndrome kindreds demonstrating a wide spectrum of mutations in WFS1. Am J Hum Genet 1999; 65:1279–1290.

39. Collier DA, Barrett TG, Curtis D, et al. Linkage of Wolfram syndrome to chromosome 4p16.1 and evidence for heterogeneity. Am J Hum Genet 1996; 59:855–863.

40. Refsum S, Salomonsen L, Skatvedt M. Heredopathia atactica polyneuritiformis in children. J Pediatr 1949; 35:335–343.

41. Kahlke W, Wagener H. Conversion of h3-phytol to phytanic acid and its incorporation into plasma lipid fractions in heredopathia atactica polyneuritiformis. Metabolism 1996; 15:687–693.

42. Oysu C, Aslan I, Basaran B, Baserer N. The site of the hearing loss in Refsum's disease. Int J Pediatr Otorhinolaryngol 2001; 61:129–134.

43. Nadal N, Rolland MO, Tranchant C, Reutenauer L. Localization of Refsum disease with increased pipecolic acidaemia to chromosome 10p by homozygosity mapping and carrier testing in a single nuclear family. Hum Mol Genet 1995; 4:1963–1966.

44. Jansen GA, Waterham HR, Wanders RJ. Molecular basis of Refsum disease: sequence variations in phytanoyl-CoA hydroxylase (PHYH) and the PTS2 receptor (PEX7). Hum Mutat 2004; 23:209–218.

5 Nonsyndromic hearing loss: cracking the cochlear code

Rikkert L Snoeckx, Guy Van Camp

Introduction

Hearing impairment (HI) is the most common sensory impairment, affecting 1/650 newborns (1). In approximately 30% of the cases, a specific syndrome can be identified, with more than 400 syndromes claiming HI as a component. The remaining 70% of cases are nonsyndromic (2,3). Prelingual HI is caused by a mutation in a single gene (monogenic) in 60% of the cases, with an autosomal-dominant (20%), autosomal-recessive (80%), X-linked (1%), and mitochondrial (<1%) inheritance pattern. The most common type of nonsyndromic HI is postlingual and affects 10% of the population by age 60 and 50% by age 80 (4). In most cases, this HI is due to an unfavourable interaction between genetic and environmental factors (multifactorial or complex disease).

The genetic factors contributing to monogenic HI have long remained unknown. The human cochlea comprises about 20,000 neurosensory hair cells that do not last a lifetime and do not regenerate when lost. Due to the low number of cells and their location in the temporal bone, which is hard to access, it is very difficult to obtain information about the function of hair cells through biochemical studies. Positional cloning of genes for genetic forms of deafness has contributed greatly to our understanding of the physiology of the inner ear. Soon after the identification of the first locus for hereditary hearing loss in 1992 (5), many other gene localisations and identifications followed. It became clear that HI could be caused by many genes, which is in accordance with the structural complexity of the inner ear. Over the years, HI has become a paradigm for genetic heterogeneity. To date, more than 90 genes have been localised for nonsyndromic HI of which 40 genes have already been identified (6).

The extraordinary progress in the identification of deafness genes has been helped greatly by the sequencing of the human and the mouse genomes and the improvement of gene annotation methods. Also, the combination of genetic research with physiological and morphological information is beginning to lead to an in-depth understanding of many complex physiological and pathophysiological mechanisms of the hearing process. However, the function of several genes is not yet elucidated and many genes for nonsyndromic HI remain to be identified.

Nonsyndromic forms of hereditary deafness can be classified by their mode of inheritance. Chromosomal loci harbouring mutations that lead to nonsyndromic HI are named with DFNA, DFNB, or DFN symbols. DFNA and DFNB symbols followed by a numerical suffix indicate that the mutant allele is segregating in an autosomal-dominant or -recessive way, respectively. Sex-linked nonsyndromic hearing loss is designated with a DFN symbol and a numerical suffix. The division between nonsyndromic and syndromic HI is, at times, not easy to define. In some syndromic forms, hearing loss is detected before the manifestations of other organ pathology. As a result, a child might be incompletely diagnosed with nonsyndromic hearing loss. Additionally, several human genes can underlie both syndromic and nonsyndromic hearing loss. Possibly, these proteins have several functions, with specific and irreplaceable functions in the inner ear and a less critical function in other tissues, which may only be compromised by certain mutations or under certain conditions. Mutations in *GJB2* cause mostly nonsyndromic HI, although some specific mutations cause additional skin abnormalities underlying keratitis-ichthyosis-deafness (KID) syndrome, Vohwinkel syndrome, and palmoplantar keratoderma (7–9). Other examples are the gene *WFS1*, which, besides autosomal-dominant nonsyndromic HI, can also cause Wolfram syndrome and the *SLC26A4* gene, which can be the cause of autosomal-recessive nonsyndromic HI as well as Pendred syndrome (10–13). Usher syndrome can be caused by mutations in *CDH23*, *MYO7A*, and *USH1C*, but these genes can also be the cause of nonsyndromic HI (14–19).

This review gives a state-of-the-art description of genes that cause nonsyndromic HI. A classification is made according their putative function. These categories include genes involved in the homeostasis of the cochlea, genes required for the morphogenesis of the hair-cell bundle, extracellular matrix components and transcription factors, and genes encoding proteins with an unknown function. Two additional categories include mitochondrial mutations and modifier genes.

Genes involved in the homeostasis of the cochlea

After the influx of K^+, the inner and outer hair cells (OHCs) are required to remove the excess of K^+ ions. A possible recycling pathway for K^+, through gap junctions and potassium channels (epithelial cell-gap junction pathway), has been proposed on the basis of physiological and morphological findings (Fig. 5.1) (21,22). Potassium ions are released basolaterally from the hair cells to the extracellular space of the organ of Corti by K^+ channels. This K^+ is taken up by the supporting cells and moves to the lower part of the spiral ligament through the epithelial-gap junction pathway. Subsequently, the ions enter the extracellular space of the spiral ligament and are then taken up by the fibrocytes (connective tissue-gap junction pathway). Finally, K^+ passes through this system towards the stria vascularis back into the endolymphatic sac (23).

Connexins

Gap junctions are channels that connect neighbouring cells and allow passive transfer of small molecules. They are made up of two hemi channels or connexons that sit in the cell membranes, and align and join to form a channel. Connexons consist of six proteins called connexins. These gap junctions are important for the electric and metabolic coupling of neighbouring cells. Connexins are expressed in many different tissues.

Connexin 26 (GJB2) and connexin 30 (GJB6)

Connexin 26 is encoded by the gap junction $\beta2$ (GJB2) gene, which is expressed in several tissues including the cochlea and skin (23). In the cochlea, GJB2 is expressed in the supporting cells, the spiral ligament, the spiral limbus, and the stria vascularis, most likely contributing to the recycling of K^+ ions (24). Recently, it has been shown that the intercellular transduction of the second messenger inositol triphosphate (IP$_3$) by gap junctions in the inner ear is also essential for the perception of sound (25). The spreading of an IP$_3$-mediated Ca^{2+} signal would be essential to the propagation of Ca^{2+} waves in cochlear-supporting cells.

In many different populations, mutations in the GJB2 gene are the major cause of autosomal-recessive nonsyndromic hearing loss at the DFNB1 locus (26–29). However, some mutations are responsible for autosomal-dominant HI, although at a much lower frequency (30). Most of these dominant mutations in GJB2 cause a syndromic form of HI, with additional skin abnormalities (keratodermas) that are clinically very heterogeneous (7–9,31,32).

In many European populations, the most frequent mutation in the GJB2 gene is the 35delG mutation (26,28,33–35). This single base-pair deletion creates a frameshift very early in the gene, most likely causing complete disruption of expression. In non-European populations, the 35delG mutation is rare, but sometimes other frequent mutations are found. These include the 235delC mutation in Japanese and Koreans (36–38), the 167delT in Ashkenazi Jews (39,40), and the R143W mutation

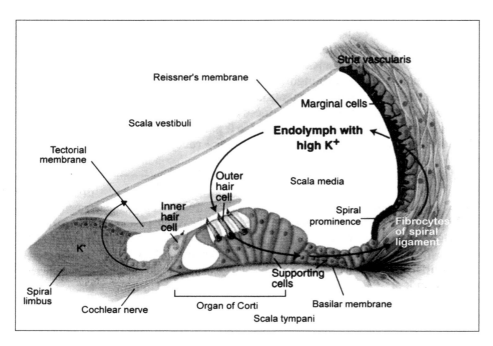

Figure 5.1 Location of the different components of the cochlea. The K^+ recycling pathway is indicated. *Source*: From Ref. 20.

in a village in eastern Ghana (41). For three of these (167delT, 35delG, and 235delC), the mutation was shown to be derived from a common founder, which in the case of 35delG was estimated to be 10,000 years old (29,33,39).

Because a general GJB2 knockout mouse is embryonically lethal (42), a tissue-specific GJB2 knockout was created using the LoxP-Cre system (43). In this way, GJB2 was disrupted only in the epithelial network of the cochlea, whereas GJB2 expression in the connective tissue network of the cochlea as well as in all other organs stayed intact. This cochlear epithelial network-specific GJB2 knockout mouse had HI, without signs of vestibular dysfunction and skin abnormalities.

Recently, two deletions near the GJB2 gene on 13q12 were detected (44, 44a). A novel 232-kb deletion involving the GJB6 gene (connexin-30) in Spanish subjects with autosomal-recessive nonsyndromic hearing impairment (submitted 2004).] These mutations, called del(GJB6-D13S1830) and del(GJB6-D13S1854), leave the GJB2 coding region intact but delete a large region close to GJB2 and truncate another connexin (CX30, GJB6) located within 50 kb of GJB2. These deletions are frequently found in compound heterozygosity with a GJB2 mutation. Coimmunostaining showed expression of CX26 (GJB2) and CX30 (GJB6) in the same gap-junction plaques (45). The del(GJB6-D13S1830) mutation was the accompanying mutation in 50% of deaf GJB2 heterozygotes in Spain, whereas the del(GJB6-D13S1854) mutation accounts for 25% of the affected GJB2 heterozygotes, which remained unexplained after screening of the GJB2 gene and the del(GJB6-D13S1830) mutation in the Spanish patients. HI in patients with both deletions is assumed to be caused by the deletion of a putative GJB2 regulatory element or by digenic inheritance. However, pure digenic inheritance seems to be unlikely because compound heterozygosity with a GJB2 mutation has not been found for other GJB6 mutations. The HI in patients with del(GJB6-D13S1830) and del(GJB6-D13S1854) is more severe than HI in patients with other GJB2 mutations (46). This may be due to the inactivation of one allele of GJB6 by the deletion. If GJB6 can partly substitute for the function of GJB2 in the inner ear, as has been suggested (45), this substitution could be less efficient with only one GJB6 gene left, leading to more severe HI. Finally, there has been only one report of a missense mutation that can cause nonsyndromic hearing loss in GJB6, i.e., T5M (47). Other mutations in the GJB6 gene can cause the Clouston syndrome, an autosomal-dominant disorder characterised by changes in the epidermis and the appendages, including diffuse palmoplantar keratoderma, nail dystrophy, and sparse scalp and body hair (48). HI of variable degree is also observed in some Clouston cases.

It is currently unknown why GJB2 mutations are a frequent cause of autosomal-recessive deafness in many ethnically diverse populations. Nevertheless, it is clear that GJB2 mutations are a major cause of deafness in most of the populations that have hitherto been studied. Generally, the most important genetic test for nonsyndromic HI is molecular screening of the GJB2 gene. A recent genotype–phenotype

correlation study for GJB2 mutations makes it possible that more accurate information about the probability of having a child with severe or profound HI can be given to couples who carry GJB2 mutations (46).

Connexin 31 (GJB3)

Another connexin that, when mutated, can cause hearing loss is Connexin 31, encoded by the GJB3 gene. This gene is localised within the DFNA2 region at chromosome 1p34, close to the KCNQ4 gene, which is also a deafness gene. GJB3 mutation analysis revealed mutations in only a few families with an autosomal-dominant or -recessive nonsyndromic HI (49,50). In the cochlea, its specific expression is restricted to the spiral limbus and spiral ligament. There is strong evidence that mutations in this gene can also cause erythrokeratoderma variabilis, an autosomal-dominant skin disorder, without HI (51). One specific dominant mutation D66H in the GJB3 gene can cause peripheral neuropathy and sensorineural HI (52). This amino acid residue at position 66 is highly conserved across species and most likely also plays a functionally important role in other connexins. In GJB2, D66H causes Vohwinkel syndrome (7), whereas 66delD in the GJB1 gene results in the peripheral neuropathy disorder X-linked Charcot-Marie-Toot disease (53). Remarkably, knockout mice with the GJB3 gene have no symptoms of hearing loss. However, a reduced embryonic viability due to placental dysmorphogenesis has been detected (54).

Claudin 14 (CLDN14)

The major role in the paracellular pathway of inner ear K^+ recycling is played by the tight junctions, which seal neighbouring cells together to prevent leakage (55). Tight junctions are composed of at least three types of membrane-spanning proteins: occludin, different members of the claudin family, and junction-adhesion molecules (56–58). Mutations in the CLDN14 gene, a member of the claudin family, can cause profound congenital recessive deafness in humans and in mice (59,60). Homozygous cldn14 knockout mice have a normal endocochlear potential, but they are deaf due to the rapid degeneration of cochlear OHCs. This is followed by a slower degeneration of inner hair cells. CLDN14 is expressed in the sensory epithelium of the organ of Corti and is probably required as a cation-restrictive barrier to maintain the ionic composition of the fluid surrounding the basolateral surface of OHCs.

Potassium channel, voltage gated, subfamily Q, member 4 (KCNQ4)

This gene encodes a voltage-gated K-channel, KCNQ4, and is responsible for the most frequent form of autosomal-dominant nonsyndromic HI (DFNA2). KCNQ proteins have six transmembrane domains and although it has not been shown directly, four KCNQ subunits probably combine to form functional potassium channels.

KCNQ4 is expressed in both inner and OHCs of the cochlea and in auditory nuclei of the brainstem. It is probably involved in basolateral K^+ secretion of hair cells (61,62). As the K^+ channel is formed by a tetramer of *KCNQ4* subunits, any given mutation with a dominant-negative effect can cause a severe reduction in K^+ channel activity. This is compatible with the autosomal-dominant inheritance pattern and complete penetrance of the progressive HI associated with *KCNQ4* mutations.

Pendrin (*SLC26A4*)

Pendred syndrome is inherited in an autosomal-recessive manner and is characterised by the association of congenital hearing loss with thyroid abnormalities (goitre). This thyroid defect can be demonstrated by the perchlorate test. Cochlear malformations are common in Pendred syndrome. All Pendred syndrome patients have enlarged vestibular aqueducts (EVA) and many have Mondini dysplasia (63). The gene responsible for this syndrome is *SLC26A4*, which encodes the chloride–iodide transporter pendrin that is expressed in both the thyroid and the cochlea (11). Pendrin has a highly discrete expression pattern throughout the endolymphatic duct and sac, in the distinct areas of the utricule and the saccule, and in the external sulcus region (64). These regions are thought to be important for endolymphatic fluid resorption in the inner ear. Some mutations in the *SLC26A4* gene can also cause nonsyndromic autosomal-recessive hearing loss with EVA but without any signs of goitre. For this reason, *SLC26A4* mutation analysis is often performed in cases with nonsyndromic HI and EVA. However, no exact genotype–phenotype correlation can be made because of the intrafamilial variability and nonpenetrance of the thyroid phenotype. Remarkably, in many patients with nonsyndromic HI and EVA, only a single *SLC26A4* mutation is found (65), suggesting common undetected mutations outside the coding region or a dominant effect in some cases.

Genes involved in the structure and function of the hair cell

Adhesion molecules

Cadherin 23 and Protocadherin 15 belong to the cadherin superfamily, most members of which play a role in calcium-dependent cell-to-cell adhesion. Cadherin 23 is located at the tips of the bundles in hair cells and is proposed to be an essential component of tip links (Fig. 5.2) (67,68). Remarkably, missense mutations of *CDH23* with presumed subtle functional defects of cadherin 23 are associated with nonsyndromic hearing loss (DFNB12), whereas Usher syndrome type 1D (USH1D) is caused by mutant alleles of *CDH23* with a more severe effect (69–71). Usher syndrome is characterised by

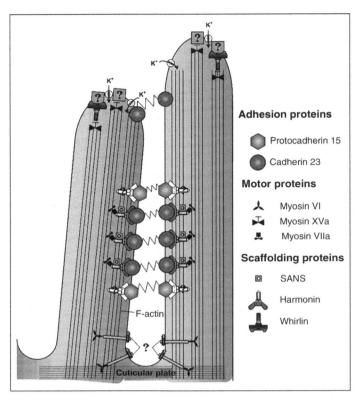

Figure 5.2 Schematised illustration of proteins that constitute adhesion complexes on the plasma membrane of stereocilia. Experimentally demonstrated interactions between myosin VIIa, harmonin, cadherin 23, and SANS are shown as well as the interaction of myosin XVa with whirlin. Cadherins and protocadherins are linked to each other, thereby constituting the lateral links. The molecules with which Myosin XVa and Whirlin may interact at the tips of the stereocilia as well as those that interact with protocadherin 15 are not yet identified. *Abbreviation*: SANS, scaffold protein containing ankyrin repeats and SAM domain. *Source:* From Ref. 66.

HI and retinitis pigmentosa and can be classified into three different types on the basis of clinical findings. To date, 11 genes have been localised for different types of Usher syndrome, of which eight genes have already been identified. In the eye, cadherin 23 is thought to play a fundamental role in the organisation of synaptic junctions. Like *CDH23*, several other genes that are required in the morphogenesis of the hair bundle have also been detected in nonsyndromic HI. Protocadherin 15 is an important protein in the morphogenesis and cohesion of stereocilia bundles through long-term maintenance of lateral connections (lateral links) between stereocilia (72). Mutations in the *PCDH15* gene are responsible for the HI in families linked to DFNB23 and for the Usher syndrome in families linked to USH1F (73,74). The two mouse strains Waltzer and Ames Waltzer have been identified as having mutations in *cdh23* and *pcdh15*, respectively. The phenotype of both mice is characterised by deafness, vestibular dysfunction, retinal dysfunction, and disorganised, splayed stereocilia in homozygous mice (70,75–77).

Scaffolding proteins

USH1C encodes a PDZ domain–containing protein called harmonin, and mutations also cause both nonsyndromic HI and Usher syndrome in families linked to the DFNB18 and the USH1C loci, respectively (14,17). PDZ domain–containing proteins are central organisers of high-order supramolecular complexes located at specific emplacements in the plasma membrane. In the cochlea, harmonin is restricted to the hair cells, where it is present in the cell body and the stereocilia. Harmonin has been shown to interact with cadherin 23 and SANS to form macromolecular complexes (78–80). The latter protein SANS is also mutated in Usher syndrome (USH1G) but not in nonsyndromic HI. An important regulator of the development of stereocilia is Whirlin, encoded by the gene *WHRN*. The protein is involved in the elongation and maintenance of stereocilia in hair cells (81). Mutations in the *WHRN* gene cause autosomal-recessive HI at the DFNB31 locus. The HI in the Whirler mouse mutant (*wi*) is caused by abnormally short but nearly normal organised stereocilia (81).

Myosins: intracellular motors

The myosin superfamily can be subdivided into 17 classes of unconventional and 1 class (class II) of conventional myosins. This conventional–unconventional dichotomy is artificial in terms of structure and evolution. However, it is operationally useful because of the historical emphasis on conventional myosins. In humans, 40 different myosin genes can be divided into 12 classes based on the relationships of their head-domain sequences and their tail structure (82). Class II consist of 15 conventional genes, including the cluster of 6 skeletal-muscle myosin heavy chains on chromosome 17, 2 cardiac myosin heavy chains, a smooth-muscle myosin heavy chain, and 3 non-muscle myosin heavy chains (83). All other myosin classes consist of a total of 25 unconventional genes. Although the role of myosin in contraction and force production in muscles is well characterised, little is known about the specific functional roles of nonmuscle myosins. They are likely to participate in motility, cytokinesis, phagocytosis, maintenance of cell shape, and particle trafficking.

Three unconventional myosins have already been extensively studied: myosin VI (MYO6), myosin VIIa (MYO7A), and myosin XVa (MYO15A). Dominant and recessive mutations in the first two myosins can cause nonsyndromic HI (DFNA22/DFNB37 and DFNA11/DFNB2, respectively) (16,19,84,85). In the MYO15A gene, only recessive mutations have been described in families linked to the DFNB3 locus (86). Additionally, mutations in the MYO7A gene have been described, which cause Usher syndrome (USH1B) (18).

Myosin VI is localised at the base of the hair bundle within the cuticular plate (87). This structure is thought to provide mechanical stability to the apex of the hair cell. The mouse strain Snell's Waltzer (*sv*) is deaf due to a mutation in the *myo6* gene that ablates all myosin VI protein in any tissue (88). The stereocilia of these mice are fused at their bases, indicating that myosin VI is required to anchor stereocilia rootlets (89,90).

Myosin VIIa binds at the lateral surface of the harmonin-cadherin 23–SANS macromolecular complexes and links them in this way to the actin filaments during hair-cell–bundle maturation. The mouse ortholog *myo7a* causes HI in the shaker-1 mouse strain (*sh1*) (91). Interestingly, two types of hair-cell anomalies have been detected in this mouse mutant. In the most severely affected mutants, the hair bundle is disorganised, with clumps of stereocilia projecting outside instead of forming the highly ordered structure. In addition, the kinocilium has an erratic position, indicating a role of myosin VIIa in the polarity of the hair bundle (92).

Myosin XVa is localised to the extreme tips of stereocilia, possibly anchored by integral membrane proteins (93). Interestingly, longer stereocilia have more myosin XVa at their tips compared to shorter stereocilia. Although not much is known about possible interactions, the PDZ domain–containing protein, whirlin, is a good candidate for HI (Fig. 5.2). The reason for this is that the myosin XVa protein has a PDZ-ligand sequence and the mouse mutants (*sh2* and *wi*) of both proteins share a similar phenotype.

Other myosins have also been shown to cause HI, although not much is known about their biological role in the cochlea. Among the conventional nonmuscle myosins, myosin IX (MYH9) and myosin XIV (MYH14) have been shown to cause autosomal-dominant HI in families linked to DFNA17 and DFNA4, respectively (94,95). The expression pattern differs between the two myosins. Myosin IX is localised specifically in the OHCs, the spiral ligament, and the Reissner's membrane, whereas myosin XIV is located in all cells of the scala media wall, except for Reissner's membrane, with a relatively higher level in the organ of Corti and the stria vascularis (94,95). Interestingly, only one mutation in the MYH9 gene has been found to cause nonsyndromic hearing loss, i.e., R705H. All other mutations cause a variety of syndromes, with a decreased number of blood platelets as a common symptom (96).

Other unconventional myosins that can cause nonsyndromic HI are myosin IIIA (MYO3A) and myosin Ia (MYO1A) in families linked to DFNB30 and DFNA48, respectively (97,98).

Genes involved in cytoskeletal formation

The cytoskeleton regulates cell shape, transport, motility, and integrity. It consists of microfilaments, intermediate filaments, and microtubules. The most abundant microfilament protein in cells is actin. In most cells, β-actin is the predominant isoform, although γ-actin, encoded by the ACTG1 gene, predominates in intestinal epithelial cells as well as in auditory hair cells, where it is found in stereocilia, the cuticular plate, and the adherens junctions (99). Auditory hair cells are highly dependent on their actin cytoskeletons (100). Mutations in *ACTG1* are the basis for hearing loss in four families affected with nonsyndromic HI (DFNA20/26) (101). Actin nucleation is accelerated through the interaction of diaphanous with the actin filaments (102). Diaphanous (*DIAPH1*) belongs to the formin protein family. Mutations in *DIAPH1* cause low-frequency HI in families linked to the DFNA1 locus (103). Another important structural element of the hair bundle of mammalian hair cells is espin, a calcium-insensitive, actin-bundling protein. A recessive mutation of the gene (*ESPN*) in the deaf jerker mouse (*je*) results in failure to accumulate detectable amounts of this protein in the hair bundle. This leads to shortening, loss of mechanical stiffness, and eventual disintegration of stereocilia (104). Remarkably, the amount of espin is proportional to the length of the stereocilium (105). In humans, recessive mutations of *ESPN* at the DFNB36 locus cause profound prelingual hearing loss and peripheral vestibular areflexia (106).

Prestin (*PRES*)

The most impressive property of OHCs in the cochlea is their ability to change their length in a voltage-dependent manner, contributing to the exquisite sensitivity and frequency-resolving capacity of the mammalian hearing organ (107,108). The contractility of their lateral cell membrane is an interesting mammalian cochlear specialisation that does not occur in inner hair cells. Prestin is a member of a gene family, solute carrier (SLC) family 26, which encodes anion transporters and related proteins. The lateral wall of OHCs has a high concentration of prestin, which is thought to be responsible for the electromotility of OHCs (104). The importance of prestin in hearing is strengthened by the detection of a 5'-UTR splice-acceptor mutation (IVS2-2A>G) in exon 3 in two unrelated families with recessive nonsyndromic deafness (109,109a). Additionally, the *pres -/-* knockout mouse model has a 40 to 60dB loss of cochlear sensitivity and their OHCs do not exhibit electromotility in vitro (110).

Extracellular matrix components

Cochlin (*COCH*)

The Coagulation Factor C Homology gene (*COCH*) encodes cochlin, a protein that is highly expressed in the cochlea (111). Cochlin comprises approximately 70% of all bovine inner ear proteins (112) and is expressed in fibrocytes of spiral limbus, spiral ligament, and fibrocytes of the connective tissue stroma underlying the sensory epithelium of the crista ampullaris in the semicircular canals (113). Sixteen different isoforms of cochlin can be classified into four groups according to their molecular weight: p63s, p44s, p40s, and CTP. Two isoforms, p63s and CTP, contain a specific limulus factor C, Coch-562 and LGL1 (LCCL) domain that is the only region in which mutations

have been found in autosomal-dominant nonsyndromic HI (DFNA9). Remarkably, DFNA9 patients also exhibit a variety of vestibular and Menière-like symptoms (including instability in the dark, imbalance, positional vertigo, tinnitus, and aural fullness). A total of six different mutations have been found in the *COCH* gene, of which P51S is the most frequent. Already 15 different families with the P51S mutation have been identified, making it the most frequent mutation in this gene. This mutation has been shown to originate from a common founder from Belgium or The Netherlands (114). The exact pathogenic mechanism of the Cochlin mutations is unknown.

Collagen XI a2 (*COL11A2*)

Collagen fibrils provide structural elements of high tensile strength in extracellular matrices. According to their function, they can be grouped into fibril-forming collagens, fibril-associated collagens, sheet-forming collagens, and anchoring collagens. Interactions between collagen fibrils, other matrix components, and cells are likely to provide the basis for the precise three-dimensional patterns of fibril arrangement in tissues. In the tectorial membrane, the fibril-forming collagen, XIa2, is an important structural component. It was not only found to cause autosomal-dominant nonsyndromic HI at the DFNA13 locus but also Stickler syndrome (STL2) (115). Mutations in two other collagens, collagen IIa1 (*COL2A1*) and collagen XIa1 (*COL11A1*), can also cause Stickler syndrome. Features of Stickler syndrome include progressive myopia, vitreoretinal degeneration, premature joint degeneration with abnormal epiphyseal development, midface hypoplasia, irregularities of the vertebral bodies, cleft palate deformity, and variable sensorineural hearing loss. Remarkably, persons with Stickler syndrome due to COL11A2 mutations do not have visual dysfunction. This can be explained by the absence of collagen XIa2 in the vitreous, where it is replaced by Collagen V (116). Electron microscopy of the tectorial membrane of homozygous col11a2 mice revealed loss of organisation of the collagen fibrils, which leads to moderate-to-severe hearing loss (115).

Otoancorin (*OTOA*) and stereocilin (*STRC*)

The attachment of inner ear acellular gels (tectorial membrane, otoconial membrane, and the cupula) to the apical surface of the underlying nonsensory cells is probably effected by otoancorin and stereocilin. These proteins share a significant similarity with 900 C-terminal amino acids (117). Stereocilin is almost exclusively expressed in the inner hair cells (118), whereas otoancorin is present on the apical surface of sensory epithelia and their overlying acellular gels (119). Based on the sequence similarity and expression pattern, it was suggested that stereocilin may have a comparable function to otoancorin, i.e., the attachment of the tectorial and otoconial membranes to sensory hair bundles at the level of hair cells. Mutations in *STRC* and *OTOA* cause nonsyndromic recessive HI at the DFNB16 and DFNB22 locus, respectively (118,119).

α-Tectorin (*TECTA*)

The tectorial membrane is an important extracellular matrix component in the cochlea that lies on top of the stereocilia. Deflection of this membrane is induced by sound and results in the generation of a receptor potential. The tectorial membrane is composed of collagens and noncollagenous glycoproteins, of which α-tectorin and β-tectorin are the most important. α-tectorin, encoded by the *TECTA* gene, is proteolytically processed into three polypeptides that are connected to each other by disulfide bridges. These polypeptides interact with β-tectorin. Several dominant and recessive mutations have already been described in the *TECTA* gene, causing HI in families linked to DFNA8/12 and DFNB21 (120,121). It was suggested that dominant mutations exert a dominant-negative effect, thereby disrupting proper interaction between the different α-tectorin polypeptides (120). Recessive mutations are functionally null alleles. Half the normal amount of α-tectorin is probably enough to preserve the auditory function, thereby explaining the lack of symptoms in heterozygous carriers. Mice homozygous for a targeted deletion in a α-tectorin have moderate-to-severe hearing loss due to the detachment of the tectorial membrane from the organ of Corti (122).

Transcription factors

Eyes absent 4 (*EYA4*)

The *EYA* gene family encodes a family of transcriptional activators that interact with other proteins in a conserved regulatory hierarchy to ensure normal embryological development. Mutations in one member, *EYA4*, can cause autosomal-dominant HI in families linked to the DFNA10 locus (123). The protein product of *EYA4* probably plays a developmental role in embryogenesis and a survival role in the mature cochlea. Its exact role in the inner ear is not yet known. Interestingly, mutations in another EYA member, *EYA1*, can cause the Branchio-Oto-Renal syndrome, an autosomal-recessive disorder that is characterised by a variable combination of branchial arch abnormalities, HI, and renal abnormalities (124).

POU genes

Pit, Oct, and Unc DNA-binding domain (*POU*) genes are members of a family of transcription-factor genes involved in development and, in particular, in terminal differentiation of neural cells (125). Mutations in two different POU-domain transcription-factor genes, *POU3F4* and *POU4F3*, are associated with nonsyndromic hearing loss in families linked to DFN3 and DFNA15, respectively (126,127). The two genes are expressed in distinct cell types and at different time points. Mice that are deficient in the transcription factor *pou3f4* have ultrastructurally abnormal fibrocytes and reduced endocochlear potential (128). *POU3F4* is likely to be important for development of inner-ear mesenchyme, which gives rise to the fibrocytes of the spiral ligament (129,130). By comparing inner ear gene expression profiles of the wild type and the *pou4f3* mutant deidler mouse strain (*ddl*), a new gene, *gfi1* (growth-factor

independence 1) was identified as a likely target gene regulated by pou4f3 (131). *Gfi1* is the first downstream target of a hair cell–specific transcription factor. The OHC degeneration in *pou4f3* mutants is thus largely or perhaps entirely a result of the loss of expression of *gfi1*.

Transcription factor cellular promoter 2 (*TFCP2L3*)

TFCP2L3 encodes a member of the transcription factor cellular promoter 2 (TFCP2) protein family that has a broad epithelial pattern of expression, including cells that line the developing cochlear duct. It shows homology to the *Drosophila* gene *grainyhead* and causes autosomal-dominant HI in families linked to the DFNA28 locus (132).

Genes with atypical or poorly understood function

The function of several deafness genes is currently not well known. No exact physiological role of these genes is known and, therefore, it is not possible to classify these genes in the previously described categories.

DFNA5 (*DFNA5*)

DFNA5 was first localised in a single, large, Dutch kindred–segregating autosomal-dominant progressive hearing loss (133). The phenotype cosegregated with an insertion/deletion in the seventh intron of a gene of unknown function that was named *DFNA5* (134). Later on, mutations were found in two other families (135,136). Although these mutations are different at the genomic DNA level, they all lead to skipping of exon 8 at the mRNA level. It is hypothesised that the HI associated with *DFNA5* is caused by a gain-of-function mutation and that mutant *DFNA5* has a deleterious new function (137). Morpholino antisense knockdown of *DFNA5* function in zebrafish leads to disorganisation of the developing semicircular canal and reduction of pharyngeal cartilage. In *DFNA5* morphants, expression of *ugdh* is absent in the developing ear and pharyngeal arches. Additionally, hyaluronic-acid (HA) levels are strongly reduced in the outgrowing protrusions of the developing semicircular canals (138). HA probably serves as a friction-reducing lubricant and molecular filter in the developing inner ear (139). It was proposed that a reduction of HA can lead to mechanical stress on hair cells and that this may lead to progressive HI (138).

Otoferlin (*OTOF*)

OTOF is a novel member of a mammalian gene family related to the *Caenorhabditis elegans* spermatogenesis factor *fer-1*. *OTOF* is expressed exclusively in adult hair cells (140). Several mutations have been found to cause hearing loss in families linked to the recessive DFNB9 locus (141,142). A founder mutation in this gene (Q829X) is a common cause of prelingual hearing loss in Spanish individuals who are not deaf due to GJB2 mutations (142). Interestingly, OTOF mutations are associated with a nonsyndromic, autosomal-recessive auditory neuropathy (143). Auditory neuropathy is a type of HI that preserves otoacoustic emissions and is not a known feature of any other autosomal-recessive phenotype. Therefore, genetic analysis of otoferlin may be indicated in cases of auditory neuropathy of presumed autosomal-recessive inheritance. However, another family with progressive, autosomal-dominant auditory neuropathy is reported by Kim et al. (144), and it maps to chromosome 13q14-21.

Transmembrane channel 1 (*TMC1*)

Mutations in this transmembrane channel–like gene are known to cause an autosomal-recessive hearing loss as well as autosomal-dominant hearing loss located at DFNB7/11 and DFNA36, respectively (145,146). TMC1 is predicted to encode a multipass transmembrane protein with no similarity to proteins of known function that is expressed in the hair cells of the postnatal mouse cochlea. TMC1 mutations were also identified in the autosomal-recessive deafness (*dn*) and autosomal-dominant Beethoven (*Bth*) mouse mutant strains segregating postnatal hair-cell degeneration (146,147). This indicates that TMC1 is required for postnatal hair-cell development or maintenance, although its exact function is not known.

Transmembrane inner ear (*TMIE*)

Mutations in the TMIE gene are a cause of vestibular and audiological dysfunction in the spinner (*sr*) mouse model. The postnatal morphological defects of the stereocilia in this mouse model suggest a role for this gene in the correct development and maintenance of stereocilia bundles (148). TMIE is expressed in many tissues and has no similarity to other known proteins (148). In humans, this gene is mutated in several consanguineous families that are linked to the autosomal-recessive DFNB6 locus (106).

Transmembrane serine protease 3 (*TMPRSS3*)

Type II transmembrane serine proteases (TTSPs) represent an emerging class of cell-surface proteolytic enzymes. Most TTSPs have been identified relatively recently and have not yet been functionally characterised. TMPRSS3 is the only protease that has so far been identified as a causative gene for HI (DFNB8/10) (149). It is expressed in the supporting cells, the stria vascularis, and the spiral ganglion (150). Although the specific role of TMPRSS3 in the development and maintenance of the cochlea is still unknown, it is reported that deafness-causing mutations in this gene disrupt the proteolytic activity of the protein (151). This will probably affect the amiloride-sensitive sodium channel (ENaC) because this could be a substrate of TMPRSS3 in the inner ear (150). This sodium channel may have a role in the maintenance of the low sodium concentration of endolymph.

Wolframin (*WFS1*)

WFS1 encodes a glycoprotein (wolframin), predominantly localised in the endoplasmic reticulum. In the cochlea, wolframin is mainly located in cells lining the scala media, in vestibular hair cells, and in spiral ganglion cells (152). Mutations in WFS1 cause the autosomal-recessive Wolfram syndrome and autosomal-dominant, low-frequency sensorineural HI DFNA6/14 (10,12,153,154). Wolfram syndrome is characterised by diabetes mellitus and optic atrophy, and, in most cases, by additional symptoms including diabetes insipidus, deafness, and urinary tract atony (155). Although not much is known about the exact function of wolframin, the gene has important diagnostic applications. Interestingly, only noninactivating WFS1 mutations that are mainly located in the C-terminal region cause nonsyndromic HI, whereas the majority of mutations in Wolfram syndrome are inactivating (156). This suggests that a loss of function of WFS1 is the cause of Wolfram syndrome. Homozygous *wfs1* knockout mice developed glucose intolerance due to insufficient insulin secretion and a subsequent progressive β-cell loss. The severity of the diabetic phenotype was dependent on the mouse background. The defective insulin secretion is accompanied by reduced cellular calcium responses (157). The auditory function of the knockout mice has not yet been studied.

Mitochondrial HI

The mtDNA molecule encodes 13 protein-coding genes as well as 2 rRNAs and 22 tRNAs, which are required for assembling a functional mitochondrial protein-synthesizing system. A cell contains several of these mitochondrial genomes. When patients with a mitochondrial disease carry the mutation in every mtDNA molecule, it is called homoplasmic. When a mixed population of normal and mutant genomes is present, the mutation is heteroplasmic. Heterogeneous tissue distribution might therefore cause large phenotypic variability in patients with heteroplasmic mutations.

mtDNA mutations are usually heteroplasmic, and most of them cause multisystem syndromes. Syndromic HI due to heteroplasmic mitochondrial mutations mostly has additional neuromuscular abnormalities (158). However, also nonsyndromic HI can be caused by mitochondrial mutations. The homoplasmic 1555A>G mutation in the mitochondrial MTRNR1 gene that encodes the 12S rRNA was the first detected in nonsyndromic HI (Table 5.1) (159). Although in many pedigrees and individual patients with this 1555A>G mutation the hearing loss occurred after aminoglycoside exposure (175–177), a significant number of pedigrees were described with HI without aminoglycoside exposure (178,160). In contrast, with the normal 12S rRNA, the mutated form has a high affinity to aminoglycosides (179). Additionally, aminoglycosides clearly

Table 5.1 Mitochondrial mutations involved in maternally inherited hearing impairment

Nonsyndromic HI gene	Mutation	Presence of additional symptoms	References
12SrRNA	1555A→G	Aminoglycoside induced/worsened	159–161
	1494C→T	Aminoglycoside induced/worsened	162
	961 (diff. mut.)	Aminoglycoside induced/worsened	163,164
tRNA$^{Ser(UCN)}$	7445A→G	Palmoplantar keratoderma	165–167
	7472insC	Neurological dysfunction	168–171
	7510T→C	None	172
	7511T→C	None	173,174

affect the protein synthesis of cells with mutated 12S rRNA (180). The phenotype of patients with the 1555A>G mutation ranges from profound congenital deafness, through progressive moderate hearing loss to completely normal hearing. This phenotypic variability is influenced by putative modifier genes of which already two have been identified. The first is the highly conserved mitochondrial protein encoded by the nuclear *MTO1* gene. It is involved in tRNA modification and may regulate the translational efficiency and accuracy of codon–anticodon base pairing on the coding region of ribosomes. It can contribute to the phenotypic variability of the 1555A>G mutation by suppressing the phenotypic manifestation of the 1555A>G mutation. The second gene encodes the mitochondrial transcription factor TFB1M (181). This methylates adenine residues in the adjacent loop of the 1555A>G mutation in the *MTRNR1* gene and its function is described as mitochondrial maintenance (181,182). Two other mutations in the *MTRNR1* gene have been reported, both of which confer susceptibility to aminoglycoside-induced ototoxicity (961delT and 1494C>T).

In another gene, *MTTS1*, which encodes the mitochondrial tRNA$^{Ser(UCN)}$, four mutations have been detected that cause nonsyndromic hearing loss (Table 5.1). Both the 7445A>G and the 7472insC mutations have been found in families with syndromic and nonsyndromic hearing loss. Additional symptoms can be palmoplantar keratoderma for the 7445A>G mutations and neurological dysfunction (ataxia and myoclonus) for the 7472insC mutation. To date, it is not fully understood how the defective tRNA$^{Ser(UCN)}$ and 12S rRNA can lead to hearing loss.

Modifier genes for HI

Phenotypic variation has been observed within both hearing-impaired families and individual patients carrying the same mutations. This variation can be attributed to either environmental or genetic factors. By interacting in the same or a parallel biological pathway as a disease gene, modifier genes can affect the phenotypic outcome of a given genotype.

In a family linked to DFNB26, several patients homozygous for the disease haplotype do not have HI. Instead, they all have a shared haplotype at the DFNM1 modifier locus at chromosome 1q24 (183). This suggests a modifier gene at the DFNM1 locus that can rescue the loss of hearing due to the pathogenic DFNB26 allele. The map location of DFNM1 was within the DFNA7 interval, suggesting that the DFNM1-suppressor phenotype and the DFNA7 hearing loss may be phenotypic variants of the same gene. To date, the responsible gene in both intervals has not been identified.

Most other identified modifier genes have a more subtle effect, affecting the age of onset, the degree of severity, or the rate of disease progression. Two examples of modifier genes detected in humans are *MTO1* and *TFB1M*. These genes can cause variability in mitochondrial deafness and were described in the previous section.

Several mouse models have already been used for detecting factors that modify the degree of hearing loss. The genetic diversity between inbred mouse strains makes them a valuable tool for studying the interaction of these factors. The CDH23^{753A} allele modifies the degree of hearing loss in the *deaf-waddler* mouse, which is caused by a mutation in the *pmca2* gene, a plasma membrane calcium pump located at chromosome 6 (184). This calcium pump helps to maintain low cytosolic Ca^{2+} by pumping Ca^{2+} out of the cell. To cause the early-onset hearing loss in *mdfw* mice, a combination of homozygosity of the cdh23^{753A} allele must coexist with haploinsufficiency of *pmca2*. Interestingly, the CDH23^{753A} allele also contributes to the susceptibility for age-related hearing loss in mice (185,186).

Diagnostic applications

To date, more than 100 loci for nonsyndromic hearing loss have been detected, and the responsible gene has been identified for 40 of them. Although this indeed represents a formidable result,

Table 5.2 Genetic testing for nonsyndromic hearing impairment[a]

Gene	Inheritance	Clinical indications
COCH	AD	Late-onset (>30 yr) progressive HI and simultaneous vestibular dysfunction
OTOF	AR	Auditory neuropathy, congenital
SLC26A4	AR	Enlarged vestibular aqueduct, congenital
MTRNR1(12S rRNA)	M	Aminoglycoside-induced HI
WFS1	AD	Low-frequency HI, early onset

[a]On the basis of specific clinical indications, routinely available in some laboratories. In the absence of specific indications, GJB2 (Cx26) testing is routinely carried out (for autosomal-recessive inheritance) in many laboratories.
Abbreviations: AD, autosomal dominant; AR, autosomal recessive; HI, hearing impairment; M, mitochondrial.

many more genes need to be discovered and many more loci probably remain unidentified. Unfortunately, this large increase in knowledge has not led to widespread diagnostic applications, as has been the case for many other hereditary diseases. The most important obstacle is the extreme genetic heterogeneity. Nonsyndromic HI gives few clinical characteristics that can be used to subclassify patients. Moreover, the few characteristics that are available are often poor indicators of the involvement of specific genes because for most genes, there is a significant clinical variability. A few exceptions exist and in some situations a clue for a possible culprit gene can be obtained from clinical data (Table 5.2). However, these exceptions only apply to a small percentage of patients with putative genetic HI. This has led to the unfortunate situation that currently a large gap exists between scientific achievements for deafness genes and diagnostic applications that result from it. With increasingly more deafness genes being found in a small number of patients, this gap widens as research progresses.

Despite these problems, there is one gene that has found widespread diagnostic applications. This gene is *GJB2*, and in several ways, it is an excellent gene for DNA diagnostics. Firstly, it is responsible for a large fraction of deafness patients in some populations, with up to 50% of patients having genetic deafness in Mediterranean countries. A second major advantage of the gene is its very small size, which makes genetic analysis affordable. However, for patients without *GJB2* mutations or for populations with a low incidence of *GJB2* mutations, the genetic causes are distributed over dozens of genes, some of which are very large in size and hence expensive to analyse. Screening all known deafness genes for mutations would be extremely expensive with current technology, prohibiting the diagnostic use of this procedure.

A promising technique for future diagnostics may be the use of DNA microarrays (also called DNA chips). Microarrays offer the possibility of performing a large number of genetic tests in parallel in a single experiment. This can either be the analysis of many known mutations or be the complete mutation analysis of one or more genes. Initiatives to use microarrays for DNA diagnostics in the deafness field are emerging. One initiative will use arrays to analyse all currently known mutations for Usher syndrome (H. Kremer, personal communication). As Usher syndrome is genetically heterogeneous, with mutations spread over several very large genes, traditional analysis is not cost effective, and DNA microarrays may yield a cost-effective alternative. A second initiative will use a DNA microarray for the complete mutation analysis of eight genes causing autosomal-recessive deafness (H. Rehm, personal communication). This method has the advantage that also currently unknown mutations can be detected, the disadvantage being that only a limited set of genes is included. However, this limitation is mainly based on the technological limitations of the array. Using several arrays, or using future more-dense arrays, the simultaneous analysis of many more genes may become a reality.

Conclusions

Over the last decade, tremendous progress has been achieved in the identification of deafness genes. As a result, our understanding of the complex mechanism of hearing has increased enormously. It is to be expected that mapping and identification of new genes will continue for years to come, with a further growing insight in to the molecular biology of hearing. Promising results have recently been reported about phenotypic variability in hearing loss caused by modifier genes. The identification and characterisation of these modifiers will definitely be a new challenge for deafness research. Despite the escalating number of genes implicated in hearing loss, only a minority of them have routinely available diagnostic tests (Table 5.2). Therefore, a promising technique for future diagnostics will be the use of robust and cost-effective DNA microarrays. Hopefully, this will help in reducing the increasing gap between scientific research and diagnostic applications for hearing loss.

References

1. Mehl AL, Thomson V. The Colorado newborn hearing screening project, 1992–1999: on the threshold of effective population-based universal newborn hearing screening. Pediatrics 2002; 109:E7.

2. Marazita ML, Ploughman LM, Rawlings B, et al. Genetic epidemiological studies of early-onset deafness in the U.S. school-age population. Am J Med Genet 1993; 46:486–491.

3. Morton NE. Genetic epidemiology of hearing impairment. Ann N Y Acad Sci 1991; 630:16–31.

4. Davis A, Wood S, Healy R, et al. Risk factors for hearing disorders: epidemiologic evidence of change over time in the UK. J Am Acad Audiol 1995; 6:365–370.

5. Leon PE, Raventos H, Lynch E, et al. The gene for an inherited form of deafness maps to chromosome 5q31. Proc Natl Acad Sci USA 1992; 89:5181–5184.

6. Hereditary Hearing Loss Homepage, http://webhost.ua.ac.be/hhh.

7. Maestrini E, Korge BP, Ocana-Sierra J, et al. A missense mutation in connexin26, D66H, causes mutilating keratoderma with sensorineural deafness (Vohwinkel's syndrome) in three unrelated families. Hum Mol Genet 1999; 8:1237–1243.

8. Alvarez A, del Castillo I, Pera A, et al. De novo mutation in the gene encoding connexin-26 (GJB2) in a sporadic case of keratitis-ichthyosis-deafness (KID) syndrome. Am J Med Genet 2003; 117A:89–91.

9. Heathcote K, Syrris P, Carter ND, et al. A connexin 26 mutation causes a syndrome of sensorineural hearing loss and palmoplantar hyperkeratosis (MIM 148350). J Med Genet 2000; 37:50–51.

10. Bespalova IN, Van Camp G, Bom SJ, et al. Mutations in the Wolfram syndrome 1 gene (WFS1) are a common cause of low frequency sensorineural hearing loss. Hum Mol Genet 2001; 10:2501–2508.

11. Everett LA, Glaser B, Beck JC, et al. Pendred syndrome is caused by mutations in a putative sulphate transporter gene (PDS). Nat Genet 1997; 17:411–422.

12. Inoue H, Tanizawa Y, Wasson J, et al. A gene encoding a transmembrane protein is mutated in patients with diabetes mellitus and optic atrophy (Wolfram syndrome). Nat Genet 1998; 20:143–148.

13. Li XC, Everett LA, Lalwani AK, et al. A mutation in PDS causes non-syndromic recessive deafness. Nat Genet 1998; 18:215–217.

14. Ahmed ZM, Smith TN, Riazuddin S, et al. Nonsyndromic recessive deafness DFNB18 and Usher syndrome type IC are allelic mutations of USHIC. Hum Genet 2002; 110:527–531.

15. Bitner-Glindzicz M, Lindley KJ, Rutland P, et al. A recessive contiguous gene deletion causing infantile hyperinsulinism, enteropathy and deafness identifies the Usher type 1C gene. Nat Genet 2000; 26:56–60.

16. Liu XZ, Newton VE, Steel KP, et al. Identification of a new mutation of the myosin VII head region in Usher syndrome type 1. Hum Mutat 1997; 10:168–170.

17. Verpy E, Leibovici M, Zwaenepoel I, et al. A defect in harmonin, a PDZ domain-containing protein expressed in the inner ear sensory hair cells, underlies Usher syndrome type 1C. Nat Genet 2000; 26:51–55.

18. Weil D, Blanchard S, Kaplan J, et al. Defective myosin VIIA gene responsible for Usher syndrome type 1B. Nature 1995; 374:60–61.

19. Weil D, Kussel P, Blanchard S, et al. The autosomal recessive isolated deafness, DFNB2, and the Usher 1B syndrome are allelic defects of the myosin-VIIA gene. Nat Genet 1997; 16:191–193.

20. Steel K. The benefits of recycling. Science 1999; 285:1363–1364.

21. Wangemann P. Comparison of ion transport mechanisms between vestibular dark cells and strial marginal cells. Hear Res 1995; 90:149–157.

22. Kikuchi T, Adams JC, Miyabe Y, et al. Potassium ion recycling pathway via gap junction systems in the mammalian cochlea and its interruption in hereditary nonsyndromic deafness. Med Electron Microsc 2000; 33:51–56.

23. Kikuchi T, Kimura RS, Paul DL, et al. Gap junctions in the rat cochlea: immunohistochemical and ultrastructural analysis. Anat Embryol (Berl) 1995; 191:101–118.

24. Lautermann J, ten Cate WJ, Altenhoff P, et al. Expression of the gap-junction connexins 26 and 30 in the rat cochlea. Cell Tissue Res 1998; 294:415–420.

25. Beltramello M, Piazza V, Bukauskas FF, et al. Impaired permeability to Ins(1,4,5)P3 in a mutant connexin underlies recessive hereditary deafness. Nat Cell Biol 2005; 7:63–69.

26. Zelante L, Gasparini P, Estivill X, et al. Connexin26 mutations associated with the most common form of non-syndromic neurosensory autosomal recessive deafness (DFNB1) in Mediterraneans. Hum Mol Genet 1997; 6:1605–1609.

27. Estivill X, Fortina P, Surrey S, et al. Connexin-26 mutations in sporadic and inherited sensorineural deafness. Lancet 1998; 351: 394–398.

28. Green GE, Scott DA, McDonald JM, et al. Carrier rates in the midwestern United States for GJB2 mutations causing inherited deafness. JAMA 1999; 281:2211–2216.

29. Ohtsuka A, Yuge I, Kimura S, et al. GJB2 deafness gene shows a specific spectrum of mutations in Japan, including a frequent founder mutation. Hum Genet 2003; 112:329–333.

30. Chaib H, Lina-Granade G, Guilford P, et al. A gene responsible for a dominant form of neurosensory non-syndromic deafness maps to the NSRD1 recessive deafness gene interval. Hum Mol Genet 1994; 3:2219–2222.

31. Kelsell DP, Wilgoss AL, Richard G, et al. Connexin mutations associated with palmoplantar keratoderma and profound deafness in a single family. Eur J Hum Genet 2000; 8:469–472.

32. Rouan F, White TW, Brown N, et al. Trans-dominant inhibition of connexin-43 by mutant connexin-26: implications for dominant connexin disorders affecting epidermal differentiation. J Cell Sci 2001; 114:2105–2113.

33. Van Laer L, Coucke P, Mueller RF, et al. A common founder for the 35delG GJB2 gene mutation in connexin 26 hearing impairment. J Med Genet 2001; 38:515–518.

34. Denoyelle F, Weil D, Maw MA, et al. Prelingual deafness: high prevalence of a 30delG mutation in the connexin 26 gene. Hum Mol Genet 1997; 6:2173–2177.

35. Kelley PM, Harris DJ, Comer BC, et al. Novel mutations in the connexin 26 gene (GJB2) that cause autosomal recessive (DFNB1) hearing loss. Am J Hum Genet 1998; 62:792–799.

36. Abe S, Usami S, Shinkawa H, et al. Prevalent connexin 26 gene (GJB2) mutations in Japanese. J Med Genet 2000; 37:41–43.

37. Park HJ, Hahn SH, Chun YM, et al. Connexin26 mutations associated with nonsyndromic hearing loss. Laryngoscope 2000; 110: 1535–1538.

38. Kudo T, Ikeda K, Kure S, et al. Novel mutations in the connexin 26 gene (GJB2) responsible for childhood deafness in the Japanese population. Am J Med Genet 2000; 90:141–145.

39. Morell RJ, Kim HJ, Hood LJ, et al. Mutations in the connexin 26 gene (GJB2) among Ashkenazi Jews with nonsyndromic recessive deafness. N Engl J Med 1998; 339:1500–1505.

40. Sobe T, Erlich P, Berry A, et al. High frequency of the deafness-associated 167delT mutation in the connexin 26 (GJB2) gene in Israeli Ashkenazim. Am J Med Genet 1999; 86:499–500.

41. Brobby GW, Muller-Myhsok B, Horstmann RD. Connexin 26 R143W mutation associated with recessive nonsyndromic sensorineural deafness in Africa. N Engl J Med 1998; 338:548–550.

42. Gabriel HD, Jung D, Butzler C, et al. Transplacental uptake of glucose is decreased in embryonic lethal connexin26-deficient mice. J Cell Biol 1998; 140:1453–1461.

43. Cohen-Salmon M, Ott T, Michel V, et al. Targeted ablation of connexin26 in the inner ear epithelial gap junction network causes hearing impairment and cell death. Curr Biol 2002; 12: 1106–1111.

44. del Castillo I, Villamar M, Moreno-Pelayo MA, et al. A deletion involving the connexin 30 gene in nonsyndromic hearing impairment. N Engl J Med 2002; 346:243–249.

44a. del Castillo FJ, Rodriguez-Ballesteros M, Alvarez A, et al. Related articles, Links a novel deletion involving the connexin-30 gene, del (GJB6d13s1854), found in trans with mutations in the GJB2 gene (connexin-26) in subjects with DFNB1 non-syndromic hearing impairment. J Med Genet 2005; 42(7):588–594.

45. Ahmad S, Chen S, Sun J, et al. Connexins 26 and 30 are co-assembled to form gap junctions in the cochlea of mice. Biochem Biophys Res Commun 2003; 307:362–368.

46. Cryns K, Orzan E, Murgia A, et al. A genotype-phenotype correlation for GJB2 (connexin 26) deafness. J Med Genet 2004; 41: 147–154.

47. Grifa A, Wagner CA, D'Ambrosio L, et al. Mutations in GJB6 cause nonsyndromic autosomal dominant deafness at DFNA3 locus. Nat Genet 1999; 23:16–18.

48. Lamartine J, Munhoz Essenfelder G, Kibar Z, et al. Mutations in GJB6 cause hidrotic ectodermal dysplasia. Nat Genet 2000; 26:142–144.

49. Xia JH, Liu CY, Tang BS, et al. Mutations in the gene encoding gap junction protein beta-3 associated with autosomal dominant hearing impairment. Nat Genet 1998; 20:370–373.

50. Liu XZ, Xia XJ, Xu LR, et al. Mutations in connexin31 underlie recessive as well as dominant non-syndromic hearing loss. Hum Mol Genet 2000; 9:63–67.

51. Richard G, White TW, Smith LE, et al. Functional defects of Cx26 resulting from a heterozygous missense mutation in a family with dominant deaf-mutism and palmoplantar keratoderma. Hum Genet 1998; 103:393–399.

52. Lopez-Bigas N, Olive M, Rabionet R, et al. Connexin 31 (GJB3) is expressed in the peripheral and auditory nerves and causes neuropathy and hearing impairment. Hum Mol Genet 2001; 10:947–952.

53. Young P, Grote K, Kuhlenbaumer G, et al. Mutation analysis in Chariot-Marie Tooth disease type 1: point mutations in the MPZ gene and the GJB1 gene cause comparable phenotypic heterogeneity. J Neurol 2001; 248:410–415.

54. Plum A, Winterhager E, Pesch J, et al. Connexin31-deficiency in mice causes transient placental dysmorphogenesis but does not impair hearing and skin differentiation. Dev Biol 2001; 231:334–347.

55. Madara JL. Regulation of the movement of solutes across tight junctions. Annu Rev Physiol 1998; 60:143–159.

56. Furuse M, Hirase T, Itoh M, et al. Occludin: a novel integral membrane protein localizing at tight junctions. J Cell Biol 1993; 123:1777–1788.

57. Tsukita S, Furuse M. The structure and function of claudins, cell adhesion molecules at tight junctions. Ann N Y Acad Sci 2000; 915:129–135.

58. Martin-Padura I, Lostaglio S, Schneemann M, et al. Junctional adhesion molecule, a novel member of the immunoglobulin superfamily that distributes at intercellular junctions and modulates monocyte transmigration. J Cell Biol 1998; 142:117–127.

59. Wilcox ER, Burton QL, Naz S, et al. Mutations in the gene encoding tight junction claudin-14 cause autosomal recessive deafness DFNB29. Cell 2001; 104:165–172.

60. Ben-Yosef T, Belyantseva IA, Saunders TL, et al. Claudin 14 knockout mice, a model for autosomal recessive deafness DFNB29, are deaf due to cochlear hair cell degeneration. Hum Mol Genet 2003; 12:2049–2061.

61. Kharkovets T, Hardelin JP, Safieddine S, et al. KCNQ4, a K+ channel mutated in a form of dominant deafness, is expressed in the inner ear and the central auditory pathway. Proc Natl Acad Sci USA 2000; 97:4333–4338.

62. Beisel KW, Nelson NC, Delimont DC, et al. Longitudinal gradients of KCNQ4 expression in spiral ganglion and cochlear hair cells correlate with progressive hearing loss in DFNA2. Brain Res Mol Brain Res 2000; 82:137–149.

63. Phelps PD, Coffey RA, Trembath RC, et al. Radiological malformations of the ear in Pendred syndrome. Clin Radiol 1998; 53: 268–273.

64. Everett LA, Morsli H, Wu DK, et al. Expression pattern of the mouse ortholog of the Pendred's syndrome gene (Pds) suggests a key role for pendrin in the inner ear. Proc Natl Acad Sci USA 1999; 96:9727–9732.

65. Naganawa S, Koshikawa T, Fukatsu H, et al. Enlarged endolymphatic duct and sac syndrome: relationship between MR findings and genotype of mutation in Pendred syndrome gene. Magn Reson Imaging 2004; 22:25–30.

66. Frolenkov GI, Belyantseva IA, Friedman TB, et al. Genetic insights into the morphogenesis of inner ear hair cells. Nat Rev Genet 2004; 5:489–498.

67. Siemens J, Lillo C, Dumont RA, et al. Cadherin 23 is a component of the tip link in hair-cell stereocilia. Nature 2004; 428:950–955.

68. Sollner C, Rauch GJ, Siemens J, et al. Mutations in cadherin 23 affect tip links in zebrafish sensory hair cells. Nature 2004; 428: 955–959.

69. Bork JM, Peters LM, Riazuddin S, et al. Usher syndrome 1D and nonsyndromic autosomal recessive deafness DFNB12 are caused by allelic mutations of the novel cadherin-like gene CDH23. Am J Hum Genet 2001; 68:26–37.

70. Di Palma F, Holme RH, Bryda EC, et al. Mutations in Cdh23, encoding a new type of cadherin, cause stereocilia disorganization in waltzer, the mouse model for Usher syndrome type 1D. Nat Genet 2001; 27:103–107.

71. Bolz H, von Brederlow B, Ramirez A, et al. Mutation of CDH23, encoding a new member of the cadherin gene family, causes Usher syndrome type 1D. Nat Genet 2001; 27:108–112.

72. Ahmed ZM, Riazuddin S, Ahmad J, et al. PCDH15 is expressed in the neurosensory epithelium of the eye and ear and mutant alleles are responsible for both USH1F and DFNB23. Hum Mol Genet 2003; 12:3215–3223.

73. Alagramam KN, Yuan H, Kuehn MH, et al. Mutations in the novel protocadherin PCDH15 cause Usher syndrome type 1F. Hum Mol Genet 2001; 10:1709–1718.

74. Ahmed ZM, Riazuddin S, Bernstein SL, et al. Mutations of the protocadherin gene PCDH15 cause Usher syndrome type 1F. Am J Hum Genet 2001; 69:25–34.

75. Alagramam KN, Zahorsky-Reeves J, Wright CG, et al. Neuroepithelial defects of the inner ear in a new allele of the mouse mutation Ames waltzer. Hear Res 2000; 148:181–191.

76. Hampton LL, Wright CG, Alagramam KN, et al. A new spontaneous mutation in the mouse Ames waltzer gene, Pcdh15. Hear Res 2003; 180:67–75.

77. Libby RT, Kitamoto J, Holme RH, et al. Cdh23 mutations in the mouse are associated with retinal dysfunction but not retinal degeneration. Exp Eye Res 2003; 77:731–739.

78. Boeda B, El-Amraoui A, Bahloul A, et al. Myosin VIIa, harmonin and cadherin 23, three Usher I gene products that cooperate to shape the sensory hair cell bundle. Embo J 2002; 21:6689–6699.

79. Siemens J, Kazmierczak P, Reynolds A, et al. The Usher syndrome proteins cadherin 23 and harmonin form a complex by means of PDZ-domain interactions. Proc Natl Acad Sci USA 2002; 99: 14946–14951.

80. Weil D, El-Amraoui A, Masmoudi S, et al. Usher syndrome type I G (USH1G) is caused by mutations in the gene encoding SANS, a protein that associates with the USH1C protein, harmonin. Hum Mol Genet 2003; 12:463–471.

81. Mburu P, Mustapha M, Varela A, et al. Defects in whirlin, a PDZ domain molecule involved in stereocilia elongation, cause deafness in the whirler mouse and families with DFNB31. Nat Genet 2003; 34:421–428.

82. Sellers JR, Goodson HV. Motor proteins 2: myosin. Protein Profile 1995; 2:1323–1423.

83. Berg JS, Powell BC, Cheney RE. A millennial myosin census. Mol Biol Cell 2001; 12:780–794.

84. Melchionda S, Ahituv N, Bisceglia L, et al. MYO6, the human homologue of the gene responsible for deafness in Snell's waltzer mice, is mutated in autosomal dominant nonsyndromic hearing loss. Am J Hum Genet 2001; 69:635–640.

85. Ahmed ZM, Morell RJ, Riazuddin S, et al. Mutations of MYO6 are associated with recessive deafness, DFNB37. Am J Hum Genet 2003; 72:1315–1322.

86. Wang A, Liang Y, Fridell RA, et al. Association of unconventional myosin MYO15 mutations with human nonsyndromic deafness DFNB3. Science 1998; 280:1447–1451.

87. Avraham KB, Hasson T, Sobe T, et al. Characterization of unconventional MYO6, the human homologue of the gene responsible for deafness in Snell's waltzer mice. Hum Mol Genet 1997; 6:1225–1231.

88. Avraham KB, Hasson T, Steel KP, et al. The mouse Snell's waltzer deafness gene encodes an unconventional myosin required for structural integrity of inner ear hair cells. Nat Genet 1995; 11:369–375.

89. Self T, Sobe T, Copeland NG, et al. Role of myosin VI in the differentiation of cochlear hair cells. Dev Biol 1999; 214:331–341.

90. Altman D, Sweeney HL, Spudich JA. The mechanism of myosin VI translocation and its load-induced anchoring. Cell 2004; 116:737–749.

91. Gibson F, Walsh J, Mburu P, et al. A type VII myosin encoded by the mouse deafness gene shaker-1. Nature 1995; 374:62–64.

92. Self T, Mahony M, Fleming J, et al. Shaker-1 mutations reveal roles for myosin VIIA in both development and function of cochlear hair cells. Development 1998; 125:557–566.

93. Belyantseva IA, Boger ET, Friedman TB. Myosin XVa localizes to the tips of inner ear sensory cell stereocilia and is essential for staircase formation of the hair bundle. Proc Natl Acad Sci USA 2003; 100:13958–13963.

94. Lalwani AK, Goldstein JA, Kelley MJ, et al. Human nonsyndromic hereditary deafness DFNA17 is due to a mutation in nonmuscle myosin MYH9. Am J Hum Genet 2000; 67:1121–1128.

95. Donaudy F, Snoeckx R, Pfister M, et al. Nonmuscle myosin heavy-chain gene MYH14 is expressed in cochlea and mutated in patients affected by autosomal dominant hearing impairment (DFNA4). Am J Hum Genet 2004; 74:770–776.

96. Toren A, Rozenfeld-Granot G, Rocca B, et al. Autosomal-dominant giant platelet syndromes: a hint of the same genetic defect as in Fechtner syndrome owing to a similar genetic linkage to chromosome 22q11–13. Blood 2000; 96:3447–3451.

97. Donaudy F, Ferrara A, Esposito L, et al. Multiple mutations of MYO1A, a cochlear-expressed gene, in sensorineural hearing loss. Am J Hum Genet 2003; 72:1571–1577.

98. Walsh T, Walsh V, Vreugde S, et al. From flies' eyes to our ears: mutations in a human class III myosin cause progressive nonsyndromic hearing loss DFNB30. Proc Natl Acad Sci USA 2002; 99:7518–7523.

99. Khaitlina SY. Functional specificity of actin isoforms. Int Rev Cytol 2001; 202:35–98.

100. Hofer D, Ness W, Drenckhahn D. Sorting of actin isoforms in chicken auditory hair cells. J Cell Sci 1997;110(Pt 6):765–770.

101. Zhu M, Yang T, Wei S, et al. Mutations in the gamma-actin gene (ACTG1) are associated with dominant progressive deafness (DFNA20/26). Am J Hum Genet 2003; 73:1082–1091.

102. Higashida C, Miyoshi T, Fujita A, et al. Actin polymerization-driven molecular movement of mDia1 in living cells. Science 2004; 303:2007–2010.

103. Lynch ED, Lee MK, Morrow JE, et al. Nonsyndromic deafness DFNA1 associated with mutation of a human homolog of the Drosophila gene diaphanous. Science 1997; 278:1315–1318.

104. Zheng L, Sekerkova G, Vranich K, et al. The deaf jerker mouse has a mutation in the gene encoding the espin actin-bundling proteins of hair cell stereocilia and lacks espins. Cell 2000; 102:377–385.

105. Loomis PA, Zheng L, Sekerkova G, et al. Espin cross-links cause the elongation of microvillus-type parallel actin bundles in vivo. J Cell Biol 2003; 163:1045–1055.

106. Naz S, Griffith AJ, Riazuddin S, et al. Mutations of ESPN cause autosomal recessive deafness and vestibular dysfunction. J Med Genet 2004; 41:591–595.

107. Brownell WE, Bader CR, Bertrand D, et al. Evoked mechanical responses of isolated cochlear outer hair cells. Science 1985; 227:194–196.

108. Dallos P, Fakler B. Prestin, a new type of motor protein. Nat Rev Mol Cell Biol 2002; 3:104–111.

109. Liu XZ, Ouyang XM, Zia XY, et al. Prestin, a cochlear motor protein, is defective in non-sndromic hearing loss. Hum Mol Genet 2003; 12:1155–1162.

109a. Tang HY, Xia A, Oghalai JS, Pereira FA, Alford RL. High frequency of the IVS2-2A>G DNA sequence variation in SLC26A5, encoding the cochler motor proein prestin, precludes its involvement in hereditary hearing loss. BMC Med Genet 2005; 6:30.

110. Liberman MC, Gao J, He DZ, et al. Prestin is required for electromotility of the outer hair cell and for the cochlear amplifier. Nature 2002; 419:300–304.

111. Robertson NG, Khetarpal U, Gutierrez-Espeleta GA, et al. Isolation of novel and known genes from a human fetal cochlear cDNA library using subtractive hybridization and differential screening. Genomics 1994; 23:42–50.

112. Ikezono T, Omori A, Ichinose S, et al. Identification of the protein product of the Coch gene (hereditary deafness gene) as the major component of bovine inner ear protein. Biochim Biophys Acta 2001; 1535:258–265.

113. Robertson NG, Resendes BL, Lin JS, et al. Inner ear localization of mRNA and protein products of COCH, mutated in the sensorineural deafness and vestibular disorder, DFNA9. Hum Mol Genet 2001; 10:2493–2500.

114. Fransen E, Verstreken M, Bom SJ, et al. A common ancestor for COCH related cochleovestibular (DFNA9) patients in Belgium and The Netherlands bearing the P51S mutation. J Med Genet 2001; 38:61–65.

115. McGuirt WT, Prasad SD, Griffith AJ, et al. Mutations in COL11A2 cause non-syndromic hearing loss (DFNA13). Nat Genet 1999; 23:413–419.

116. van Steensel MA, Buma P, de Waal Malefijt MC, et al. Oto-spondylo-megaepiphyseal dysplasia (OSMED): clinical description of three patients homozygous for a missense mutation in the COL11A2 gene. Am J Med Genet 1997; 70:315–323.

117. Jovine L, Park J, Wassarman PM. Sequence similarity between stereocilin and otoancorin points to a unified mechanism for mechanotransduction in the mammalian inner ear. BMC Cell Biol 2002; 3:28.

118. Verpy E, Masmoudi S, Zwaenepoel I, et al. Mutations in a new gene encoding a protein of the hair bundle cause non-syndromic deafness at the DFNB16 locus. Nat Genet 2001; 29:345–349.

119. Zwaenepoel I, Mustapha M, Leibovici M, et al. Otoancorin, an inner ear protein restricted to the interface between the apical surface of sensory epithelia and their overlying acellular gels, is defective in autosomal recessive deafness DFNB22. Proc Natl Acad Sci USA 2002; 99:6240–6245.

120. Verhoeven K, Van Laer L, Kirschhofer K, et al. Mutations in the human alpha-tectorin gene cause autosomal dominant non-syndromic hearing impairment. Nat Genet 1998; 19:60–62.

121. Mustapha M, Weil D, Chardenoux S, et al. An alpha-tectorin gene defect causes a newly identified autosomal recessive form of sensorineural pre-lingual non-syndromic deafness, DFNB21. Hum Mol Genet 1999; 8:409–412.

122. Legan PK, Lukashkina VA, Goodyear RJ, et al. A targeted deletion in alpha-tectorin reveals that the tectorial membrane is required for the gain and timing of cochlear feedback. Neuron 2000; 28:273–285.

123. Wayne S, Robertson NG, DeClau F, et al. Mutations in the transcriptional activator EYA4 cause late-onset deafness at the DFNA10 locus. Hum Mol Genet 2001; 10:195–200.

124. Abdelhak S, Kalatzis V, Heilig R, et al. Clustering of mutations responsible for branchio-oto-renal (BOR) syndrome in the eyes absent homologous region (eyaHR) of EYA1. Hum Mol Genet 1997; 6:2247–2255.

125. Wegner M, Drolet DW, Rosenfeld MG. POU-domain proteins: structure and function of developmental regulators. Curr Opin Cell Biol 1993; 5:488–498.

126. de Kok YJ, van der Maarel SM, Bitner-Glindzicz M, et al. Association between X-linked mixed deafness and mutations in the POU domain gene POU3F4. Science 1995; 267:685–688.

127. Vahava O, Morell R, Lynch ED, et al. Mutation in transcription factor POU4F3 associated with inherited progressive hearing loss in humans. Science 1998; 279:1950–1954.

128. Minowa O, Ikeda K, Sugitani Y, et al. Altered cochlear fibrocytes in a mouse model of DFN3 nonsyndromic deafness. Science 1999; 285:1408–1411.

129. Phippard D, Heydemann A, Lechner M, et al. Changes in the subcellular localization of the Brn4 gene product precede mesenchymal remodeling of the otic capsule. Hear Res 1998; 120:77–85.

130. Phippard D, Lu L, Lee D, et al. Targeted mutagenesis of the POU-domain gene Brn4/Pou3f4 causes developmental defects in the inner ear. J Neurosci 1999; 19:5980–5989.

131. Hertzano R, Montcouquiol M, Rashi-Elkeles S, et al. Transcription profiling of inner ears from Pou4f3(ddl/ddl) identifies Gfi1 as a target of the Pou4f3 deafness gene. Hum Mol Genet 2004; 13:2143–2153.

132. Peters LM, Anderson DW, Griffith AJ, et al. Mutation of a transcription factor, TFCP2L3, causes progressive autosomal dominant hearing loss, DFNA28. Hum Mol Genet 2002; 11:2877–2885.

133. van Camp G, Coucke P, Balemans W, et al. Localization of a gene for non-syndromic hearing loss (DFNA5) to chromosome 7p15. Hum Mol Genet 1995; 4:2159–2163.

134. Van Laer L, Huizing EH, Verstreken M, et al. Nonsyndromic hearing impairment is associated with a mutation in DFNA5. Nat Genet 1998; 20:194–197.

135. Yu C, Meng X, Zhang S, et al. A 3-nucleotide deletion in the polypyrimidine tract of intron 7 of the DFNA5 gene causes nonsyndromic hearing impairment in a Chinese family. Genomics 2003; 82:575–579.

136. Bischoff AM, Luijendijk MW, Huygen PL, et al. A novel mutation identified in the DFNA5 gene in a Dutch family: a clinical and genetic evaluation. Audiol Neurootol 2004; 9:34–46.

137. Van Laer L, Vrijens K, Thys S, et al. DFNA5: hearing impairment exon instead of hearing impairment gene? J Med Genet 2004; 41:401–406.

138. Busch-Nentwich E, Sollner C, Roehl H, et al. The deafness gene dfna5 is crucial for ugdh expression and HA production in the developing ear in zebrafish. Development 2004; 131:943–951.

139. Anniko M, Arnold W. Hyaluronic acid as a molecular filter and friction-reducing lubricant in the human inner ear. ORL J Otorhinolaryngol Relat Spec 1995; 57:82–86.

140. Yasunaga S, Grati M, Cohen-Salmon M, et al. A mutation in OTOF, encoding otoferlin, a FER-1-like protein, causes DFNB9, a nonsyndromic form of deafness. Nat Genet 1999; 21:363–369.

141. Houseman MJ, Jackson AP, Al-Gazali LI, et al. A novel mutation in a family with non-syndromic sensorineural hearing loss that disrupts the newly characterised OTOF long isoforms. J Med Genet 2001; 38:E25.

142. Migliosi V, Modamio-Hoybjor S, Moreno-Pelayo MA, et al. Q829X, a novel mutation in the gene encoding otoferlin (OTOF), is frequently found in Spanish patients with prelingual non-syndromic hearing loss. J Med Genet 2002; 39:502–506.

143. Rodriguez-Ballesteros M, del Castillo FJ, Martin Y, et al. Auditory neuropathy in patients carrying mutations in the otoferlin gene (OTOF). Hum Mutat 2003; 22:451–456.

144. Kim TB, Isaacson B, Sivakumaran TA, et al. A gene responsible for autosomal dominant auditory neuropathy (AUNA1) maps to 13q14–21. J Med Genet 2004; 41:872–876.

145. Scott DA, Carmi R, Elbedour K, et al. An autosomal recessive nonsyndromic-hearing-loss locus identified by DNA pooling using two inbred Bedouin kindreds. Am J Hum Genet 1996; 59:385–391.

146. Kurima K, Peters LM, Yang Y, et al. Dominant and recessive deafness caused by mutations of a novel gene, TMC1, required for cochlear hair-cell function. Nat Genet 2002; 30:277–284.

147. Vreugde S, Erven A, Kros CJ, et al. Beethoven, a mouse model for dominant, progressive hearing loss DFNA36. Nat Genet 2002; 30:257–258.

148. Mitchem KL, Hibbard E, Beyer LA, et al. Mutation of the novel gene Tmie results in sensory cell defects in the inner ear of spinner, a mouse model of human hearing loss DFNB6. Hum Mol Genet 2002; 11:1887–1898.

149. Scott HS, Kudoh J, Wattenhofer M, et al. Insertion of beta-satellite repeats identifies a transmembrane protease causing both congenital and childhood onset autosomal recessive deafness. Nat Genet 2001; 27:59–63.

150. Guipponi M, Vuagniaux G, Wattenhofer M, et al. The transmembrane serine protease (TMPRSS3) mutated in deafness DFNB8/10 activates the epithelial sodium channel (ENaC) in vitro. Hum Mol Genet 2002; 11:2829–2836.

151. Lee YJ, Park D, Kim SY, et al. Pathogenic mutations but not polymorphisms in congenital and childhood onset autosomal recessive deafness disrupt the proteolytic activity of TMPRSS3. J Med Genet 2003; 40:629–631.

152. Cryns K, Thys S, Van Laer L, et al. The WFS1 gene, responsible for low frequency sensorineural hearing loss and Wolfram syndrome, is expressed in a variety of inner ear cells. Histochem Cell Biol 2003; 119:247–256.

153. Young TL, Ives E, Lynch E, et al. Non-syndromic progressive hearing loss DFNA38 is caused by heterozygous missense mutation in the Wolfram syndrome gene WFS1. Hum Mol Genet 2001; 10:2509–2514.

154. Strom TM, Hortnagel K, Hofmann S, et al. Diabetes insipidus, diabetes mellitus, optic atrophy and deafness (DIDMOAD) caused by mutations in a novel gene (wolframin) coding for a predicted transmembrane protein. Hum Mol Genet 1998; 7:2021–2028.

155. Wolfram DJ, Wagener HP. Diabetes mellitus and simple optic atrophy among siblings: report of four cases. Mayo Clin Proc 1938; 13:715–718.

156. Cryns K, Sivakumaran TA, Van den Ouweland JM, et al. Mutational spectrum of the WFS1 gene in Wolfram syndrome, nonsyndromic hearing impairment, diabetes mellitus, and psychiatric disease. Hum Mutat 2003; 22:275–287.

157. Ishihara H, Takeda S, Tamura A, et al. Disruption of the WFS1 gene in mice causes progressive beta-cell loss and impaired stimulus-secretion coupling in insulin secretion. Hum Mol Genet 2004; 13:1159–1170.

158. Fischel-Ghodsian N. Mitochondrial deafness mutations reviewed. Hum Mutat 1999; 13:261–270.

159. Prezant TR, Agapian JV, Bohlman MC, et al. Mitochondrial ribosomal RNA mutation associated with both antibiotic-induced and non-syndromic deafness. Nat Genet 1993; 4:289–294.

160. Estivill X, Govea N, Barcelo E, et al. Familial progressive sensorineural deafness is mainly due to the mtDNA A1555G mutation and is enhanced by treatment of aminoglycosides. Am J Hum Genet 1998; 62:27–35.

161. Usami S, Abe S, Kasai M, et al. Genetic and clinical features of sensorineural hearing loss associated with the 1555 mitochondrial mutation. Laryngoscope 1997; 107:483–490.

162. Zhao H, Li R, Wang Q, et al. Maternally inherited aminoglycoside-induced and nonsyndromic deafness is associated with the novel C1494T mutation in the mitochondrial 12S rRNA gene in a large Chinese family. Am J Hum Genet 2004; 74:139–152.

163. Bacino C, Prezant TR, Bu X, et al. Susceptibility mutations in the mitochondrial small ribosomal RNA gene in aminoglycoside induced deafness. Pharmacogenetics 1995; 5:165–172.

164. Casano RA, Johnson DF, Bykhovskaya Y, et al. Inherited susceptibility to aminoglycoside ototoxicity: genetic heterogeneity and clinical implications. Am J Otolaryngol 1999; 20:151–156.

165. Fischel-Ghodsian N, Prezant TR, Fournier P, et al. Mitochondrial mutation associated with nonsyndromic deafness. Am J Otolaryngol 1995; 16:403–408.

166. Reid FM, Vernham GA, Jacobs HT. A novel mitochondrial point mutation in a maternal pedigree with sensorineural deafness. Hum Mutat 1994; 3:243–247.

167. Sevior KB, Hatamochi A, Stewart IA, et al. Mitochondrial A7445G mutation in two pedigrees with palmoplantar keratoderma and deafness. Am J Med Genet 1998; 75:179–185.

168. Jaksch M, Klopstock T, Kurlemann G, et al. Progressive myoclonus epilepsy and mitochondrial myopathy associated with mutations in the tRNA(Ser(UCN)) gene. Ann Neurol 1998; 44:635–640.

169. Schuelke M, Bakker M, Stoltenburg G, et al. Epilepsia partialis continua associated with a homoplasmic mitochondrial tRNA(Ser(UCN)) mutation. Ann Neurol 1998; 44:700–704.

170. Tiranti V, Chariot P, Carella F, et al. Maternally inherited hearing loss, ataxia and myoclonus associated with a novel point mutation in mitochondrial tRNASer(UCN) gene. Hum Mol Genet 1995; 4:1421–1427.

171. Verhoeven K, Ensink RJ, Tiranti V, et al. Hearing impairment and neurological dysfunction associated with a mutation in the mitochondrial tRNASer(UCN) gene. Eur J Hum Genet 1999; 7:45–51.

172. Hutchin T. Sensorineural hearing loss and the 1555G mitochondrial DNA mutation. Acta Otolaryngol 1999; 119:48–52.

173. Gluckman E, Broxmeyer HA, Auerbach AD, et al. Hematopoietic reconstitution in a patient with Fanconi's anemia by means of umbilical-cord blood from an HLA-identical sibling. N Engl J Med 1989; 321:1174–1178.

174. Sue CM, Tanji K, Hadjigeorgiou G, et al. Maternally inherited hearing loss in a large kindred with a novel T7511C mutation in the mitochondrial DNA tRNA(Ser(UCN)) gene. Neurology 1999; 52:1905–1908.

175. Matthijs G, Claes S, Longo-Mbenza B, et al. Non-syndromic deafness associated with a mutation and a polymorphism in the mitochondrial 12S ribosomal RNA gene in a large Zairean pedigree. Eur J Hum Genet 1996; 4:46–51.

176. Pandya A, Xia X, Radnaabazar J, et al. Mutation in the mitochondrial 12S rRNA gene in two families from Mongolia with matrilineal aminoglycoside ototoxicity. J Med Genet 1997; 34:169–172.

177. Gardner JC, Goliath R, Viljoen D, et al. Familial streptomycin ototoxicity in a South African family: a mitochondrial disorder. J Med Genet 1997; 34:904–906.

178. el-Schahawi M, Lopez de Munain A, Sarrazin AM, et al. Two large Spanish pedigrees with nonsyndromic sensorineural deafness and the mtDNA mutation at nt 1555 in the 12s rRNA gene: evidence of heteroplasmy. Neurology 1997; 48:453–456.

179. Hamasaki K, Rando RR. Specific binding of aminoglycosides to a human rRNA construct based on a DNA polymorphism which causes aminoglycoside-induced deafness. Biochemistry 1997; 36:12323–12328.

180. Guan MX, Fischel-Ghodsian N, Attardi G. A biochemical basis for the inherited susceptibility to aminoglycoside ototoxicity. Hum Mol Genet 2000; 9:1787–1793.

181. Bykhovskaya Y, Mengesha E, Wang D, et al. Human mitochondrial transcription factor B1 as a modifier gene for hearing loss associated with the mitochondrial A1555G mutation. Mol Genet Metab 2004; 82:27–32.

182. Seidel-Rogol BL, McCulloch V, Shadel GS. Human mitochondrial transcription factor B1 methylates ribosomal RNA at a conserved stem-loop. Nat Genet 2003; 33:23–24.

183. Riazuddin S, Castelein CM, Ahmed ZM, et al. Dominant modifier DFNM1 suppresses recessive deafness DFNB26. Nat Genet 2000; 26:431–434.

184. Street VA, McKee-Johnson JW, Fonseca RC, et al. Mutations in a plasma membrane Ca2+ -ATPase gene cause deafness in deafwaddler mice. Nat Genet 1998; 19:390–394.

185. Zheng QY, Johnson KR, Erway LC. Assessment of hearing in 80 inbred strains of mice by ABR threshold analyses. Hear Res 1999; 130:94–107.

186. Nemoto M, Morita Y, Mishima Y, et al. Ahl3, a third locus on mouse chromosome 17 affecting age-related hearing loss. Biochem Biophys Res Commun 2004; 324:1283–1288.

6 Age-related hearing impairment: ensemble playing of environmental and genetic factors

Lut Van Laer, Guy Van Camp

Introduction

The next 50 years will witness a significant increase in ageing in the European Union, the United States, and Japan, with the number of people aged 65 and above growing significantly. The most common sensory impairment among the elderly is age-related hearing impairment (ARHI), also called presbyacusis. In its most typical presentation, ARHI is mid to late adult-onset, progressive, bilaterally symmetrical, sensorineural, and most pronounced in the high frequencies, leading to a moderately sloping pure tone audiogram. Thirty-seven percent of people aged between 61 and 70 have a significant hearing loss of at least 25 dB (1). This prevalence increases further at older ages. Sixty percent of 71- to 80-year-olds are affected by ARHI (1). Considering the ageing of the population in large parts of the Northern hemisphere, the number of people affected by ARHI will steadily increase in the future.

ARHI patients often experience difficulty adjusting to their sensory loss. In addition, hearing loss may have a major influence on their quality of life and their feeling of well-being. Hearing impairment has a deleterious impact on social life; reduced communication skills frequently result in poor psychosocial functioning and consequently in isolation of the ageing individual. In addition, ARHI grossly limits independence and may contribute to depression, anxiety, lethargy, and possibly cognitive decline (2).

Currently, hearing aids are the only possibility for therapeutic intervention in ARHI. Unfortunately, these are only suitable for a limited number of people. Although hearing aids succeed in sufficient amplification of sound, the gain in speech recognition is often experienced as poor, especially in noisy environments. In addition, many do not accept hearing aids because of social stigmatisation. Future therapies for hearing impairment will have to rely on basic rather than on symptomatic approaches. This requires a thorough knowledge of the aetiological factors leading to ARHI. Up to now, little research has been performed on ARHI. This is, at least partly, due to the misconception that hearing impairment is an inevitable burden of ageing, rather than a potentially preventable or even curable disease. This chapter will give an overview of the current status of knowledge on ARHI and will outline future research aiming at the identification of the genetic risk factors involved in ARHI.

Epidemiology

ARHI is the most frequent sensory disability of the elderly. Between the ages of 61 and 70, the prevalence of clinically significant hearing loss (25 dB and over) for the general British population was approximately 37%, increasing to 60% between the ages of 71 and 80 (pure tone thresholds averaged for 0.5, 1,

2, and 4 kHz in the better ear) (1). These figures are comparable with those obtained in a U.S. population-based cross-sectional study—the Beaver Dam Epidemiology of Hearing Loss Study in Wisconsin. The latter study revealed prevalence figures of 44% for the age range 60 to 69 years and 66% for the 70 to 79 age range (pure tone thresholds averaged for 0.5, 1, 2, and 4 kHz in the worse ear) (3). The same population was investigated five years later. Twenty-one percent of subjects with normal hearing abilities during the first investigation showed a significant hearing loss in the follow-up examination, indicating that older adults (between 48 and 92 years) have a high risk of developing ARHI (4).

The prevalence of ARHI is gender related, in general, men being more severely affected (1,3). Using data from the extended Baltimore Longitudinal Study of Ageing, it was concluded that hearing thresholds increase more than twice as fast in men as in women for all ages and frequencies, that the age of onset is later in women than in men, and that men hear better than women at lower frequencies, while women hear better than men at frequencies above 1000 Hz (5). Interestingly, gender-related differences were also detected in mouse models for age-related hearing loss (AHL). In CBA mice, a model for late-onset AHL, distortion product otoacoustic emissions (DPOAEs) decreased in middle-aged and old males, while in females, the decline in outer hair cell (OHC) function was only initiated at older, postmenopausal ages (6). Another study confirmed the younger age of onset for male hearing loss in CBA mice, while in a model for early-onset hearing loss (C57BL/6J), it was found that females tend to lose their hearing capabilities earlier than males (7).

On average, ARHI thresholds increase approximately 1 dB per year for individuals aged 60 and over (8). However, ARHI shows extensive variation; the age at onset, the progression, and the severity of the hearing loss vary considerably among the elderly. The International Organisation for Standardisation (ISO) 7029 standard perfectly illustrates this variation (9). These norms were recorded by the ISO in 1984 and represent the median thresholds for otologically normal persons and the spread around this median, for each age and each frequency, both in men and in women (9). The largest spread is found at high frequencies and at older ages. For instance, at 60 years of age, the best hearing 10% of the population display high frequency thresholds better than 10 dB, while the worst hearing 10% suffer from a hearing loss of 55 to 75 dB at the high frequencies (9). This significant variation was seen as an indication of the involvement of hereditary factors in the development of ARHI.

Age-related pathological changes in the inner ear

Based on correlations between audiometric data and histological findings, Schuknecht proposed a classification scheme of human ARHI (10). Schuknecht's framework involves three cochlear components: the afferent neurons, the organ of Corti, and the stria vascularis, which can all degenerate independently. In "sensory" ARHI, the primary degeneration involves the organ of Corti, while in "strial" ARHI and in "neural" ARHI, the stria vascularis and the spiral ganglion, respectively, are the major affected structures (10,11). According to Schuknecht, audiometric or speech discrimination data may reflect degeneration of only one of the three structures. A fourth hypothetical category, "cochlear-conductive" ARHI, comprises a gradually decreasing, linear audiometric pattern without pathological correlate. Schuknecht speculated that this type of hearing loss is caused by alterations in the physical characteristics of the cochlear duct (10,11). The most common type is sensory ARHI with predominantly high-frequency hearing loss. Less common is the "metabolic" or strial type of ARHI, which is characterised by an audiogram that is flat across the low frequencies with variable degrees of high-frequency hearing loss. A combination of pathologies affecting many cell types ("mixed" ARHI) is often found. In addition, 25% of all cases cannot be classified according to Schuknecht's scheme. These cases are designated as "indeterminate" ARHI (10,11).

In humans, preferential loss of OHCs was observed, most prominent in the first half of the basal turn (12,13). This correlates tonotopically with the high-frequency hearing loss present in sensory ARHI. In another study, human temporal bones of seven individuals with sensory ARHI were investigated. Approximately 80% of the OHCs, mainly in the apical parts of the cochlea, were lost. Apart from the expected reduction in hair cells, the most significant change in the cochlea was an age-related loss of nerve fibres. The latter had most probably occurred secondary to the hair cell loss (14). Using electron microscopy, further ultrastructural changes were detected in these specimens, including changes in the cuticular plate, the stereocilia, the pillar cells, the stria vascularis, and the spiral ligament (15). Finally, in a study on human temporal bones selected for their typical strial type of audiometry (i.e., flat), only one out of six had significant atrophy of the stria vascularis. The most prominent changes in these specimens were OHC loss in combination with inner hair cell (IHC) or spiral ganglion cell (SGC) loss (16). Pathologic changes in the inner ear as a direct function of age remain, therefore, controversial (17).

Correlations between audiometric data and inner ear pathology are difficult to obtain in humans. Mouse ARHI models can help to validate the classification scheme proposed by Schuknecht and clarify the underlying cellular changes. Table 6.1 gives an overview of some recent findings in the inner ear of C57BL/6J inbred mice, the early-onset model for AHL.

The most prominent changes in this mouse model were OHC and SGC loss in addition to atrophy of the stria vascularis, leading to a mixed type of AHL. Only a few data exist for other inbred strains. In contrast to the early start of hair cell loss in C57BL/6J mice (one to two months of age), mice of the CBA/Ca strain, the model for late-onset AHL, show relatively little hair cell loss until late in life (18). In the senescence-accelerated mouse (SAMP1), loss of IHCs and OHCs and atrophy of the stria vascularis were demonstrated. Areas of degeneration were concentrated in the apex and the base (25). In CD-1 mice, the changes were similar to those observed in C57BL/6J mice (26). In BALB/cJ mice, AHL seemed to be best correlated with changes in the supporting cells of the basal half of the cochlea and with alterations in the spiral limbus in the apical part of the cochlea (27). Finally, in the 129S6/sV strain, high-frequency hearing loss seemed to correlate with basal loss of OHCs and type IV fibrocytes of the spiral ligament and with alterations in the supporting cells at the cochlear base (28). In addition, apical neuronal loss was accompanied by abnormalities in pillar cells and the Reissner's membrane and loss of fibrocytes in the spiral limbus at the apical cochlear turn (28). Other animals that have been studied include the monkey, rat, rabbit, gerbil, dog, and guinea pig. For instance, in house dog cochleas, loss of SGCs, atrophy of the organ of Corti and the stria vascularis, and thickening of the basilar membrane were observed. The changes were most prominent at the base of the cochlea. The advantage of studying house dogs instead of laboratory animals is that they have been kept in a similar environment as humans (29).

Central auditory dysfunction—auditory neuropathy

In the ageing population, speech discrimination scores often decrease without a parallel loss in pure tone thresholds (30–32). This indicates that in addition to peripheral pathology,

degenerative changes in the central auditory pathway are involved in the development of ARHI. In the Framingham cohort, a relation between auditory and cognitive dysfunction was observed. Moreover, aberrant test results for central auditory function could predict the onset of senile dementia (33). In the C57BL/6J mouse model, a disruption of the central representation of frequency (i.e., the tonotopic organisation) was observed (34). In addition, it was shown that many normally responding neurons survive alongside slowly responding neurons in older mice, indicating that wastage of individual neurons and not a general decline seems to accompany the ageing process (34). Finally, an increase in the spontaneous activity of inferior colliculus neurons in older animals might suggest a change in the physiological signal-to-noise ratio, contributing to presbyacusis as well as tinnitus (34). More recently, additional studies gathered different types of evidence of the role of the central auditory pathway in presbyacusis. The contralateral suppression of DPOAEs was tested in humans and in CBA mice. Contralateral suppression is the phenomenon that white noise stimulation of one ear typically reduces the magnitude of the DPOAEs measured in the opposite ear. This contralateral suppression is due to activation of the medial olivocochlear system, which, in turn, inhibits the cochlear OHCs. Both DPOAE levels and contralateral inhibition decreased with age in humans as well as in mice. Moreover, the decline in contralateral inhibition preceded the decline in DPOAE levels, indicating that a functional decline of the medial olivocochlear system with age precedes OHC degeneration (35,36).

Table 6.1 Age-related changes in the inner ear of the C57BL/6J mouse model for early-onset age-related hearing loss

Cell type or structure	Age-related effect	References
OHC	Preferential loss of OHCs	18, 19
	Base-to-apex gradient of OHC loss	18, 19–22
	Regionalised patterns of OHC loss correlated with changes in hearing thresholds	21
IHC	Less affected than OHCs	19, 20
SGC	Loss of SGCs; retrograde degeneration	20, 22, 23
Stria vascularis	Atrophy	23
Organ of Corti	Disorganisation	23
Spiral ligament	Degeneration of type IV fibrocytes	22
	Reduced density of Cx26 staining	23
	Na-K-ATPase immunolabelling increased	23
Spiral limbus	Changes in the apical part of the cochlea	24
Pillar cells	Apical-to-basal progression of pathology	24
Reissner's membrane	Apical-to-basal progression of pathology	24

Abbreviations: IHC, inner hair cell; OHC, outer hair cell; SGC, spiral ganglion cell.

Heritability of ARHI

Heritability in human subjects

The spectrum of human diseases forms a continuum between purely genetic and purely environmental conditions. Nearly all frequent diseases that are important for public health such as diabetes, heart disease, and cancer are complex in aetiology, involving the interaction of several genes and environmental factors. The relative importance of the genetic and the environmental factors in the aetiology of the disease is often expressed as the heritability of a disease. The hypothesis that ARHI has a genetic basis has been put forward for many years in many publications, but the scientific basis for this claim has only recently been laid. Three separate studies have estimated heritability values for ARHI and have shown that ARHI is a complex disorder with genetic as well as environmental aetiological factors.

In a first study, a Swedish male twin population, comprising 250 monozygotic and 307 dizygotic twins aged between 36 and 80 years, was studied using a combination of audiometric and questionnaire data (37). This study clearly indicated that the variation in hearing ability in the high frequencies is due to an interaction of genetic and environmental effects. Moreover, the relative influence of the environment becomes more important with increasing age. The heritability estimate for the age group above 65 years was 0.47, indicating that approximately half of the population variance for high-frequency hearing ability above the age of 65 is caused by genetic differences, and half by environmental differences (37).

A second study analysed audiometric data from families who participated in the Framingham Heart and the Framingham Offspring Study. The auditory status in genetically unrelated (spouse pairs) and genetically related people (sibling pairs, parent-child pairs) was compared. This study showed a clear familial aggregation for age-related hearing levels, although the aggregation levels were stronger in women than in men. The heritability estimates of this study suggested that 35% to 55% of the variance of the sensory type of ARHI and 25% to 42% of the variance of the strial type of ARHI is attributable to the effects of genes (38).

More recently, a Danish twin study evaluated the self-reported reduced hearing abilities in 3928 twins of 75 years of age and older. Calculations of concordance rates, odds ratios, and correlations resulted in consistently higher values for monozygotic twin pairs when compared to dizygotic twin pairs across all age and sex categories. This indicates the involvement of genetic risk factors. The heritability value was estimated at 40% in this study (39). Because self-assessment of hearing loss only partly corresponds to audiometric measures of hearing loss and frequently results in misclassification (30), this heritability value may represent an underestimate of the involvement of genetic factors in ARHI. Although it has been proven in three separate studies that ARHI is a complex disease caused by an interaction of environmental and genetic factors,

so far nothing is known about the genes that contribute to ARHI in humans.

Heritability in mouse models for AHL

Evidence for a substantial genetic basis for ARHI was not only gathered from studies on human subjects. An important contribution involves research performed in inbred mouse strains with AHL. These mouse strains may represent valuable models and may be used for the investigation of genetic factors in human ARHI.

Through the study of hearing loss in 5 inbred strains and the 10 possible combinations of F1 hybrids, Erway et al. found evidence that supports a genetic model for recessive alleles contributing to AHL at three different loci (40). A first major, recessive gene affecting AHL in C57BL/6J mice (designated Ahl) was localised to chromosome 10, near D10Mit5, using a C57BL/6J × CAST/Ei backcross (41). Ahl was associated with degeneration of the organ of Corti, the stria vascularis, and the spiral ligament and with loss of SGCs, suggesting that it promotes a "mixed" type of AHL (mixed sensory/neural/strial type, according to Schuknecht's typology). In subsequent studies, the Ahl gene was shown to be a major contributor to the hearing loss present in nine other inbred mouse strains—129P1/ReJ, A/J, BALB/cByJ, BUB/BnJ, C57BR/cdJ, DBA/2J, NOD/LtJ, SKH2/J, and STOCK760 (42)—and to be allelic with the modifier of deaf waddler gene (mdfw) (43). The gene responsible was identified in 2003; in exon 7 of cadherin 23 (Cdh23), a hypomorphic single-nucleotide polymorphism (753A), leading to in-frame skipping of exon 7, showed significant association with Ahl and mdfw (44). The AHL of inbred strains homozygous for this polymorphism may be due to altered adhesion properties or reduced stability of the CDH23 protein lacking exon 7 (44). Using a congenic strain with genomic DNA derived completely from C57BL/6J, except in the Ahl-chromosome 10 region, where the genomic material was derived from CAST/Ei (B6.CAST-+Ahl), it has recently been shown that additional loci, besides the Ahl locus, may contribute to the differences in hearing loss between C57BL/6J × CAST/Ei mice (45).

A second locus affecting AHL (Ahl2) was mapped to chromosome 5 using a C57BL/6J × NOD/LtJ backcross. Johnson and Zheng demonstrated that the hearing loss attributable to Ahl2 is dependent on a predisposing Ahl genotype (46). Using a C57BL/6J × MSM backcross, a third locus (Ahl3) was positioned on chromosome 17 (47).

Nongenetic risk factors for ARHI

As illustrated above, ARHI is a complex disease caused by a combination of environmental and genetic factors. ARHI excludes hearing loss caused by factors such as exposure to excessive noise, intrinsic otological disease (including otosclerosis, chronic otitis media, Ménière's disease), and some underlying medical conditions. ARHI might, however, reflect the cumulative effects of disease, ototoxic agents, and other environmental (including noise) and dietary factors that act together with hereditary factors to influence the cochlear ageing process.

Environmental risk factors

Several environmental risk factors have been put forward as being involved in the development of ARHI (noise, drugs, organic solvents, etc.). However, considerable controversy exists concerning the role of many of the risk factors. The best known and the most studied risk factor for hearing loss is noise exposure. In general, ageing and noise exposure lead to similar physiological and anatomical changes (27). Although exposure to excessive occupational noise should be excluded as a causative factor, constant low-level noise (the noise of every day life in our industrialised and urbanised environment, also called "acoustic smog") is regarded as an environmental risk factor for ARHI. This is best illustrated by the absence of ARHI in some isolated African tribes in the Kalahari Desert and the Sudan, who live in relatively noise-free environments (48,49). Also, noise exposure due to leisure activities (rock, classical or jazz music, personal listening devices, e.g., walkmans, and "household" noise) should be taken into consideration, although the most serious assault on hearing capabilities results from recreational hunting or target shooting (50). From experiments in a mouse strain carrying the *Ahl* gene (C57BL/6J, see above), it became clear that a genetic predisposition to ARHI might be revealed sooner in life due to noise exposure. In other words, genes that are associated with ARHI might render the cochlea more susceptible to noise (51,52). It has been a point of debate whether ageing and noise act in an additive or in an interactive way to produce permanent hearing loss. If the latter is more important, the question remains whether they amplify each other or tone each other down (53). The assumption of an additive effect has been most widely accepted. However, recently an interesting interaction between ageing and noise has been proposed (54). Using data from the Framingham cohort, it was shown that noise-induced hearing loss reduces the effects of ageing at noise-associated frequencies but accelerates the deterioration of hearing at adjacent frequencies. The rate of ARHI seems to differ in noise-damaged ears when compared to non–noise-damaged ears (54). In general, there is agreement on the fact that age-related changes exceed noise-induced changes for the 0.5, 1, 2, and 3 KHz pure-tone average (55).

Besides noise, several other environmental factors have been implicated in the aetiology of ARHI, an overview of which is given in Table 6.2.

Ototoxic medication as a risk factor for hearing loss is well documented. Especially in the elderly, ototoxic medication can become problematic because they usually take more medication and for longer periods compared to other age groups, and because they have altered liver and renal functions, which can cause blood levels of drugs to rise above certain critical levels (56–59). The detrimental effects of some chemicals on hearing

levels are indisputable (60,61). The effect of tobacco smoking and of alcohol (ab)use on hearing loss remains controversial (57,62–67). Hearing loss due to head trauma could possibly be caused by disruption of the membranous portion of the cochlea, by disturbance in the cochlear microcirculation, or by haemorrhage into the fluids of the cochlea (68). The nutritional status also seems to have importance (69), while caloric-restriction does not seem to have much effect (70). Finally, even socioeconomic status has been implicated as a contributory factor. Interestingly, this effect remained even when noise exposure was taken into account (71). Clearly, it will be very difficult to assess what the contribution of all separate factors will be on the final outcome, i.e., the level of hearing loss.

Medical risk factors

Several medical conditions have been postulated as risk factors for ARHI. A possible relation between ARHI and cardiovascular disease (coronary heart disease, stroke, and intermittent claudication) and cardiovascular disease risk factors (including hypertension, diabetes, smoking, weight, and serum lipid levels) was investigated in the Framingham cohort (65). Cardiovascular disease was associated with ARHI, although predominantly in the low-frequency range and in women. Of the cardiovascular disease risk factors, hypertension and systolic blood pressure were related to hearing thresholds both in men and in women, while high-density lipoprotein and blood glucose levels were associated with low-frequency pure-tone averages only in women (65). Brant et al. later confirmed the relationship between ARHI and systolic blood pressure for speech frequencies (66), while Lee et al. could confirm the effect of high-density lipoproteins on ARHI in women (72). Classically, low-frequency ARHI has been associated with microvascular disease, leading to atrophy of the stria vascularis. Another indication that vascular abnormalities might be important in the development of ARHI has recently been obtained in an animal model for ARHI (C57BL/6J mice), where a significantly reduced expression of cochlear vascular endothelial growth factor (VEGF) was observed as a function of age (73).

Patients who suffer from chronic renal failure and undergo dialysis are also at risk of developing high-frequency hearing loss. Either the disease itself (due to uraemic neuropathy, electrolyte imbalance, premature cardiovascular disease, shared antigenicity between cochlea and kidney) or the treatment (chronic dialysis most often followed by kidney transplantation and an accompanied use of ototoxic medication) might be responsible for the increased risk in renal patients (74). Demineralisation of the cochlear capsule in conjunction with age-related bone mass loss may lead to ARHI. This was reported by Clark et al., who could demonstrate that the femoral neck bone mass, but not the radial bone mass, was associated with ARHI in a population of rural women aged 60 to 85 years (75). Another study could not demonstrate a relation between hip-bone mineral density and hearing abilities (76). Several investigators have observed an association between diabetes mellitus

Table 6.2 Environmental risk factors for ARHI

Factor	Effect[a]	References
Ototoxic medication	Salicylate	56, 57
	β-adrenergic drugs	58
	Aminoglycosides	59
	Loop diuretics	59
Chemicals	Organic solvents	60, 61
	Heavy metals	60
Smoking	Causing hearing loss	57, 62–64
	Having no effect	65, 66
	Passive smoking: causing hearing loss	63
Alcohol	Abuse causing hearing loss	57, 67
	Abuse having no effect	62
	Moderate use: protective effect	62, 67
Head trauma	Whiplash	68
Nutrition status	Low vitamin B-12	69
	Low folate	69
Caloric-restricted diet	No, or a very small, protective effect	70
Socioeconomic	Low social class	71
	Lower level of education	71

[a]Unless indicated otherwise the environmental factors listed here cause hearing loss.

and high-frequency hearing loss. This association might be explained either by microangiopathic lesions in the inner ear (cochlear loss) or by primary neuropathy of the acoustic nerve (retrocochlear loss) (77).

Finally, a role for the immune system in the development of ARHI has been suggested. When SAMP1 mice were bred in a specific pathogen-free environment, the age-related diseases typically observed in these mice (including AHL) were delayed in onset, when compared to mice bred in pathogenic environments. The involvement of autoimmune mechanisms was excluded (78). It was argued that the stress that a host experiences due to pathogen-induced infections impairs the immune functions, preceding a general decline in various physical functions (78).

Genetic risk factors for ARHI

In contrast to the huge quantity of information regarding environmental and medical risk factors involved in the development of ARHI, only a minimal amount of information regarding genetic risk factors can be found in existing literature. Most of the studies describe work on animal models. Up to the

present time, only few studies have attempted to identify ARHI genes in human, and none have been identified so far.

In the section on heritability in mouse models for AHL (see above), the localisation of three mouse AHL loci (*Ahl*) (41,46,47) and the identification of a first mouse AHL gene (*CDH23*) (44) were described. Another gene that has been implicated in the development of AHL in mice is *VEGF* (also described above), for which a significant reduction in expression was observed as a function of age (73). Recently, it has been shown that mice susceptible to AHL have a significant decrease in expression of the β2 subunit of the high-affinity nicotinic acetylcholine receptor (nAChR). In addition, in mice lacking the β2 nAChR subunit, a significant hearing loss and reduction in the number of SGCs has been observed, indicating a requirement for the β2 nAChR subunit in the maintenance of SGCs during ageing (79).

An important causative role for oxidative stress and consequently also for mitochondrial deletions has been postulated. Both aspects are further elaborated in the following paragraphs.

Oxidative stress

Reactive oxygen species (ROS) have been implicated in hearing loss associated with ageing and noise exposure. ROS are a normal by-product of cellular metabolism, in particular of the oxidative phosphorylation process. ROS are potentially toxic and can cause DNA, cellular and tissue damage if not inactivated by cellular antioxidant protection systems (glutathione and glutathione-related enzymes, superoxide dismutases and catalase). ROS can cause direct damage to mitochondrial DNA. Hypoperfusion leads to the formation of ROS. As a reduction in blood flow to several tissues, including the cochlea, has been associated with ageing, this might mean that hypoperfusion of the cochlea is an important causative factor of ROS formation and subsequent hearing loss (80).

Significantly decreased glutathione levels have been observed in the auditory nerve, but not in other cochlear parts, in 24-month-old rats (81). Cytosolic copper/zinc superoxide dismutase (SOD1) is highly expressed in the cochlea. SOD1-deficient mice displayed a more pronounced AHL than wild-type mice (82,83). However, SOD1 overexpression did not protect against AHL, indicating that the oxidative metabolism may be more complex than previously assumed (84). Antioxidants, which block and scavenge ROS, thereby reducing the deleterious impact of ROS at the molecular level, might attenuate ARHI. This has been demonstrated with oversupplementation of vitamins E and C (85), and with two mitochondrial metabolites (acetyl-1-carnitine and alpha-lipoic acid) (86). Animals treated with these nutritional supplements demonstrated an overall reduction in mitochondrial deletions, less OHC loss, and the best preservation of hearing abilities. Caloric restriction, which is also thought to reduce levels of oxidative stress, reduced the rate of AHL (85), although in previous studies in humans no, or only a very small, effect had been observed for caloric restriction (Table 6.2) (70). Supplementation with lecithin, a polyunsaturated phophatidylcholine that plays a role in SOD activation, also resulted in significant protection (80).

Mitochondrial deletions

Mitochondrial DNA has a high mutation rate. This might be due to the fact that mitochondrial DNA is in the close vicinity of the mitochondrial inner membrane, which is the major source of ROS. When sufficient mitochondrial DNA damage accumulates, the affected cell will become bioenergetically deficient. The most vulnerable cells are found in muscle and nerve tissue (including the cochlea) because these cells require high energy levels. In addition, cochlear cells are terminally differentiated; damaged cells will not be replaced. As a result, cochlear tissues are very sensitive to mitochondrial damage caused by oxidative stress.

Specific acquired mitochondrial mutations have been proposed as one of the causes of ARHI. They occur more frequently with increasing age and with the progression of ARHI. The so-called common ageing mitochondrial deletion involves 4977 bp in humans (87–89), 4834 bp in rats (87,90), and 3867 bp in mice (91). An accumulation of many different acquired mitochondrial mutations was detected in auditory tissues of at least a proportion of ARHI patients (92). Clinical expression of mitochondrial mutations is dependent both on environmental factors and on nuclear-encoded modifier genes (93).

How genes involved in ARHI can be identified

Up to now, no ARHI susceptibility genes have been identified in humans. Since it was clearly demonstrated that ARHI has an important genetic component (see the section on the Heritability of ARHI), the use of extended genetic association and linkage studies aiming at the identification of ARHI susceptibility genes seems justified. However, the late onset of the ARHI phenotype and the numerous confounding nongenetic factors complicate human genetic studies for ARHI.

How genes involved in complex diseases can be identified

The dissection of complex traits in humans has been particularly problematic. However, presently, many of the initial problems have been overcome by new technological developments (both statistical and laboratory methods). In general, two possible study designs can be used for the identification of susceptibility genes for complex diseases: linkage studies on one hand and association studies on the other hand. Both types of studies rely on the analysis of genetic polymorphisms. These can be microsatellites (polymorphic tandem repeat consisting of small repeat units of 2 to 5 bp) or single nucleotide polymorphisms (SNPs). SNPs are variations that occur at a single nucleotide position at a frequency of over 1 per 1000 bp throughout the entire genome. SNPs are a by-product of the Human Genome Project and are thought to be a main source of variation among individuals. According to the "common variant, common disease" hypothesis, some of these SNPs might also be causative factors for complex diseases. All currently identified SNPs (more than 4 million) are entered in a SNP-database [(dbSNP; (94)]. By taking into account linkage disequilibrium between neighbouring SNPs, which is being determined for the complete human genome by the international HapMap project (95), efficient SNP selection strategies are now possible. Most typically, microsatellites are used for linkage studies and SNPs for association studies. But this is certainly not a general rule. In fact, due to the development of high throughput SNP genotyping methods, linkage studies using SNPs have become increasingly popular.

Linkage studies try to identify regions of the genome that harbour susceptibility genes on the basis of the inheritance pattern of the disease and genetic markers. If marker alleles from a certain region are coinherited with the disease more than can be expected by chance, this region is said to be linked to the disease under investigation. Typically for complex diseases, nonparametric linkage analysis is performed on a large collection of small families. The nonparametric methods, also called model-free methods, make no assumptions about the mode of inheritance, the disease frequency, or other parameters. Association studies on the other hand analyse genetic variations in unrelated individuals and try to identify those variations that are more frequent in affected individuals compared to unaffected individuals. The ultimate in association studies is a genome-wide association study. In that case, hundreds of thousands of SNPs across the entire genome are analysed in unrelated individuals. Although genome-wide association studies have become technically feasible very recently, they remain prohibitively expensive, and usually association studies are limited to a carefully selected set of candidate genes.

Extended sample collections, preferably containing thousands of samples, are a prerequisite for genetic studies of complex diseases. The nature of the sample collections depends on the study design. Linkage studies require large sets of small families, while association studies are usually done using large sets of unrelated individuals.

Description of the ARHI phenotype

A first requirement for undertaking genetic studies for ARHI is a clear description of the phenotype. ARHI can be treated as a dichotomous trait. In this case, a group of patients affected with ARHI (cases) will be compared with unaffected individuals (controls). This subdivision is usually based upon audiometric values. On the other hand, ARHI can also be regarded as a quantitative trait—an approach that should have advantages over the dichotomous approach, since the dichotomisation of a quantitative trait leads to loss of statistical power (96). If ARHI is described as dichotomous trait, a genetic variant that is associated with ARHI would be more frequent among affected individuals (cases) than among unaffected individuals (controls). When ARHI is treated as a quantitative trait, samples will be grouped according to the genotype of a particular polymorphism under investigation, and the differences in the quantitative values between the groups will be statistically analysed.

Recently, a novel Z-score-based method has been published that allows ARHI to be described as a quantitative trait (97). The Z-score, which is based on the ISO7029 standard (9), gives an indication of the affection status of an individual independent of age and gender. Z-scores are calculated for each frequency as units of standard deviations from the median value for a particular age and gender. A negative Z-score indicates a person with better than median hearing, while a positive Z-score indicates hearing that is worse than the median value of otologically normal persons (97).

Association studies for ARHI

As explained above, association studies compare the presence of variations in candidate genes in predefined groups. The selection of candidate genes is based upon physiological, functional, and expression information. The genes identified for monogenic hearing loss are excellent candidate ARHI susceptibility genes (see Box).

MONOGENIC FORMS OF HEARING LOSS ARE CANDIDATE ARHI SUSCEPTIBILITY GENES

Up to now, genetic research into hearing impairment has mainly focused on monogenic forms of hearing loss. Using classic positional cloning approaches and provided that extended families are available, the localisation and identification of genes for monogenic types of hearing impairment is relatively easy and straightforward, especially since the completion of the human genome sequence. At the moment, 54 loci for nonsyndromal autosomal dominant (DFNA), 59 loci for nonsyndromal autosomal recessive (DFNB), and 8 loci for X-linked (DFN) hearing loss, in addition to two modifier loci (DFNM), have been reported. More than 40 genes for monogenic nonsyndromal hearing impairment and even more for syndromal hearing impairment have been identified. These genes belong to very different gene families with various functions, including transcription factors, extracellular matrix molecules, cytoskeletal components, and ion channels and transporters. For an overview of the current state of the art, see Chapter 5. In addition, the Hereditary Hearing Loss Homepage (http://webhost.ua.ac.be/hhh/) is a regularly updated online source of information on monogenic hearing impairment in humans.

As the most frequent type of ARHI is progressive, sensorineural, and most pronounced in the high frequencies, genes causing monogenic hearing impairment with phenotypic similarities to ARHI, although with a much younger age at onset, are excellent candidate ARHI susceptibility genes. KCNQ4 (DFNA2), DFNA5 (DFNA5), COCH (DFNA9), MYH9 (DFNA17), and TMC1 (DFNA36) are examples of such genes. Notably, all these genes are autosomal dominant hearing loss genes. This does not mean that autosomal recessive genes cannot be candidates for ARHI. Because some genes are responsible for autosomal recessive as well as autosomal dominant hearing loss, or for syndromal as well as nonsyndromal hearing loss, one might argue that all genes involved in monogenic hearing loss are excellent ARHI candidate genes.

Molecular knowledge of the genetics of nonsyndromal hearing impairment has been obtained only relatively recently. Before 1994, only a single gene localisation had been reported, and until 1997 only one single gene had been identified. The increasing knowledge regarding these purely genetic, albeit rare forms of monogenic deafness, is in sharp contrast with the lack of knowledge regarding genes leading to ARHI. Hopefully, a similar increase in knowledge of the complex forms of hearing loss can be realised in the near future.

Only a few association studies have been published for ARHI. Van Laer et al. studied the involvement of the DFNA5 gene in a Flemish set (using the quantitative Z-score method) and in a set derived from the Framingham cohort (using the dichotomous method) (98). DFNA5 was selected as a candidate ARHI susceptibility gene because mutations in DFNA5 cause a type of hearing loss that closely resembles the most typical type of ARHI (i.e., high-frequency, progressive, sensorineural hearing loss). Two SNPs leading to an amino acid substitution in DFNA5 were analysed. However, no significant association was detected in either sample collection (98). Recently, a second study has been published. To investigate the hypothesis that variations in gluthathione-related antioxidant enzyme levels are associated with the risk of ARHI, Ates et al. analysed three glutathione S-transferase polymorphisms (GSTM1, GSTT1, and GSTP1) using a case–control association study (99). This study could not demonstrate a significant association either.

Linkage studies for ARHI

A huge problem in collecting families for linkage studies of ARHI is the late onset of the disease, which means that the parents from the required pedigrees are frequently deceased. In a first study using the Framingham cohort, this problem was overcome by collecting DNA and audiological information for the parents in a first phase (between 1973 and 1975), and for the children in a second phase (between 1995 and 1999). Pure tone averages of medium and low frequencies were adjusted for cohort, sex, age, age squared, and age cubed, and a genome-wide linkage scan was performed. This led to the identification of several chromosomal regions that showed suggestive evidence for linkage: 11p, 11q13.5, and 14q (100).

In complex diseases, several genome-wide scans need to be performed on independent sample sets in order to confirm previously published candidate regions and to identify new regions that might be linked to ARHI. Preferably, after the completion of a handful of such studies, a meta-analysis should be performed that will define the ultimate candidate regions. Because currently only one genome scan has been published, there is still a lot of work to be done to unravel the genetic basis of ARHI.

Future prospects

Although a great deal of work has been done already, in particular, the unravelling of the genetic basis of ARHI will demand further joint efforts. Genetic analysis will clarify the influence of genetic variations in ARHI susceptibility genes: which variations in these genes increase the risk for ARHI and which do not. By integrating information on genetic and environmental risk factors, it may become clear how the vulnerability of a person's hearing system correlates with his genetic background. It might be that certain environmental risk factors are potentially harmful only in a limited number of individuals, depending on their genetic background. By means of genetic testing for susceptibility genes in an individual, personalised guidelines for ARHI prevention may be designed.

Future therapies for hearing impairment will have to rely on basic rather than on symptomatic approaches. To achieve this, a better understanding of the basic molecular and cellular processes involved in ARHI is a prerequisite. Ultimately, a pharmacogenomic (i.e., adapting drugs to an individual's genetic background) approach to ARHI may become feasible.

References

1. Davis A. Prevalence of Hearing Impairment. In: Davis A, ed. Hearing in Adults. London: Whurr Publishers Ltd, 1994:43–321.
2. Dalton DS, Cruickshanks KJ, Klein BE, et al. The impact of hearing loss on quality of life in older adults. Gerontologist 2003; 43:661–668.
3. Cruickshanks KJ, Wiley TL, Tweed TS, et al. Prevalence of hearing loss in older adults in Beaver Dam, Wisconsin. The Epidemiology of Hearing Loss Study. Am J Epidemiol 1998; 148:879–886.
4. Cruickshanks KJ, Tweed TS, Wiley TL, et al. The 5-year incidence and progression of hearing loss: the epidemiology of hearing loss study. Arch Otolaryngol Head Neck Surg 2003; 129:1041–1046.
5. Pearson JD, Morrell CH, Gordon-Salant S, et al. Gender differences in a longitudinal study of age-associated hearing loss. J Acoust Soc Am 1995; 97:1196–1205.
6. Guimaraes P, Zhu X, Cannon T, et al. Sex differences in distortion product otoacoustic emissions as a function of age in CBA mice. Hear Res 2004; 192:83–89.
7. Henry KR. Males lose hearing earlier in mouse models of late-onset age-related hearing loss; females lose hearing earlier in mouse models of early-onset hearing loss. Hear Res 2004; 190:141–148.
8. Lee FS, Matthews LJ, Dubno JR, et al. Longitudinal study of pure-tone thresholds in older persons. Ear Hear 2005; 26:1–11.
9. International Organization for Standardization. Acoustics-threshold of hearing by air conduction as a function of age and sex for otologically normal persons. International Standard ISO7029 1984.
10. Schuknecht HF. Further observations on the pathology of presbycusis. Arch Otolaryngol 1964; 80:369–382.
11. Schuknecht HF, Gacek MR. Cochlear pathology in presbycusis. Ann Otol Rhinol Laryngol 1993; 102:1–16.
12. Johnsson LG, Felix H, Gleeson M, et al. Observations on the pattern of sensorineural degeneration in the human cochlea. Acta Otolaryngol Suppl 1990; 470:88–96.
13. Soucek S, Michaels L, Frohlich A. Evidence for hair cell degeneration as the primary lesion in hearing loss of the elderly. J Otolaryngol 1986; 15:175–183.
14. Felder E, Schrott-Fischer A. Quantitative evaluation of myelinated nerve fibres and hair cells in cochleae of humans with age-related high-tone hearing loss. Hear Res 1995; 91:19–32.

15. Scholtz AW, Kammen-Jolly K, Felder E, et al. Selective aspects of human pathology in high-tone hearing loss of the aging inner ear. Hear Res 2001; 157:77–86.

16. Nelson EG, Hinojosa R. Presbycusis: a human temporal bone study of individuals with flat audiometric patterns of hearing loss using a new method to quantify stria vascularis volume. Laryngoscope 2003; 113:1672–1686.

17. Ohlemiller KK. Age-related hearing loss: the status of Schuknecht's typology. Curr Opin Otolaryngol Head Neck Surg 2004; 12:439–443.

18. McFadden SL, Ding D, Salvi R. Anatomical, metabolic and genetic aspects of age-related hearing loss in mice. Audiology 2001; 40:313–321.

19. Mizuta K, Nozawa O, Morita H, et al. Scanning electron microscopy of age-related changes in the C57BL/6J mouse cochlea. Scanning Microsc 1993; 7:889–896.

20. White JA, Burgess BJ, Hall RD, et al. Pattern of degeneration of the spiral ganglion cell and its processes in the C57BL/6J mouse. Hear Res 2000; 141:12–18.

21. Francis HW, Ryugo DK, Gorelikow MJ, et al. The functional age of hearing loss in a mouse model of presbycusis. II. Neuroanatomical correlates. Hear Res 2003; 183:29–36.

22. Hequembourg S, Liberman MC. Spiral ligament pathology: a major aspect of age-related cochlear degeneration in C57BL/6 mice. J Assoc Res Otolaryngol 2001; 2:118–129.

23. Ichimiya I, Suzuki M, Mogi G. Age-related changes in the murine cochlear lateral wall. Hear Res 2000; 139:116–122.

24. Ohlemiller KK, Gagnon PM. Apical-to-basal gradients in age-related cochlear degeneration and their relationship to "primary" loss of cochlear neurons. J Comp Neurol 2004; 479:103–116.

25. Saitoh Y, Hosokawa M, Shimada A, et al. Age-related cochlear degeneration in senescence-accelerated mouse. Neurobiol Aging 1995; 16:129–136.

26. Wu T, Marcus DC. Age-related changes in cochlear endolymphatic potassium and potential in CD-1 and CBA/CaJ mice. J Assoc Res Otolaryngol 2003; 4:353–362.

27. Ohlemiller KK. Reduction in sharpness of frequency tuning but not endocochlear potential in aging and noise-exposed BALB/cJ mice. J Assoc Res Otolaryngol 2002; 3:444–456.

28. Ohlemiller KK, Gagnon PM. Cellular correlates of progressive hearing loss in 129S6/SvEv mice. J Comp Neurol 2004; 469:377–390.

29. Shimada A, Ebisu M, Morita T, et al. Age-related changes in the cochlea and cochlear nuclei of dogs. J Vet Med Sci 1998; 60:41–48.

30. Matthews LJ, Lee FS, Mills JH, et al. Audiometric and subjective assessment of hearing handicap. Arch Otolaryngol Head Neck Surg 1990; 116:1325–1330.

31. Boettcher FA. Presbyacusis and the auditory brainstem response. J Speech Lang Hear Res 2002; 45:1249–1261.

32. Pichora-Fuller MK, Souza PE. Effects of aging on auditory processing of speech. Int J Audiol 2003; 42(suppl 2):2S11–2S16.

33. Gates GA, Cobb JL, Linn RT, et al. Central auditory dysfunction, cognitive dysfunction, and dementia in older people. Arch Otolaryngol Head Neck Surg 1996; 122:161–167.

34. Willott JF. Central physiological correlates of ageing and presbycusis in mice. Acta Otolaryngol Suppl 1991; 476:153–156.

35. Jacobson M, Kim S, Romney J, et al. Contralateral suppression of distortion-product otoacoustic emissions declines with age: a comparison of findings in CBA mice with human listeners. Laryngoscope 2003; 113:1707–1713.

36. Kim S, Frisina DR, Frisina RD. Effects of age on contralateral suppression of distortion product otoacoustic emissions in human listeners with normal hearing. Audiol Neurootol 2002; 7:348–357.

37. Karlsson KK, Harris JR, Svartengren M. Description and primary results from an audiometric study of male twins. Ear Hear 1997; 18:114–120.

38. Gates GA, Couropmitree NN, Myers RH. Genetic associations in age-related hearing thresholds. Arch Otolaryngol Head Neck Surg 1999; 125:654–659.

39. Christensen K, Frederiksen H, Hoffman HJ. Genetic and environmental influences on self-reported reduced hearing in the old and oldest old. J Am Geriatr Soc 2001; 49:1512–1517.

40. Erway LC, Willott JF, Archer JR, et al. Genetics of age-related hearing loss in mice: I. Inbred and F1 hybrid strains. Hear Res 1993; 65:125–132.

41. Johnson KR, Erway LC, Cook SA, et al. A major gene affecting age-related hearing loss in C57BL/6J mice. Hear Res 1997; 114:83–92.

42. Johnson KR, Zheng QY, Erway LC. A major gene affecting age-related hearing loss is common to at least ten inbred strains of mice. Genomics 2000; 70:171–180.

43. Zheng QY, Johnson KR. Hearing loss associated with the modifier of deaf waddler (mdfw) locus corresponds with age-related hearing loss in 12 inbred strains of mice. Hear Res 2001; 154:45–53.

44. Noben-Trauth K, Zheng QY, Johnson KR. Association of cadherin 23 with polygenic inheritance and genetic modification of sensorineural hearing loss. Nat Genet 2003; 35:21–23.

45. Keithley EM, Canto C, Zheng QY, et al. Age-related hearing loss and the Ahl locus in mice. Hear Res 2004; 188:21–28.

46. Johnson KR, Zheng QY. Ahl2, a second locus affecting age-related hearing loss in mice. Genomics 2002; 80:461–464.

47. Nemoto M, Morita Y, Mishima Y, et al. Ahl3, a third locus on mouse chromosome 17 affecting age-related hearing loss. Biochem Biophys Res Commun 2004; 324:1283–1288.

48. Rosen S, Bergman M, Plester D, et al. Presbycusis study of a relatively noise-free population in the Sudan. Ann Otol Rhinol Laryngol 1962; 71:727–743.

49. Jarvis JF, van Heerden HG. The acuity of hearing in the Kalahari Bushmen . A pilot survey. J Laryngol Otol 1967; 81:63–68.

50. Clark WW. Noise exposure from leisure activities: a review. J Acoust Soc Am 1991; 90:175–181.

51. Erway LC, Shiau YW, Davis RR, et al. Genetics of age-related hearing loss in mice. III. Susceptibility of inbred and F1 hybrid strains to noise-induced hearing loss. Hear Res 1996; 93:181–187.

52. Ohlemiller KK, Wright JS, Heidbreder AF. Vulnerability to noise-induced hearing loss in 'middle-aged' and young adult mice: a

dose-response approach in CBA, C57BL, and BALB inbred strains. Hear Res 2000; 149:239–247.

53. Corso JF. Support for Corso's hearing loss model. Relating aging and noise exposure. Audiology 1992; 31:162–7.

54. Gates GA, Schmid P, Kujawa SG, et al. Longitudinal threshold changes in older men with audiometric notches. Hear Res 2000; 141:220–228.

55. Dobie RA. The relative contributions of occupational noise and aging in individual cases of hearing loss. Ear Hear 1992; 13:19–27.

56. Stypulkowski PH. Mechanisms of salicylate ototoxicity. Hear Res 1990; 46:113–145.

57. Rosenhall U, Sixt E, Sundh V, et al. Correlations between presbyacusis and extrinsic noxious factors. Audiology 1993; 32:234–243.

58. Mills JH, Matthews LJ, Lee FS, et al. Gender-specific effects of drugs on hearing levels of older persons. Ann N Y Acad Sci 1999; 884:381–388.

59. Aran JM, Hiel H, Hayashida T. Noise, aminoglycosides, diuretics. In: Dancer A, Henderson D, Salvi R, Hamernik R, eds. Noise Induced Hearing Loss. St. Louis: Mosby, 1992:175–187.

60. Rybak LP. Hearing: the effects of chemicals. Otolaryngol Head Neck Surg 1992; 106:677–686.

61. Johnson AC, Nylen PR. Effects of industrial solvents on hearing. Occup Med 1995; 10:623–640.

62. Itoh A, Nakashima T, Arao H, et al. Smoking and drinking habits as risk factors for hearing loss in the elderly: epidemiological study of subjects undergoing routine health checks in Aichi, Japan. Public Health 2001; 115:192–196.

63. Cruickshanks KJ, Klein R, Klein BEK, et al. Cigarette smoking and hearing loss: the epidemiology of hearing loss study. J Am Med Ass 1998; 279:1715–1719.

64. Uchida Y, Nakashimat T, Ando F, et al. Is there a relevant effect of noise and smoking on hearing? A population-based aging study. Int J Audiol 2005; 44:86–91.

65. Gates GA, Cobb JL, D'Agostino RB, et al. The relation of hearing in the elderly to the presence of cardiovascular disease and cardiovascular risk factors. Arch Otolaryngol Head Neck Surg 1993; 119:156–161.

66. Brant LJ, Gordon-Salant S, Pearson JD, et al. Risk factors related to age-associated hearing loss in the speech frequencies. J Am Acad Audiol 1996; 7:152–160.

67. Popelka MM, Cruickshanks KJ, Wiley TL, et al. Moderate alcohol consumption and hearing loss: a protective effect. J Am Geriatr Soc 2000; 48:1273–1278.

68. Fitzgerald DC. Head trauma: hearing loss and dizziness. J Trauma 1996; 40:488–496.

69. Houston DK, Johnson MA, Nozza RJ, et al. Age-related hearing loss, vitamin B-12, and folate in elderly women. Am J Clin Nutr 1999; 69:564–571.

70. Willott JF, Erway LC, Archer JR, et al. Genetics of age-related hearing loss in mice. II. Strain differences and effects of caloric restriction on cochlear pathology and evoked response thresholds. Hear Res 1995; 88:143–155.

71. Sixt E, Rosenhall U. Presbyacusis related to socioeconomic factors and state of health. Scand Audiol 1997; 26:133–140.

72. Lee FS, Matthews LJ, Mills JH, et al. Analysis of blood chemistry and hearing levels in a sample of older persons. Ear Hear 1998; 19:180–190.

73. Picciotti P, Torsello A, Wolf FI, et al. Age-dependent modifications of expression level of VEGF and its receptors in the inner ear. Exp Gerontol 2004; 39:1253–1258.

74. Antonelli AR, Bonfioli F, Garrubba V, et al. Audiological findings in elderly patients with chronic renal failure. Acta Otolaryngol Suppl 1990; 476:54–68.

75. Clark K, Sowers MR, Wallace RB, et al. Age-related hearing loss and bone mass in a population of rural women aged 60 to 85 years. Ann Epidemiol 1995; 5:8–14.

76. Purchase-Helzner EL, Cauley JA, Faulkner KA, et al. Hearing sensitivity and the risk of incident falls and fracture in older women: the study of osteoporotic fractures. Ann Epidemiol 2004; 14:311–318.

77. Kurien M, Thomas K, Bhanu TS. Hearing threshold in patients with diabetes mellitus. J Laryngol Otol 1989; 103:164–168.

78. Iwai H, Lee S, Inaba M, et al. Correlation between accelerated presbycusis and decreased immune functions. Exp Gerontol 2003; 38:319–325.

79. Bao J, Lei D, Du Y, et al. Requirement of nicotinic acetylcholine receptor subunit ß2 in the maintenance of spiral ganglion neurons during aging. J Neurosci 2005; 25:3041–3045.

80. Seidman MD, Khan MJ, Tang WX, et al. Influence of lecithin on mitochondrial DNA and age-related hearing loss. Otolaryngol Head Neck Surg 2002; 127:138–144.

81. Lautermann J, Crann SA, McLaren J, et al. Glutathione-dependent antioxidant systems in the mammalian inner ear: effects of aging, ototoxic drugs and noise. Hear Res 1997; 114:75–82.

82. McFadden SL, Ding D, Burkard RF, et al. Cu/Zn SOD deficiency potentiates hearing loss and cochlear pathology in aged 129,CD-1 mice. J Comp Neurol 1999; 413:101–112.

83. McFadden SL, Ding D, Reaume AG, et al. Age-related cochlear hair cell loss is enhanced in mice lacking copper/zinc superoxide dismutase. Neurobiol Aging 1999; 20:1–8.

84. Coling DE, Yu KCY, Somand D, et al. Effect of SOD1 overexpression on age- and noise-related hearing loss. Free Radic Biol Med 2003; 34:873–880.

85. Seidman MD. Effects of dietary restriction and antioxidants on presbyacusis. Laryngoscope 2000; 110:727–738.

86. Seidman MD, Khan MJ, Bai U, et al. Biologic activity of mitochondrial metabolites on aging and age-related hearing loss. Am J Otol 2000; 21:161–167.

87. Seidman MD, Bai U, Khan MJ, et al. Association of mitochondrial DNA deletions and cochlear pathology: a molecular biologic tool. Laryngoscope 1996; 106:777–783.

88. Bai U, Seidman MD, Hinojosa R, et al. Mitochondrial DNA deletions associated with aging and possibly presbycusis: a human archival temporal bone study. Am J Otol 1997; 18:449–453.

89. Dai P, Yang W, Jiang S, et al. Correlation of cochlear blood supply with mitochondrial DNA common deletion in presbyacusis. Acta Otolaryngol 2004; 124:130–136.

90. Seidman MD, Bai U, Khan MJ, et al. Mitochondrial DNA deletions associated with aging and presbyacusis. Arch Otolaryngol Head Neck Surg 1997; 123:1039–1045.

91. Zhang X, Han D, Ding D, et al. Cochlear mitochondrial DNA3867 bp deletion in aged mice. Chin Med J (Engl) 2002; 115:1390–1393.

92. Fischel-Ghodsian N, Bykhovskaya Y, Taylor K, et al. Temporal bone analysis of patients with presbycusis reveals high frequency of mitochondrial mutations. Hear Res 1997; 110:147–154.

93. Fischel-Ghodsian N. Mitochondrial deafness. Ear Hear 2003; 24:303–313.

94. http://www.ncbi.nlm.nih.gov/

95. http://www.hapmap.org

96. Page GP, Amos CI. Comparison of linkage-disequilibrium methods for localization of genes influencing quantitative traits in humans. Am J Hum Genet 1999; 64:1194–1205.

97. Fransen E, Van Laer L, Lemkens N, et al. A novel Z-score-based method to analyze candidate genes for age-related hearing impairment. Ear Hear 2004; 25:133–141.

98. Van Laer L, DeStefano AL, Myers RH, et al. Is DFNA5 a susceptibility gene for age-related hearing impairment? Eur J Hum Genet 2002; 10:883–886.

99. Ates NA, Unal M, Tamer L, et al. Glutathione S-transferase gene polymorphisms in presbycusis. Otol Neurotol 2005; 26:392–397.

100. DeStefano AL, Gates GA, Heard-Costa N, et al. Genomewide linkage analysis to presbycusis in the Framingham Heart Study. Arch Otolaryngol Head Neck Surg 2003; 129:285–289.

7 Noise-related hearing impairment

Ilmari Pyykkö, Esko Toppila, Jing Zou,
Howard T Jacobs, Erna Kentala

Introduction

The economic basis of our society—the way the people make their livelihoods—has undergone fundamental changes during the last half of the twentieth century. The important changes include dependency on communication skills and increase of environmental noise exposure. In the past, we depended largely on manual labour. Today we depend upon communication skills—hearing, speech, and language. This, in turn, has a profound effect on definition of illness and society's expectation and demands placed on the medical profession. About 13% of European citizens have a communication disorder that almost exclusively depends on being hard of hearing. In 1853, Robert Koch stated "now when we have won the battle over tuberculosis, we have to conquer the next great problem—noise-induced hearing loss (NIHL)." This statement is still valid, and the riddle of NIHL has not been solved.

In Europe, around 50 million subjects are exposed to hazardous levels of environmental noise, creating a risk for NIHL and tinnitus. The losses in economic terms are substantial, at a minimum level 0.2% of national net income. This equals about 400 billion Euros annually at European Community level. This amount includes direct and indirect costs related to production. The indirect costs do not include factors related to reduced quality of life. The factors affecting quality of life include social isolation, increased unemployment, and difficulties in family life due to communication difficulties related to hearing handicap. Needless to say, NIHL is still one of the leading health-related problems in industrialised countries.

NIHL is insidious and progressive in nature and is invisible. At no time is there a sudden noticeable change in hearing. The loss of frequency resolution is unknown to people and the inability to hear sounds against background noise is attributed to other causes and not to hearing loss in the workplace. The affected workers attribute their difficulties to fatigue, lack of interest or concentration, poor articulation of the talkers, and excessive background noise. Interaction with these people reveals inconsistent behaviour and is attributed to an unwillingness to communicate.

Definition of NIHL

NIHL refers to sensory-neural hearing loss (SNHL) in subjects exposed to environmental noise, when other reasons for SNHL are excluded. Causes such as head trauma, ototoxic medication, hereditary hearing loss, and various inner ear diseases should be excluded. In estimation of the specific noise-related hearing loss, the subject's age is used as a correction term in most models (1,2). For example in the ISO 1999 (1990) database (2), age correction is used when the subject is older than 18 years. According to the ISO 1999 database A (1) model for NIHL, an exposure of 100 dB for 8 hours a day over 30 years gives a median NIHL of 45 dB, with variation of 60 dB (10th–90th percentiles) at 4 kHz. Several confounding factors have been cited to attempt to explain the variance, such as inadequate evaluation of the noise exposure, pitfalls in the equal energy principle, prevalence of combined exposure, and individual susceptibility to noise. Due to unknown factors for SNHL, exact risk prediction for NIHL is difficult in individual cases (Fig. 7.1) (3,4).

Age is regarded as a contributing factor for NIHL but has been subjected to criticism. The age correction provided in most proposed NIHL standards may not be an accurate estimate

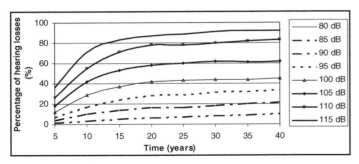

Figure 7.1 Noise–exposure curves for the development of noise-induced hearing loss based on ISO 1999 (1976).

of deterioration of hearing in individual cases and may cause variation in estimating NIHL (5,6). A deeper analysis of confounding factors might reduce the uncertainty in evaluation of NIHL. Another problem in the evaluation of NIHL is the shortage of information on free-time noise and on the individual use of hearing protectors. In the estimation of noise dose, evaluation of free-time noise exposure and the type of hearing protector and its attenuation profile and use should be included (7). A database should include all this information if its purpose is to evaluate total exposure for assessing hearing loss risk in individual cases.

Historical databases used in evalution of NIHL

One of the first criteria for the risk of damage based on exposure to steady-state noise was proposed by Kryter (8). The damage risk criterion is derived from a group of curves that were based on laboratory experiments on the development of temporary threshold shift (TTS). Data collected during 1955 to 1956 on permanent threshold shifts (PTS) in workers exposed to industrial noise was also included. The committee on hearing, bioacoustics, and biomechanics (9) used the data to express the hearing level contour as a function of exposure. This was the first norm proposed for evaluation of hazardous noise.

The first large epidemiological study of the relationship between noise exposure and hearing loss was made by Baughn (10). His studies from the early 60s involved a large worker population (n = 6835) at stable work locations and under conditions with stable noise exposure (10,11). The exposure durations went up to 45 years, with average noise exposure levels of 78, 86, and 92 dB(A). Baughn (10) recommended that the hearing loss of subjects exposed to the 78 dB(A) noise should be considered as typical of non–noise-exposed males. According to his data, it is possible that factory workers suffer more socioacusis and nosoacusis than the general population.

Burns and Robinson (12) studied 759 subjects, of whom 422 males were exposed to four classes of noise ranging from 87

to 97 dB(A). The maximum exposure was about 49 years. As controls 97 subjects not exposed to noise were included in the study. The population was shown to be otologically normal. The authors developed a mathematical generalisation of the predicted hearing loss (13,14). This model introduced the energy principle to enable the combination of different sound levels (15). Hearing loss was divided into two parts: age-dependent hearing loss (presbyacusis) and NIHL. After correcting the model for age and gender, the distribution of hearing loss was calculated by using the specific formulas. The separation of presbyacusis from NIHL leads to a predicted hearing loss that is smaller than that found in other models, partly because the material was rigorously screened for otologically healthy subjects (16).

Passchier-Vermeer (17) summarised the results of 19 smaller studies, 12 of which have 50 or fewer cases. The data agree well with Robinson's data at some frequencies, but, at other frequencies, large differences were found. One reason was the variation in the definition of audiometer zero level used in some of the studies (18).

Johnson (19) prepared a report for the U.S. Environmental Protection Agency on the prediction of NIHL from exposure to continuous noise. This report is based on the data of Burns and Robinson (12) and Passchier-Vermeer (17). The data of Baughn (10,11) was also used in evaluating hearing loss in the nonexposed population. For this reason, the hearing loss of the nonexposed population is somewhat less in this report than in the work by Burns and Robinson (12) or Passchier-Vermeer (17).

The National Institute for Occupational Safety and Health (NIOSH) in the United States conducted a study on industrial workers exposed to noise levels of approximately 85, 90, and 95 dB(A) and control subjects exposed to levels below 80 dB(A) (NIOSH 1974). The study consisted of an otologically screened normal population of 792 noise-exposed subjects and 380 controls. Hearing loss was tabulated by a function determined by exposure level and duration. Using these tables, the occurrence of NIHL could be calculated by subtracting the control values from hearing threshold values measured in noise-exposed subjects.

In 1975 the ISO published a standard for assessing occupational noise exposure for hearing conservation [ISO 1999 (1975)] (20). The information on which this standard is based is not identified, but, according to Suter (16), the data of Baughn (10,11) form the basis of this standard. The ISO standard adopted the equal-energy principle for the combination of different exposure levels from the Robinson model. According to ISO tables, 5% of non–noise-exposed people have a hearing loss, whereas Robinson and Sutton (21) demonstrated a 10% and U.S. public health services study (22,23) a 20% prevalence of hearing loss for non-noise–exposed people. The ISO model was corrected, and a mathematical formula for the hearing loss was given in order to produce the present standard model [ISO 1999 (1990)] (2).

The problem with historical data is that subjects were not screened for genetic factors and with few exceptions the workers were exposed to the same type of noise. In today's society, the noise exposure sources vary and free-time noise has become an important source for NIHL. Therefore, the ISO standard [ISO 1999 (1990)] has frequently been criticised.

Demands set by new European union directives

The European Union (EU) has set a directive for protection of workers against occupational hazards (Council Directive on the Introduction of Measures to Encourage Improvements in the Safety and Health of Workers at Work, No 89/391/EC). Based on this framework directive, a new directive (2003/10/EC) was introduced on protection against noise. In this directive, the need to evaluate all factors affecting the development of NIHL is recognised. This includes noise characteristics (duration, impulsiveness, and level) and the effect of combined exposure with vibration and ototoxic chemicals. Finally, the employer must give particular attention when carrying out risk assessment

on workers belonging to particularly sensitive risk groups during their whole working career. To deal with this, a database should include all environmental and health related factors that may be cause of hearing loss in NIHL. In prevention work the focus in early diagnosis of NIHL. The following table (Table 7.1) shows the limit values set by the directive and their relation to the ISO 1999 (1990) international standard.

Evaluation of noise exposure history

In one study, Pyykkö et al. (24) recorded accurate work histories from 675 of 682 workers in different occupations. For data collection, an expert program (NoiseScan ver 1.0) was used (25). For all subjects, noise immission of individual working places (machines) or working tasks (grinding and welding) was measured by determining the environmental noise and thereafter by performing noise dosimetry in selected workers. The noise immission in forest work was evaluated by determining the average noise level of the chain saws and by performing noise dosimetry in selected forest workers. The collected immission

Table 7.1 Relationship between EU noise directive (EN-10/2003/EU) and ISO 1999 (1990)

Noise level[a]–Daily equivalent level and peak level	Relevance in regulation (Directive EN-10/2003/EU)	Reference to ISO 1999
75 dB(A)	Not defined	No changes in hearing thresholds
80 dB(A) and 135 dB(C)[b]	*Lower exposure action level* Preventive efforts to reduce noise should be attempted Worker has access to hearing protectors Workers have right to test their hearing Workers should receive information on noise risks and benefit of the use of hearing protectors	No hearing loss in speech frequencies (500–2000 Hz)
85 dB(A) and 137 dB(C)[b]	*Upper exposure action level* Preventive efforts to reduce noise should be done Employer must establish a noise control program and provide hearing protectors Employer must promote the use of hearing protectors by all possible means Workers must use hearing protectors Noise areas must be identified and marked and access to these areas should be restricted	5% of workers will get NIHL
87 dB(A) and 140 dB(C)[c]	Exposure limit value must not be exceeded	8% of workers will get NIHL

[a]Weekly equivalent level may be used if there is a large variation in daily noise exposure.
[b]The effect of hearing protectors is not taken into account.
[c]The effect of hearing protectors is taken into account.
Abbreviations: EU, European Union; NIHL, noise-induced hearing loss.

data was used in the estimation of noise exposure for each worker by determining their daily exposure to noise. The immission data gave noise level outside the hearing protective device (HPD). Noise immission remained relatively constant in all workplaces. In a paper mill, the mean noise immission level was 91 to 94 dB (A), in a shipyard, it was 93 to 95 dB (A), and in forest work, it was 95 to 97 dB (A).

To obtain the noise level inside the protector, the mean attenuation performance of the HPD was measured with miniature microphone techniques (26). Noise measurements were taken simultaneously inside and outside the HPD. Inside the HPD, a miniature microphone was attached at the middle of the ear canal entrance. The microphone signal was fed to a signal analyser by a thin (0.3 mm) cable to minimise leakage between the skin and the HPD cushion ring. At different work sites, 10 minute samples were recorded for the analysis of A-weighted noise equivalent level and impulsiveness (27). The measurements showed that the protector attenuation is about 15 dB among forest workers, 17 dB among paper mill workers, and 20 dB in the shipyard workers (more impulsive noise).

For the calculation of lifetime exposure to noise, the results from a questionnaire on occupational history and use of hearing protectors were included. Noise levels were used to calculate the A-weighted noise immission level (L_{ANO}) outside the HPD and emission level (L_{ANI}) inside the HPD for each worker according to the following formulae:

$$L_{ANO} = \sum (L_{AEqi} + 10 \cdot LOG(T)),$$
$$L_{ANI} = \sum (L_{AEqi} - A' - 10 \cdot LOG(T_i)), \qquad (1)$$

where L_{AEqi} is the A-weighted equivalent noise level during ith exposure period, A' is the effective attenuation of hearing protectors, T_i is the length of the ith work period in years, and LOG is base 10 logarithm. The effective attenuation (A') of HPDs was calculated using the following formula, which takes into account the use rates:

$$A' = L - L' = L - 10 \cdot LOG(10^{L/10} \cdot (1 - c)$$
$$+ 10^{((L-A)/10)} \cdot c), \qquad (2)$$

where L = noise level outside the HPD, L' = noise level inside the HPD, A = attenuation of the HPD, and c = usage rate/100. Use rates were elicited for all work periods in steps 0, 25, 50, 75, and 100, where 0 means no use at all and 100 means regular use.

The contribution of occupational, free-time, and military noise and use of hearing protectors can also be evaluated. Although the 3 dB equal-energy rule is not universally accepted as a method for characterising exposures that consist of both impulsive and continuous-type noises, the evaluation of cumulative lifetime noise exposure might be based on the concept of "the noise immission level" (in dB).

After some modification, the total noise immission level that takes into consideration occupational, free-time, and military noises can be expressed using following formula:

$$L_{1A,total} = 10 \log \left(\frac{E_{A,tot,occup} + E_{A,tot,freetime} + E_{A,tot,military}}{p_0^2 \cdot T_0} \right) \qquad (3)$$

where $E_{A,tot,occup}$ is the total occupational A-weighted sound exposure, $E_{A,tot,freetime-totalfreetime}$ is the weighted sound exposure, and $E_{A,tot,militaryp}$ the total military A-weighted sound exposure, T_0 reference duration (=one year), and ρ_0 reference sound pressure, in Pa ($\rho_0 p = 20 \, \mu$Pa). $E_{At0,x} = 10^{L_{ANI}/10}$ and x refers to occupational, free-time, or military exposure.

Accuracy of measurement

The detailed noise exposure measurements are necessary to improve the understanding of exposure–response relationships. Factors such as the calibration of instruments, validity of measurement periods, and the site of the measurement may affect the measurement by as much as ±8 dB [ISO 9612 (1997)] (28).

Steady-state vs. impulsive noise

The equal energy principle provides a good approximation for the vulnerability of the ear in steady-state noise as in the process industry. However, the time domain characteristics of noise have been shown to affect the harmfulness of noise; the risk of NIHL is higher in occupations where workers are exposed to impulse noise. In several occupations, the impulses are so rapid that they contribute only a minimal amount to the energy content of noise. For example, in impulsive noise among shipyard workers, the hearing loss was 10 dB greater than could be predicted by the model. The observed hearing levels were very consistent with the model for forest workers, where the noise was not impulsive. Pauses in exposure allow for some recovery, and the resulting hearing loss is not as great as is proposed by the equal energy principle in animal experiments (29). Among paper mill workers, the hearing loss among those who used HPDs on average 50% of the time was less than the hearing loss among those who never used HPD. The difference could not be explained by the small change in exposure. The conclusion was that even temporary use of HPDs may provide relatively good protection against hearing loss.

Free-time and military noise exposure

The most frequent exposure to noise in free time is exposure to loud music. The highest music exposure rates are from rock music. Noise levels in a concert or a disco often exceed 100 dB (30). Thus, only one attendance a week causes an exposure exceeding the occupational exposure limit value. Similar levels are reported in the users of portable cassette recorders (31). In classical music, the levels are lower, but the musicians still have a risk of hearing loss (32). The role of music in NIHL is not well understood. In studies conducted among young people, exposure to loud music causes no changes in the audiogram. It has been suggested that the effect of music exposure would show up later. This is in accordance with recent studies showing that people exposed to loud music had more frequent and severe tinnitus than people with less exposure to music (33).

Free-time and military noise

The A-weighted sound exposure for free-time and military noise, excluding shooting noise and impulse noise from military sources, will be determined in a similar way. In this case $L_{ex,8h_i}$ should be replaced with the equivalent continuous A-weighted sound pressure level. Effective time exposure per day (or week or year) will be also taken into consideration.

In the case of shooting noise (hunting as a hobby) or impulse noise from military sources, the A-weighted sound exposure EA_{imp} (in Pa^2s) might be calculated from the equation (4):

$$E_{AImpi} = E_0 \sum_{i=1}^{M} N_i \cdot 10^{(L_{EAm1s_u} - K_{HDi})/10} ,\qquad (4)$$

where N_i is number of impulses, $L_{EA,1s_i}$ is the A-weighted sound exposure level of single impulse [averaged over one second; see ISO 1999 (1990)], E_0 the reference sound exposure ($E_0 = 4\cdot10^{-10} Pa^2s$), K_{HDi} is a hearing protector correction, in dB, and M is the total number of various sources of impulse noise.

Apart from assessment of the total lifetime noise exposure, each type of exposure (occupational, free-time, and military) will be considered separately. Additionally, in the case of occupational exposure, the noise spectrum will be evaluated for audible, ultrasonic, and infrasonic frequencies [see ISO 9612 (1997)].

In the case of shooting noise and impulse noise from military exposure, evaluations based on the number of shots or explosions and C-weighted or unweighted peak sound pressure level will be incorporated (e.g., see Regulations for Shooting Noise in the Netherlands) (Fig. 7.2).

Nonoccupational noise exposure interacts with occupational noise exposure by enhancing the risk of NIHL. At present, this interaction is not taken into account in assessing risk criteria for NIHL in industry. In addition to occupational noise, other noise sources such as military noise, vehicle noise, and, especially, exposure to free-time noise have become increasingly important for the development of NIHL. The nonoccupational noise exposure confounds the NIHL and, in many cases, overrules the occupational noise exposure.

Evaluation of the use of HPDS

The use of HPDs started in the early 1970s in most workplaces and since then has increased over time. In Nordic countries, in 1990s, about 60% of paper mill workers, 90% of shipyard workers, and 97% of forest workers reported that they used HPDs during the whole working time (7).

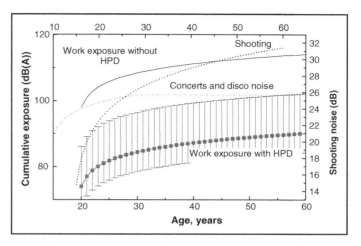

Figure 7.2 Example of prediction of hearing loss when environmental factors are included. The shipyard worker starts working at the age of 20 years in an impulsive noise environment of 98dB(A). The nominal attenuation of HPD is 24dB. He attends weekly discos and concerts with a mean sound pressure level of 98dB(A) for six hours. He starts visiting the discos at the age of 15 and stops at the age of 30. His hobby is hunting with annually 30 shots in the forest without HPD and 100 shots for targeting with HPDs. Abbreviation: HPD, hearing protective device.

Although the use rate is now at a very high level in some branches of industry, there is still room for improvement in other branches. The nominal attenuation, recommended by the manufacturers, varies from 11 to 35 dB, depending on the HPD and the frequency content of the noise. Whether this nominal attenuation is obtained is often questioned (34,35). For maximum attenuation, a use rate of over 99% is needed (EN 458-1993) and the HPD needs to be in good condition. The real protection provided by HPDs depends on the use rate. A case study among paper mill workers demonstrated that hearing loss among those who used HPDs on average 50% of the time was less than the hearing loss among those who never used HPDs. The difference could not be explained by the small change in exposure. Thus, even temporary use of HPDs provides some protection against hearing loss. However, the use of manufacturers' data for the evaluation of attenuation has been questioned by the several studies, suggesting that 3 to 18 dB should be subtracted from the protection values given by the manufacturer. At present, a proposal under preparation in Europe is that for custom-moulded HPDs 3 dB should be subtracted, for ear muffs 5 dB, and for ear plugs 8 dB. The HPDs attenuate industrial impulse noise even more effectively than steady-state continuous noise. This is due to the high content of high frequencies in impulses (36) that are attenuated effectively by earmuffs. Even though earmuffs reduce the impulse noise rate, workers in the metal industry are still exposed to more impulsive noise than workers in paper mills and forestry.

The use of HPDs gives best results with motivated users. Low motivation to wear HPDs is manifested as low use rates and low true attenuation values (37). Successful motivation can be obtained via appropriate education and training. The users must be informed about the effects of noise and the risks at work (2003/10/EC). Best results are obtained if personal audiometric data is used (38). This means that the education must be given privately. Users need training on the maintenance, installation, and use of HPDs. The attenuation of HPDs works well only if the HPDs are well maintained (EN 458-1993). Good maintenance consists of cleaning, changing of replaceable parts such as cushions, and overall monitoring of the state of the HPD. Installation must be done before entering the noisy area (EN 458-1993). If earplugs are used, special attention must be paid to the proper installation technique (34,37).

In branches of the military where large calibre weapons are used, recruiters face a high risk of developing NIHL. HPDs have shown to be less effective due to the nonlinearity of the attenuation against very high peak levels and the low frequency components of large calibre weapons. According to one study, workers exposed to occupational noise showed on average 5 dB greater hearing loss if during their conscript period they were exposed to the noise of large calibre weapons (39).

Although it is possible to obtain highly motivated users with proper education and training, the motivation tends to decrease over time. To avoid this, the education and training must be repeated consistently (38).

Measurement of hearing and evaluation of hearing Loss

Audiometry

Calibration of the audiometer, background noise in the measurement booth, instructions given to test subjects, and possible contamination with TTSs should be considered in the measurement protocol and included in the evaluation of hearing threshold. In practice, we recommend that the audiometry test starts at 1 kHz and that the tester evaluates the threshold in descending order. The hearing threshold is set when the subject correctly hears two out of three tone peeps at the lowest thresholds. Thereafter lower frequencies are tested, then the 1 kHz test frequency is repeated, and after that higher frequencies of 2, 3, 4, 6, and 8 kHz are tested. Measurement errors as much as 10 dB can occur in audiometric data if each of the items mentioned before is not controlled. In practice, the examiner should screen the accuracy of the audiometry each day by listening to the sound before making any evaluation of test subject's hearing level. The type of audiometer used (clinical, Bekesy, screening, bone conducting, or automatic) should be noted in the evaluation. This is because screening audiometry measures hearing at 20 dB HL level at best, whereas other audiometers are able to measure hearing threshold values at 0 dB level. The automatic audiometer has a step accuracy of 1 dB, in contrast to clinical audiometry that has a step width of 5 dB (Fig. 7.3). These all cause variability in the audiometric database and should be noted in the measurement protocol.

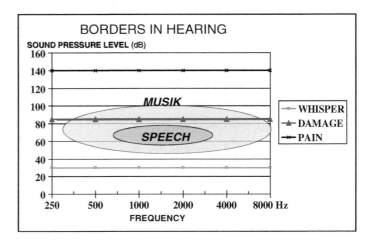

Figure 7.3 Thresholds for hearing and whisper; hearing damage limit and pain limit shown as a function of sound pressure level. Also sound pressure levels for speech and music are indicated.

Otoacoustic emission

The term otoacoustic emission (OAE) refers to sounds emitted by the ear (40). The emitted sounds originate from the electrical activation of outer hair cells that leads to mechanical contraction of the organ of Corti and may be helpful in the early identification of SNHL caused by occupational noise exposure. It must be stressed that OAE provides a statistical measure based on a large hair cell population. Three forms of OAE exist, all of which are evoked by particular stimuli. In the normal ear, spontaneous OAEs (SPOEAs) are present in the absence of acoustic stimulation among 70% of subjects. After even subtle lesions, the spontaneous oto-acoustic emissions (SOAE) seems to disappear (41). Thus absence of previously identified SOAE indicates a lesion in the contractile properties of the outer hair cells.

Transient-evoked OAEs (TOEAS) are elicited by brief stimuli such as clicks or tone pips. When two signals are averaged and compared, the repeatability of the signal can be ascertained. As parameters for hair cell damage, the amplitude of the signal over a specified frequency range and its repeatability can be used. Transient emissions are normally present when hearing loss is 20 dB or less. Thereafter transient oto-acoustic emissions (TOAEs) decrease in a nonlinear manner and are absent when the sound pressure level (SPL) is about 40 dB. This nonlinearity in the response and the absence of any early indication of incipient hearing loss limit the use of TOAE in diagnosis of SNHL (42,43).

Distortion product OAEs (DPOAEs) are elicited by a nonlinear interaction of two simultaneous long-lasting pure tones. The evoking tones are referred to as the f1 and f2 primaries in humans. The largest DPOAEs occur at a frequency equivalent to $2f_1$ to f_2. DPOAEs are widely used as a screening method for SNHL, and there is a moderately good correlation between SNHL and the output of DPOAE. In the assessment, the amplitudes at different frequencies are used for comparison (44). However, there is no physiological evidence to support the expectation that normal DPOAEs can predict pure tone thresholds directly. There are various ways by which the recording and interpretation of DPOAE can be improved. In comparing pure tone audiometry with DPOAE, Kimberley et al. (44) demonstrated a significant probability of false responses when the DPOAE amplitude is less than 6 dB above the noise floor.

Contralateral inhibition of the distortion product is recognised as a reduction in the amplitude of evoked OAE upon stimulation of the opposite ear.

OAEs are vulnerable to noxious agents such as ototoxic drugs, intense noise, and hypoxia, which are all known to affect the cochlea. They are absent with cochlear hearing loss greater than 35 dB. The type of OAE most commonly used for clinical purposes is TOAE. These are attractive for use as a screening procedure as the test procedure is short and no cooperation of the subject is needed. DPOAE may be more sensitive than TEOAE to discriminate subjects with NIHL (45). However, the value and accuracy of OAE in assessing NIHL have not yet been evaluated. So far few databases exist with data on OAE.

Assessment of NIHL

According to ISO 1999 (1990) (2), noise vulnerability is linked to the A-weighted sound energy entering to the ear. No changes in the audiogram are to be expected at speech frequencies if the A-weighted equivalent noise level is less than 80 dB. However, in most countries, if compensation is to be awarded, a higher level of 85 or 90 dB(A) is required. Although the new EU Directive (46) recognised that 80 dB can cause NIHL to the most susceptible people, a higher limit may be used for compensation. The criteria of NIHL outside the EU are country dependent and may include other criteria than those related to the audiogram, such as speech intelligibility. In clinical work, NIHL is acknowledged when the mean hearing loss exceeds 25 dB across speech frequencies and starts to cause problems with communication. Although this limit is arbitrary, it closely follows the normal threshold values for hearing defined by the World Health Organisation. Usually NIHL starts in the 3 to 6 kHz area where a typical notch in the audiogram can be observed. When the noise damage increases the notch becomes wider and deeper and the audiogram starts to flatten, indicating damage at speech frequencies. With prolonged and very severe noise exposure, the NIHL levels out across the high frequencies at 60 to 80 dB HL, but commonly low frequencies are less affected than high frequencies. Usually both ears are involved to the same extent, and if the interaural difference at speech frequencies exceeds 10 dB HL, inner ear damage should be assumed to be confounded by factors other than noise.

Often the occupational assistants who carry out industrial audiometry have little experience and education in the field of audiology. Earwax may not be removed and the ears may not have been inspected. We not infrequently observe workers with wax-blocked ear canals or with noise protection cotton left in the ear canal, and such situations may cause biased deterioration in the hearing threshold shift. On certain occasions, the subject may not understand the instructions and provides inaccurate responses, resulting in an unreliable audiogram. Instructions should be simple and given verbally before the test. Importantly the noise-free period should be 16 hours to allow hearing threshold measurement that is free from TTSs caused by environmental or occupational noise. Therefore, the audiometry test should be done as the first thing in the morning and the subject should not have been exposed to noise in the previous evening. Attention should be paid to the background noise in the audiometry booth, and this noise should be measured, as even at low frequencies it may mask the tone pips in the tested frequencies. In these instances, the 0-dB threshold values cannot be measured. As a rule, the background should not exceed 30 dB(A) in the booth to allow 0-dB threshold values to be measured. In industry, screening audiometry is performed for 20-dB hearing level at any frequency. For this purpose, background noise should not exceed 40 dB(A) in the booth.

For audiogram evaluation, the Occupational Safety and Health Administration (OSHA) uses the occurrence of a "standard threshold shift" (STS), defined as 10 dB or greater worsening over time in the average hearing threshold levels for 2, 3, and 4 kHz tones in either ear. NIOSH recommended an improved criterion for the detection of significant threshold shifts in workplace audiometric monitoring, the "15 dB twice" criterion. This is defined as 15 dB worsening at any frequency, 0.5 through 6 kHz, remaining present in two consecutive annual audiograms. Daniell et al. (47) evaluated a relatively large population in a longitudinal retrospective study of eight years with consecutive audiograms. None of the criteria used was accurate, and all the criteria produced significant numbers of false-positive audiograms. Based on the OSHA criteria, 36% of workers had at lest one threshold shift in seven years, and it was estimated by other criteria that the true value was 18%. The respective figures for NIOSH criteria were 54% and 35%.

Who then should be referred to an otologist? A worker with a 10 dB hearing change at two frequencies between the last two audiograms should be referred, as the change may indicate NIHL or an ear disorder. Also if the threshold shift is greater than 25 dB at any single frequency, the worker should be referred to an otologist. Also any subjects with possible conductive or inner ear disorders other than NIHL should be referred. Some inner ear diseases such as idiopathic tinnitus, Ménière's disease, otosclerosis, and sudden deafness may begin with a pure inner ear component affecting only hearing or masking the hearing as tinnitus may do. Infectious ear diseases such as chronic otitis media or tympanosclerosis cause hearing loss and should be identified.

In addition to a complete exposure history and audiograms, the case history must document other factors that may cause SNHL. These include head traumas, explosives, and use of vibrating tools. The possible use of ototoxic drugs such as streptomycin and cisplatin should be queried. Heavy use of anti-inflammatory agents as salicylates and indomethacin-type analgesics may cause reversible or nonreversible hearing loss and aggravate the NIHL (48).

Early detection of problems

Although individual models for the development of NIHL have been provided in a few of them (49,50), the studies have not been very successful so far. One reason may be inaccuracies in the evaluation of exposure data, in the use rate of hearing protectors or in estimations of sosioacusis and of socioacusis, especially in the detection of genetic factors.

One of the most confounding factors in assessing damage risk criteria for noise is the large variation, often exceeding 60 dB, in expected NIHL. This large variation means that in assessing the risk of noise damage in the workplace, a large number of subjects are needed before any conclusions can be reached. In order to reduce the number of subjects there are two possibilities:

1. Removal from the study sample of subjects having a non-NIHL
2. Taking into account the effect of individual risk factors for NIHL

Both these methods are disadvantageous. In the former alternative, a large number, perhaps a majority of subjects, are excluded from the analysis. In the latter alternative, the risk factors may play variable roles in the aetiology of hearing loss in different subjects and at different ages.

By taking a population having similar risk profiles the variation of results is reduced. In subjects with practically no risk factors, the effect of noise on hearing is evident (27). When subjects have a large number of risk factors for hearing loss, the effect of noise is severely masked by these risk factors. In the case of interaction of a chemical and noise, this effect may easily be masked in small populations unless the risk profile of the workers is taken into account.

Age as a confounder for NIHL

Several factors have been suspected as being the underlying cause of age-related hearing loss (presbyacusis), including hypertension, dietary habits, drugs, and social noise exposure. For example, Rosen and Olin (5) and Hincliffe (6) suggest that if all environmental and disease processes could be controlled, no prominent age-related hearing impairment could be demonstrated. Driscol and Royster (51) concluded in their study on the aetiology of age-dependent SNHL that existing databases are contaminated by environmental noise, leading to overestimation of the effect that age has on hearing. Stephens (52) examined consecutive presbyacusis patients seeking rehabilitation and found that in 93%, there was an underlying cause for presbyacusis. A prospective study of the causes of hearing loss in the elderly by Lim and Stephens (53) showed that in 83% of cases, a disease condition was associated with a hearing loss. About 30% of the subjects took ototoxic medications. Humes (54), in a critical review of the causes of hearing loss, found several confounding factors affecting age-related hearing loss.

To compare people of different ages, an age correction is usually made. The interaction of NIHL and presbyacusis does not yet seem to be well established (55). The uncertainty in the age correction might be diminished by selecting an internal control group. Usually a group that would be otologically screened and exposed to similar environmental stressors other than noise is not available. Robinson (13) focused on the problem of evaluating NIHL in an industrial population. He concluded that it is not generally realistic to compare such a population with an age-matched "otologically normal" baseline, since a noise-exposed population will include adventitious hearing loss as well as noise-related components. The lack of a well-documented baseline for data comparison makes it difficult to estimate hearing loss in different geographic areas by using standard forms. In baseline data adopted by Robinson and Sutton (21), the importance of age-related hearing loss in the context of industrial noise exposure is documented and also provides the basis of age-related changes in hearing loss. Although aging gives a crude estimate of the effect these biological factors have on hearing, age correction for individual cases can be misleading. In Robinson's study aging alone seems to influence NIHL to a smaller extent than would be expected in the ISO 1999 model.

Individual risk factors

Figure 7.4 demonstrates factors affecting noise susceptibility in man. The reciprocal connections and the weight of each factor vary from subject to subject. In order to prevent NIHL, all these factors should be analysed and documented, and based on the individual model, prevention should be commenced.

Several biological factors have been studied as possible aggravating factors for NIHL. In population surveys, advanced hearing loss in nonexposed populations has been attributed to biological (3,56) and environmental factors (6). Factors such as elevated blood pressure (57,58), altered lipid metabolism (5), the vibration syndrome (58,59), and genetic factors (60) are associated with NIHL.

An association between elevated blood pressure and NIHL has been described by some researchers (61–63), but the relationship has not been found in all studies (64). Animal studies have indicated that arterial hypertension accelerates age-related hearing loss (57,65). An antihypertensive medication may partly mask the effect of elevated blood pressure on NIHL (3). The effect of hypertension on hearing is promoted by other factors. Toppila et al. (27) showed among noise-exposed workers that age alone explained about 18% of the variance of NIHL in a linear model. Cholesterol levels correlated significantly with age, as did hypertension treatment and smoking. The older subjects also suffered more often from pain than the younger subjects and consequently used more analgesics. Therefore, presbyacusis was contaminated by several factors, each of which could affect hearing but mediated by somewhat

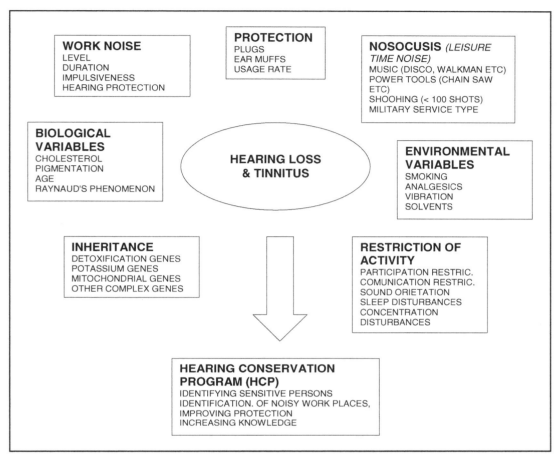

Figure 7.4 Summary diagram of factors influencing noise-induced hearing loss and outcome measures. *Abbreviation*: HCP, hearing conservation program.

different mechanisms. There is not sufficient evidence to show whether the effects of noise and hypertension are additive or synergistic. Smoking together with hypertension heightens the role of smoking in causing NIHL (66). Pyykkö et al. (3) studied noise-exposed workers and proposed that the predicted hearing loss at 4000 Hz should be corrected with the following factors: smoking 1.5 dB (23), cholesterol 1 dB at 4000 Hz (24), and hypertension 2 dB at 4000 Hz (6). The cholesterol-linked hearing loss is age dependent and is observed in subjects aged 40 years or over (67). Synergism occurs also between noise and solvents. In animal experiments, noise combined with a high level of styrene (600 ppm/m³) caused a threshold shift in hearing that is 30 dB greater than when the animals were exposed to noise or styrene alone (68). Such a high level of styrene is seldom encountered in industry, and solvent-linked NIHL is significantly less likely in man than demonstrated in this animal experiment.

Skin pigmentation seems to affect the vulnerability to NIHL. A study among African-Americans showed a somewhat better average hearing threshold levels than among Caucasians (49). This has been attributed to higher levels of melanocytes

and their capability to protect the inner ear against noise damage (69,70).

Many authors have found a significant and relatively large difference in vulnerability between men and women (2,71). These results may be explained by women's smaller exposure to free-time noise, especially to gunfire. In a recent study where these factors were controlled more accurately, no difference was found (33).

Evidence for genetic factors

There are insufficient data available on the relationship between NIHL and genetic background. Such data would be crucial in explaining the great variability of noise vulnerability in population studies. Several studies have estimated the heritability (the proportion of the population variance attributable to genetic variation) of age-related hearing loss. An extension of the Framingham Heart Study examined the heritability of human age-related hearing impairment and tried to identify the chromosomal regions involved (72). Audiometric examinations were conducted on 2263 original cohort members and 2217 offspring. Of these, 1789 individuals were members of 328 extended pedigrees used for linkage analysis. DeStefano et al. (72) found heritability of age-adjusted pure-tone average at medium and low frequencies to be 0.38 and 0.31, respectively. A good correlation was found with early onset of hearing loss and extent of presbyacusis within the family. In men, the relationship was not as evident as in females. In men, the exposure to environmental noise was a significant confounding factor.

Christensen et al. (73) conducted a population survey on the genetic influence on presbyacusis in twins aged 70 and older identified in Danish Twin Registry. In total, 2778 twins aged 70 to 76 were studied, and hearing was evaluated by questionnaire. The heritability was estimated using structural-equation analyses. Concordance rates, odds ratios, and correlations were consistently higher for monozygotic twin pairs than for dizygotic twin pairs in all age and sex categories, indicating heritable effects. The heritability of self-reported reduced hearing was 40% (95%, CI = 19–53%). The remaining variation could be attributed to individuals' nonfamilial environments.

Kaksonen et al. (74) studied a large pedigree with late-onset nonsyndromic hearing loss. They found weak evidence for a correlation between noise exposure and hearing loss among affected family members, but the levels of occupational and free-time noise exposures were quite low, seldom exceeding 90 dB. Those subjects who had passed military service demonstrated worse hearing, but this association could be biased by sex as women did not perform military service. They also found an association between the use of analgesics and hearing loss. The strongest association was with the use of non-steroid anti-inflammatory drugs (NSAID) analgesics, confirming the findings of some other studies (3,24). In the pedigree, the patients more often had vertigo with tinnitus than their normal hearing relatives. It is likely that a similar degeneration in the vestibular end organ occurs, similar to that in the cochlea that can be measured with audiograms. This may explain the presence of vertigo in some genetic disorders, for example, in DFNA9. Although case histories indicate that some vestibular disorders such as Meniere's disease can arise by extensive noise trauma, the evidence of linkage between NIHL and vestibular deficit is still not documented.

Identifying the genetic susceptibility factors

Many genes have been identified that when mutated cause mendelian forms of hearing impairment (see Chap. 5). Genetically induced hearing loss in nonsyndromic form is often difficult to separate from NIHL. It is often age dependent and worsens with aging. Therefore, genes identified as causing mendelian forms of hearing loss have been good candidate

susceptibility factors for age-related and noise-induced loss. Mutations of large effect might cause the mendelian forms, whereas mutations with much smaller functional effects could act as susceptibility factors. The scientific basis of the linkage and association methods used is described in Chapter 6.

In the extended Framingham study, quantitative measures from audiometric examinations were tested for linkage to markers from a genome-wide scan in this population-based sample ascertained without respect to hearing status. The outcome traits for linkage analysis were pure-tone average at medium (0.5, 1.0, and 2.0 kHz) and low (0.25, 0.5, and 1.0 kHz) frequencies adjusted for cohort, sex, age, age squared, and age cubed. The analysis did not identify any statistically significant lod scores, but several locations showed suggestive evidence of linkage. Of particular interest are the regions 11p [maximum multipoint lod score (MLOD), 1.57], 11q13.5 (MLOD, 2.10), and 14q (MLOD, 1.55), which overlap with genes known to cause congenital deafness, for example, Usher syndrome. In this study, there was evidence that genetic and environmental factors contribute to hearing loss in the mature human population. However, the study was inconclusive as to whether the same genes cause presbyacusis and congenital hearing loss.

Of particular interest are genes where the mutants show inner ear structural changes similar to those seen in age-related or noise-induced loss. It is notable that actin structures appear to be structurally damaged as a consequence of noise exposure and aging (75). Actin is one of the major proteins responsible for providing the structural basis for hair cell shape, and Chan et al. (76) have demonstrated that acoustic overstimulation causes reversible reduction in the stiffness of the outer hair cells. Zhu et al. (77) have determined that mutations in g-actin are the basis for hearing loss in four families affected with DFNA20/26. Persons affected with the DFNA20/26 disorders display sensorineural hearing loss that, like age related hearing loss gene (AHL), begins in high frequencies and steadily progresses to include all frequencies. DPOAE data are consistent with a cochlear site of lesion. Thus people with minor abnormalities in the actin genes may be more susceptible to NIHL.

Genetic analysis in mice has identified three loci (Ahl, Ahl2, and Ahl3) involved in age-related hearing loss, as described in Chapter 6. Several functional studies have reported that the Ahl gene renders mice more susceptible to NIHL than strains that do not carry this gene (78–80). Harding and Bohne (81) exposed the mice to 4 kHz octave band noise for four hours. They observed sizeable variation in the magnitude of TTSs, PTS, and hair-cell loss among mice of the same genetic strain. The congenic B6.CAST ± Ahl male mice had significantly less TTS immediately postexposure than C57BL/6J males or females but not less PTS or hair-cell losses at 20 days postexposure. These results indicate that, at one month of age, mice carrying two copies of the Ahl gene have an increased susceptibility to TTS from low-frequency noise before they have any indication of age-related hearing or hair-cell loss. However, this appeared not to be the case for PTS. The Ahl gene appears to play a role in susceptibility to NIHL, but the authors point out that other genes as well as systemic and local factors are involved. Because of the similarities between the human and mouse auditory systems, the genes causing AHL in mice may also identify homologous human genes. The mouse *Ahl* allele is a single-nucleotide variant in the *Cdh23* (*cadherin 23*) gene; it is not clear whether a similar functional variant exists in humans, and if so whether it can explain any of age related or NIHL.

Recent studies have shed light on the genetic background on caspase activation, including mitogen-activated protein kinases and p53. Cheng et al (82) suggested that p53 is activated by noise oppoture initiating apoptous. Also genes involved in potassium recycling in the exmer ear are respected to cause nubnerclarity to noise (83).

Mitochondrial genes

It is also possible that mitochondrial gene defects may cause NIHL, as hearing in noise is a high-energy consuming process. The prevalence of these mutations in the population and their association with NIHL has not been documented yet. Most studies are difficult to interpret, either because the patient selection criteria are too imprecise or because they focus only on families with probable maternal inheritance of hearing impairment, or else only a subset of possible mutations was investigated. In addition, virtually all previous studies have been conducted in localised populations, so that their wider relevance is unclear.

Many previous reports in the literature have identified matrilineal pedigrees in which mitochondrial DNA mutations are associated with isolated nonsyndromic deafness. The most commonly reported such mutations are *A1555G* (84), *A7445G* (85,86), *7472insC* (87,88), and *A3243G* (89,90); the latter mutation is also found in families with more severe, syndromic disease. Assignment of these mutations as pathological is based upon their absence from unaffected families, their ability to produce a biochemical phenotype in cultured cell models such as rho-zero cybrids, and demonstrable effects on mitochondrial protein synthesis (91–96). A number of other mutations in tRNA$^{Ser(UCN)}$, i.e., *T7510C* (97,98), *T7511C* (99,100), and *T7512C* (101), as well as another mutation in 12S rRNA, *C1494T* (102), have been reported in cases of similar phenotypes (syndromic hearing impairment in the case of *T7512C*). This tRNA as well as tRNA$^{Leu(UUR)}$ may be hotspots for such mutations, although other tRNAs have not been systematically excluded.

According to Jacobs et al. (103), the specific case of the *A1555G* mutation presents additional problems. It was originally reported in matrilineal pedigrees and singleton cases with acute aminoglycoside ototoxicity, as well as in some families with nonsyndromic deafness but no known aminoglycoside exposure (84,86). More recent studies have revealed the mutation in a substantial proportion (up to approximately 25%) of cases of late-onset, familial, sensorineural deafness in Spain (104–106). However, studies in other populations, including other European countries, have reported it only at a much lower frequency, typically 1% to 2% of cases (107,108), although the groups of patients studied were not always identically defined. The majority of Spanish A1555G patients have no recorded history of aminoglycoside use. Such use is very rare in, for example, Nordic countries today. Since the mutation is found on diverse haplogroup backgrounds amongst Spanish patients (105), founder effects seem an unlikely explanation. Multiple founder effects in a population that is otherwise not untypical of the European norm would have to be invoked. This leaves two other plausible explanations. Either there is some systematic difference in the way patients have been recruited or defined in Spain versus other countries or else environmental factors such as unrecorded aminoglycoside exposure or local dietary components may account for the difference. Lehtonen et al. (109) reported that in Northern Finland, the prevalence of A1555G was 2.6% in a highly selected population with sensorineural hearing loss. Confirming their findings, in our recent study, we found A1555G mutations in 3/500 subjects visiting a tertiary referral centre for hearing loss (Jacobs H. unpublished observation). Thus in Nordic countries mutations linked to A1555G seem not to be important in the aetiology of NIHL (103).

Mitochondrial haplogroup affiliations and hearing impairment

The background and emigration of populations can be traced according to their membership of ancient matrilineal clans defined by founder polymorphisms in mtDNA. These haplogroups and their sub-branches [haplogroup clusters (HVs)] show subtle differences between populations (110), for example, east–west and north–south clines within Europe (western Eurasia). Previously, associations between specific haplogroups or HVs have been reported with a variety of disorders, including male infertility (111), Parkinson's Disease (112), Alzheimer's and other types of dementia (113,114), and multiple sclerosis (115), as well as with longevity in different populations (116,117). Not all these studies are congruent, however, and virtually no evidence is available to support a specific functional role in the pathogenesis of polymorphisms characteristic of, or unique to, specific haplogroup backgrounds. Nevertheless, a general trend is evident, in that the most common European haplogroup H, or the HV to which it belongs, is associated more frequently than expected, given its overall population frequency, with disease or short lifespan (103). So far, it is not known whether specific haplogroups are linked to any hearing loss or increase in susceptibility to NIHL. However, studies conducted on identical twins favour the idea of genetic background for increased vulnerability or predisposition.

Jacobs et al. (103) have recently focused on the assessment of possible associations between the haplogroups and hearing loss. Lehtonen (109) found an increased number of rare polymorphisms amongst Finnish patients with sensorineural hearing impairment, compared with controls, consistent with at least some of them being mildly deleterious mutations contributing collectively to the phenotype. Several recent papers have suggested that mitochondrial haplogroup can influence the disease phenotype of patients carrying other mtDNA mutations. Thus, the A12308G polymorphism, diagnostic for the U.K. HV, seems to be associated with a more severe phenotype, including retinopathy, short stature, and cardiac defects, amongst patients with mtDNA deletions (118). However, Torroni et al. (119) failed to find any haplogroup associations underlying phenotypic variability of A3243G patients.

The data of Jacobs et al. (103) suggest a distortion towards HV amongst patients with early-onset but postlingual hearing impairment, at least compared with population controls or patients with presbyacusis. The fact that this applies to two geographically distinct populations supports it as being meaningful, but it is of only borderline statistical significance. A recent study demonstrated statistically significant haplogroup differences between adult Finnish controls and a healthy cohort of individuals aged 90 to 91 from the same geographical area, on the basis of which they proposed a haplogroup association with healthy aging. Whatever the underlying cause of this phenomenon, it suggests that "population controls" may not be rigorous enough to demonstrate haplogroup associations with hearing loss, and that tightly age-matched controls might be needed. The bias in HV would suggest that polymorphisms that have arisen uniquely on the HV background may contribute to hearing loss (103).

The need for further research

There is an urgent need for population studies in the EU to clarify the role of genetic factors in the aetiology of NIHL. It has been suggested that as much as 60% of NIHL may be linked to genetic factors (120). A modern database should therefore include possible indications of a genetic background for NIHL. The complete case history should include questions on possible hard-of-hearing relatives in the pedigree. This is also the aim in the new EU-based noise control directive.

We are currently performing a study of a number of gene loci known to cause mendelian forms of hearing loss in a large sample of EU citizens with hearing loss. So far no significant clusters of gene mutations have been found that would indicate increased noise sensitivity [EU age related hearing impairment (ARHI) project, 2005]. It seems likely that the genes currently identified through family studies are not the major loci responsible for noise vulnerability or aging.

Hearing conservation program

The primary goal of an industrial hearing conservation program (HCP) is prevention (or, at least, limitation) of NIHL associated with exposure to industrial noise (121). Other goals

may be formulated in addition to this primary goal, such as reduction of employees' stress and absenteeism and reduction of workplace accidents. An HCP is costly and demands resources and personnel. Often due to these factors only selected personnel who are in high risk for the development of NIHL are tested audiologically, whereas newly employed persons are not tested. If a hearing test is not carried out before starting to work, it may be difficult later to show that the hearing loss is of preemployment origin. It is strongly recommended that all person entering jobs with a risk of developing NIHL should be tested.

Several HCPs have been launched in order to better understand the effect of occupational noise on the human ear (49,122–124). Some recent HCPs utilise database analysis programs comparing data on the noise emission level and including evaluation of factors other than workplace noise (50,125). These programs may take into consideration, for instance, the association of aging, nonoccupational noise, and medical history (125). Other researchers use models based on risk analysis in which the relative importance of various factors as well as workplace noise is considered (3,59). Only few programs actively monitor the use of personal hearing protectors and their attenuation efficacy. The OSHA (126) requires employers with excessively noisy jobs to maintain a continuing and effective HCP, providing personal hearing protecting devices, annual training, and annual audiometric monitoring for exposed workers. The employer must monitor individuals' audiograms for occurrence of STS, defined as 10 dB or greater worsening over time in the average hearing threshold levels of 2, 3, and 4 kHz tones in either ear. When STS is documented, the employer is required to notify the individual worker, provide retraining and refitting of hearing protectors, and make any necessary referral for otological evaluation.

One major problem in HCPs is establishing individual baseline values. Royster and Royster (50) demonstrated a significant improvement of age-corrected audiograms when the subjects were annually tested over six years. The improvement was interpreted as due to the training effect but depended on the noise emission level. Also, those with prominent hearing loss had less training effect. Royster and Royster (50) proposed that the audiogram showing the best hearing at frequencies of 500 to 6000 Hz should form the baseline level. Thus any audiometric evaluation used in a HCP should be based on a serial audiogram, and the database should include some expert programs to validate the data in order to establish baseline values for hearing and also to calculate hearing loss.

The components of an effective HCP are as follows (127):

1. Measurement of work-area noise levels
2. Identification of overexposed employees
3. Reduction of hazardous noise exposure to the extent possible through engineering and administrative control
4. Provision of HPD if other controls are inadequate
5. Initial and periodic education of workers and management
6. Motivation of workers to comply with HCP policies

7. Professional audiogram review and recommendations
8. Follow-up for audiometric changes
9. Detailed record-keeping system for the entire HCP
10. Professional supervision of HCP

One observes that many of these above-mentioned tasks are not well defined. The exposure evaluation is not a simple straightforward task, and comparison of audiograms is not easy, due to large variations in NIHL and the strong effect of age.

The use of HPDs gives best results with motivated users. Low motivation to wear HPDs is seen as low usage rates and low true attenuation values (37). A successful motivation can be obtained via appropriate education and training. The users must be informed about the effects of noise and the risks at work (89/188/EEC, 2003/10/EC). Best results are obtained if personal audiometric data is used (38). This means that the education must be given privately. Users need training on maintenance, installation, and the use of HPDs. The attenuation of protectors works well only if they are well maintained (EN 458-1993). Good maintenance consists of cleaning, changing of replaceable parts such as cushions, and overall monitoring of the state of the HPD. Installation must be done before entering the noisy area (EN 458-1993). If earplugs are used, special attention to the proper installation technique must be paid (37).

Although it is possible to obtain highly motivated users with proper education and training, the motivation tends to decrease over time. To avoid this, the education and training must be repeated consistently (38).

The data should preferably refer to a large international database of individual worker information to include the individual susceptibility factors and thereby provide personalised HCP.

The approach to the protection of workers described in the directive 2003/10/EC is based on the identification of the risks in the workplace. The identification includes the effect of impulse noise, interaction with vibration and ototoxic chemicals, and effect noise and hearing protection of risk of accident. Also the groups susceptible to noise must be identified. If there is risk of NIHL, the employer must develop a HCP (Fig. 7.5). In HCP, the first task is to evaluate the sources of noise and the possibilities to reduce the levels by technical means. If reduction of the noise source is not possible, the workers should be provided with HPDs and the workers should be informed about the risks and the correct use of the selected HPDs in an appropriate way.

These guidelines are not sufficient for practical purposes. The following problems must be solved:

- How to guarantee that the HPDs are used properly
- How to discover risky workplaces or tasks
- Addressing protective measures against the relevant noise source, especially if the greatest exposure occurs in free time is difficult.

By solving these questions, the minimal legal requirements of a HCP will be achieved. A good HCP contains additional

elements. These elements are added to increase the power of the HCP.

Objectives of the database

The database should be multidisciplinary, and the extent of hearing loss should be studied as a function of environmental noise exposure, individual sensitivity factors, interacting diseases, and genetic background, as indicated with the recent EU-based noise directive. In assessment of these factors, artificial intelligence may be used to create a complete HCP valid for individual subjects. The database should include the following components:

1. Information on separate and combined exposures for occupational noise
2. Information on use of hearing protecting device and type
3. Information on separate and combined effects of free-time noise
4. Information of human (risk) factors on hearing impairment
5. Information of interaction of diseases on hearing impairment
6. Information of genetic factors in the aetiology of hearing impairment
7. Relevant audiological test results
8. Otologic history and examination
9. The impact of hearing impairment on the quality of life

A functionally customer friendly database program should contain three major parts: the database, inference engine, and interface. The purpose of the interface is to provide easy access for the user to view the data or add new cases. The inference engine assists the user to combine different noise sources to generate a single index of exposure and determine the efficacy of hearing protectors against noise. It also should warn against excessive noise sensitivity and print out the risk factors for NIHL at individual level.

The inference engine should be based on knowledge and decision-making rules, because the purpose of HCP is to assist in minimising the risk of developing hearing loss. Usually the executive part is composed from abstract grammar or algorithms (e.g., genetic algorithms, neural networks, and decision trees). The engine calculates different ways of classifying the data, based on a set of training examples. The risk models should by preference be based on the ISO model; new models may emerge from the analysis. In a sophisticated form, the database can be used to formulate individual HCPs.

Quality of life

The psychosocial consequences of environmental noise are widespread, in addition to measurable hearing loss. Thus,

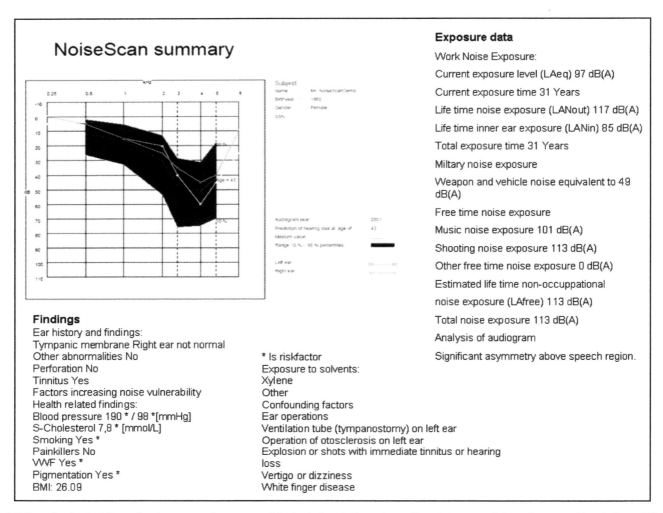

Figure 7.5 Example of output from a hearing conservation program data sheet given to the customer. Note that a copy of the audiogram and its relation to ISO standard, lifetime noise dose, environmental and work dose, and individual risk factors are displayed.

reduced oral communication is a social handicap. NIHL also reduces the perception of warning signals, exposing to subjects to unwanted events such as accidents and distortion of environmental sounds fields or music. Consequently, NIHL may lead to social isolation, decreased worker productivity and morale, and an increase in job-related accidents. The effects of NIHL are often misperceived. On first questioning, most workers do not associate their listening and communication difficulties with their hearing loss as assessed by audiometry.

Below is the diagram of International Classification of Function that describes the dimensions causing the handicap in NIHL (Fig. 7.6). NIHL is insidious and progressive in nature and is invisible. At no time is there a sudden noticeable change in hearing. The loss of frequency resolution is unknown to people. Affected workers attribute their difficulties to fatigue, lack of interest or concentration, poor articulation of speakers, and excessive background noise. Interaction with these people reveals inconsistent behaviour and is attributed to an unwillingness to communicate.

The awareness of hearing difficulties is further hampered by the stigma associated with deafness. The experience of hearing difficulties has a strong negative impact on self-image, which manifests itself as a sense of being incompetent, perceiving oneself as abnormal, physically diminished, prematurely old, or having a defect (128). Any sign of impairment is seen as a sign of weakness, thus concealment is adopted as a strategy. When NIHL is moderate to severe, it leads to speech distortion, reduced word discrimination, noise intolerance, and tinnitus. NIHL may be a limiting factor of quality of life, and in short inventories hearing loss–related problems are reflected in reduced mobility and in mood of the subject [for example in European quality of life (EQoL) 5D (129) and in 15D (130)]. Therefore a database should by some means also record factors related to quality of life. In Europe, one instrument that is relatively simply to use and needs only a few questions answering is EQoL 5D. Other instruments used in Europe are the quality-of-life instruments 15D and SF 12 (131) that also include a question on hearing ability.

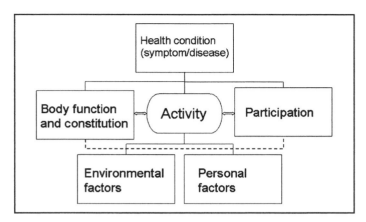

Figure 7.6 Components of international classification of function in evaluating effect of disorder on the performance of the subject in society.

Construction of a modern database program

The interface between the subject and database may be interactive as was previously common when the nurse or doctor took the exposure history (4,25). It may be based on questionnaires that can be scanned later or an interview with a person with direct access to a database or can be interactive when the person fills the database by himself through the computer (4). The modern possibility to operate the questionnaire through Internet is useful in large surveys as in recruiting persons in military bases or in assessing hearing loss in large factories. Interactive questioning with direct input into the database is most commonly used by midsize and small industries where the occupational nurse will feed the data in of the case histories (25). Paper-based questionnaires are mostly used in field studies and in cross-sectional studies. Commonly the questionnaires are scanned in with a text scanner and screened for possible error. Specific software and text scanners reduce the rate of input errors. An example of a questionnaire for NIHL is documented in Appendix I. We have recently launched an Internet-based questionnaire, where the subject can input the data at home or in the office. Security is guaranteed and the subject has the right to fill in the questionnaire and correct it up to the point when it is ready to be submitted. This model is available for demonstration at www.equicare.fi (132).

Summary

NIHL is insidious and progressive in nature and is invisible. At no time is there a sudden noticeable change in hearing. To prevent workers from hearing loss several efforts have been made: regulation of noise exposure, use of personal hearing protectors, and establishment of HCP among others. These efforts may be useful on a large scale, but still sensitive subjects may become affected by noise injury. Several important questions remain to be solved, including genetic susceptibility to noise trauma, individual risk factors and their role, and age factors. One of the approaches that should be applied to all workplaces is to establish a common database for hearing conservation. This should include (i) screening of workers who may be at a risk of developing NIHL in selected work tasks or sites, (ii) warning against excessive noise pollution in selected work tasks or sites, (iii) allowing comparative assessment of success among various HCPs, and finally (iv) calling to attention individual susceptibility. To fulfil these demands, the common database must include all known factors that affect hearing loss. Such factors are audiometric testing methods, the testing environment, the type and use of hearing protectors, and exposure to military and leisure time noise. It must provide accurate data from lifetime noise exposure in various jobs or work tasks. Finally, confounding factors must be controlled, such as genetic inheritance, elevated blood pressure, the presence of vibration-induced white finger syndrome, elevated serum cholesterol level, and use of various ototoxic drugs. Such factors can explain a significant part of the variation in the extent of hearing loss in individual cases. In the present database, we have attempted to include such factors known to be relevant for HCP.

References

1. Robinson DW. Estimating the risk of hearing loss due to continuous noise. In: Robinson DW, ed. Occupational Hearing Loss. London: Academic Press, 1971.
2. ISO 1999 (1990). Acoustics—Determination of occupational noise exposure and estimation of noise induced hearing impairment. International Organization for Standardization, Geneva.
3. Pyykkö I, Koskimies K, Starck J, Pekkarinen J, Färkkilä M, Inaba R. Risk factors in the genesis of sensorineural hearing loss in Finnish forestry workers. Br J Ind Med 1989; 46:439–446.
4. Toppila E, Pyykkö I, Starck J, Kaksonen R, Ishizaki H. Individual risk factors in the development of noise-induced hearing loss. Noise Health 2000; 8:59–70.
5. Rosen S, Olin P. Hearing loss and coronary heart disease. Arch Otolaryngol 1965; 82:236–243.
6. Hincliffe R. Epidemiology of sensory-neural hearing loss. Audiology 1973; 12:446–452.
7. Toppila E, Pyykkö I, Starck J. The use of hearing protectors among forest, shipyard and paper mill workers in Finland - a longitudinal study. Noise Health 2005; 7(26):3–9.
8. Kryter KD. Damage risk criterion and contours based on permanent and temporary hearing loss data. J Am Ind Hyg Assoc 1965; 26:34–44.
9. Kryter KD, Ward WD, Miller JD, Eldredge DH. Hazardous exposure to intermittent and steady-state noise. J Acoust Soc Am 1966; 39:451–464.
10. Baughn W. Relation between daily exposure and hearing loss based on evaluation of 6835 industrial noise exposure cases. US Air Force 1973; Rep. AMRL-TR-7353.
11. Baughn W. Noise control—Percent of population protected. Int Audiol 1966; 5:331–338.

12. Burns W, Robinson DW. Hearing and noise in industry. Her Majesty's Stationery Office 1970.

13. Robinson DB, Shipton MS. Tables for the estimation of noise-induced hearing loss. NPL Acoustics Rep Ac 61. 2nd ed. British A.R.C., 1977.

14. Robinson DW. The relationship between hearing loss and noise exposure. NPL Aero Rep Ac 32. British A.R.C., 1968.

15. Burns W, Permanents effects of noise on hearing. In: Burns W, eds. Noise and Man. 2nd ed. John Murray London, 1973.

16. Suter A. The development of federal noise standards and damage risk criteria. In: Lipscomb D, ed. Hearing Conservation in Industry, Schools and the Military. San Diego: Singular publishing Group, 1994.

17. Passchier-Vermeer W. Hearing loss due to continuous exposure to steady-state broad-band noise. J Acoust Soc Am 1974; 46(5):1585–1593.

18. Glorig A, Nixon J. Distribution of hearing loss in various populations. Ann Otol Rhinol Laryngol 1960; 69(2):497–516.

19. Johnson D. Prediction of NIPTS due to continuous noise exposure. US Air Force 1973; Rep. AMRL-TR-73-91.

20. ISO 1999 (1975). Acoustics - Determination of occupational noise exposure and estimation of noise induced hearing impairment. International Organization for Standardization, Geneva.

21. Robinson DW, Sutton GJ. Age effects in hearing—a comparative analysis of published threshold data. Audiology 1979; 18:320–334.

22. Glorig A, Roberts JJ. Hearing levels of adults by age and sex: United States 1960–1962, Rep. PHS-PUB-100-SER-11-11, Nat Cent health serv res dev, Oct 1965.

23. Rowland M. Basic data on hearing levels of adults 25–74 years. DHEW Publ no (PHS) 80-1663, series 11, no 215 US dep Health, Educ and Welfare, Jan 1980.

24. Pyykkö I, Starck J, Toppila E, Juhola M, Auramo Y, Ishizaki H. Motivation for the hearing program-factors explaining the variability in hearing losses. In: Prasher D, Luxon L, Pyykkö I, eds. Advances in Noise Research: Protection against noise. Vol. 2. London: Whurr Publishers Ltd, 1998:224–230.

25. Pyykkö I, Toppila E, Starck J, Juhola M, Auramo Y. Database for a hearing conservation program. Scand Audiol 2000; 29:52–58.

26. Liu Chang-Chun, Pekkarinen J, Starck J. Application of the probe microphone method to measure attenuation of hearing protectors against high impulse sound levels. Appl Acoustics 1989; 27:13–25.

27. Toppila E, Pyykkö I, Starck J. Age and noise-induced hearing loss. Scand J Audiol 2001; 30:236–244.

28. ISO 9612.2 (1997) Acoustics—Guidelines for the measurements and assessments of exposure to noise in working environment, International Organization for Standardization, Geneva.

29. Campo P, Lataye PR. Intermittent noise and equal energy hypothesis. In: Dancer, et al., eds. Noise-Induced Hearing Loss. Mosby year Book. St. Louis: publ, 1992:456–466.

30. Smith P, Davis A, Ferguson M, Lutman M. The prevalence and type of social noise exposure in young adults. Noise Health 2000; 6:41–56.

31. Airo E, Pekkarinen J, Olkinuora P. Listening to music with earphones: an assessment of noise exposure. Acustica united with acta acustica, 1996; 82, 8:885–894.

32. Laitinen H, Toppila E, Olkinuora P, Kuisma K. Sound exposure among the Finnish national opera personnel. Appl Occup Environ Hyg 2003; 18(3):177–182.

33. Davis AC, Lovell EA, Smith PA, Ferguson MA. The contribution of social noise to tinnitus in young people—a preliminary report. Noise Health 1998; 1(1):40–46.

34. Berger E, Franks J, Lindgren F. International review of field studies of hearing protector attenuation. In: Axelsson A, Borchgrevink H, Hamenik RP, Hellström P, Hendersson D, Salvi RJ, eds. Scientific Basis of Noise-Induced Hearing loss. New York: Thieme Medical Publication, 1983.

35. Toppila E. What kind of protectors are used in the EU and is their use mandatory? In: Prasher D, Luxon L, Pyykkö I, eds. Advances in Noise Research: Protection Against Noise. Vol. 2. London: Whurr Publishers Ltd, 1998:164–166.

36. Starck J, Pekkarinen J, Pyykkö I. Impulse noise and hand-arm vibration in relation to sensory neural hearing loss. Scand J Environ Health 1988; 14:265–271.

37. Foreshaw S, Cruchley J. Hearing protector problems in military operations. In: Alberti P, ed. Personal Hearing Protection in Industry. New York: Raven Press, 1981 (sivut).

38. Lipscomb DM. The employee education program. In: Lipscomb DM, ed. Hearing Conservation in Industry, Schools and the Military. San Diego: Singular publishing group inc., 1994:81–230.

39. Pekkarinen J, Iki M, Starck J, Pyykkö I. Hearing loss risk from exposure to shooting impulses in workers exposed to occupational noise. Br J Audiol 1993; 27:175–182.

40. Kemp DT. Evidence of mechanical nonlinearity and frequency selective wave amplification in the cochlea. Arch Otorhinonlaryngol 1979; 224:37–45.

41. Furst M, Reshef J, Attias J. Manifestations of intense noise stimulations on spontanous emissios and threshold microstucture: experiment and model. J Acoust Soc Am 1992; 91:1003–1013.

42. Avan P, Bonfils P. Frequency specifity of human distortion product otoacoustic emissions. Audiology 1993; 32:12–26.

43. Harris FP, Probst R. Otoaucoustic emissions and audiometric outcomes. In: Robinette MS, Glattke TJ, eds. Otoacoustic Emissions: Clinical Applications. New York: Thieme, 1997:151–180.

44. Kimberley BP, Brown DK, Allen JB. Distortion product emissions aqnd sensorineural hearing loss. In: Robinette MS, Glattke TJ, eds. Otoacoustic Emissions: Clinical Applications. New York: Thieme, 1997:180–204.

45. Oeken J. Typical findings of distortion product otoacoustic emissions (DPOAE). In: Prasher D, ed. Occupational Noise-Induced Hearing Loss. Vol. 1. Biological Effects of Noise. London: Luxon L, Whurr I Publisher Ltd, 1998:193–204.

46. 2003/10/EC Council directive on the minimum health and safety requirements regarding the exposure of workers to the risks arising from physical agents (noise), Brussels 2003.

47. Daniell WE, Stover BD, Takaro TK. Comparison of criteria for significant threshold shift in workplace hearing conservation programs. J Occup Environ Med 2003; 45:295–304.

48. Grifo S. Aspirin ototoxicity in the Guinea pig. ORL 1975; 37:27–34.

49. Royster LH, Lilley LT, Thomas WG. Recommended criteria for evaluating effectiveness of hearing conservation program. Am Ind Hyg Assoc 1980; 41:40–48.

50. Royster JD, Royster LH. Using audiometric data base analysis. J Occup Med 1986; 28:1055–1068.

51. Driscoll DP, Royster L. Comparisons between the median hearing threshold levels for an black non-industrial noise exposed population (NINEP) and four presbycusis data bases. Am Ind Hyg Assoc J 1984; 45:577–593.

52. Stephens SGD. Clinical investigation of hearing loss in the elderly. In: Stephens SGD, ed. Adult Audiology, Part II Scott-Brown's Otolaryngology. London: Butterworths, 1982:142–143.

53. Lim D, Stephens SGD. Clinical investigation of hearing loss in the elderly. In: Stephens D, ed. Causes of Hearing Loss in Adults. Adult Audiology. Scott-Brown's otolaryngology. London: Butterworths, 1987.

54. Humes LE. Noise-induced hearing loss as influenced by other agents and by some physical characteristics of the individual. J Acoust Soc Am 1984; 76:1318–1329.

55. Rössler G. Progression of hearing loss caused by occupational noise. Scand Audiol 1994; 23:13–37.

56. Chung DY, Willson GN, Cannon RP, Mason K. In: Hammernik RP, Henderson D, Salvi R, eds. Individual Susceptibility to Noise. New Perspectives on Noise-Induced Hearing Loss. New York: Raven Press, 1982:511–519.

57. McCormic G, Harris DT, Hartley CB, Lassiter RBH. Spontaneous genetic hypertension in the rat and its relationship to reduced cochlear potentials: implications for preservation of human hearing. Proc Natl Acad Sci USA 1982; 79:26–68.

58. Pyykkö I, Koskimies K, Starck J, Pekkarinen J, Inaba R. Evaluation of factors affecting sensory neural hearing loss. Acta otolaryngol (Stockh) 1988; 449:155–160.

59. Pyykkö I, Pekkarinen J, Starck J. Sensory-neural hearing loss in forest workers. An analysis of risk factors. Int Arch Occup Environ Health 1986; 59:439–454.

60. Gates GA, Couropmitree NN, Meyers RH. Genetic associations in age-related hearing thresholds. Arch Otol Head Neck Surg 1999; 125:654–659.

61. Johansson A, Hansson L. Prolonged exposure to a stressful stimulus (noise) as a cause of raised blood pressure in man. Lancet 1977; 1:86–87.

62. Andren L, Lindstedt G, Bjorkman M, Borg KO, Hansson L. Effect of noise on blood pressure and stress hormones. Clin Sci (Lond) 1982; 62(2):137–141.

63. Talbott E, Helmkamp J, Matthews K, Kuller L, Cottington E, Redmont G. Occupational noise exposure, noise-inclued hearing loss, and the epidemiology of high blood pressure. Am J Epidemiol 1985; 121: 501–514.

64. Drettner B, Hedstrand H., Klockhoff I, Svedberg A. Cardiovascular risk factors and hearing loss. Acta Otolaryngol 1975; 79:366–371.

65. Borg E. Noise-induced hearing loss in normotensive and spontaneously hypertensive rats. Hear Res 1982; 8:117.

66. Starck J, Toppila E, Pyykko I. Smoking as a risk factor in sensory neural hearing loss among workers exposed to occupational noise. Acta Otolaryngol 1999; 119(3):302–305.

67. Nieminen O, Pyykkö I, Starck J, Toppila E, Iki M. Serum cholesterol and blood pressure in the genesis of noise induced hearing loss. In: Olofsson J, ed. Transactions of the XXV Congress of the Scandinavian Oto-Laryngological Society. Bergen, Norway: Daves Tryckeri, 2000:48–50.

68. Mäkitie A. The ototoxic effect of styrene and its interactions with an experimental study in rats. Helsinki: Academic dissertation University of Helsinki, Helsinki University Hospital, 1997.

69. Barrenäs M, Lindgren F. The influence of eye color on susceptibility to TTS in humans. Br J Audiol 1991; 25:203–207.

70. Barrenäs M. Pigmentation and noise-induced hearing loss: is the relationship between pigmentation and noise-induced hearing loss due to an ototoxic pheolaminin interaction or to otoprotective eumelan effects. In: Prasher D, ed. Advances in Noise Research. Vol. 1. Biological Effects of Noise. London: L Luxon, Whurr Publisher Ltd, 1998:59–70.

71. Berger E, Royster L, Thomas W. Presumed noise-induced permanent threshold shift resulting from exposure to an A-weighted Leq of 89 dB. J Acoust Soc Am 1978; 64(1):192–197.

72. DeStefano AL, Gates GA, Heard-Costa N, Myers RH, Baldwin CT. Genomewide linkage analysis to presbyacusis in the Framingham Heart Study. Arch Otolaryngol Head Neck Surg 2003; 129(3):285–289.

73. Christensen K, Frederiksen H, Hoffman HJ. Genetic and environmental influences on self-reported reduced hearing in the old and oldest old. J Am Geriatr Soc 2001; 49(11):1512–1517.

74. Kaksonen R, Widen E, Cormand B, et al. Autosomal dominant midfrequency hearing impairment. Scandinavian Audiology, Taylor and Francis Ltd 2001; 30(1):85–87.

75. Hu BH, Henderson D. Changes in F-actin in the outer hair cell and the Deiters cell in the chinchilla cochlea following noise exposure. Hear Res 1997; 110:209–218.

76. Chan E, Suneson A, Ulfendahl M. Acoustic trauma causes reversible stiffness changes in auditory sensory cell. Neuroscience 1998; 83:961–968.

77. Zhu M, Yang T, Wei S. Mutations in the gamma-actin gene (ACTG1) are associated with dominant progressive deafness (DFNA20/26). Am J Hum Genet 2003; 73(5):1082–1091.

78. Davis RR, Newlander JK, Ling X-B, Cortopassi GA, Krieg EF, Erway LC. Genetic basis for susceptibilty to noiseinduced hearing loss in mice. Hear Res 2001; 155:82–90.

79. Davis RR, Newlander JK, Ling X-B, Cortopassi GA, Krieg EF, Erway LC. Genetic basis for susceptibility to noiseinduced hearing loss in mice. Hear Res 2001; 155:82–90.

80. Jimenez AM, Stagner BB, Martin GK, Lonsbury-Martin BL. Susceptibility of DPOAEs to sound overexposure in inbred mice with AHL. J Assoc Res Otolaryngol 2001; 2:233–245.

81. Harding GW, Bohne BA, Vos JD. The effect of an age-related hearing loss gene (Ahl) on noise-induced hearing loss and cochlear damage from low-frequency noise. Hear Res 2005; 204(1–2):90–100.

82. Cheng AG, Cunningham LL, Rubel EW. Mechanisms of hair cell death and protection. Curr Opin Otolaryngol Head Neck Surg 2005; 13(6):343–348.

83. Van Lear L, CarlssonPI, Ottschytsch N, et al. The contribution of genes involved in potassium-recyling in the inner ear to noise-induced hearing loss. Hum Mutat 2006; 27(8):786–795.

84. Prezant TR, Agapian JV, Bohlman MC, et al. Mitochondrial ribosomal RNA mutation associated with both antibiotic-induced and non-syndromic deafness. Nature Genet 1993; 4: 289–294.

85. Reid FM, Vernham GA, Jacobs HT. Complete mtDNA sequence of a patient in a maternal pedigree with sensorineural deafness. Hum Mol Genet 1994; 3:1435–1436.

86. Fischel-Ghodsian N, Prezant TR, Chaltraw WE, et al. Mitochondrial gene mutation is a significant predisposing factor in aminoglycoside ototoxicity. Am J Otolaryngol 1997; 18:173–178.

87. Tiranti V, Chariot P, Carella F, et al. Maternally inherited hearing loss, ataxia and myoclonus associated with a novel point mutation in mitochondrial tRNASer(UCN) gene. Hum Mol Genet 1995; 4:1421–1417.

88. Verhoeven K, Ensink RJ, Tiranti V. Hearing impairment and neurological dysfunction associated with a mutation in the mitochondrial tRNASer(UCN) gene. Eur J Hum Genet 1999; 7:45–51.

89. van den Ouweland JM, Lemkes HH, Ruitenbeek W, et al. Mutation in mitochondrial tRNA(Leu)(UUR) gene in a large pedigree with maternally transmitted type II diabetes mellitus and deafness. Nature Genet 1992; 1:368–371.

90. Majamaa K, Moilanen JS, Uimonen S, et al. Epidemiology of A3243G, the mutation for mitochondrial encephalomyopathy, lactic acidosis, and strokelike episodes: prevalence of the mutation in an adult population. Am J Hum Genet 1998; 63:447–454.

91. Reid FM, Rovio A, Holt IJ, Jacobs HT. Molecular phenotype of a human lymphoblastoid cell-line homoplasmic for the np 7445 deafness-associated mitochondrial mutation. Hum Mol Genet 1997; 6:443–449.

92. El Meziane A, Lehtinen SK, Hance N, et al. A tRNA suppressor mutation in human mitochondria. Nature Genet 1998; 18:350–353.

93. Guan MX, Enriquez JA, Fischel-Ghodsian N, et al. The deafness-associated mitochondrial DNA mutation at position 7445, which affects tRNASer(UCN) precursor processing, has long-range effects on NADH dehydrogenase subunit ND6 gene expression. Mol Cell Biol 1998; 18:5868–5879.

94. Guan MX, Fischel-Ghodsian N, Attardi G. Nuclear background determines biochemical phenotype in the deafness-associated mitochondrial 12S rRNA mutation. Hum Mol Genet 2001; 10:573–580.

95. Chomyn A, Enriquez JA, Micol V, Fernandez-Silva P, Attardi G. The mitochondrial myopathy, encephalopathy, lactic acidosis, and stroke-like episode syndrome-associated human mitochondrial tRNALeu(UUR) mutation causes aminoacylation deficiency and concomitant reduced association of mRNA with ribosomes. J Biol Chem 2000; 275:19198–19209.

96. Toompuu M, Yasukawa T, Suzuki T, et al. The 7472insC mitochondrial DNA mutation impairs the synthesis and extent of aminoacylation of tRNASer(UCN) but not its structure or rate of turnover. J Biol Chem 2002; 277:22240–22250.

97. Hutchin TP, Cortopassi GA. Mitochondrial defects and hearing loss. Cell Mol Life Sci 2000; 57(13–14):1927–1937.

98. del Castillo FJ, Villamar M, Moreno-Pelayo MA, et al. Maternally inherited non-syndromic hearing impairment in a Spanish family with the 7510T > C mutation in the mitochondrial tRNA (Ser(UCN)) gene. J Med Genet 2002; 39:82.

99. Sue CM, Tanji K, Hadjigeorgiou G, et al. Maternally inherited hearing loss in a large kindred with a novel T7511C mutation in the mitochondrial DNA tRNA(Ser(UCN)) gene. Neurology 1999; 52:1905–1908.

100. Chapiro E, Feldmann D, Denoyelle F, et al. Two large French pedigrees with non syndromic sensorineural deafness and the mitochondrial DNA T7511C mutation: evidence for a modulatory factor. Eur J Hum Genet 2002; 10:851–856.

101. Jaksch M, Klopstock T, Kurlemann G, et al. Progressive myoclonus epilepsy and mitochondrial myopathy associated with mutations in the tRNA(Ser(UCN)) gene. Ann Neurol 1998; 44:635–640.

102. Zhao H, Li R, Wang Q, et al. Maternally inherited aminoglycoside-induced and nonsyndromic deafness is associated with the novel C1494T mutation in the mitochondrial 12S rRNA gene in a large Chinese family. Am J Hum Genet 2004; 74:139–152.

103. Jacobs HT, Hutchin TP, Kappi T, et al. Mitochondrial DNA mutations in patients with postlingual, nonsyndromic hearing impairment. Eur J Hum Genet 2005; 13(1):26–33.

104. Estivill X, Govea N, Barcelo E, et al. Familial progressive sensorineural deafness is mainly due to the mtDNA A1555G mutation and is enhanced by treatment of aminoglycosides. Am J Hum Genet 1998; 62:27–35.

105. Torroni A, Cruciani F, Rengo C, et al. The A1555G mutation in the 12S rRNA gene of human mtDNA: recurrent origins and founder events in families affected by sensorineural deafness. Am J Hum Genet 1999; 65:1349–1358.

106. Gallo-Teran J, Morales-Angulo C, del Castillo I, et al. Genetic associations in age-related hearing thresholds. Arch Otol Head Neck Surg 1999; 125:654–659.

107. Ostergaard E, Montserrat-Sentis B, Gronskov K, Brondum-Nielsen K. The A1555G mtDNA mutation in Danish hearing-impaired patients: frequency and clinical signs. Clin Genet 2002; 62:303–305.

108. Tekin M, Duman T, Bogoclu G, et al. Maternally inherited hearing loss, ataxia and myoclonus associated with a novel point mutation in mitochondrial tRNASer(UCN) gene. Hum Mol Genet 1995; 4:1421–1417.

109. Lehtonen MS, Uimonen S, Hassinen IE, Majamaa K. Frequency of mitochondrial DNA point mutations among patients with familial sensorineural hearing impairment. Eur J Hum Gene 2000; 8:315–318.

110. Richards M, Macaulay V, Torroni A, Bandelt HJ. In search of geographical patterns in European mitochondrial DNA. Am J Hum Genet 2002; 71:1168–1174.

111. Ruiz-Pesini E, Lapena AC, Diez-Sanchez C, et al. Human mtDNA haplogroups associated with high or reduced spermatozoa motility. Am J Hum Genet 2000; 67:682–696.

112. van der Walt JM, Nicodemus KK, Martin ER, et al. Mitochondrial polymorphisms significantly reduce the risk of Parkinson disease. Am J Hum Genet 2003; 72:804–811.

113. Chinnery PF, Taylor GA, Howell N, et al. Mitochondrial DNA haplogroups and susceptibility to AD and dementia with Lewy bodies. Neurology 2000; 55:302–304.

114. Carrieri G, Bonafe M, De Luca M, et al. Mitochondrial DNA haplogroups and APOE4 allele are non-independent variables in sporadic Alzheimer's disease. Hum Genet 2001; 108:194–198.

115. Kalman B, Li S, Chatterjee D, et al. Large scale screening of the mitochondrial DNA reveals no pathogenic mutations but a haplotype associated with multiple sclerosis in Caucasians. Acta Neurol Scand 1999; 99:6–25.

116. De Benedictis G, Rose G, Carrieri G, et al. Mitochondrial DNA inherited variants are associated with successful aging and longevity in humans. FASEB J 1999; 13:1532–1536.

117. Niemi AK, Hervonen A, Hurme M, Karhunen PJ, Jylha M, Majamaa K. Mitochondrial DNA polymorphisms associated with longevity in a Finnish population. Hum Genet 2003; 112:29–33.

118. Crimi M, Del Bo R, Galbiati S, et al. Mitochondrial A12308G polymorphism affects clinical features in patients with single mtDNA macrodeletion. Eur J Hum Genet 2003; 11:896–898.

119. Torroni A, Campos Y, Rengo C, et al. Mitochondrial DNA haplogroups do not play a role in the variable phenotypic presentation of the A3243G mutation. Am J Hum Genet 2003; 72:1005–1012.

120. Pyykkö I, Starck J, Toppila E, Johnson A-C. Methodology and value of databases. Henderson D, Prasher D, Kopke R, Salvi R, Hamernik R, eds. Noise Induced Hearing Loss Basic Mechanisms, Prevention and Control. London: Noise Research Network Publications, 2001:387–399.

121. Royster LH, Royster JD, Berger EH. Guidelines for developing an effective hearing conservation program. Sound Vib 1982; 16:22–25.

122. Melnick W. Evaluation of industrial hearing conservation programs: a review and analysis. Am Ind Hyg Assoc J 1984; 45:459–467.

123. Dement JM, Pompeii LA, Ostbye T, et al. An integrated comprehensive occupational surveillance system for health care workers. Am J Ind Med 2004; 45:528–538.

124. Starck J, Toppila E, Pyykkö I. Do we have unnecessary hearing loss - Can we improve the efficiency of hearing conservation programs? In: Henderson D, Prasher D, Kopke R, Salvi R, Hamernik R, eds. Noise Induced Hearing Loss a Basic Mechanisms, Prevention and Control. London: Noise Research Network Publication, 2001:197–202.

125. Franks JR, Davis RR, Kreig EF. Analysis of hearing conservation program data base: factors other than work place noise. Ear hear 1989; 10:273–280.

126. Occupational Health and Safety Administration (OSHA). Occupational injury and illness record keeping and reporting requirements; final rule. Occupational Safety and Health Administration. Federal Register 2002; 67:44037–44048.

127. Stewart AP. The comprehensive hearing conservation program. In: Lipscomb DM, ed. Hearing Conservation in Industry, Schools and the Military. San Diego: Singular Publishing Group Inc, 1994:81–230.

128. Stephens D. Audiological rehabilitation. In: Luxon LM et al., eds. Audiological Medicine. Clinical Aspects of Hearing and Balance. London: Martin Dunitz Taylor & Francis Group, 2003:513–532.

129. Szende A, Williams A, ed. Measuring Self-reported Population Health: An International Perspective based on EQ-5D. Spring MED Publishing, 2004.

130. Sintonen H, Pekurinen M. A fifteen-dimensional measure of health-related quality of life (15 D) and its applications. In: Walker SR, Rosser RM, eds. Quality of Life Assessment. Key Issues in the 1990s. Dordrecht: Kluwer Academic Publishers, 1993.

131. Stewart AL, Hays RD, Ware JE Jr. The MOS short-form general health survey. Reliability and validity in a patient population. Med Care 1988; 26(7):724–735.

132. www.equicare.fi

8 Otosclerosis: a genetic update

Frank Declau, Paul Van De Heyning

Introduction

Otosclerosis (OTSC) is a disorder of the bony labyrinth and stapes known to affect only humans. It affects the bone homeostasis of the labyrinthine capsule, resulting in abnormal resorption and redeposition of bone. This bone dysplasia limited to the otic capsule originates in the endochondral bone layer. OTSC neither affects other endochondral bones in humans nor is found in animals. OTSC is the most important cause of chronic progressive conductive hearing loss in adults and a significant cause of progressive sensorineural hearing loss as well (1). Conductive hearing loss develops when otosclerotic foci invade the stapediovestibular joint (oval window) or round window region and interfere with the free motion of the stapes. Although the sensorineural hearing loss cannot be corrected, stapes microsurgery has proven to be a highly successful means to restore normal ossicular conduction and improve hearing thresholds.

Here we present an analysis of the literature concerning the phenotypic expression, mode of inheritance, prevalence, age of onset, sex ratio, and sporadic cases of OTSC.

Phenotypic expression

The diagnostic criteria for OTSC consist of conductive hearing loss unrelated to known causes such as the sequelae of Eustachian tube dysfunction, trauma, or congenital cholesteatoma. The magnitude of the conductive hearing loss is directly related to the degree of fixation of the stapes footplate (2,3). The otolaryngologist must take into account the physical examination, pure tone audiogram, and admittance findings as well as the past medical and surgical history. As a rule, the tympanoscopy is normal. Sporadically, the otospongiotic focus reveals itself otoscopically as a pink or violaceous hue on the promontory (known as Schwartz's sign). Tympanometry demonstrates a normal type A or a type As.

The progression of the hearing loss in OTSC may be described as follows. At first, only the low frequencies are diminished ("stiffness tilt") due to an enhanced stiffness of the tympano-ossicular system. Then, the ossicular chain becomes heavier, which gives rise to a flat conductive hearing loss. Often an elevation of bone conduction thresholds can be seen, known as the Carhart notch. The elevation of the bone conduction thresholds is approximately 5 dB at 500 Hz, 10 dB at 1000 Hz, 15 dB at 2000 Hz, and 5 dB at 4000 Hz. Acoustic stapedial reflexes are usually absent in full blown OTSC. However, in the initial stage of the disease, a biphasic response may be seen, known as the on-off effect. The offset in particular is pathologic (the onset may be seen in 40% of the normal population).

The foci of otosclerotic bone are symptomatically quiescent until the movement of the stapes is impaired by invasion of the stapedovestibular joint (4). Fixation of the stapes as a cause of hearing loss was first recognised by Valsalva as early as 1704 (5). In 1894, Politzer (6) called this type of ankylosis "OTSC." In 1912, Siebenmann's microscopic examinations (7) showed that the lesion apparently began as a spongification of the bone; hence, the term "otospongiosis." In commenting on OTSC, Guild (8) emphasised the importance of distinguishing between clinical and histological OTSC. "Histological OTSC" refers to the disease process without clinical symptoms or manifestations that only can be discovered by sectioning of the temporal bone at autopsy. "Clinical OTSC" concerns the presence of OTSC at a site where it causes conductive hearing loss by interfering with the motion of the stapes or of the round window membrane. Many otologists believe that OTSC also damages the inner ear to cause progressive sensorineural hearing loss (9,10). Although Guild (8) failed to establish a correlation between OTSC and sensorineural hearing loss, Topsakal et al. recently found a statistically significant additional perceptive hearing loss component in otosclerotic patients as compared to a normal population (1). In a histopathological survey of 248 temporal bones with OTSC, Kelemen and Alonso (10) found an otosclerotic focus involving the cochlear endost in 40% of patients with clinical OTSC. Any encroachment of the membranous labyrinth usually occurs in the lateral arcs of each cochlear turn (4). In these areas, the inner periosteal layer is deformed, and subjacent atrophy of the spiral ligament may be seen (11). However, severe alterations in the bony labyrinth and spiral ligament may occur with no observable histological alterations in the structures of the cochlear duct (4). There does not appear to be a consistent spatial relationship between areas of atrophy of the spiral ligament and atrophy of the organ of Corti. Several reports correlate the degree of cochlear endosteal involvement with the magnitude of the sensorineural hearing loss (12–14). According to Hueb et al. (15), there is a relation between the size of the foci and the degree of sensorineural hearing loss.

The concept of "cochlear OTSC," that is, pure sensorineural hearing loss caused by OTSC of the bony labyrinth without stapes fixation, has been the subject of much debate (16). Causse and Causse (17) believe that a number of cases with low-, mid-, and high-frequency sensorineural hearing loss and a dominant mode of inheritance, described as separate syndrome entities by Königsmark and Gorlin (18), actually represent cochlear OTSC. On the other hand, a temporal bone study of patients with pure sensorineural deafness of unknown cause has failed to show otosclerotic foci of significant incidence or size to explain the inner ear changes (4,15).

OTSC usually involves both ears. However, Morrison (19) and Cawthorne (20) found unilateral OTSC in 13% and Larsson (21) in 15%. Guild (8) reported histologically unilateral OTSC in 30%.

Usually low-pitch tinnitus is present. Vertiginous spells or dizziness are quite common (25–55%). Three types of vertigo may exist: (i) attacks of dizziness and mild instability (20 minutes–6 hours) with a normal caloric response and no visible nystagmus, (ii) postural instability, and (iii) Menièriform attacks with acute rotatory vertigo with tinnitus enhancement and fluctuating hearing loss; the caloric test may be normal or diminished and the rotatory chair test is abnormal. Virolainen (22) found objective disturbances, in order of frequency, were caloric hypoexcitability and elevated thresholds of angular acceleration and deceleration, directional preponderance, and positional nystagmus. At the initial stages, paracusis Willisii or the ability to hear better in a crowd, may be present.

Histopathological appearance

Histologically, distinct sites of predilection of this dysplasia within the otic capsule exist. The most common site is the anterior margin of the oval window [80% according to Guild (8)]. Other areas of predilection are the round window niche, the anterior wall of the internal auditory canal, and within the stapedial footplate (4). OTSC was restricted to the footplate in 12% of a series reported by Guild (8), and 5% of those studied by Rüedi and Spoendlin (23).

The otosclerotic lesion is pleomorphic, varying from spongiotic to dense sclerotic bone. The progression of OTSC may be divided into four stages (4,24): the common factor is total disorganisation of the lesion that replaces normal bone.

Resorptive phase (= *otospongiosis*): The focus of resorption arises in the endochondral bone of the otic capsule. The bone is replaced with a highly vascular cellular and fibrous tissue. This resorption occurs through osteoclastic bone destruction, perhaps by vascular obliteration, or by lysosomal enzymes secreted by macrophages (25). According to Jorgensen and Kristensen (26), the smallest focus that can be detected by light microscopy is about 80 μm in diameter: only at this size is a medullary space and vascularised connective demonstrable.

Early new bone formation: Osteoid and mucopolysaccharide deposits within the fibrous tissue matrix produce a dysplastic, immature basophilic bone.

Remodelling: Repetition of the remodelling process of resorption and new bone formation: the basophilic bone becomes more acidophilic. The bone demonstrates a disordered lamellar appearance and is less vascular than in the earlier phases.

Mature phase: Formation of a highly acidophilic bone having a mosaic-like appearance because of irregular patterns of resorption and new bone formation associated with the deposition of fatty tissue in the marrow spaces.

These various phases may occur simultaneously in adjacent areas of the same focus, or various stages may be found in separate foci within the temporal bone.

Based on micromorphological studies of the normal development of the human otic capsule in the prenatal period, it has been concluded that its bony tissue is highly specialised and unique in the human body (27). The otic capsule is completely formed at term and the micromorphological organisation of its bone undergoes hardly any changes throughout subsequent life. The otic capsule differs in this respect from other bones, where bone remodelling is continuous and characterised by repetitive cycles of resorption and redeposition. According to Frisch et al. (28), the otic capsule bone remodelling is spatially organised into a distinct perilabyrinthine pattern. All bones within this narrow perilabyrinthine zone are completely inactive, including most of the primary endochondral bone. Outside this "no-remodelling zone," capsular bone remodelling units are distributed centrifugally in relation to inner ear spaces. Since OTSC can be defined as a defect in the physiologic inhibition of bone turnover at this narrow perilabyrinthine zone of "no-remodelling," the search for otosclerotic foci has to be restricted to this area (29).

Aetiology

OTSC is generally accepted to be a hereditary disorder, with segregation analyses most consistent with autosomal dominant inheritance with reduced penetrance (25–40%). OTSC represents a heterogeneous group of heritable diseases in which different genes may be involved in regulating the bone homeostasis of the otic capsule. It is hypothesised that various gene defects allow the physiologic inhibition of bone turnover in the otic capsule to be overruled by environmental factors, resulting in the localised bone dysplasia known as OTSC (30). Many different environmental factors have been implicated in the aetiology of OTSC, including infectious causes such as measles virus (31), hormones (related to puberty, pregnancy, and menopause) (32), and nutritional factors (fluoride intake) (33). About 50% of patients with OTSC report a positive family history, with the remainder considered sporadic.

No gene responsible for OTSC has yet been cloned. However, six genetic loci, OTSC1 (OMIM 166800), OTSC2 (OMIM 605727), OTSC3, OTSC4, OTSC5, and OTSC7, have been identified to date, supporting the hypothesis that mutations in any of a number of genes may be capable of causing the OTSC phenotype (34). Such genetic heterogeneity has been well demonstrated for nonsyndromic sensorineural hearing loss. OTSC1 was mapped to chromosome 15q25-q26 in an Indian family in which hearing loss began in childhood and penetrance appeared to be complete (35). The OTSC2 locus was mapped to a 16 cM region on chromosome 7 in a large Belgian family (36). More recently, the OTSC3 locus was mapped on chromosome 6 in a large Cypriot family (37). The defined OTSC3 interval covers the human leukocyte antigen (HLA) region, consistent with reported associations between HLA-A/HLA-B antigens and OTSC (38). The localisation of OTSC4 at chromosome 16q21-23.2 in an Israeli family was also recently reported (39). OTSC5 has been localised on chromosome 3q22–24 in a Dutch family (40). OTSC7 has recently been localized on chromosome 6q13–16.1 in a large Greek pedigree (40a).

The pooled data from two families segregating with the OTSC2 locus demonstrated quite variable audiometric configurations with only a limited contribution of age. Even in this monogenic form of OTSC, it seems that other modifying factors are implicated in the mechanism that triggers the osseous change (41). McKenna et al. (42) suggest that mutations in COL1A1, similar to those that occur in type-I osteogenesis imperfecta, may account for a small percentage of cases of OTSC, and that the majority of cases of clinical OTSC are related to other genetic abnormalities yet to be identified. Also some cases of OTSC and osteoporosis could share a functionally significant polymorphism in the Sp1 transcription factor binding site in the first intron of the COL1A1 gene (43). However, Rodriguez et al. (44) found no evidence supporting the putative link of COL1A1 and COL1A2 genes with OTSC.

Although genetic and basic histologic patterns have been identified in OTSC, there is no definite agreement as to aetiology and pathogenesis. Various hypotheses implicate one or more environmental factors including (i) viral involvement, (ii) enzymatic and cellular reactions, (iii) vascular changes, (iv) infection, radiation, trauma, or exposure to toxic substances, (v) an autoimmune phenomenon, and (vi) metabolic changes.

1. Studies suggest that mumps and measles vaccines may reduce the incidence of OTSC. Particles of viruses have been found in the inner ear bone of those affected by the disorder. Niedermeyer et al. (45) used a very sensitive polymerase chain reaction technique in assessing the association between viruses and OTSC. Evidence showed that the disorder was a measles virus–associated disease. It was concluded that the viral infection acts as at least one factor in the development of the spongy tissue. Arnold and Friedmann (46) and McKenna and Mills (31) found expression of viral antigens within otosclerotic foci. McKenna and Mills (31) showed ultrastructural and immunohistochemical evidence of measles virus type A (nucleocapsid in osteoblasts and pre-osteoblasts) in active OTSC. However isolation and characterisation of virus from otosclerotic bone has not yet been successful. It is not clear if this material came from isolated or familial cases. However, an inflammatory response to an inciting antigen is proposed (46).

2. The enzymatic concept of otospongiotic disease has been put forward by Chevance et al. (47) in 1972. These authors postulated that lysosomal (cytotoxic) enzymes diffusing from histiocytes and some osteoclasts into the perilymph are the cause of the sensorineural loss as a result of their direct effect on the organ of Corti. Fluorides are known to be potent inhibitors of lysosomal enzymes (48). They also reduce osteoclastic bone resorption and at the same time promote osteoblastic bone formation (49). The use of sodium fluoride as an enzyme inhibitor to stabilise otosclerotic foci was first recommended by Shambaugh and Scott (50) in 1964. Fluoridation of drinking water has been found to have a beneficial effect on nonoperated otosclerotic ears (51).

3. Radiation of the cochlear bone induces a lesion similar to OTSC and causes recruitment of similar cells in this process (52).

4. Yoo (53) showed the presence of elevated antibody titers to type-II collagen and proposed that OTSC is a consequence of an autoimmune process against collagen molecules. According to this author, cartilage rests in the globuli interossei become autoantigenic and the response would be genetically controlled by the Ir-genes in the major histocompatibility loci. Bujia et al. (54) found significant elevated levels of antibodies to collagen type II and IX. Both research groups claim an autoimmune process as the aetiology for OTSC.

5. Gordon et al. (55) found a significantly lower level of mRNA production for stromelysin (an activator of tissue collagenase) among individuals with OTSC as compared to controls. According to these authors, OTSC could be a more generalised connective tissue disorder.

Epidemiology

Clinical OTSC is a quite frequent hearing disorder, although its exact incidence is unknown. Knowing this however is important for health planning. In Sweden, the clinical incidence has recently been estimated (56) as 6.1/100 000. This figure is lower than others reported previously: [12/100 000: Stahle et al. (57); 13.7/100 000: Pearson et al. (58)]. Levin's estimate (56) was based on the number of patients admitted in hospital for stapedectomy due to OTSC. The recent decline of OTSC operations and hence of the incidence calculations can be explained by the overwhelming publicity for stapedectomy and stapedotomy operations during the fifties, sixties, and seventies. However, McKenna (Personal communication, Harold Schuknecht meeting, Boston, 1994.) argues that systematic vaccination for measles also accounts for the decreased incidence of OTSC.

Elucidation of the prevalence of OTSC is befogged by the differentiation of clinical and histological OTSC (59). The prevalence of clinical OTSC in the white population has been studied by different authors (Table 8.1). In the early studies (2,20,60), no attempt has been made to relate the clinical condition to a known population at a given time. Clinical OTSC has a reported prevalence of 0.3% among white adults, making it the single most common cause of hearing impairment in this population (17).

The prevalence of histological OTSC has also been studied by different authors (Table 8.2). Although its prevalence has been estimated as high as 8.3% among white adults (64), in a prospective study of Declau et al. (65), only 6 of 236 temporal bones (2.5%) or 4 of 118 autopsy cases (3.4%) revealed otosclerotic foci. Although histology remains the gold standard for the evaluation of OTSC, a multitechnique method was used to screen for otosclerotic lesions in a cost-effective and less time-consuming way. Lesions as small as 1.4 mm could be detected. There had been no selection of the material in the present study that would favour OTSC. On the contrary, previous publications were all based on existing laboratory collections, which may have contained results biased by the presence of cases with hearing loss or other otological diseases. This is witnessed by the fact that many of these publications included audiometric data recorded during life, questioning the unselected character of these temporal bone banks. Also many of these authors candidly admit that a certain selection had taken place when ascertaining the reasons for which the various institutions had sent them the temporal bones for histological investigation (65). Having made some allowance for this possible error, there is no doubt that histological OTSC (phenotype) occurs in the absence of clinical OTSC (genotype).

According to the figures of Guild (7), 15% of temporal bones with histological OTSC showed ankylosis of the stapediovestibular articulation. In Altmann's review on histological OTSC (64), 12% of the temporal bones with histological OTSC had stapedial fixation. Although the prevalence figure of 2.5% is strikingly lower than previously published figures on histological OTSC, it correlates well with the extrapolated data based on clinical studies of otosclerotic families. If this prevalence figure is used to calculate by extrapolation the prevalence of clinical OTSC, the calculated figure of 0.30 to 0.38% correlates well with the clinical data of otosclerotic families (clinical prevalence = 0.3%).

The female-to-male ratio was approximately 7 to 6.

OTSC is predominantly a Caucasian disease and follows their geographic distribution throughout the world. OTSC is quite rare among Blacks, Orientals, and American Indians (64).

One possible exception is that of the Todas, an isolate in South India. The prevalence of what appears to be OTSC (there is no histological confirmation) in these people is about 17% (64a).

Age of onset

The age of onset of OTSC varies from the first through fifth decades of life, most commonly presenting in the third decade. About 90% of affected persons are under 50 years of age at the time of diagnosis. The exact age of onset is difficult to determine, since a patient may not become aware of a hearing impairment for a number of years. Based on the similar findings of Davenport (60), Larsson (21), and Morrison (19), the greatest

Table 8.1 Prevalence of clinical otosclerosis in the white population

Author	Prevalence (%)
Davenport et al. (60)	0.1–0.25
Shambaugh (2)	0.5–1
Cawthorne (20)	0.5
Morrison (19)	0.2
Hall (61)	0.3
Pearson et al. (58)	0.28
Gapany-Gapanavicius (62)	0.044–0.1
Ben Arab et al. (63)	0.6

Table 8.2 Prevalence of histological otosclerosis in the white population

Author	Number of temporal bones studied	Number of cadavers	Prevalence (%)
Weber (66)	?	200	11
Engström (67)	145	100	12
Guild (7)	?	518	8.3
Jorgensen and Kristensen (26)	237	155	11.4
Schuknecht and Kirchner (68)	734	?	4.4
Hueb et al. (15)	144	?	12.75
Declau et al. (65)	236	118	2.5

period of risk can be determined between 11 and 45 years. Cawthorne (20) reported that 70% of patients with clinical OTSC first noticed the hearing losses between the age of 11 and 30. Deafness interpreted as OTSC and beginning as early as age five in some cases was described by Kabat (69). The age of onset is similar in males and females. There is also a striking similarity within families and especially within sibships. On the other hand, Morrison (19) found a tendency towards an earlier age of onset with succeeding generations (anticipation).

Mode of inheritance

The first pedigrees in which the transmission of OTSC from generation to generation was demonstrated were published by Hammerschlag (70), Körner (71), Albrecht (72), and Bauer and Stein (73). Albrecht (72) concluded that OTSC is due to a simple dominant factor, but Bauer and Stein (73), with larger material and more sophisticated statistical methods, postulated a double autosomal recessive mode of inheritance. These early 20th century studies show a lot of bias due to inadequate otologic diagnosis, especially in secondary cases, and improper selection strategies.

The majority of the more recent studies on OTSC (17,19,21,62) indicate an autosomal dominant mode of inheritance. The monogenic forms of OTSC also demonstrate an autosomal dominant mode. These studies have included all patients without regard to family history, age, or prior therapy. A firm clinical diagnosis was made by otoscopic and audiometric analysis and also to a large extent by surgery. Exclusion of phenotypes has also been done. Bias of ascertainment has been corrected using Weinberg's proband method (74) (omission of the proband and inclusion of the sibship each time it is ascertained) for correcting incomplete multiple ascertainment. The expected frequencies of affected individuals for autosomal dominant traits were compared with the observed frequencies for relatives of otosclerotics. Many families had transmission of OTSC through three or more generations. Analysis of families with secondary cases outside the sibship of the proband revealed that they inherited the gene from only one side of the family. In the offspring of two affected parents, no accelerated or early onset cases were detected. There is no evidence for a phenotypical difference between the heterozygous and homozygous state.

The assumption of autosomal dominant inheritance is based on the existence of particular pedigrees. However, it may be difficult to draw definite conclusions from isolated pedigrees for the following reasons (75): (*i*) Individual families may demonstrate exceptions to the rule. They may have attracted attention by noteworthy accumulations of secondary cases or particularly serious cases (21). (*ii*) Individual pedigrees may mimic a mode of inheritance, especially if a carrier state, incomplete penetrance, or variable expressivity exists. (*iii*) More than one mode of inheritance may be responsible for a given disease (as in retinitis pigmentosa). (*iv*) A given entity may actually represent a heterogeneous group of diseases.

Modifying genes and environmental factors are likely to play a role in the expression or penetrance of OTSC and may be responsible for the high degree of variability between families. This is in no way inconsistent with the accepted autosomal dominant mode of inheritance (19). Ben Arab et al. (63) postulated an autosomal dominant major gene with a high polygenic component.

Other modes of inheritance are highly unlikely as can be concluded from the detailed mathematical analyses of Larsson (21) and Gapany-Gapanavicius (62). Autosomal recessive inheritance is unlikely given the presumed degree of penetrance, but cannot absolutely be ruled out. Digenic inheritance has been claimed by several authors: two autosomal recessive genes (73), an autosomal dominant and an X-linked dominant gene (60), or an autosomal recessive and an X-linked dominant gene (76). It is relatively easy to create an ad hoc hypothesis to fit existing data with such models, but this type of inheritance is quite uncommon in humans and the models do not convincingly explain the overall epidemiology of OTSC.

Penetrance

Larsson (21) and Morrison and Bundey (77) explained that the degree of penetrance represents the percentage of patients with histologic OTSC in whom the otosclerotic foci interfere with the hearing mechanism. In the monogenic forms, a high degree of penetrance can be found (41): 50% for OTSC 1 and 100% for OTSC 2. In pedigree studies however, the degree of penetrance is much lower. Two methods for determining the degree of penetrance of OTSC have appeared in the literature. Morrison (19) and Causse and Causse (17) calculated the difference between observed and expected ratios in relatives of otosclerotics. In both cases, the authors concluded that penetrance approximated 40%. Larsson (21) calculated a penetrance of 25% by applying a formula devised by Weinberg (74) to Guild's postmortem material (7). His study has been criticised by Gordon (75), who pointed to a number of unwarranted assumptions in the method and deficiencies in the data.

Sporadic cases

According to most studies (Table 8.3), the percentage of isolated cases ranges from 40% to 50%.

According to Morrison and Bundey (77), the presence of isolated cases can be explained as follows:

1. Isolated cases of OTSC may be phenocopies of the disease. Without surgical exploration, it may be difficult to exclude acquired or congenital ossicular fixations or defects.
2. New mutations may account for a small fraction of these isolated cases [Morrison (19) suggested the mutation rate is: 50×10^{-6}].

Table 8.3 Frequency of sporadic cases with clinical otosclerosis

Author	% Isolated cases
Nager (78)	42
Cawthorne (20)	46
Shambaugh (2)	44.5
Larsson (21)	49
Morrison (19)	30
Gapany-Gapanavicius (62)	48.4

3. Given the reduced penetrance of 25% to 40%, it would seem reasonable to suppose that sporadic cases are due to nonpenetrance in other family members (though they might be expected to have histological OTSC). However, the incidence of histologic OTSC exceeds the incidence of clinical OTSC by far more than can be accounted for by accepted penetrance figures alone. Therefore, Morrison and Bundey (77) proposed that these isolated cases might have an alternate mode of inheritance, so that clinical OTSC could be explained by more than one genetic mechanism. They calculated the theoretical prevalence of histological OTSC on the assumption that isolated cases follow recessive inheritance, while the familial cases follow dominant inheritance. According to their theory, the homozygous state would produce clinical OTSC, while the heterozygous "carrier" state might result in areas of histological OTSC without stapedial ankylosis. The frequency of histological OTSC was the sum of the heterozygous recessive state, the dominant genotype (as seen in pedigrees), and (the less significant) mutation rates for each mode of inheritance. It was estimated as 6.145%, close to the frequency recorded by Guild (7) (8.3%).

There is no evidence that the hearing loss in sporadic OTSC is of greater severity than in the obvious hereditary cases (19). However, in contrast to familial cases, there is a consistent tendency for later birth ranks to be associated with more cases of OTSC. Both maternal and paternal ages do not differ from the expected. So this tendency must be due to either parity or environmental factors. The sex ratio in sporadic cases is exactly equal. According to Larsson (21), there is a lower morbidity risk for siblings of probands. He explains this finding as follows: (i) There exists a lower degree of penetrance, owing to modifying genes. (ii) It is also possible that they follow a different mode of inheritance. (iii) An admixture of environmental factors can also not be excluded.

Sex ratio

Investigations of the occurrence of histological OTSC have not shown any significant sex disparity (7,66,67), whereas it is common knowledge among otologists that clinical OTSC is encountered more frequently in females than in males. Interestingly, as regards the occurrence of stapes ankylosis in those cases of histological OTSC, the males predominate (21). A sex ratio in clinical OTSC of about 2F:1M has been noted by many authors (2,19–21,60,73,78,79). This circumstance may indicate that OTSC manifests itself clinically in a higher percentage of females than males (21). This impression is partly given by the increasing proportion of females in any population of advancing years, coupled with the increasing disability of otosclerotic deafness with the passage of time. There is no obvious difference in the age of onset between males and females nor their hearing loss at the time of consultation. However the progression of the hearing loss is greater in females than in males during the first 20 years of the disease (21) (10 dB +). Also at surgical intervention, the pathological process of ankylosis of the stapes is more advanced (19). Unilateral OTSC is more common in males [20% in men vs. 9% in women (19)]. The apparent sex disparity has been ascribed to hormonal factors, particularly pregnancy (20,78,79). On the other hand, the partial sex limitation with regard to clinical OTSC mainly relates to probands, while among unselected secondary cases, the sex ratio becomes exactly equal (77). If Weinberg's ascertainment method is used to cope with the ascertainment bias, than the sex ratio in complete sibships becomes almost equal. Gristwood and Venables (80) calculated the likelihood that female patients with bilateral OTSC would report worsening of their hearing during pregnancy. Their results ranged from 33% after one pregnancy to 63% after six pregnancies. Schaap and Gapany-Gapanavicius (81) found in the Lithuanian population another explanation for the observed increase in frequency of clinical OTSC in females. They found a distorted sex ratio of offspring (both affected and normal) in the matings of a normal parent with a parent with OTSC. Moreover, a considerably higher frequency of OTSC was found in the female than in the male offspring (36.5% vs. 20.2%). Schaap and Gapany-Gapanavicius (81) explained this finding as an intrauterine selection against heterozygous or hemizygous males. In the families with at least one affected male, however, the morbidity risk was again equal. However, James (82) does not accept this hypothesis because a disparity in sex ratio should be present in sibs as well as in the offspring. Since it is not, there has to be another explanation. According to this author, the familial pattern of female selection could be related to steroid hormone metabolism. This distorted sex ratio in the offspring is not a universal finding: both Larsson (21) and Morrison (19) found an almost equal sex ratio after applying Weinberg's correction.

Conclusion

We suggest that OTSC represents a heterogeneous group of heritable diseases in which different genes may be involved in regulating the bone homeostasis of the otic capsule. It is hypothesised that in response to various gene defects, the physiologic inhibition of bone turnover in the otic capsule is overruled due to a greater susceptibility to environmental factors, resulting in a localised bone dysplasia known as OTSC. Search for huge OTSC families with at least 12 positively identified cases is warranted, so that a genome search within each family becomes possible. However, such families are rare. Since the age of onset of OTSC is delayed, multiple generations of subjects with clinical OTSC are usually not available for study. Consequently, it has been difficult to identify large families with a sufficient number of affected persons to allow adequate statistical power for genetic linkage analysis. Nonparametric methods (e.g., affected sibling pair or affected pedigree member) could be employed, but under an assumption of genetic heterogeneity, it is likely that hundreds of relative pairs affected with OTSC would be required to have sufficient power. Smaller families may only be informative if OTSC patients are present with associated chromosomal or additional abnormalities.

A candidate gene approach, while feasible, would be quite labour-intensive, given the large number of candidate genes with a large number of exons. Even if DNA analysis of the exons revealed no mutations, it may be impossible to rule out a gene. A mutation in an intron may interfere with mRNA splicing, or a mutation in a remote enhancer may otherwise reduce expression. Moreover, the diagnosis of OTSC is befogged by the differentiation of clinical and histological OTSC: Clinically unaffected members cannot be considered as genetically unaffected due to the limited penetrance and the variable expression. A genetic susceptibility may be harder to recognise when penetrance is reduced, syndromic features are subtle, and, by chance, all siblings and/or children may be unaffected. Also in family members with only perceptive hearing loss, we fail to discriminate these individuals with cochlear OTSC from those with other types of genetic hearing loss.

References

1. Topsakal V, Fransen E, Schmerber S, et al. Audiometric analyses confirm a cochlear component, disproportional to age, in stapedial otosclerosis. Otol Neurotol 2006; 27(6):781–787.
2. Shambaugh GE. Fenestration operation for otosclerosis. Acta Otolaryngol Suppl (Stockh) 1949; 79:1–101.
3. Arnold W, Friedmann I. Presence of viral specific antigens (measles, rubella) around the active otosclerotic focus. Ann Rhinol Laryngol 1987; 66:167–171.
4. Schuknecht HF. Pathology of the Ear. Cambridge: Harvard University Press, 1974.
5. Valsalva AM. De aure humana tractatus. Utrecht 1704.
6. Politzer A. Uber primare Erkrankung der Knochernen Labyrinthkapsel. Z Ohrenheilkd 1894; 25:309.
7. Siebenmann F. Totaler knocherner Verschluss beider Labyrinthfester und Labyrinthitis serosa infolge progressiver Spongiosierung. Verh Dtsch Otol Ges 1912; 21:267.
8. Guild SR. Histologic otosclerosis. Ann Otol Rhinol Laryngol 1944; 53:246–267.
9. Ramsay HAW, Linthicum FH Jr. Mixed hearing loss in otosclerosis: indication for long-term follow-up. Am J Otol 1994; 15(4):536–538.
10. Kelemen G, Alonso A. Penetration of the cochlear endost by the fibrous component of the otosclerotic focus. Acta Otolaryngol 1980; 89:453–458.
11. Friedmann I. Pathology of the Ear. Oxford: Blackwell, 1974.
12. Lindsay JR, Beal DD. Sensorineural deafness in otosclerosis: observations on histopathology. Ann Otol Rhinol Laryngol 1966; 75:436–457.
13. Linthicum FH. Pathology and pathogenesis of sensorineural deafness in otosclerosis. EENT Digest 1967; 29:51–56.
14. Linthicum FH, Filipo R, Brody S. Sensorineural hearing loss due to cochlear otospongiosis: theoretical considerations of etiology. Ann Otol Rhinol Laryngol 1975; 85:544–551.
15. Hueb MM, Goycoolea MV, Paparella MM, Oliveira JA. Otosclerosis: the University of Minnesota temporal bone collection. Otolaryngol Head Neck Surg 1991; 105(3):396–405.
16. Shambaugh GE. Clinical diagnosis of cochlear (labyrinthine) otosclerosis. Laryngoscope 1965; 75:1558.
17. Causse JR, Causse JB. Otospongiosis as a genetic disease. Am J Otol 1984; 5(3):211–223.
18. Königsmark BW, Gorlin RJ. Genetic and metabolic deafness. Philadelphia: WB Saunders, 1976.
19. Morrison AW. Genetic factors in otosclerosis. Ann R Coll Surg Eng 1967; 41:202–237.
20. Cawthorne T. Otosclerosis. J Laryngol Otol 1955; 69:437–456.
21. Larsson A. Otosclerosis: a genetic and clinical study. Acta Otolaryngol Suppl (Stockh) 1960; 154:1–86.
22. Virolainen E. Vestibular disturbances in clinical otosclerosis. Acta Otolaryngol Suppl (Stockh) 1972; 306.
23. Rüedi L, Spoendlin H. Die Histologie der otosklerotischen Stapesankylose im Hinblick auf die chirurgische Mobilisation des Steigbügels. Bibl Otol rhinol laryngol Fasc 1957; 4:1.
24. Arnold WJ, Laissue JA, Friedmann I, Naumann HH. Diseases of the Head and Neck. An Atlas of Histopathology. New York: Thieme Medical Publishers, 1987.
25. Chevance LG, Bretlau P, Jorgensen MB, Causse J. Otosclerosis. An electron microscopic and cytochemical study. Acta Otolaryngol Suppl (Stockh) 1970; 272:1–44.
26. Jorgensen MB, Kristensen HK. Frequency of histological otosclerosis. Ann Otol Rhinol Laryngol 1967; 76:83–88.
27. Declau F. Morfologische organisatie van het beenweefsel in het otische kapsel van de humane foetus. Ph. D. Thesis. University of Antwerp, Belgium, 1991.
28. Frisch T, Sorensen MS, Overgaard S, Bretlau P. Predilection of otosclerotic foci related to the bone turnover in the otic capsule. Acta Otolaryngol Suppl 2000; 543:111–113.
29. Declau F, Scheuermann W, Somers T, Van de Heyning P. Scanning electron microscopy of normal and otosclerotic bone in the region of the oval window. In: Lurato S, Veldman J, eds. Progress in Human Auditory and Vestibular Histopathology. New York: Kugler Publications, 1997:31–39.

30. Declau F, Van de Heyning P, Van Camp G. The GENDEAF otosclerotic database. Bulletin of the European network on genetic deafness 2003; 2:5–7.

31. McKenna M, Mills BG. Ultrastructural and immunohistochemical evidence of measles virus in active otosclerosis. Acta Otolaryngol Suppl (Stockh) 1990; 470:130–140.

32. Weber BP, Zenner HP. Otosclerosis and estrogen-gestagen substitution in the menopause. Dtsch Med Wochenschr 1991; 116:1292.

33. Shambaugh GE Jr, Petrovic A. The possible value of sodium fluoride for inactivation of the otosclerotic bone lesion. Experimental and clinical studies. Acta Otolaryngol 1967; 63:331–339.

34. Van den Bogaert K, Govaerts PJ, De Leenheer EMR, et al. Otosclerosis: a genetically heterogeneous disease involving at least 3 different genes. Bone 2002; 30:624–630.

35. Tomek MS, Brown MR, Mani SR, et al. Localization of a gene for otosclerosis to chromosome 15q25-q26. Hum Mol Genet 1998; 7:285–290.

36. Van den Bogaert K, Govaerts PJ, Schatteman I, et al. A second gene for otosclerosis, OTSC2, maps to chromosome 7q34-36. Am J Hum Genet 2001; 68:495–500.

37. Chen W, Campbell CA, Green GE, et al. Linkage of otosclerosis to a third locus (OTSC3) on human chromosome 6p21.3-22.3. J Med Genet 2002; 39:473–477.

38. Singhal SK, Mann SB, Datta U, et al. Genetic correlation in otosclerosis. Am J Otolaryngol 1999; 20:102–105.

39. Brownstein Z, Frydman M, Avraham KB. Identification of a New Gene for Otosclerosis, OTSC4. ARO Meeting. Daytona Beach, Florida, USA, 2004.

40. Van den Bogaert K, de Leenheer EMR, Chen W, et al. A fifth locus for otosclerosis, OTSC5, maps to chromosome 3q22-24. J Med Genet 2004; 4:1450–1453.

40a. Thys M, Van Den Bogaert K, Iliadou V, et al. A Seventh locus for otosclerosis, OTSC7, maps to Chromosome 6q13–161. Eur J Hum Genet 2007; 15(3): 362–368.

41. Declau F, Van den Bogaert K, Van De Heyning P, et al. Phenotype-genotype correlations in otosclerosis: clinical features of OTSC2. In: Häusler R, ed. Advances in ORL. Otosclerosis and Stapes Surgery. 2007; 65:114–118.

42. McKenna MJ, Kristiansen AG, Tropitzsch AS. Similar COL1A1 expression in fibroblasts from some patients with clinical otosclerosis and those with type I osteogenesis imperfecta. Ann Otol Rhinol Laryngol 2002; 111(2):184–189.

43. McKenna MJ, Nguyen-Huynh AT, Kristiansen AG. Association of otosclerosis with Sp1 binding site polymorphism in COL1A1 gene: evidence for a shared genetic etiology with osteoporosis. Otol Neurotol 2004; 25(4):447–450.

44. Rodriguez L, Rodriguez S, Hermida J, et al. Proposed association between the COL1A1 and COL1A2 genes and otosclerosis is not supported by a case-control study in Spain. Am J Med Genet A 2004; 128(1):19–22.

45. Niedermeyer H, Arnold W, Neubert WJ, Hofler H. Evidence of measles virus RNA in otosclerotic tissue. J Otorhinolaryngol Relat Spec 1994; 56(3):130–132.

46. Arnold W, Friedmann I. Immunohistochemistry of otosclerosis. Acta Otolaryngol Suppl (Stockh) 1990; 470:124–129.

47. Chevance LG, Causse J, Jorgensen MB, Bergés J. Hydrolytic activity of the perilymph in otosclerosis. A preliminary report. Acta Otolaryngol (Stockh) 1972; 74:23–28.

48. Parahy CH, Linthicum FH. Otosclerosis. Relationship of spiral ligament hyalinization to sensorineural hearing loss. Laryngoscope 1983; 93:717–720.

49. Petrovic A, Shambaugh GE Jr. Promotion of bone calcification by sodium fluoride: short-term experiments on newborn rats using tetracycline labeling. Arch Otolaryngol 1966; 83:104–122.

50. Shambaugh GE Jr, Scott A. Sodium fluoride for arrest of otosclerosis. Arch Otolaryngol 1964; 80:263–270.

51. Vartianen E, Karjalainen S, Nuutinen J, et al. Effect of drinking water fluoridation on hearing of patients with otosclerosis in a low fluoride area: a follow-up study. Am J Otol 1994; 15(4): 545–548.

52. Mendoza D, Rius M, De Stefani E, Leborgne F Jr. Experimental otosclerosis. Its causation by ionizing radiations. Acta Otolaryngol (Stockh) 1969; 67(1):9–16.

53. Yoo TJ. Etiopathogenesis of otosclerosis: a hypothesis. Ann Otol Rhinol Laryngol 1984; 93(1):28–33.

54. Bujia J, Alsalameh S, Jerez R, et al. Antibodies to the minor cartilage collagen type IX in otosclerosis. Am J Otol 1994; 15(2):222–224.

55. Gordon MA, McPhee JR, Van De Water TR, Ruben RJ. Aberration of the tissue collagenase system in association with otosclerosis. Am J Otol 1992; 13(5):398–407.

56. Levin G, Fabian P, Stahle J. Incidence of otosclerosis. Am J Otol 1988; 9(4):299–301.

57. Stahle J, Stahle CH, Arenberg JK. Incidence of Meniere's disease. Arch Otolaryngol 1978; 104:99–102.

58. Pearson RD, Kurland LT, Cody DTR. Incidence of diagnosed clinical otosclerosis. Arch Otolaryngol 1974; 99:288–291.

59. Declau F, Van De Heyning PH. In: Martini A, Read A, Stephens D, eds. Genetics and Hearing Impairment. London: Whurr Publishers, 1996:221–235.

60. Davenport CB, Milles BL, Frink LB. The genetic factor in otosclerosis. Arch Otolaryngol 1933; 17:135–170, 340–383, 503–548.

61. Hall JG. Otosclerosis in Norway. A geographical and genetical study. Acta Otolaryngol Suppl 1974; 324:1–20.

62. Gapany-Gapanavicius B. Otosclerosis: Genetics and Surgical Rehabilitation. Jerusalem: Keter, 1975.

63. Ben Arab S, Bonaiti-Pellie C, Belkahia A. A genetic study of otosclerosis in a population living in the north of Tunisia. Ann Genet 1993; 36:111–116.

64. Altmann F, Glasgold A, Mcduff JP. The incidence of otosclerosis as related to race and sex. Ann Otol Rhinol Laryngol 1967; 76(2):377–392.

64a. Kapur YP, Patt AJ. Hearing in Todas of South India. Arch Otolarngol 1967; 85(4): 400–406.

65. Declau F, Van Spaendonck M, Timmermans JP, et al. Prevalence of otosclerosis in an unselected series of temporal bones. Otol Neurotol 2001; 22:596–602.

66. Weber M. Otosklerose und Umbau der Labyrinthkapsel. Leipzig: Poeschel and Trepte, 1935.

67. Engström H. On the frequency of otosclerosis. Acta Otolaryngol 1939; 27:608–614.
68. Schuknecht HF, Kirchner JC. Cochlear otosclerosis: fact or fantasy? Laryngoscope 1974; 84:766–782.
69. Kabat C. A family history of deafness. J Hered 1943; 34:377–378.
70. Hammerschlag V. Zur Frage der Vererbbarkeit der "Otosklerose." Wien Klin Rundschau 1905; 19:5–7.
71. Körner O. Das Wesen der Otosklerose im Lichte der Vererbungslehre. Ztschr Ohrenheilk 1905; 50:98.
72. Albrecht W. Uber der Vererbung der konstitutionellen sporadischen Taubstummheit und der Otosclerose. Arch Ohren Nasen Kehlkopfheilkd 1922; 110:15–48.
73. Bauer J, Stein C. Verbung und Konstitution bei Ohrenkrankheiten. Ztchr ges Anat 1925; 10:483.
74. Weinberg W. Methoden und Technik der Statistik mit besonderer Berücksichtigung der Sozialbiologie. In: Gottstein A, Schlossmann A, Teleky L, eds. Handbuch der sozialem. Berlin: Springer, 1925.
75. Gordon MA. The genetics of otosclerosis: a review. Am J Otol 1989; 10(6):426–438.
76. Hernandez-Orozco F, Courtney GT. Genetic aspects of clinical otosclerosis. Ann Otol Rhinol Laryngol 1964; 73:632–644.
77. Morrison AW, Bundey SE. The inheritance of otosclerosis. J Laryngol Otol 1970; 84:921–932.
78. Nager F. Zur klinik und pathologischen Anatomie der Otosklerose. Acta Otolaryngol 1939; 27:542.
79. Schmidt E. Erblichkeit und Gravidität bei der Otosklerose. Arch Ohr Nas Kehlheilk 1933; 136:188.
80. Gristwood RE, Venables WN. Pregnancy and otosclerosis. Clin Otolaryngol 1983; 8:205–210.
81. Schaap T, Gapany-Gapanavicius B. The genetics of otosclerosis: distorted sex ratio. Am J Hum Genet 1978; 30:59–64.
82. James WH. Sex ratios in otosclerotic families. J Laryngol Otol 1991; 103:1036–1039.

9 Mitochondrial DNA, hearing impairment, and ageing

Kia Minkkinen, Howard T Jacobs

Introduction

In recent years, inherited mutations in mitochondrial DNA (mtDNA) have been discovered to be associated with a variety of human diseases. mtDNA mutations can be thought of as forming a continuous spectrum from neutral (or even advantageous) polymorphisms through mildly or moderately deleterious changes to clearly pathological mutations, with devastating disease phenotypes. Supposedly neutral mtDNA polymorphisms, which have accumulated sequentially along radiating maternal lineages as the result of mtDNA evolution, define the mtDNA haplotypes of modern-day populations. In the recent years, haplogroup-defining polymorphisms have been suggested to contribute to the multifactorial aetiologies of many late-onset degenerative disorders by acting as "risk factors" that predispose individuals of certain mtDNA haplogroups to these diseases. Deleterious mtDNA mutations, on the other hand, have been found to be directly responsible for a wide range of phenotypes, most often by compromising the function of the mitochondrial oxidative phosphorylation (OXPHOS) system in individual cell types, tissues, or whole organisms. In addition to inherited mtDNA mutations, somatically acquired mutations and rearrangements have been shown to accumulate within many tissues during ageing. Such accumulation may lead to a progressive decline in energy production and the overall function of the tissue, thereby precipitating the onset of many age-related degenerative diseases. Lastly, mtDNA mutations rarely act alone, and the clinical presentation of a mitochondrial disease is often the result of the interplay between the mitochondrial and the nuclear genomes as well as various environmental factors.

Among this diverse spectrum of diseases, mtDNA mutations are recognised as one of the most frequent causes of familial hearing disorders. Inherited mtDNA mutations have been identified in both syndromic and nonsyndromic hearing loss as well as in predisposition to aminoglycoside-induced ototoxicity (1). However, most of the previous studies have been limited to cases of early-onset deafness, which has been recently shown to be genetically distinct from age-related hearing impairment (ARHI) (2). The possible involvement of the mtDNA genotype in ARHI, one of the most common age-related sensorineural defects, remains controversial.

In this review, we briefly summarise current knowledge concerning the mitochondrial genetic system, discuss the relationship between mtDNA genotype and defined hearing disorders, and evaluate the evidence for possible mtDNA involvement in ARHI.

mtDNA and disease

Mitochondria

Structure and organisation

Mitochondria are cytoplasmic organelles that have a variety of functions in the cell, the most important being the synthesis of adenosine triphosphate (ATP) by OXPHOS. Mitochondria are present in all cell types except mature erythrocytes. A typical human cell has several hundred up to a thousand mitochondria, the exact number depending on the metabolic activity and energy requirements of the tissue. Mitochondria can also vary in shape, size, and location depending on the cell type and tissue function. Rather than isolated individual entities, mitochondria are thought to exist in the cell as a dynamic network, with constant fusion and fission events.

A mitochondrion has two membranes, the outer membrane that surrounds the organelle and the inner membrane that is folded into structures called cristae to maximize its surface area. The compartment between the outer and the inner membranes is called the intermembrane space (IMS). The outer membrane contains large transmembrane channels composed of the protein porin, and the membrane is readily permeable to ions and most molecules smaller than 5 kDa. The inner membrane in turn is impermeable to most small ions and molecules including protons and specific transporters are required for these species to cross the inner membrane. Embedded in the inner membrane are the enzymes involved in OXPHOS, namely, the complexes of the respiratory chain (I to IV), the ATP synthase (complex V), and the adenine nucleotide translocator (ANT). Enclosed by the inner membrane is the mitochondrial matrix, which is an aqueous solution containing a number of metabolic enzymes including those involved in the tricarboxylic acid cycle (TCA cycle), the β-oxidation pathway, the pathways of amino acid oxidation, and the oxidation of pyruvate (the pyruvate dehydrogenase complex), as well as a multitude of different intermediates of energy metabolism. Also found in the matrix are several copies of the circular mtDNA, the mitochondrial ribosomes, the transfer RNAs (tRNAs), and the various enzymes required for the maintenance, transcription, and translation of the mitochondrial genome. Many of these components of the matrix are, however, intimately associated with the inner membrane.

The role of mitochondria in energy metabolism

The most important function of mitochondria in the cell is the production of ATP by OXPHOS. In aerobic organisms, OXPHOS is the final stage of energy-yielding metabolism, where all oxidative steps in the degradation of carbohydrates, fats, and amino acids converge. The mitochondrial matrix contains all the pathways of substrate oxidation except glycolysis, which takes place in the cytosol. Specific transporters carry pyruvate (produced from carbohydrates by glycolysis), fatty acids (from triglycerides), and amino acids or their α-keto derivatives (from protein breakdown) into the matrix to be further converted into the two-carbon acetyl group of acetyl-CoA by the pyruvate dehydrogenase complex, the β-oxidation pathway and the pathways of amino acid oxidation, respectively. The acetyl groups are taken up by the TCA cycle, which enzymatically oxidizes them to CO_2. The energy released by the oxidation is conserved in the reduced forms of freely diffusible electron carriers, nicotinamide adenine dinucleotide (NADH) and flavin adenine dinucleotide, reduced form (FADH$_2$), which in turn can pass the high-energy electrons to the respiratory chain (3).

The protein complexes of the respiratory chain are located within the inner membrane. Each of the complexes is assembled from multiple subunits, which, apart from complex II, include subunits encoded by both the mitochondrial and the nuclear genomes. Subunits of the complexes include proteins with prosthetic groups capable of accepting and donating either one or two electrons, thus forming a series of sequentially acting electron carriers. High-energy electrons are first transferred

from NADH to complex I (NADH dehydrogenase) and then to ubiquinone (Q), whereas the electrons from succinate are passed to ubiquinone via complex II (succinate dehydrogenase), the only membrane-bound enzyme of the TCA cycle. Similarly, the glycerol 3-phosphate dehydrogenase on the outer face of the inner membrane and the FAD-containing enzymes of the fatty acid oxidation, both bypass complex I by delivering the reducing equivalents directly to ubiquinone. From the reduced form of ubiquinone, QH$_2$, the electrons are transferred to complex III (ubiquinone:cytochrome c oxidoreductase), which carries them to cytochrome c. Complex IV (cytochrome c oxidase) completes the process by transferring the electrons from cytochrome c to molecular oxygen, which is reduced to H$_2$O.

The oxygen consumption of the electron transport chain (ETC) is coupled with the phosphorylation of adenosine diphosphate (ADP) through an electrochemical gradient (4). The energy released in the process of electron transfer is efficiently conserved in the form of a proton gradient across the inner mitochondrial membrane. Protons are pumped from the matrix to the IMS by complexes I, III, and IV. For each pair of electrons that are transferred to O$_2$, 4H$^+$ are pumped out by complex I, 4H$^+$ by complex III, and 2H$^+$ by complex IV, resulting in the formation of an electrochemical gradient ($\Delta\Psi$) across the inner membrane. The flow of protons down this gradient back to the matrix side creates a proton-motive force, which is used to drive the synthesis of ATP from ADP and inorganic phosphate (P$_i$). This reaction is catalysed by the enzyme complex ATP synthase, which has two multimeric components, an integral membrane component F$_O$, which forms the proton channel, and a peripheral membrane protein F$_1$, providing the active sites for the ATP synthesis.

In addition to providing the energy for ATP synthesis, the proton-motive force is also responsible for driving the transport of substrates, ADP and P$_i$ into the mitochondrial matrix, and the product, ATP, out to the cytosol. The exchange of the ionic forms of ADP^{3-} and ATP^{4-} is carried out by the antiporter, ANT, dissipating some of the electrical gradient. The P$_i$ in turn is imported by a membrane symporter phosphate translocase in the form of H$_2$PO$_4^-$. For each H$_2$PO$_4^-$, one proton is moved into the matrix, thereby consuming the proton gradient. A summary of the components essential for the process of OXPHOS is shown in Figure 9.1.

The mitochondrial genome

Compelling evidence exists for the theory that the energy-converting organelles of present-day eukaryotes evolved from aerobic bacteria in an endosymbiotic process about two to three billion years ago (5,6). The structure and lipid composition of the mitochondrial double membrane as well as the existence of the circular mitochondrial genome and tRNAs and ribosomal RNAs (rRNAs) of the mitochondria-specific transcription and translation systems that resemble those of prokaryotes support the hypothesis that mitochondria originate from aerobic

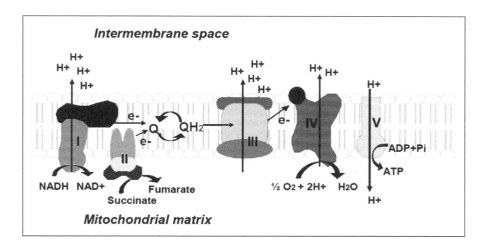

Figure 9.1 Electron transport chain complexes (I–IV) and the ATP synthase (V). *Abbreviations*: Q, ubiquinone; QH_2, reduced form of ubiquinone; ADP, adenosine diphosphate; ATP, adenosine triphosphate.

bacteria, which were engulfed by primitive eukaryotic cells (7). Being capable of aerobic energy production, the endosymbiont can be assumed to have provided an obvious metabolic advantage to the host. The initial uptake event has been followed over time by sequential transfer of the genes of the organelle to the developing nucleus of the host cell. As a consequence, present day mitochondria have lost much of their own genome and become heavily dependent on the nucleus for its gene products. In fact, out of the estimated 1500 polypeptides of the mitochondrial proteome (8), only 13 are encoded by their own DNA. Despite their small number, however, the gene products of mtDNA have fundamental and essential functions in the energy metabolism of eukaryotic cells.

Each mitochondrion contains 1 to 11 copies of the circular, double-stranded mtDNA molecule, the average being estimated at about two genomes per organelle (9). In humans, each mtDNA molecule is 16,569 base pairs long and contains 13 genes-encoding subunits of the OXPHOS system as well as the genes for the two (12S and 16S) rRNAs and 22 tRNAs essential for the mitochondrial protein synthesis machinery. The human mtDNA Cambridge Reference Sequence, published in 1981, was the first component of the human genome to be completely sequenced (10). The two strands of the mtDNA differ in base composition and can be separated by denaturing cesium chloride gradient centrifugation. The guanine-rich strand encoding 12 of the 13 polypeptide encoding genes, 14/22 of the *tRNA* genes, and both of the *rRNA* genes is named the heavy strand, while the other, cytosine-rich strand is called the light strand. Due to the absence of introns and the contiguous organisation of the coding sequences, the human mtDNA is a very small and compact genome. Some genes overlap each other, and some of the termination codons are not even encoded in the genome but are generated posttranscriptionally by polyadenylation (11). The only substantial noncoding segment of the mtDNA is the displacement loop (D-loop) region (nt 16104–16191), which is thought to contain the proposed origin of replication as well as the promoters for heavy- and light-strand transcription (P_H, P_L) (Fig. 9.2).

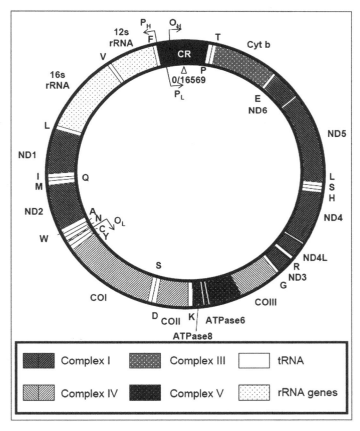

Figure 9.2 Organisation of the human mitochondrial genome. Transfer RNA genes are denoted by the single letter abbreviation for the amino acid they carry. *Source*: From Ref. 12.

mtDNA exists as protein–DNA complexes called nucleoids, which can be detected by confocal microscopy as distinct spots within the mitochondrial networks (13). Each nucleoid is believed to contain several copies of the mtDNA as well as proteins required for the maintenance and replication of the genome. They have also been suggested to be the unit of mtDNA inheritance (14). However, the exact role, molecular composition, and dynamics of the nucleoids remain to be elucidated.

mtDNA is replicated and transcribed within the mitochondrion but it is completely reliant on nuclear-encoded proteins for its maintenance and propagation. Replication of the mitochondrial genome continues throughout the lifespan of an organism, in both proliferating and postmitotic cells. The mtDNA had originally been thought to replicate by a bidirectional and asynchronous mechanism (15) in which the synthesis of DNA initiates at two distinct origins. According to this model, heavy strand synthesis starts from the so-called origin of heavy-strand, O_H, and proceeds two-thirds of the way around the circular molecule, displacing the parental strand until the light-strand origin, O_L, is exposed. Light-strand synthesis is then initiated and proceeds in the opposite direction along the heavy-strand template.

However, evidence from the analysis of two-dimensional agarose gel electrophoresis of replication intermediates has suggested an alternative model in which two mechanisms of DNA replication may exist simultaneously (16). In addition to the asymmetric asynchronous mechanism, another more conventional mechanism has been proposed, where the synthesis of the leading and lagging strand are coupled. In this case, the synthesis would start from a single origin and proceed unidirectionally around the circular genome, and the lagging strand would have to be synthesised in short Okazaki-like fragments. Unlike the strand-asynchronous replication, which is thought to work mainly in the maintenance of a constant-copy number of the mitochondrial genome, the synchronous mechanism would involve frequent lagging-strand initiation and be the predominant mode of replication in conditions for which efficient mtDNA amplification is required (16). Recent data suggests, however, that instead of a single origin of replication, the replication of mtDNA may initiate from multiple origins across a broader initiation zone, proceed first bidirectionally, and only after fork arrest near O_H, be restricted to one direction only (17).

The machinery responsible for mtDNA replication is known to include several nuclear-encoded proteins, only four of which have been well characterised: the actual DNA polymerase of mtDNA called DNA polymerase gamma (POLG) and its accessory subunit (18,19), the mitochondrial single-stranded DNA-binding protein (20), and the transcription factor A of mitochondria (TFAM) (21,22). Other proteins with a suggested role in mtDNA replication and maintenance include Twinkle, a putative mtDNA helicase (23).

The human mitochondrial genome is transcribed by the mitochondrial RNA polymerase (24), assisted by mitochondrial transcription factors, all of which are nuclear-encoded proteins. mtDNA is transcribed as long polycistronic transcripts from two heavy-strand promoters (P_H) and one light-strand promoter (P_L) (25). tRNA sequences, which are scattered around the genome, provide structural signals for RNA processing. They fold within the transcripts and are cleaved out, after which the precursors of tRNAs and released mRNAs and rRNAs undergo posttranscriptional processing (11). An RNA transcript from the P_L is also proposed to act as a primer for the mtDNA synthesis (26), thus functionally coupling mtDNA

transcription with replication of the genome and explaining why defective mtDNA transcription may also affect replication (27).

The 13 mitochondrially encoded mRNAs are translated into polypeptides on the mitochondrial ribosomes, using a mitochondrion-specific genetic code, which differs slightly from that used in the nucleus. These proteins, assembled into functional complexes together with more than 60 nuclear-encoded subunits, form four of the five enzyme complexes that are required for OXPHOS (complex II consists solely of subunits encoded by nuclear genes). In addition to the majority of subunits of the OXPHOS complexes, all the metabolic enzymes, ribosomal proteins, DNA and RNA polymerases, and other proteins involved in mtDNA maintenance, RNA synthesis and translation, as well as protein import and turnover are encoded by nuclear genes, synthesised on cytoplasmic ribosomes, and imported posttranslationally into mitochondria.

Special features of mitochondrial genetics

Due to the cytoplasmic location and high copy number of the mitochondrial genome, mitochondrial genetics has several unique features that are essential for understanding the origin and transmission of mitochondrial diseases. Some of these characteristic features are discussed below.

Maternal inheritance

mtDNA is transmitted exclusively through the maternal line (28). The sperm cell contributes a small number of mitochondria to the fertilised egg but these mitochondria seem to be eliminated at the early stages of embryogenesis by a mechanism that is not currently well known but is suspected to involve the ubiquitin-proteosome pathway (29). Apart from one reported exception, a patient with severe mitochondrial disease, there is no evidence of paternal inheritance of mtDNA under normal conditions of fertilisation (30). Maternal inheritance is therefore a characteristic feature of mitochondrial disease pedigrees. In addition, it is one of the factors that make mtDNA a particularly useful tool in human evolutionary studies.

High mutation rate

Mitochondria are suspected to lack some of the efficient DNA-repair mechanisms that are present in the nucleus. There may also be a lack of proteins to physically package and protect mtDNA in a manner analogous to the histones in the nucleus, although the TFAM could fulfill such a role, at least to some extent. If the mtDNA is exposed to the deleterious effects of various mutagenic agents, including the endogenous reactive oxygen species (ROS), which are generated as a by-product of OXPHOS, it could be especially susceptible to damage. Furthermore, mtDNA molecules are attached to or located in close proximity with the inner mitochondrial membrane, which is the primary site of oxygen radical generation. These reasons are proposed to account for the unusually high mutation rate of the mtDNA, which has been estimated to be up to 10 to 20 times as fast as that of the nuclear DNA (31). Because of the highly compact organisation and lack of introns and intergenic regions in the mtDNA, the relative mutation frequency affecting the coding regions can be thought to be even higher. As well as a variety of pathological mutations identified in the mtDNA, the fast mutation rate has also resulted in the accumulation of neutral polymorphisms throughout the genome. Most of these sequence variants are located within the fast-evolving, noncoding region of the mtDNA (the D-loop), and the rate of accumulation of mtDNA point mutations can be used as a "molecular clock" when determining evolutionary events and relationships.

Heteroplasmy and replicative segregation

In human cells, mtDNA is present in 10^3 to 10^4 copies per cell (32), depending on the cell type, and generally, all of these copies are identical. When an mtDNA mutation arises, however, an intracellular mixture of mutated and nonmutated mtDNA molecules is created. This condition is referred to as heteroplasmy as opposed to homoplasmy in which the individual shows only a single mitochondrial genotype with respect to a given nucleotide (nt) position. At each mitotic or meiotic cell division, the individual mitochondria and mtDNAs are believed to be randomly distributed to the daughter cells, and the percentage of mutant versus normal molecules in a cellular lineage may drift toward either pure mutant or pure wild type over many cell generations, a process known as replicative segregation (33). However, at least in some cell types, the process has been suggested to be constrained in some way (14).

Replicative segregation in the female germ line can result in variable proportions of mutant mtDNA being transmitted from the mother to the offspring, and the genetic drift may be quite rapid. Large variations in the percentage of mutant mtDNA between generations are believed to be due to a so-called "genetic bottleneck," which occurs during early embryogenesis (34). In the first cell divisions of a fertilised zygote, prior to blastocyst formation, there is no biogenesis of mitochondria. Instead, the existing pool of mitochondria and mtDNA (about $1–2 \times 10^5$ copies) is distributed along with the cytoplasm to the daughter cells, resulting in a dramatic reduction in the mtDNA copy number in the cells of the blastocyst, including those destined to become the female germ line (35). At later stages of oogenesis, this pool is amplified up to 1000 times to reach the normal high copy number of a mature oocyte. Because of this bottleneck, the resulting mtDNA pool originates from a very small number of mtDNA molecules, introducing a large in vivo sampling error. If a mutant mtDNA is acquired by the germ-line progenitors, the proportion of the mutant mtDNA may increase dramatically. If such an oocyte ends up being fertilised, this increased proportion of mutant mtDNA is passed on to the offspring, and the mtDNA genotype can shift to virtually pure mutant in just a few generations.

Mitochondrial disease

A growing number of human diseases can be attributed to mutations in mtDNA. These mutations can affect any of the 13 mitochondrially encoded polypeptides of the OXPHOS system or the rRNAs and tRNAs required for the mitochondrial protein synthesis. In addition to the over 50 different pathological mtDNA point mutations that have been identified to date, large-scale rearrangements of mtDNA have been found in tissues of patients suffering from neuromuscular disorders of varying severity. These include both sporadically occurring heteroplasmic deletions and duplications such as those seen in the Kearns–Sayre syndrome (KSS) (36) as well as the rare forms of inherited diseases in which the multiple mtDNA deletions are due to a nuclear defect, for example, POLG mutations in progressive external ophthalmoplegia (PEO) (37). A large number of other mitochondrial diseases are due to mutations in the nuclear genes, encoding either the subunits of the respiratory chain complexes or the large number of proteins involved in the maintenance and expression of the mitochondrial genome (38). Many of these defects are not yet characterised at the molecular level but can be defined in terms of the biochemical consequences and distinguished from mtDNA defects by the Mendelian transmission of the phenotypes. In addition to causative mutations, supposedly neutral polymorphisms defining the mtDNA haplotype have been proposed as genetic risk factors or possible modifiers of the phenotypic expression of various disorders. Finally, somatic point mutations in the mtDNA are known to accumulate with age and have been linked to the pathogenesis of many degenerative diseases.

Pathological mtDNA mutations

Except where arising as new mutations, pathological mtDNA mutations are invariably inherited through the maternal line and can occur in genes encoding the mitochondrial tRNAs, rRNAs, or the mitochondrially encoded subunits of the respiratory chain complexes. Because of the biochemical and genetic complexity of the OXPHOS system, the mitochondrial disorders can present with an exceptionally wide spectrum of clinical symptoms, making systematic classification of mitochondrial diseases very challenging. The phenotypes range from lesions of single tissues or structures such as the optic nerve in Leber hereditary optic neuropathy (LHON) or the cochlea in maternally inherited nonsyndromic deafness to more widespread lesions including myopathies, encephalomyopathies, cardiomyopathies, or complex multisystem syndromes (39). The molecular background of some syndromes is fairly well established, whereas others are defined only on the basis of clinical, morphological, or biochemical findings. Curiously, the same mutation can lead to entirely different phenotypes in different individuals and, on the other hand, very similar phenotypes can be produced by different mutations. Moreover, some of the mitochondrial mutations might lead to disease only when a specific nuclear/mitochondrial genotype or environmental agent is present, further adding to the complexity of these diseases.

The threshold effect

As described above, many (although not all) pathological mtDNA mutations are heteroplasmic. The penetrance and severity of the disease phenotype is often dependent on the ratio of the mutant versus wild-type mitochondrial genotype, i.e., the level of heteroplasmy. There is generally a certain critical proportion of the mutant mtDNA, a threshold level above which the deleterious effects of the mutation can no longer be complemented by the coexisting wild-type mtDNA, and the mutation therefore becomes relevant in terms of cellular dysfunction and pathology. However, the degree of heteroplasmy that is tolerated without clinical presentation of the disease is known to vary greatly depending on the nature of the mutation as well as other coexisting genetic and environmental factors.

Tissue specificity

Although the pathological mtDNA mutation is usually present in all tissues of the body, the clinical symptoms of the disease are often tissue specific. Possible explanations for the highly tissue-specific phenotypes seen in mitochondrial diseases include varying levels of heteroplasmy in different tissues, differential expression of the nuclear components of the mitochondrial genetic system, or variable sensitivity of different cell or tissue types to the deleterious effects of the decreased respiratory chain function and energy-generating capacity. Different tissues and organs have their own tissue-specific energetic thresholds, and the organs that are commonly involved and severely affected by mitochondrial disease include many of the ones with the highest aerobic energy demands, such as the central nervous system, the heart, and the skeletal muscle. Not all tissues with high ATP demands are as severely affected, however (40). For example, tissues as highly energy dependent as the liver and the kidney do not seem to be affected by OXPHOS deficiency to the same extent as nerve or muscle.

It has been suggested that because cells with continuous lack of ATP would inevitably die and thereby compromise the viability of the whole organism (creating an in utero lethal phenotype), the cells most severely affected by mtDNA mutations are perhaps the ones with varying ATP demands (41). Such cells are predicted to function relatively normally until their ATP demand is stimulated above the basal level. The lack of ATP under such conditions would compromise the primary function of the cells as well as increase their susceptibility to apoptosis. This idea would apply particularly well to muscle and neuronal cells in which the energy demand is known to be uneven and might also provide an explanation for the selective loss of some specific cells such as the optic nerve or cochlear hair cells, which are continuously having to respond to rapidly changing environmental stimuli.

Mitochondrial sequence variation and disease

mtDNA sequence variation in human populations

Due to the lack of protective histones, the possibly inefficient DNA repair systems, and the continuous exposure to mutagenic effects of oxygen radicals, the mutation rate in the mtDNA is approximately 10 to 20 times higher than that of the nuclear

genome (31) and varies between different regions of the mtDNA, with the hypervariable sequences in the noncoding D-loop evolving much more rapidly than the coding regions (42). Occasionally, genetic drift allows selectively neutral base substitutions to reach polymorphic frequencies. Over time, the high mutation rate has resulted in a wide range of neutral population-specific polymorphisms in the mitochondrial genome, and it has been estimated that the mtDNA sequence of any one person in the world today differs from that in another person by an average of 25 base substitutions (43).

mtDNA as a phylogenetic tool

The mtDNA polymorphisms have accumulated sequentially along radiating maternal lineages, which have diverged as human populations have colonised different geographical regions of the world (44). The mode of inheritance of the mtDNA, i.e., the maternal transmission and the relative lack of recombination makes it a particularly useful tool in human evolutionary studies. Phylogenetic analyses of mtDNAs, in conjunction with the calibrated mutation rates for the analysed sequences, have in fact allowed the clarification of several controversial issues concerning the origin of humans, the time and colonisation pattern of the various regions of the world, and some of the genetic relationships of modern human populations (45).

mtDNA sequencing and restriction fragment length polymorphism (RFLP) analysis of mtDNAs from a wide range of modern human populations have revealed a number of single-nucleotide polymorphisms that have presumably originally arisen in our early ancestors who migrated out of Africa about 130,000 years ago to become dispersed among the different continents (Fig. 9.3). Since those days, these founder polymorphisms have increased in frequency to a considerable level of prevalence and have characterised the present-day human populations in different geographical regions. Based on different combinations of these sequence variants, modern populations can be stratified into a variety of related groups of mtDNAs called haplogroups.

Haplogroups show subtle differences between populations, and the majority of them have been shown to be continent specific (44). According to the scheme proposed by Macaulay and Richards (Fig. 9.4) (47–49), the root of the human mtDNA sequences from which all others descend, the so-called "mitochondrial Eve," belongs to the L1 cluster of the African haplogroups. There are two other major African clusters, L2 and L3, but all non-African sequences appear to have descended from the L3 branch. The non-African subclusters of L3 include M and N. Asian and Native American haplogroups map to both of these clusters, whereas all European haplogroups belong to the N branch of the tree.

Haplogroup associations of clinical disorders

Haplogroup analysis can be used in conjunction with disease data to reveal a possible correlation between a certain haplogroup and an increased disease susceptibility. Polymorphisms

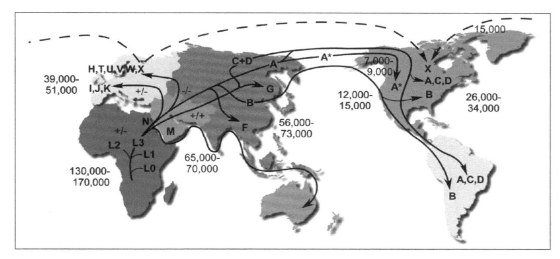

Figure 9.3 The major events of the migratory history of the human mitochondrial DNA haplogroups. Figures are number of years before present; letters represent the various mt-DNA haplogroups. *Source*: From Ref. 46.

in the coding regions of the mtDNA, although often termed "neutral," may cause subtle changes in the mitochondrially encoded polypeptides or the components of the mitochondrial translation system required for their expression, thereby affecting the function of the OXPHOS. It has been suggested that due to defective respiration and the consequent increase in the production of deleterious free radicals, individuals with a certain mitochondrial haplotype may be predisposed to a variety of degenerative cellular processes (51). Alternatively, polymorphisms characteristic of a given mitochondrial haplotype may themselves play no role in the disease susceptibility but merely serve as markers of the genetic background upon which some more recent pathological variant(s) may have arisen.

A considerable body of literature has recently emerged, reporting the association of certain haplogroups or haplogroup clusters with a variety of disorders including male infertility (52), Parkinson's disease (53,54), multiple sclerosis (55), Alzheimer's disease (AD) (56,57), Lewy body dementia (35), and occipital stroke (58). Some of these results remain inconclusive, however, due to small sample cohorts, the use of subpopulations from very limited geographical areas or, in case of multiple studies, the failure to reproduce previous findings.

An association of certain mtDNA haplogroups with successful ageing and longevity has also been suggested in two different populations (51,59). These associations have, however, been shown to be population specific and even discrepant between populations (60,61). An underrepresentation of haplogroup H and a corresponding excess of haplogroups J and U was reported in Finnish individuals older than 90 years compared with both middle-aged and infant controls from the same population, supporting the view that mitochondrial genotype may be one of the factors affecting ageing. Based on these results, two possibilities were suggested by the authors: that mildly deleterious polymorphisms may cause a subtle decrease in OXPHOS activity and thereby shorten lifespan, or conversely, that there are certain advantageous polymorphisms in

haplotypes J and U, which may actually contribute to the longevity of these individuals (51).

Polymorphisms characteristic of a certain mtDNA haplogroup have also been shown to modulate the clinical expression of some disease phenotypes in individuals carrying other primary mtDNA mutations. For example, the degree of penetrance of the pathological mtDNA mutations in LHON (62–64), or a large-scale mtDNA deletion in mitochondrial encephalomyopathies (65), has been reported to depend on the mtDNA background on which they occur. Conversely, the expression of mitochondrial myopathy, encephalopathy, lactic acidosis, and stroke-like episodes (MELAS), although very complex and varied, does not seem to be affected significantly by the haplogroup background (66,67).

mtDNA and deafness

mtDNA and hearing impairment

It has been estimated that up to 67% of patients with mtDNA disorders also manifest sensorineural hearing loss (68). The majority of the deafness-associated mitochondrial mutations have been found in families with severe systemic neuromuscular diseases such as KSS, myoclonic epilepsy with ragged red fibres (MERRF), or the MELAS syndrome, hearing loss being only one of the symptoms of the general neuromuscular dysfunction associated with these disease phenotypes. The causative mutations are often heteroplasmic and the disease shows great phenotypic variability. As an example, the consequences of a heteroplasmic point mutation at np 3243 of the *tRNA-Leu(UUR)* gene have been shown to range from diabetes and hearing loss when present at 10% to 30% of total mtDNA (69) to most severe forms of the MELAS syndrome at heteroplasmy levels higher than 70% (70).

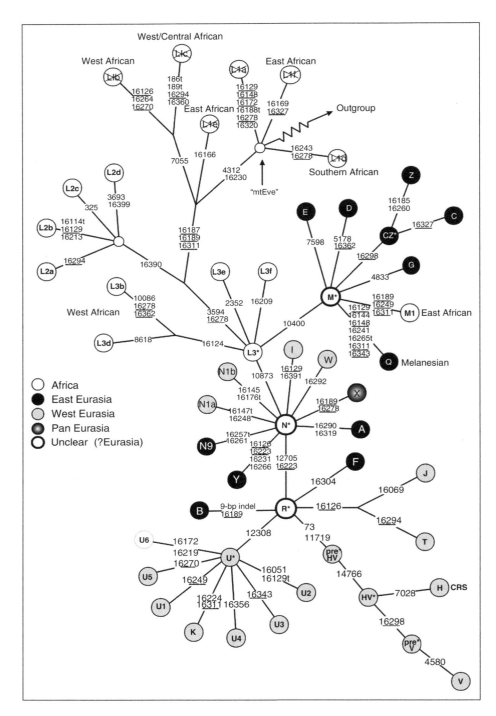

Figure 9.4 The Macaulay and Richards phylogenetic tree of human mtDNA sequences. *Abbreviation*: mt, mitochondrial. Numbers refer to the position of the nucleotide change. *Source*: From Ref. 50.

In addition, a multitude of different mtDNA mutations has been reported in maternal pedigrees, with isolated sensorineural hearing impairment (SHI). The term nonsyndromal deafness is used in this case to distinguish the phenotype from those linked to other syndromal diseases. Although these mutations give rise to a severe tissue-specific auditory phenotype, they do not seem to have such deleterious effects on other tissues or on development in general. These mutations have been found to be generally homoplasmic, suggesting that the highly tissue-specific phenotype is not a result of different levels of heteroplasmy but

rather the complex interactions between the mitochondrial genotype, the nuclear genotype, and the environmental factors (71).

Previously identified mutations in nonsyndromal SHI

The most commonly reported mtDNA mutations associated with nonsyndromal hearing impairment (NSHI) include A1555G in the *12S rRNA* gene (72), A7445G (73,74) and 7472insC (75,76) in the gene for tRNA-Ser(UCN), and A3243G (77,78) in tRNA-Leu(UUR), which, however, has also been found in families with diabetes mellitus and MELAS, showing that the distinction between the syndromal and the nonsyndromal forms of SHI is not always clear-cut.

Interestingly, most of the mtDNA mutations found in association with nonsyndromal SHI appear to be located in a few distinct regions, namely the *tRNA* genes Leucine (UUR) and Serine (UCN) and the gene for the 12S rRNA. Several other mutations in the tRNA-Ser, including T7510C (79,80), T7511C (81,82), and T7512C (83), as well as another mutation in the 12S rRNA, C1494T (84), have also been reported with similar phenotypes.

The molecular consequences of the SHI-associated mutations are complex and only partially understood. It has been suggested that some of the mutations in the *tRNA* genes interfere with the pre-tRNA processing or the translational properties of the mature tRNAs such as their aminoacylation (85,86). The resulting imbalance in the ratio of different functional tRNAs may lead to defects in the mitochondrial protein synthesis, such as misincorporation of amino acids or premature translation termination. Accumulation of abnormal translation products has in fact been proposed as one of the key mechanisms involved in the pathology of SHI.

The rRNA mutations on the other hand are known to affect the translational accuracy centre of the mitoribosome and increase its susceptibility to antibiotics, which further impair the translational fidelity. Such relaxation of the stringency of translation is also suspected to promote the accumulation of abnormal translation products, leading to a unifying hypothesis linking mtDNA mutations to SHI (71). Based on this hypothesis, any genes whose products have a role in the mitochondrial protein quality control may be considered candidates for involvement in SHI, including the components of the mitoribosomal accuracy centre, tRNA processing, and aminoacylation, as well as any of the nuclear-encoded proteins involved in the delivery and discrimination of the charged tRNAs, the correct folding and subunit assembly of the released polypeptides, and the turnover of mistranslated or misfolded proteins in the mitochondria.

Whether the above hypothesis is fully accurate remains to be answered as does the question as to why the clinical defect remains confined to the cochlea rather than affecting every tissue of the body. One proposed explanation for the tissue specificity is the possible existence of cochlear-specific isoforms or splice variants of the nuclear proteins involved in mitochondrial RNA processing or translation. The abnormal interaction of such tissue-specific proteins with the mutated rRNAs, tRNAs, or polycistronic mRNA transcripts is suggested to lead to qualitative or quantitative changes in the mitochondrial protein products (1).

Deafness-associated mtDNA mutations and ARHI

An interesting aspect of mitochondrial SHI is its striking similarity to ARHI in terms of audiometrical findings. Both these forms of hearing loss initially present with elevation in the high-frequency thresholds. Based on the similarities, mitochondrial SHI could perhaps be hypothesised to represent an acceleration of the more gradual process of age-related hearing loss, raising the possibility of a common underlying cause. However, this view was seemingly contradicted by the results of a previous study in which we screened patients with postlingual SHI from two different populations (United Kingdom and Italy) for the most common previously reported deafness-associated mtDNA mutations. Causative mutations were found in approximately 5% of patients in both the populations, representing almost 10% of the cases that were clearly familial (2). The age of onset of hearing loss in these patients was generally childhood or early adulthood. In contrast, no instances of any of the previously reported mtDNA mutations were found in patients with late-onset hearing loss (Table 9.1), indicating that at least in terms of mtDNA mutations, ARHI seems to be genetically distinct from early-onset, nonsyndromal deafness.

A1555G transition and aminoghycoside-induced ototoxicity

The A-to-G transition in the gene for the 12S rRNA is a remarkable example of how the auditory phenotype caused by mtDNA mutations can be affected by the complex interactions between the mtDNA genotype, the nuclear genotype, and environmental agents. Individuals carrying the homoplasmic A1555G mutation are known to be abnormally sensitive to aminoglycoside antibiotics (72). When exposed to aminoglycosides, these patients typically experience a sharp loss of hearing within a short period of time due to acute ototoxicity.

However, this mutation has also been found in families with hearing loss in the absence of known exposure to aminoglycosides (87), suggesting the involvement of a possible nuclear modifier, which has also been supported by genetic and biochemical evidence (88,89). A candidate locus has been identified on chromosome 8 (90) but no definite modifier genes have been detected so far. In contrast to the acute severe aminoglycoside-induced deafness, in the absence of aminoglycoside

Table 9.1 Causative mitochondrial DNA mutations found among patients with postlingual nonsyndromal hearing impairment and age-related hearing impairment

	United Kingdom (postlingual)	S. Italy (postlingual)	Finland (ARHI)
A1555G	2/80	2/128	0/138
A3243G	1/80	0/110	0/221
A7445G	1/80	2/115	0/313
7472insC	1/80	1/115	0/313
T7510C	1/80	0/115	0/313
T7511C	0/80	0/115	0/313
T7512C	0/80	0/115	0/313
Total frequency (%)	7.5%	4.2%	0%

Abbreviation: ARHI, age-related hearing impairment.
Source: From Ref. 2.

exposure, the *A1555G* mutation typically results in milder, late-onset, progressive sensorineural hearing loss (87,91), suggesting that the mutation may have an age-dependent penetrance, which is enhanced by treatment with aminoglycosides. Conversely, aminoglycoside-induced deafness is also seen in the absence of the *A1555G* mutation, especially in the Asian populations (92), suggesting that in some cases, the interaction of the nuclear genotype and the medication alone can account for the ototoxic effect.

Consistent with the endosymbiosis theory (5,6), the mitochondrial ribosomes more closely resemble bacterial ribosomes than those found in the cytosol of eukaryotes, although almost half of the rRNA contained in the bacterial ribosome is replaced with proteins in the mitoribosome (93). Many of the functionally important proteins of the translational accuracy centre show structural similarity to their bacterial homologs as well as resemblance in terms of sensitivity of the ribosomes to certain antibiotics (94). There is relatively little primary sequence conservation between the bacterial and the mitochondrial rRNAs; yet, the major secondary structures have been preserved. The np 1555 site maps to a phylogenetically highly conserved domain of the small subunit (SSU) rRNA and is equivalent to the position 1491 in the 16S rRNA of *Escherichia coli* (95). The biochemical basis for the pathology of the A1555G transition is thought to lie in the change of the small subunit rRNA to a secondary structure that more closely resembles that of the bacterial equivalent in a region that is known to have a key role in translational fidelity (96).

The mutated nt A at np 1555 is predicted to form a novel base pair with a cytosine at np 1494 and thereby lengthen the base-paired stem region of the 12S rRNA molecule by one nt pair (Fig. 9.5), rendering it more similar to the bacterial SSU rRNA than the wild type. The antibacterial effect of the aminoglycoside antibiotics is based on their ability to bind the decoding site of the bacterial SSU rRNA, thereby causing translational infidelity. The G-C base pair is expected to create a new binding site for these drugs in the 12S rRNA structure,

thus promoting aminoglycoside sensitivity (96). Consistent with this model are the findings that the C-to-T mutation at np 1494, which facilitates the equivalent base pairing of the 1494U with the wild-type 1555A, is also associated with aminoglycoside-induced hearing loss (84).

The frequency of the *A1555G* mutation in patients with nonsyndromal deafness varies considerably between different countries, being exceptionally high in Spain, where it has been shown to account for up to 20% to 30% of all cases with familial NSHI (87,97) as opposed to about 1% to 3% in other European populations (2,98,99). However, the general population prevalence has been shown to be surprisingly similar in different European populations (Jacobs et al., unpublished data), suggesting that the high frequency of deafness caused by the A1555G in Spain is likely to be due to high levels of aminoglycoside exposure, either via therapeutic use or via dietary exposure.

The typical late onset of the hearing loss in patients in the absence of aminoglycoside exposure prompts the question as to whether the *A1555G* mutation could account for some proportion of the unexplained ARHI cases. Although none of the ARHI patients in the initial screen was found to carry this mutation, these results may be considered inconclusive because of the relatively small sample number ($n = 138$).

mtDNA and ageing

The role of mitochondria in ageing

Ageing is a complex multifactorial process, characterised by the progressive decline in physiological capacity and the reduced ability to respond to environmental stresses (100). These time-dependent changes lead to increased vulnerability to various age-associated diseases, accompanied by an exponential increase in mortality with age. Although a universal and widely studied process, no unifying theory of ageing exists, owing to the obvious complexity of the phenomenon. At least a dozen different hypotheses have been proposed in the last few decades, however, including both stochastic and developmental genetic theories. Among the proposed mechanisms, the so-called free-radical theory, or its more refined version, the mitochondrial theory of ageing, have perhaps attracted the most attention. According to these hypotheses, ageing is associated with an impairment of bioenergetic function due to the accumulation of mtDNA mutations and the resulting increase in the production of ROS.

ROS and oxidative stress

ROS are oxygen-derived species that contain an unpaired electron and are therefore highly unstable. These free radicals react readily with other nearby molecules to capture the missing electron and become chemically stable. As a consequence, more free radicals are formed out of the attacked molecules, which subsequently create more free radicals, starting a chain reaction

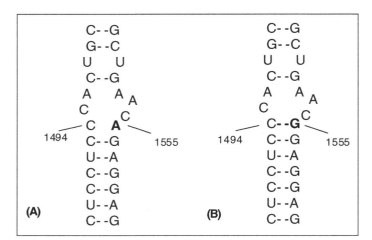

Figure 9.5 The decoding region of the human mitochondrial 12S rRNA. (A) Wild type, (B) containing the *A1555G* mutation. *Source*: From Ref. 96.

and amplifying the effects of the initial attack (100). It has been well established that the major intracellular source of free radicals is the mitochondrial ETC, which has been estimated to generate more than 90% of the intracellular ROS. The nature of the one-electron oxidation–reduction reactions within the mitochondrial ETC makes the electron carriers prone to side reactions with molecular oxygen. Complexes I and III are thought to be the predominant sites of ROS production (101). The high-energy electrons react with O_2 to form the superoxide anion O_2^-, which is converted to hydrogen peroxide, H_2O_2 by the manganese superoxide dismutase (MnSOD). H_2O_2 is usually detoxified by glutathione peroxidase but in the presence of reduced transition metals, it can be converted to the highly reactive hydroxyl radical, OH, by the Fenton reaction.

It has been estimated that approximately 0.4% to 4% of all oxygen consumed by the mitochondria is converted to ROS in normal human tissues (102). ROS have the capacity to oxidize cellular macromolecules, causing irreversible damage to the mitochondrial and cellular proteins, lipids, and nucleic acids. Each of the different species of ROS has its own mechanisms of production, detoxification, and reactions with their biological targets, and the exact pathological effects thus vary, depending on the species involved. The free-radical theory of ageing, first proposed by Harman (103), states that ageing is caused by the mitochondrial production of ROS and the resulting accumulation of damage to biological macromolecules, which eventually overwhelms the self-repair capacity of the biological systems, leading to an inevitable functional decline.

Ironically, the mitochondria, as well as being the major generators of ROS, also seem to be the direct victims of the deleterious effects of these species. Because mtDNA lies in immediate proximity to the major sites of ROS production and is unprotected by histones, it is considered an especially sensitive target for ROS attack. Compared with nuclear DNA, the level of oxidatively modified bases in mtDNA has been found to be 10- to 20-fold higher (104). The different types of lesions detected in the mtDNA include base modifications, abasic sites, and point mutations, as well as strand breaks and rearrangements. One of the most commonly used markers of oxidative damage of DNA is the content of the oxidised nucleoside, 8-hydroxy2′-deoxyguanosine (8-OHdG), which has been shown to increase in mtDNA of various ageing tissues (105–107). 8-OHdG is premutagenic because it is capable of pairing with both adenine and cytosine with almost equal efficiency and can therefore induce mutations during DNA replication (108).

Because all the gene products of the mtDNA are either polypeptides of the ETC or components required for their synthesis, any random mutation in the coding regions of mtDNA is likely to affect the OXPHOS system in one way or another. Accumulation of mutations in the mtDNA can be expected to lead to the synthesis of increasingly dysfunctional mitochondrially encoded subunits that are incorporated into the respiratory chain complexes. The defective or incorrectly assembled complexes are predicted to allow greater interaction between oxygen and redox active electron carriers, increasing the

production of ROS. ROS generation can be thought to increase in proportion to the general rate of respiratory chain electron flow in a given cell or tissue, leading to differential accumulation of oxidative stress between tissues and organs, and possibly explaining the differences in their functional decline in human ageing (109). It has also been suggested that since the disturbed synthesis of mitochondrial polypeptides most severely affects the assembly and/or function of those complexes of the ETC with the highest content of mitochondrial subunits, the chain ends up being "disproportionate." Such partial defects within the chain are predicted to block the electron flow near the site of the defect and increase the half-lives of the upstream redox active components, increasing the level of ROS production above the critical threshold for toxicity (110).

ROS are not exclusively detrimental for the cells, however. They also take part in various critical cellular functions, for example, as secondary messengers in signalling pathways regulating differential gene expression, replication, and differentiation, ion transport, calcium mobilisation, and apoptotic program activation (111). Under normal conditions, an array of different antioxidant enzymes takes care of the disposal of ROS. The MnSOD and copper/zinc superoxide dismutases (Cu/ZnSOD) can convert the superoxide anion to less dangerous and diffusible H_2O_2, which is further converted to H_2O by reactions catalysed by glutathione peroxidase and catalase. With the help of some smaller molecular weight antioxidants such as glutathione and vitamins C and E, these enzymes enable the cell to cope with the normal production of ROS. However, complete or partial deficiency of these enzymes has been shown to lead to a rapid accumulation of oxidative damage, induction of apoptosis, and shorter lifespan (112). Oxidative stress can thus be thought to result from any imbalance between the ROS-generating mechanisms and the protective mechanisms, and ageing can be attributed to not only increasing levels of ROS but also decreasing capacity of the intracellular antioxidant and damage-repair systems with advancing age.

The "mitochondrial theory of ageing"
The extension of the initial free-radical theory (103) has led to the development of several different ageing theories such as the "altered protein theory," "the waste accumulation theory," and the "mitochondrial theory." According to the mitochondrial theory of ageing, mtDNA mutations accumulate progressively during life and are directly responsible for the deficiency in the function of the OXPHOS system. Defects in the respiratory chain are proposed to cause increased production of ROS, which in turn leads to the accumulation of further mtDNA damage (113,114). The ageing process has therefore been suggested to be a self-perpetuating vicious cycle (Fig. 9.6) of exponentially increasing oxidative damage, which eventually leads to a bioenergetic crisis, various age-associated metabolic and physiologic changes, as well as activation of apoptosis and the loss of specific cell types, tissue dysfunction, and an increased susceptibility to disease.

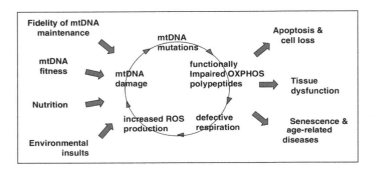

Figure 9.6 The vicious cycle proposed by the mitochondrial theory of ageing. *Abbreviations*: mtDNA, mitochondrial DNA; ROS, reactive oxygen species; OXPHOS, oxidative phosphorylation.

There is a substantial amount of indirect evidence supporting various aspects of the mitochondrial theory of ageing, including the proposed role of the increasing burden of mtDNA mutations in ageing and degenerative disease. Both point mutations and rearrangements (deletions and/or duplications) of the mtDNA have been reported to accumulate with age in a variety of tissues in both humans and experimental animals. The occurrence of a specific 4977 bp deletion, previously found among patients with the rare mitochondrial diseases KSS and PEO, has been shown to increase in the postmitotic tissues also during normal ageing (115). Accumulation of certain pathological mtDNA mutations such as those associated with MELAS (116) or MERRF (117) has also been reported in normally ageing individuals, albeit to a very low level and in a highly tissue-specific manner (118). Similarly, specific point mutations in the noncoding region of the mtDNA, such as A189G and T408A in skeletal muscle (119), T414G in fibroblasts (120), or T150C in leukocytes (121) have been reported to accumulate in aged individuals but have also been shown to be restricted to specific tissues.

Besides systematic accumulation of specific mutations, the abundance of different types of somatic mtDNA rearrangements (deletions and partial duplications), detected by semiquantitative polymerase chain reaction (PCR) assay, has also been shown to increase with age in the human heart, although a considerable variation in their levels was detected at all ages (122). In addition, sequencing of the D-loop region, and, more recently, also certain coding regions, has revealed an age-dependent increase in the total point-mutation load in mtDNA from mouse liver (123) as well as human brain (124,125) and, based on preliminary results, possibly also heart (Vahvaselkä et al., unpublished results).

The reported mutation levels are typically in the range of one to two mutations per 10 kb of sequence and can therefore be estimated to affect only a few percent of the total mtDNA. According to model cell systems, levels of 60% to 80% of mutant mtDNA are required in vitro to observe deleterious biochemical effects (126), and relatively high heteroplasmic levels are also often tolerated by patients with mtDNA mutations without detectable clinical presentation of the disease. Therefore, it seems unlikely that the low levels of mutations detected in the above-mentioned studies could actually result in any

biochemical defect, assuming they were distributed randomly among cells. This assumption is also supported by previous observations from cultured human cells expressing 3' to 5' proofreading-deficient mtDNA polymerase (127). Cells with the "POLG mutator"-accumulated mtDNA mutation loads higher than 5/10 kb after two to three months were yet associated with only a very modest respiratory chain deficiency, indicating that the threshold level for OXPHOS deficiency is considerably higher than the mutation loads generally observed in ageing tissues.

The possibility that needs to be considered, however, is that low levels of mutated mtDNA may clonally expand in a small subset of cells due to mitotic segregation or genetic drift in postmitotic cells during ageing. High proportions of clonal mutant mtDNA, presumably expanded from a single initial mutant mtDNA molecule, have been detected in single-cell analysis of tissues as diverse as buccal epithelium and heart muscle (128). Clonal expansion of mtDNA-point mutations or deletions within individual skeletal muscle-cell fibres has been shown to lead to very high levels of specific mtDNA mutations, causing defects in the mitochondrial OXPHOS complex cytochrome-c-oxidase (COX) in single-muscle fibres (129,130). Similar COX-deficient cells have been detected in other aged tissues including the human heart (131) as well as brain tissue of patients with AD (132), indicating high levels of mutant mtDNA in individual cells. Although it is unclear whether such a mosaic pattern of respiratory chain deficiency is able to actually compromise the function of the whole tissue or organ, it has nevertheless been hypothesised that clonal expansion of mutations may be actively involved in ageing and degenerative disease (128), and pathological consequences have been suggested particularly if the affected cells perform an integral role in a complex network, as is often the case in the central nervous system (133).

Although a considerable number of studies support the idea that mtDNA mutations accumulate during ageing, it is impossible to conclude from such correlative data alone that this accumulation actually has a causal role in ageing rather than just being an epiphenomenon of the process. The first direct, experimental link between the increased levels of somatic mtDNA mutations, the respiratory chain dysfunction, and the accelerated ageing phenotype was established by creating a homozygous knock-in mouse expressing a proofreading-deficient mitochondrial polymerase POLG (134). These mice developed a three- to fivefold increase in the levels of somatic mtDNA mutations compared with wild-type animals, and the substantial burden of mutations was associated with reduced lifespan and premature onset of many age-related changes such as weight loss, reduced subcutaneous fat, alopecia, kyphosis, osteoporosis, anaemia, reduced fertility, and heart hypertrophy, suggesting a causative link between mtDNA mutations and ageing phenotypes in mammals. Although the mutation loads found in the oldest POLG-mutator mice were of the order of 10 to 15 mutations per 10 kb, their premature ageing was accompanied by only a moderate OXPHOS deficiency, consistent with the previous observations in cultured human cells with a similar mutator (127). These results initially suggested that rather than bioenergetic insufficiency alone, the accumulation of mtDNA mutations is likely to promote ageing via some kind of toxic mechanism or via extensive mitotic segregation and genetic drift.

The most obvious candidate for a toxic mechanism is the increased production of ROS, as suggested by the mitochondrial theory of ageing. Recent results show, however, that contrary to the vicious cycle theory, which would predict an exponential accumulation of mtDNA mutations, the mtDNA-mutator mice accumulate mtDNA mutations in an approximately linear manner over their lifetime (135). Despite the respiratory chain deficiency, the amount of ROS production was shown to be normal, as were the levels of the studied biomarkers of oxidative stress and the expression levels of antioxidant defence enzymes. Based on these observations, it was proposed that rather than a vicious cycle of increasing oxidative stress and exponential accumulation of mtDNA mutations, the accelerated ageing of the mtDNA mutator mice is after all induced primarily by the respiratory chain dysfunction itself via a variety of possible mechanisms, including a bioenergy deficit in physiologically crucial cells, decreased signal thresholds for apoptosis, or induction of replicative senescence in stem cells.

ARHI

Deterioration of hearing ability is one of the inevitable consequences of advancing age. Because of its high prevalence, ARHI is a significant socioeconomic health problem. In Finland, for example, ARHI represents one of the most common age-associated sensorineural defects, estimated to affect one-third of the adults between the ages of 65 and 75 and as much as two-thirds of the Finnish population older than 75 years (136).

ARHI, also known as presbyacusis, is a multifactorial process that shows variation in age of onset and progression and can range in severity from mild to substantial. Clinically, the disorder is characterised by a progressive, bilateral high-frequency hearing loss that is demonstrated by a moderately sloping audiogram. The symptoms include reduced hearing sensitivity and speech discrimination, especially in environments with background noise, slowed central processing of acoustic information as well as impaired localisation of sound sources (137). With time, the hearing loss usually extends also to the lower frequencies, further impairing the comprehension of speech and the overall communication abilities of the affected individuals.

Despite extensive research attempting to determine the underlying causes of presbyacusis, understanding of the exact pathophysiology still remains incomplete. The process of sound perception follows a complex pathway, and age-related changes in several of its components can contribute to the loss of hearing sensitivity. Most often, the hearing loss can be attributed to degeneration or loss of the sensory cells (inner and outer cochlear hair cells), neural damage of the spiral ganglion, and/or atrophy of the stria vascularis (138), although it is currently not clear to what extent each of these contributes.

Clinical classification

The aetiology of age-related hearing loss is still not understood. Most current knowledge comes from animal models, epidemiological studies, clinical experience, and human temporal-bone research. According to early studies of Schuknecht et al. (139), presbyacusis can be divided to four main subcategories, based on the histological changes in the cochleae and the corresponding premortem clinical symptoms and auditory test results (140). These classic types of the disorder—sensory, neural, strial, and mechanical—can occur alone or in combination.

Sensory presbyacusis is characterised by atrophy of the sensory hair cells and supporting cells in the organ of Corti, originating in the basal turn of the cochlea and progressing toward the apex. The consequence of these changes is an abrupt high-frequency hearing loss, usually beginning after middle age.

Neural presbyacusis, on the other hand, refers to the degeneration of the spiral ganglion nerve cells and central neural pathways. Even without noticeable elevation in hearing thresholds, the neural form often leads to a severe decrease in speech discrimination, especially in the presence of background noise.

The third category, named strial presbyacusis, involves atrophic changes of the stria vascularis. Because the normal function of these cells is critical to the maintenance of the endocochlear potential as well as the metabolic health of the sensory cells, this form of presbyacusis is also sometimes called metabolic presbyacusis. The loss of threshold sensitivity begins in the high-frequency region but progresses to the lower frequencies as the metabolic function of the strial cells declines. Because the entire cochlea is eventually affected, the hearing loss in strial presbyacusis is typically represented by a flat or slightly descending audiogram.

The last form is the mechanical presbyacusis, which is thought to result from changes in the vibrational properties of the basilar membrane, thereby affecting the conductivity of the cochlea. Hearing loss due to mechanical stiffness of the basilar membrane results in a linear, gradually sloping audiogram, with the highest frequencies being the most affected.

Regardless of the above division, in the majority cases of ARHI, simultaneous changes occur at multiple sites, making such a classification difficult. In fact, Schuknecht et al. also later added two more categories: mixed and indeterminate, the latter of which they proposed to account for 25% of all cases (139).

Heritability of ARHI

Heritability studies indicate that ARHI is a complex disorder influenced by both genetic and environmental factors. The relative importance of the genetic component of a disease can be expressed as the fraction of the phenotypic variance that is due to the effect of genes (141). Recent studies on monozygotic and dizygotic twins (142) as well as cohort studies of genetically related and unrelated individuals (143) show a clear familial aggregation, indicating that as much as half of the variance in ARHI may be due to heritable factors.

Much of the past and current research has focused on finding some of the underlying genetic abnormalities, which may cause, contribute to, or predispose to the development of ARHI. However, unravelling the genetics of complex diseases is far from straightforward. Since the number of causative variants and risk factors and their relative contributions to the phenotype and complex interactions with each other are not known, classic positional cloning strategies are not applicable to complex disorders. As a consequence, very little is known about the genetic component of ARHI. Up to now, almost 130 loci have been reported for monogenic nonsyndromal hearing impairment, and about 50 of these genes have been identified. Conversely, there are only a few candidate loci for late-onset or progressive hearing loss, and no true susceptibility genes have been identified so far (144).

Two of the most powerful strategies for searching for genetic determinants of ARHI are association studies and linkage analysis. Association studies search for DNA variants associated with the trait using unrelated samples, based on the assumption that if a certain variant confers increased susceptibility to a complex disease, it should be more frequent among the affected individuals compared to a control group. Linkage studies, on the other hand, attempt to identify the regions harbouring the susceptibility genes by nonparametric linkage analysis on a large collection of small families. In the case of ARHI, collecting families can be difficult due to the late onset of the disorder because samples from higher generations are generally not available.

Due to the similarities between the monogenic forms of NSHI and ARHI, the genes causing NSHI comprise a well-defined set of candidate genes to be tested for involvement in ARHI. Possible candidate genes have also been derived from murine models of age-related hearing loss. Inner ear function is similar between mice and humans, which suggests that the pathways to hearing loss may also be shared, and the human orthologs of genes identified to be associated with ARHI in mice are therefore justifiable candidates to be tested in humans. The most interesting of such mouse loci is the Ahl locus in chromosome 10 (145), which has been described to contain several candidate genes for possible predisposition to ARHI. Because of the suspected interplay between genetic and environmental factors, the genetic risk factors of interest also include those that may increase the susceptibility to noise, ototoxicity, or ageing.

Environmental risk factors

ARHI is often regarded as the consequence of accumulating auditory stresses during life, superimposed upon the natural ageing process. The involvement of environmental factors is implied, for example, by the fact that hearing levels are generally poorer in industrialised than in isolated or agrarian societies (137). Apart from family history, the most commonly studied risk factors of age-related hearing loss include noise-induced damage, otological, and other disorders as well as exposure to ototoxic agents. It is unclear, for the most part, whether these factors act on specific physiological pathways or just somehow speed up the rate of the normal ageing of the cochlea. Complex interactions between the effects of various factors are likely to affect the overall susceptibility to hearing loss, although the evidence of such interactions remains incomplete.

Noise exposure is the most studied environmental factor causing hearing loss. Very high–intensity acoustic overstimulation is known to cause mechanical damage to the cochlea (146), whereas at lower noise levels, the cochlear damage is predominantly metabolic, suggested to be mediated by increased production of free radicals (147), glutamate excitotoxicity (148), impaired mitochondrial function (149), and/or glutathione (GHS) depletion (150). Based on animal models, the primary histopathological sign of noise exposure is loss of the outer hair cells, but with continuous overexposure for a long time, the inner hair cells will also disappear (151). Excitotoxicity may also cause swelling of the afferent nerve endings and disruption of the postsynaptic structures, leading to neuronal death in the spiral ganglion (148). Histological as well as audiometric changes in noise-induced hearing loss are often indistinguishable from those of age-related hearing loss.

Certain prescribed drugs, namely aminoglycoside antibiotics, are well known ototoxins and account for approximately 3% to 4% of hearing loss in developing countries and a smaller but still significant number of adults in developed countries (152). The problem has been suggested to be even more pronounced among the elderly, who often use more medication compared to people in other age groups (141). Aminoglycoside-induced ototoxicity is usually dose dependent, and in the elderly, the blood levels of medication may also be more likely to rise above the critical levels due to altered renal or liver functions. Other major classes of drugs known to cause permanent hearing loss are the platinum-based chemotherapeutic agents such as Cisplatin, used in the treatment of cancer. Both these groups of drugs are known to damage the hair cells in a pattern similar to noise-induced damage, causing nonreversible, high-frequency hearing loss. In spite of the differences in the nature of the insult, the hearing loss from ototoxic drugs and noise exposure share a number of similarities in cochlear pathology, and similar mechanisms including increased oxidative stress and glutathione depletion have been suggested to mediate the hair-cell death (150). Aminoglycosides have also been reported to intensify the ototoxic effects of noise exposure and vice versa (141). Another example of the complex interactions between the various genetic and environmental factors contributing to hearing loss is the fact that three mtDNA mutations have been reported to confer an increased susceptibility to aminoglycoside ototoxicity.

Cardiovascular disease and its risk factors have been shown to affect hearing to some extent (153). Stroke, myocardial infarction, claudication, hypertension, hyperlipidaemia, and diabetes mellitus have all been previously associated with excessive hearing loss (154–156). In some studies, long-term smoking (157) and excessive alcohol intake (158) have been shown to correlate with hearing loss in the elderly, although the effects of smoking still remain controversial. A variety of work-place chemicals are known as potentially ototoxic if exposure exceeds a certain level (159), and there is accumulating evidence that many of these toxins may be able to potentiate the ototoxicity of noise through oxidative stress mechanisms (1). The effects of diet on age-related hearing loss have been extensively studied, and high-lipid diets have been associated with poor hearing (154). Potential benefits of low-calorie diets or consumption of antioxidant agents in preventing auditory ageing have been suggested (160), but the existing evidence remains inconclusive.

Prevention and therapy

Based on the current knowledge of the risk factors, the most essential preventive strategies include avoidance of hazardous noise exposure and ototoxic agents as well as maintenance of good general health and fitness. Because of the presumed involvement of ROS in several of the mechanisms triggering hearing loss, one suggested strategy to protect the inner ear from ototoxicity would be the administration of antioxidant drugs to scavenge ROS and thereby prevent the activation of cell-death pathways. Downstream prevention of apoptosis with any possible drug-based therapy would in turn require interruption of the already activated cell-death cascades, for which a much more detailed knowledge of these pathways and the key cellular targets is needed.

There is no cure currently available for ARHI. Because the hearing loss is irreversible, the existing treatment strategies are mainly focused on functional improvement, i.e., compensating for the disability as much as possible. Hearing aids are usually recommended when the impaired hearing causes a significant disadvantage in the everyday life of the patient. Even though the hearing aids and assistive listening devices cannot restore hearing to normal, they can, in many cases, improve the patient's ability to communicate. The benefits are, however, very individual. In very severe cases, where hearing aids no longer provide benefit, cochlear implantation may be considered.

In order to actually restore hearing, it would have to become possible to successfully replace the lost hair cells and/or spiral ganglion neurons. However, even such strategies would probably turn out to be inefficient, unless the actual cause of the cell death is known and can be treated. Overall, the future development of efficient treatment strategies will clearly require a more detailed knowledge of the molecular mechanisms underlying the cell loss.

The proposed role of mtDNA in ARHI

One of the key molecular mechanisms suggested to underlie cell loss in ARHI is mitochondrial dysfunction due to mtDNA mutations (68). Mitochondria have several important roles in cells, their primary function being the production of ATP by OXPHOS. Mutations in the mtDNA can affect either components of the OXPHOS system directly or the rRNAs and tRNAs required for their synthesis. Their deleterious effects on cell function can thus be mediated via a variety of different mechanisms, including impaired mitochondrial protein synthesis, accumulation, and defective turnover of abnormal translation products, bioenergy insufficiency, oxidative stress, calcium dyshomeostasis, and activation of apoptotic cell death (41). Inherited mtDNA mutations have been linked to a diverse spectrum of human disorders. In addition, polymorphic variants associated with certain mtDNA haplotypes have been reported to act as predisposing factors to a variety of disorders.

A considerable amount of evidence also supports the involvement of mtDNA in sensorineural hearing loss. Mutations in the mtDNA have been identified in both syndromal and nonsyndromal hearing loss as well as in predisposition to aminoglycoside induced to ototoxicity (1), therefore, also comprising an obvious set of candidates for possible involvement in ARHI. Moreover, it has been proposed that somatic mtDNA mutations accumulate during ageing, especially in postmitotic tissues and are responsible for the age-related decline in bioenergetic function and tissue viability. Accumulation of somatically acquired mtDNA mutations has therefore been suggested to play a role in many age-related degenerative processes including cochlear cell degeneration that causes decreased auditory sensitivity in ARHI (161).

Does mtDNA mutation accumulation play a role in ARHI?

Evidence of increased levels of mtDNA damage has not only been reported in normally ageing individuals but also in various tissues of patients with age-related degenerative diseases. For example, increased levels of mtDNA rearrangements, namely the 4977 bp deletion, have been found in different regions of the brain of patients with AD (162) and Parkinson's disease (163) compared with age-matched controls. The aggregate burden of mtDNA-point mutations has also been reported to increase in the brain mtDNA of AD patients with age (124). In contrast, other studies have failed to detect any signs of mtDNA-point mutation accumulation in the brains of either normal elderly individuals or patients with age-related neurodegenerative disease (164).

ARHI is a common aspect of ageing. Similar to many classical neurodegenerative diseases, functional deficits in ARHI are also associated with irreversible loss of specific cell types, namely the cochlear hair cells, the cells of the stria vascularis, or the spiral ganglion neurons. It has thus been suggested that the accumulation of mtDNA mutations, and the subsequent impairment of mitochondrial function, could also play a role in the age-related degeneration of auditory tissue in ARHI (161). In support of this idea, increased levels of mtDNA mutations (165) as well as the common 4977 bp ageing deletion (166) have been detected in mtDNA from archived human temporal bones of patients with presbyacusis compared with controls, suggesting that at least some proportion of ARHI patients have significant loads of mtDNA mutations in the auditory tissue. However, these findings can hardly be considered conclusive due to the very small number of samples studied.

The deleterious physiological effects of mtDNA mutations on the acoustic neural system could be thought to result from a general deficiency of OXPHOS or be mediated via other cumulative toxic mechanisms such as excessive generation of ROS. Significantly reduced blood supply in the ageing cochlea has been suggested to lead to ischaemia and increased generation of ROS in the cochlear tissue (160,167). The resulting oxidative stress has been proposed to adversely affect the inner-ear neural structures and contribute to the decline in cellular viability and cochlear function during the ageing process. Based on animal studies, treatment with antioxidant compounds known to either block or scavenge ROS has been suggested to have a protective effect on age-related hearing loss (160).

Lastly, and perhaps most interestingly, very recent results from the analysis of the POLG-mutator mice show that, along with all the above-listed consequences of premature ageing, the mice also develop a progressive impairment of hearing with auditory system pathology strikingly similar to that found in humans with ARHI (Aleksandra Trifunovic, personal communication). In these mice, the progressive loss of hearing is accompanied by apoptotic loss of cells of the stria vascularis as well as neurons of the spiral ganglion and the central cochlear nuclei, suggesting that elevation of somatic mtDNA mutation levels does indeed result in progressive degeneration of the auditory system and leads to age-related hearing loss in the mice. The cell loss in the auditory system was observed to progress in an approximately linear fashion, which is congruent with the previously reported linear accumulation of mtDNA mutations and respiratory chain deficiency in these mice (135) but contradicts the idea of the vicious cycle of exponential deterioration of mitochondrial function due to mtDNA mutation accumulation.

Despite the recent findings indicating that mitochondrial dysfunction due to increased levels of somatic mtDNA mutations has the capacity to cause pathology closely resembling the physiological and anatomical changes seen in human ARHI, no direct evidence exists so far that mtDNA mutations do actually accumulate in excessive amounts in patients with ARHI.

Acknowledgements

Our work is supported by the Academy of Finland, Juselius Foundation, Tampere University Medical Research Fund, and the European Union (GENDEAF QLG1-CT-2001-01429, MitAGE QLK6-CT-2000-00054, MitEURO QLG1-CT-2001-00966, and EUMITOCOMBAT LSHM-CT-2004-503116 projects). We are very grateful to Marie Lott (Mitomap.org), Vincent Macaulay, Martin Richards, and Anja Rovio for providing pictures and to Ilmari Pyykkö, Anu Wartiovaara, Hans Spebrink, and many other colleagues for stimulating discussions and suggestions.

References

1. Fischel-Ghodsian N, Kopke RD, Ge X. Mitochondrial dysfunction in hearing loss. Mitochondrion 2004; 4:675–694.
2. Jacobs HT, Hutchin TP, Käppi T, et al. Mitochondrial DNA mutations in patients with postlingual, nonsyndromic hearing impairment. EJHG 2005; 13:26–33.
3. Nelson DL, Cox MM. Lehninger Principles of Biochemistry. 3rd ed. New York: Worth Publishers, 2000:659–690.
4. Mitchell M. Coupling of phosphorylation to electron and hydrogen transfer by a chemiosmotic type of mechanism. Nature 1961; 191:144–148.
5. Margulis L. Symbiosis in Cell Evolution. San Fransisco: WH Freeman, 1981.
6. Gray MW, Berger G, Lang BF. Mitochondrial evolution. Science 1999; 283:1476–1481.
7. Gray MW. The endosymbiont hypothesis revisited. Intl Rev Cytol 1992; 141:233–357.
8. Taylor SW, Fahy E, Ghosh SS. Global organellar proteomics. Trends Biotech 2003; 2182–2188.
9. Cavelier L, Johannisson A, Gyllensten U. Analysis of mtDNA copy number and composition of single mitochondrial particles using flow cytometry and PCR. Exp Cell Res 2000; 259:79–85.
10. Anderson S, Bankier AT, Barrell BG, et al. Sequence and organization of the human mitochondrial genome. Nature 1981; 290:357–465.
11. Ojala D, Montoya J, Attardi G. tRNA punctuation model of RNA processing in human mitochondria. Nature 1981; 290:470–474.
12. MITOMAP: A Human Mitochondrial Genome Database. http://www.mitomap.org, 2006—mitomapgenome.pdf.
13. Garrido N, Griparic L, Jokitalo E, et al. Composition and dynamics of human mitochondrial nucleoids. Mol Biol Cell 2003; 14:1483–1496.
14. Jacobs HT, Lehtinen SK, Spelbrink JN. No sex please, we are mitochondria: a hypothesis on the somatic unit of inheritance of mammalian mtDNA. Bioessays 2000; 22:564–572.
15. Clayton DA. Replication of animal mitochondrial DNA. Cell 1982; 28:693–705.
16. Holt IJ, Lorimer HE, Jacobs HT. Coupled leading- and lagging-strand synthesis of mammalian mitochondrial DNA. Cell 2000; 100:515–524.
17. Bowmaker M, Yang MY, Yasukawa T, et al. Mammalian mitochondrial DNA replicates bidirectionally from an initiation zone. J Biol Chem 2003; 278:50961–50969.
18. Ropp PA, Copeland WC. Cloning and characterization of the human mitochondrial DNA polymerase, DNA polymerase γ. Genomics 1996; 36:449–458.
19. Lim SE, Longley MJ, Copeland WC. The mitochondrial p55 accessory subunit enhances DNA binding, promotes processive DNA synthesis, and confers NEM resistance to human DNA polymerase. J Biol Chem 1999; 274:38197–38203.
20. Tiranti V, Rocchi M, DiDonato S, et al. Cloning of human and rat cDNAs encoding the mitochondrial single-stranded DNA-binding protein (SSB). Gene 1993; 126:219–225.

21. Parisi MA, Clayton DA. Similarity of human mitochondrial transcription factor 1 to high mobility group proteins. Science 1991; 252:965–969.

22. Parisi MA, Xu B, Clayton DA. A human mitochondrial transcriptional activator can functionally replace a yeast mitochondrial HMG-box protein both in vivo and in vitro. Mol Cell Biol 1993; 13:1951–1961.

23. Spelbrink JN, Li FY, Tiranti V, et al. Human mitochondrial DNA deletions associated with mutations in the gene encoding Twinkle, a phage T7 4-like protein localized in mitochondria. Nat Genet 2001; 28:223–231.

24. Tiranti V, Anna Savoia A, Forti F, et al. Identification of the gene encoding the human mitochondrial RNA polymerase (h-mtRPOL) by cyberscreening of the expressed sequence tags database. Hum Mol Genet 1997; 6:4615–4625.

25. Montoya J, Christianson T, Levens D, et al. Identification of initiation sites for heavy-strand and light-strand transcription in human mitochondrial DNA. Proc Natl Acad Sci USA 1982; 79:7195–7199.

26. Chang DD, Clayton DA. Priming of human mitochondrial DNA replication occurs at the light-strand promoter. Proc Natl Acad Sci USA 1985; 82:351–355.

27. Clayton DA. Transcription and replication of mitochondrial DNA. Hum Reprod 2000; 15:11–17.

28. Giles RE, Blanc H, Cann HM, et al. Maternal inheritance of human mitochondrial DNA. Proc Natl Acad Sci USA 1980; 77:6715–6719.

29. Manfredi G, Thyagarajan D, Papadopoulou LC, et al. The fate of human sperm-derived mtDNA in somatic cells. Am J Hum Genet 1997; 61:953–960.

30. Schwartz M, Vissing J. No evidence for paternal inheritance of mtDNA in patients with sporadic mtDNA mutations. J Neurol Sci 2004; 218:99–101.

31. Wallace DC, Ye JH, Neckelmann SN, et al. Sequence analysis of cDNAs for the human and bovine ATP synthase beta subunit: mitochondrial DNA genes sustain seventeen times more mutations. Curr Genet 1987; 12:81–90.

32. Lightowlers RN, Chinnery PF, Turnbull DM, et al. Mammalian mitochondrial genetics: heredity, heteroplasmy and disease. Trends Genet 1997; 13:450–455.

33. Wallace DC. Mitochondrial DNA sequence variation in human evolution and disease. Proc Natl Acad Sci USA 1994; 91:8739–8746.

34. Marchington DR, Macaulay V, Hartshorne GM, et al. Evidence from human oocytes for a genetic bottleneck in an mtDNA disease. Am J Hum Genet 1998; 63:769–775.

35. Chinnery PF, Taylor GA, Howell N, et al. Mitochondrial DNA haplogroups and susceptibility to AD and dementia with Lewy bodies. Neurol 2000; 55:302–304.

36. Poulton J, Morten KJ, Marchinton D, et al. Duplications of mitochondrial DNA in Kearns-Sayre syndrome. Muscle Nerve 1995; 3:S154–S158.

37. Zeviani M, Bresolin N, Gellera C, et al. Nucleus-driven multiple large-scale deletions of the human mitochondrial genome: a new autosomal dominant disease. Am J Hum Genet 1990; 47:904–914.

38. Suomalainen-Wartiovaara A. Multiple mitochondrial DNA deletions and mitochondrial DNA depletion. In: Holt IJ. Genetics of Mitochondrial Disease. Oxford University Press, 2003:165–180.

39. Zeviani M, Tiranti V, Piantadosi C. Mitochondrial disorders. Medicine (Baltimore) 1998; 77:59–72.

40. Inoue K, Nakada K, Ogura A, et al. Generation of mice with mitochondrial dysfunction by introducing mouse mtDNA carrying a deletion into zygotes. Nature Genet 2000; 26:176–181.

41. James AM, Murphy MP. The effects of mitochondrial DNA mutations on cell function. In: Holt IJ. Genetics of Mitochondrial Disease. Oxford University Press, 2003:209–228.

42. Howell N, Kubacka I, Mackey DA. How rapidly does the human mitochondrial genome evolve? Am J Hum Genet 1996; 59:501–509.

43. Chinnery PF, Howell N, Andrews RM, et al. Mitochondrial DNA analysis: polymorphisms and pathogenicity. J Med Genet 1999; 36:505–510.

44. Torroni A, Huoponen K, Francalacci P, et al. Classification of European mtDNAs from an analysis of three European populations. Genetics 1996; 144:1835–1850.

45. Torroni A, Wallace DC. Mitochondrial DNA variation in human populations and implications for detection of mitochondrial DNA mutations of pathological significance. J Bioenerg Biomembr 1994; 26:261–271.

46. MITOMAP: A Human Mitochondrial Genome Database. http://www.mitomap.org, 2006—WorldMigrations.pdf.

47. Macaulay V, Richards M, Hickey E, et al. The emerging tree of West Eurasian mtDNAs: a synthesis of control region sequences and RFLPs. Am J Hum Genet 1999; 64:232–249.

48. Richards M, Macaulay V, Hickey E, et al. Tracing European founder lineages in the Near Eastern mtDNA pool. Am J Hum Genet 2000; 67:1251–1276.

49. Richards M, Macaulay V, Torroni A, et al. In search of geographical patterns in European mitochondrial DNA. Am J Hum Genet 2002; 71:1168–1174.

50. www.stats.gla.ac.uk/~vincent/images/skeleton07-08-02.jpg.

51. Niemi AK, Hervonen A, Hurme M, et al. Mitochondrial DNA polymorphisms associated with longevity in a Finnish population. Hum Genet 2003; 112:29–33.

52. Ruiz-Pesini E, Lapena AC, Diez-Sanchez C, et al. Human mtDNA haplogroups associated with high or reduced spermatozoa motility. Am J Hum Genet 2000; 67:682–696.

53. van der Walt JM, Nicodemus KK, Martin ER, et al. Mitochondrial polymorphisms significantly reduce the risk of Parkinson disease. Am J Hum Genet 2003; 72:804–811.

54. Ross OA, McCormack R, Maxwell LD, et al. mt4216C variant in linkage with the mtDNA TJ cluster may confer a susceptibility to mitochondrial dysfunction resulting in an increased risk of Parkinson's disease in the Irish. Exp Gerontol 2003; 38:397–405.

55. Kalman B, Li S, Chatterjee D, et al. Large scale screening of the mitochondrial DNA reveals no pathogenic mutations but a haplotype associated with multiple sclerosis in Caucasians. Acta Neurol Scand 1999; 99:16–25.

56. Chagnon P, Gee M, Filion M, et al. Phylogenetic analysis of the mitochondrial genome indicates significant differences between patients with Alzheimer disease and controls in a French-Canadian founder population. Am J Med Genet 1999; 85:20–30.

57. Carrieri G, Bonafe M, De Luca M, et al. Mitochondrial DNA haplogroups and APOE4 allele are non-independent variables in sporadic Alzheimer's disease. Hum Genet 2001; 108:194–198.

58. Majamaa K, Finnila S, Turkka J, et al. Mitochondrial DNA haplogroup U as a risk factor for occipital stroke in migraine. Lancet 1998; 352:455–456.

59. De Benedictis G, Rose G, Carrieri G, et al. Mitochondrial DNA inherited variants are associated with successful aging and longevity in humans. FASEB J 1999; 13:1532–1536.

60. Ross OA, McCormack R, Curran MD, et al. Mitochondrial DNA polymorphism: its role in longevity of the Irish population. Exp Gerontol 2001; 36:1161–1178.

61. Dato S, Passarino G, Rose G, et al. Association of the mitochondrial DNA haplogroup J with longevity is population specific. Eur J Hum Genet 2004; 12:1080–1082.

62. Brown MD, Sun F, Wallace DC. Clustering of Caucasian Leber hereditary optic neuropathy patients containing the 11778 or 14484 mutations on an mtDNA lineage. Am J Hum Genet 1997; 60:381–387.

63. Torroni A, Petrozzi M, D'Urbano L, et al. Haplotype and phylogenetic analyses suggest that one European-specific mtDNA background plays a role in the expression of Leber hereditary optic neuropathy by increasing the penetrance of the primary mutations 11778 and 14484. Am J Hum Genet 1997; 60:1107–1121.

64. Howell N, Herrnstadt C, Shults C, et al. Low penetrance of the 14484 LHON mutation when it arises in a non-haplogroup J mtDNA background. Am J Med Genet 2003; 119:147–151.

65. Crimi M, Del Bo R, Galbiati S, et al. Mitochondrial A12308G polymorphism affects clinical features in patients with single mtDNA macrodeletion. Eur J Hum Genet 2003; 11:896–898.

66. Hofmann S, Jaksch M, Bezold R, et al. Population genetics and disease susceptibility: characterization of central European haplogroups by mtDNA gene mutations, correlation with D loop variants and association with disease. Hum Mol Genet 1997; 6:1835–1846.

67. Torroni A, Campos Y, Rengo C, et al. Mitochondrial DNA haplogroups do not play a role in the variable phenotypic presentation of the A3243G mutation. Am J Hum Genet 2003; 72:1005–1012.

68. Seidman MD, Ahmad N, Bai U. Molecular mechanisms of age-related hearing loss. Ageing Res Rev 2002; 1:331–343.

69. van den Ouweland JM, Lemkes HH, Trembath RC, et al. Maternally inherited diabetes and deafness is a distinct subtype of diabetes and associates with a single point mutation in the mitochondrial tRNA(Leu(UUR)) gene. Diabetes 1994; 43:746–751.

70. Goto Y, Nonaka I, Horai S. A mutation in the tRNA(Leu)(UUR) gene associated with the MELAS subgroup of mitochondrial encephalomyopathies. Nature 1990; 348:651–653.

71. Jacobs HT. Mitochondrial deafness. Ann Med 1997; 29:483–491.

72. Prezant TR, Agapian JV, Bohlman MC, et al. Mitochondrial ribosomal RNA mutation associated with both antibiotic-induced and non-syndromic deafness. Nat Genet 1993; 4:289–294.

73. Reid FM, Vernham GA, Jacobs HT. A novel mitochondrial point mutation in a maternal pedigree with sensorineural deafness. Hum Mutat 1994; 3:243–247.

74. Fischel-Ghodsian N, Prezant TR, Fournier P, et al. Mitochondrial mutation associated with nonsyndromic deafness. Am J Otolaryngol 1995; 16:403–408.

75. Tiranti V, Chariot P, Carella F, et al. Maternally inherited hearing loss, ataxia and myoclonus associated with a novel point mutation in mitochondrial tRNASer(UCN) gene. Hum Mol Genet 1995; 4:1421–1427.

76. Verhoeven K, Ensink RJ, Tiranti V, et al. Hearing impairment and neurological dysfunction associated with a mutation in the mitochondrial tRNASer(UCN) gene. Eur J Hum Genet 1999; 7:45–51.

77. van den Ouweland JM, Lemkes HH, Ruitenbeek W, et al. Mutation in mitochondrial tRNA(Leu)(UUR) gene in a large pedigree with maternally transmitted type II diabetes mellitus and deafness. Nat Genet 1992; 1:368–371.

78. Majamaa K, Moilanen JS, Uimonen S, et al. Epidemiology of A3243G, the mutation for mitochondrial encephalomyopathy, lactic acidosis, and stroke-like episodes: prevalence of the mutation in an adult population. Am J Hum Genet 1998; 63:447–454.

79. Hutchin TP, Parker MJ, Young ID, et al. A novel mutation in the mitochondrial tRNA(Ser(UCN)) gene in a family with non-syndromic sensorineural hearing impairment. J Med Genet 2000; 37:692–694.

80. del Castillo FJ, Villamar M, Moreno-Pelayo MA, et al. Maternally inherited non-syndromal hearing impairment in a Spanish family with the 7510T > C mutation in the mitochondrial tRNA(Ser(UCN)) gene. J Med Genet 2002; 39:e82.

81. Sue CM, Tanji K, Hadjigeorgiou G, et al. Maternally inherited hearing loss in a large kindred with a novel T7511C mutation in the mitochondrial DNA tRNA(Ser(UCN)) gene. Neurol 1999; 52:1905–1908.

82. Chapiro E, Feldmann D, Denoyelle F, et al. Two large French pedigrees with nonsyndromic sensorineural deafness and the mitochondrial DNA T7511C mutation: evidence for a modulatory factor. Eur J Hum Genet 2002; 10:851–856.

83. Jaksch M, Klopstock T, Kurlemann G, et al. Progressive myoclonus epilepsy and mitochondrial myopathy associated with mutations in the tRNA(Ser(UCN)) gene. Ann Neurol 1998; 44:635–640.

84. Zhao H, Li R, Wang Q, et al. Maternally inherited aminoglycoside-induced and nonsyndromic deafness is associated with the novel C1494T mutation in the mitochondrial 12S rRNA gene in a large Chinese family. Am J Hum Genet 2004; 74:139–152.

85. Reid FM, Rovio A, Holt IJ, et al. Molecular phenotype of a human lymphoblastoid cell-line homoplasmic for the np 7445 deafness-associated mitochondrial mutation. Hum Mol Genet 1997; 6:443–449.

86. Toompuu M, Yasukawa T, Suzuki T, et al. The 7472insC mitochondrial DNA mutation impairs the synthesis and extent of aminoacylation of tRNASer(UCN) but not its structure or rate of turnover. J Biol Chem 2002; 277:22240–22250.

87. Estivill X, Govea N, Barcelo E, et al. Familial progressive sensorineural deafness is mainly due to the mtDNA A1555G mutation and is enhanced by treatment of aminoglycosides. Am J Hum Genet 1998; 62:27–35.

88. Bu X, Shohat M, Jaber L, et al. A form of sensorineural deafness is determined by a mitochondrial and an autosomal locus: evidence from pedigree segregation analysis. Genet Epidemiol 1993; 10:3–15.

89. Guan MX, Fischel-Ghodsian N, Attardi G. Biochemical evidence for nuclear gene involvement in phenotype of non-syndromic deafness associated with mitochondrial 12S rRNA mutation. Hum Mol Genet 1996; 5:963–971.

90. Bykhovskaya Y, Yang H, Taylor K, et al. Modifier locus for mitochondrial DNA disease: linkage and linkage disequilibrium mapping of a nuclear modifier gene for maternally inherited deafness. Genet Med 2001; 3:177–180.

91. Yamasoba T, Goto Y, Oka Y, et al. Atypical muscle pathology and a survey of cis-mutations in deaf patients harboring a 1555 A-to-G point mutation in the mitochondrial ribosomal RNA gene. NMD 2002; 12:506–512.

92. Fischel-Ghodsian N, Prezant TR. Mitochondrial ribosomal RNA analysis in patients with sporadic aminoglycoside ototoxicity. Am J Hum Genet 1993; 53:1158.

93. Suzuki T, Terasaki M, Takemoto-Hori C, et al. Structural compensation for the deficit of rRNA with proteins in the mammalian mitochondrial ribosome. Systematic analysis of protein components of the large ribosomal subunit from mammalian mitochondria. J Biol Chem 2001; 276:21724–21736.

94. Scheffler IE. Evolutionary origin of mitochondria. In: Mitochondria. San Diego: University of California, Wiley-Liss, Inc. 1999:7–13.

95. Hamasaki K, Rando RR. Specific binding of aminoglycosides to a human rRNA construct based on a DNA polymorphism which causes aminoglycoside-induced deafness. Biochemistry 1997; 36:12323–12328.

96. Guan MX, Fischel-Ghodsian N, Attardi G. A biochemical basis for the inherited susceptibility to aminoglycoside ototoxicity. Hum Mol Genet 2000; 9:1787–1793.

97. Gallo-Teran J, Morales-Angulo C, del Castillo I, et al. Familial susceptibility to aminoglycoside ototoxicity due to the A1555G mutation in the mitochondrial DNA. Med Clin (Barc) 2003; 121:216–218. [Article in Spanish]

98. Ostergaard E, Montserrat-Sentis B, Gronskov K, et al. The A1555G mtDNA mutation in Danish hearing-impaired patients: frequency and clinical signs. Clin Genet 2002; 62:303–305.

99. Tekin M, Duman T, Bogoclu G, et al. Frequency of mtDNA A1555G and A7445G mutations among children with prelingual deafness in Turkey. Eur J Pediatr 2003; 162:154–158.

100. Troen BR. The biology of aging. Mt Sinai J Med 2003; 70:3–22.

101. Balaban RS, Nemoto S, Finkel T. Mitochondria, oxidants, and aging. Cell 2005; 120:483–495.

102. Golden TR, Melov S. Mitochondrial DNA mutations, oxidative stress, and aging. Mech Ageing Dev 2001; 122:1577–1589.

103. Harman D. Aging: a theory based on free radical and radiation chemistry. J Gerontol 1956; 11:298–300.

104. Richter C, Park JW, Ames BN. Normal oxidative damage to mitochondrial and nuclear DNA is extensive. Proc Natl Acad Sci USA 1988; 85:6465–6467.

105. Hayakawa M, Torii K, Sugiyama S, et al. Age-associated accumulation of 8-hydroxydeoxyguanosine in mitochondrial DNA of human diaphragm. Biochem Biophys Res Comm 1991; 179:1023–1029.

106. Hayakawa M, Hattori K, Sugiyama S, et al. Age-associated oxygen damage and mutations in mitochondrial DNA in human hearts. Biochem Biophys Res Comm 1992; 189:979–985.

107. Mecocci P, MacGarvey U, Kaufman AE, et al. Oxidative damage to mitochondrial DNA shows marked age-dependent increases in human brain. Ann Neurol 1993; 34:609–616.

108. Cheng KC, Cahill DS, Kasai H, et al. 8-Hydroxyguanine, an abundant form of oxidative DNA damage, causes G—T and A—C substitutions. J Biol Chem 1992; 267:166–172.

109. Wei YH. Oxidative stress and mitochondrial DNA mutations in human aging. Proc Soc Exp Biol Med 1998; 217:53–63.

110. Szibor M, Holtz J. Mitochondrial ageing. Basic Res Cardiol 2003; 98:210–218.

111. Finkel T. Oxidant signals and oxidative stress. Curr Opin Cell Biol 2003; 15:247–254.

112. Melov S, Schneider JA, Day BJ, et al. A novel neurological phenotype in mice lacking mitochondrial manganese superoxide dismutase. Nat Genet 1998; 18:159–163.

113. Harman D. The biologic clock: the mitochondria? J Am Geriatr Soc 1972; 20:145–147.

114. Linnane AW, Marzuki S, Ozawa T, et al. Mitochondrial DNA mutations as an important contributor to ageing and degenerative diseases. Lancet 1989; I(8639):642–645.

115. Cortopassi GA, Shibata D, Soong NW, et al. A pattern of accumulation of a somatic deletion of mitochondrial DNA in aging human tissues. Proc Natl Acad Sci USA 1992; 89:7370–7374.

116. Liu VW, Zhang C, Linnane AW, et al. Quantitative allele-specific PCR: demonstration of age-associated accumulation in human tissues of the A > G mutation at nucleotide 3243 in mitochondrial DNA. Hum Mutat 1997; 9:265–271.

117. Muenscher C, Rieger T, Mueller-Hoecker J, et al. The point mutation of mitochondrial DNA characteristic for MERRF disease is found also in healthy people of different ages. FEBS Lett 1993; 317:27–30.

118. Murdock DG, Christacos NC, Wallace DC. The age-related accumulation of a mitochondrial DNA control region mutation in muscle, but not brain, detected by a sensitive PNA-directed PCR clamping based method. Nucl Acids Res 2000; 28:4350–4355.

119. Wang Y, Michikawa Y, Mallidis C, et al. Muscle-specific mutations accumulate with aging in critical human mtDNA control sites for replication. Proc Natl Acad Sci USA 2001; 98:4022–4027.

120. Michikawa Y, Mazzucchelli F, Bresolin N, et al. Aging-dependent large accumulation of point mutations in the human mtDNA control region for replication. Science 1999; 286:774–779.

121. Zhang J, Asin-Cayuela J, Fish J, et al. Strikingly higher frequency in centenarians and twins of mtDNA mutation causing remodeling of replication origin in leukocytes. Proc Natl Acad Sci USA 2003; 100:1116–1121.

122. Kajander OA, Karhunen PJ, Jacobs HT. The relationship between somatic mtDNA rearrangements, human heart disease and aging. Hum Mol Genet 2002; 11:317–324.

123. Khaidakov M, Heflich RH, Manjanatha MG, et al. Accumulation of point mutations in mitochondrial DNA of aging mice. Mutat Res 2003; 526:1–7.

124. Lin MT, Simon DK, Ahn CH, et al. High aggregate burden of somatic mtDNA point mutations in aging and Alzheimer's disease brain. Hum Mol Genet 2002; 11:133–145.

125. Simon DK, Lin MT, Zheng L, et al. Somatic mitochondrial DNA mutations in cortex and substantia nigra in aging and Parkinson's disease. Neurobiol Aging 2004; 25:71–81.

126. Hayashi J, Ohta S, Kikuchi A, et al. Introduction of disease-related mitochondrial DNA deletions into HeLa cells lacking mitochondrial DNA results in mitochondrial dysfunction. Proc Natl Acad Sci USA 1991; 88:10614–10618.

127. Spelbrink JN, Toivonen JM, Hakkaart GA, et al. In vivo functional analysis of the human mitochondrial DNA polymerase POLG expressed in cultured human cells. J Biol Chem 2000; 275:24818–24828.

128. Nekhaeva E, Bodyak ND, Kraytsberg Y, et al. Clonally expanded mtDNA point mutations are abundant in individual cells of human tissues. Proc Natl Acad Sci USA 2002; 99:5521–5526.

129. Brierley EJ, Johnson MA, Lightowlers RN, et al. Role of mitochondrial DNA mutations in human aging: implications for the central nervous system and muscle. Ann Neurol 1998; 43:217–223.

130. Fayet G, Jansson M, Sternberg D, et al. Ageing muscle: clonal expansions of mitochondrial DNA point mutations and deletions cause focal impairment of mitochondrial function. NMD 2002; 12:484–493.

131. Muller-Hocker J. Cytochrome-c-oxidase deficient cardiomyocytes in the human heart - an age-related phenomenon. A histochemical ultracytochemical study. Am J Pathol 1989; 134:1167–1173.

132. Cottrell DA, Blakely EL, Johnson MA, et al. Mitochondrial enzyme-deficient hippocampal neurons and choroidal cells in AD. Neurol 2001; 57:260–264.

133. Elson JL, Samuels DC, Turnbull DM, et al. Random intracellular drift explains the clonal expansion of mitochondrial DNA mutations with age. Am J Hum Genet 2001; 68:802–806.

134. Trifunovic A, Wredenberg A, Falkenberg M, et al. Premature ageing in mice expressing defective mitochondrial DNA polymerase. Nature 2004; 429:417–423.

135. Trifunovic A, Hansson A, Wredenberg A, et al. Somatic mtDNA mutations cause aging phenotypes without affecting reactive oxygen species production. Proc Natl Acad Sci USA 2005; 102:17993–17998.

136. www.kuulonhuoltoliitto.fi.

137. Gates GA, Mills JH. Presbycusis. Lancet 2005; 366:1111–1120.

138. Spicer SS, Schulte BA. Pathologic changes of presbycusis begin in secondary processes and spread to primary processes of strial marginal cells. Hear Res 2005; 205:225–240.

139. Schuknecht HF, Gacek MR. Cochlear pathology in presbycusis. Ann Otol Rhinol Laryngol 1993; 102:1–16.

140. Schuknecht HF. Presbycusis. Laryngoscope 1955; 65:402–419.

141. Fransen E, Lemkens N, Van Laer L, et al. Age-related hearing impairment (ARHI): environmental risk factors and genetic prospects. Exp Gerontol 2003; 38:353–359.

142. Karlsson KK, Harris JR, Svartengren M. Description and primary results from audiometric study of male twins. Ear Hear 1997; 18:114–120.

143. Gates GA, Couropmitree NN, Myers RH. Genetic associations in age-related hearing thresholds. Arch Otolaryngol Head Neck Surg 1999; 125:654–659.

144. Hereditary Hearing-loss Homepage http://webhost.ua.ac.be/hhh/.

145. Johnson KR, Zheng QY, Erway LC. A major gene affecting age-related hearing loss is common to at least ten inbred strains of mice. Genomics 2000; 70:171–180.

146. Mulroy MJ, Henry WR, McNeil PL. Noise-induced transient microlesions in the cell membranes of auditory hair cells. Hearing Res 1998; 115:93–100.

147. Yamasoba T, Nuttall AL, Harris C, et al. Role of glutathione in protection against noise-induced hearing loss. Brain Res 1998; 784:82–90.

148. Pujol R, Puel JL. Excitotoxicity, synaptic repair, functional recovery in mammalian cochlea: a review of recent findings. Ann N Y Acad Sci 1999; 884:249–254.

149. Hyde GE, Rubel EW. Mitochondrial role in hair cell survival after injury. Otolaryngol Head Neck Surg 1995; 113:530–540.

150. Henderson D, Hu B, McFadden S, et al. Evidence of a common pathway in noise-induced hearing loss and carboplatin ototoxicity. Noise Health 1999; 2:53–70.

151. Emmerich E, Richter F, Reinhold U, et al. Effects of industrial noise exposure on distortion product otoacoustic emissions (DPOAEs) and hair cell loss of the cochlea: long term experiments in awake guinea pigs. Hearing Res 2000; 148:9–17.

152. Rybak LP, Whitworth CA. Ototoxicity: therapeutic opportunities. Drug Discov Today 2005; 10:1313–1321.

153. Torre P III, Cryickshanks KJ, Klein BE, et al. The association between cardiovascular disease and cochlear function in older adults. J Speech Lang Hear Res 2005; 48:473–481.

154. Gates GA, Cobb JL, D'Agostino RB, et al. The relation of hearing in the elderly to the presence of cardiovascular disease and cardiovascular risk factors. Arch Otolaryngol Head Neck Surg 1993; 119:156–161.

155. Brant LJ, Gordon-Salant S, Pearson JD, et al. Risk factors related to age-associated hearing loss in the speech frequencies. J Am Acad Audiol 1996; 7:152–160.

156. Kurien M, Thomas K, Bhanu TS. Hearing threshold in patients with diabetes mellitus. J Laryngol Otol 1989; 103:164–168.

157. Mellström D, Rundgren A, Jagenburg R, et al. Tobacco smoking, ageing and health among the elderly: a longitudinal population study of 70-year-old men and an age cohort comparison. Age Ageing 1982; 11:45–58.

158. Rosenhall U, Sixt E, Sundh V, et al. Correlations between presbyacusis and extrinsic noxious factors. Audiology 1993; 32:234–243.

159. Rybak LP. Hearing: the effects of chemicals. Otolaryngol Head Neck Surg 1992; 106:677–686.

160. Seidman MD. Effects of dietary restriction and antioxidants on presbyacusis. Laryngoscope 2000; 110:727–738.

161. Seidman MD, Ahmad N, Joshi D, et al. Age-related hearing loss and its association with reactive oxygen species and mitochondrial DNA damage. Acta Otolaryngol Suppl 2004; 552:16–24.

162. Corral-Debrinski M, Horton T, Lott MT, et al. Marked changes in mitochondrial DNA deletion levels in Alzheimer brains. Genomics 1994; 23:471–476.

163. Ikebe S, Tanaka M, Ohno K, et al. Increase of deleted mitochondrial DNA in the striatum in Parkinson's disease and senescence. Biochem Biophys Res Comm 1990; 170:1044–1048.

164. Chinnery PF, Taylor GA, Howell N, et al. Point mutations of the mtDNA control region in normal and neurodegenerative human brains. Am J Hum Genet 2001; 68:529–532.

165. Fischel-Ghodsian N, Bykhovskaya Y, Taylor K, et al. Temporal bone analysis of patients with presbycusis reveals high frequency of mitochondrial mutations. Hearing Res 1997; 110:147–154.

166. Han W, Han D, Jiang S. Mitochondrial DNA4977 deletions associated with human presbycusis. Zhonghua Er Bi Yan Hou Ke Za Zhi 2000; 35:416–419. [Article in Chinese].

167. Seidman MD, Khan MJ, Dolan DF, et al. Age-related differences in cochlear microcirculation and auditory brain stem response. Arch Otolaryngol Head Neck Surg 1996; 122:1221–1226.

Part II
Current management

10 Psychosocial aspects of genetic hearing impairment

Dafydd Stephens

Introduction

There is an extensive literature on the psychosocial impact of hearing impairment and much of this literature has been recently reviewed (1). The present chapter will address those elements of such a psychosocial impact due to genetic disorders, which may be superimposed on such general effects of the hearing impairment per se.

Over the years, genetic hearing impairment has been found to account for a larger and larger proportion of individuals with hearing difficulties, now widely regarded as being responsible for at least 50% of permanent hearing loss both in young children and in elderly people (2,3). In certain isolated communities, a particular genetic cause of prelingual hearing impairment may achieve a high prevalence and result in a different set of attitudes towards deafness in that society. This mirrors, in some ways, the attitudes towards people with acquired hearing impairment in certain communities with a long history of employment in a particularly noisy industry, such as the jute weavers of Dundee (4).

Probably the best known example of a high prevalence of congenital deafness affecting societal attitudes was the case of Martha's Vineyard, an island off the coast of Massachusetts, vividly described by Norma Groce in her book "Everyone here spoke sign language" (5). The population, in that case, had a high prevalence of a nonsyndromal recessive condition, which appeared to have originated in Southeast England. The high prevalence of the condition resulted in "deafness" being regarded as a normal state and the hearing population using sign language to communicate with their deaf family and neighbours in a natural way.

Such communities have been found elsewhere in the world (6), and one of the most interesting examples is found in the northern part of the island of Bali. Here there is a village called Bengkala where some 2% to 3% of the population has congenital deafness caused by DFNB3, a recessive mutation involving the *Myosin 15A* gene (7,8). The social interactions within this community, where both the deaf and hearing people communicate using sign language, with the deaf people well adjusted and integrated within the community have been described (9). However, even within this community, the great majority of deaf children receive no formal education.

Elsewhere, in the general population, there have been a number of anecdotal reports of people denying genetic factors as a cause of hearing loss in their children, of being unaware of such hearing loss in their parents and siblings, and attributing it merely to age, noise, or other factors. Thus parents of a deaf child with a clearly dominant family history may insist that the child was deafened as a result of a pertussis infection. Eighty-year-old patients have reported that their parents' hearing loss was due to "old age" even though it began at the age of 60 and their own hearing loss dated back to such an age or younger.

There has been little attempt to explore any effects of genetic or familial hearing loss in a systematic way, and the present chapter sets out to do that under the aegis of Working Party 6 of the European Union GENDEAF project within the fifth framework. The present author is particularly indebted to the contributions in this respect of Sylviane Chéry-Croze, Lionel Collet, Berth Danermark, Lesley Jones, Sophia Kramer, Kerstin Möller, Wanda Neary, and Hung Thai Van. An additional group member, who contributed widely to the discussions, was Anna Middleton, author of the next chapter in the present book. The aim of the working group was to provide an interface between the molecular and clinical geneticists and those people facing the real world problems caused by genetic disorders affecting the auditory system.

This chapter deals fairly briefly with hearing disorders in children, an area in which it was difficult to obtain participants in either qualitative or quantitative studies. Hearing disorders affecting working age and older adults are studied using both epidemiological approaches and clinic-based studies, and this provides the main focus for the chapter. The first studies in this respect are based on secondary analyses of epidemiological investigations. These are followed by a qualitative analysis of people's perception of the impact of their family history on themselves. That, in turn, leads to investigations of such an impact on activity limitations and participation restrictions, motivation for seeking rehabilitative help, and on rehabilitative outcomes. This is followed by a consideration of the influence of a family history on the impact of tinnitus and finally by two specific genetic disorders. These are otosclerosis, one of the few causes of genetic hearing impairment amenable to surgical intervention, and neurofibromatosis 2 (NF2) in which premature death may occur and which generally presents with a hearing loss.

The background to this work has been presented in some detail in the literature review produced by the working party (1) and details of most of the experimental studies presented here will be found in the second publication (10).

Overall, in nonsyndromal hearing impairment, it would seem that a family history with role models available is what has had the greatest effect on people affected themselves, rather than the genetic hearing loss per se. The total impact of that from a psychosocial standpoint is also relatively modest compared with other factors such as the severity of the impairment and the age of its onset.

Family history influences in children

These studies date back to the 1940s, but two important investigations were conducted in the 1970s in the United States (11) and in the United Kingdom (12). These, together with a number of related investigations, have been discussed in some detail elsewhere (13), but may be summarised as indicating that it is the fact of having deaf parents, which is important, rather than having a specific genetic disorder. Thus, it was found that, among a group of children with genetic disorders, the children of deaf parents who signed to them performed better on a number of educational parameters in the Stanford Achievement test than did those without deaf parents (11).

Deaf school leavers from throughout the United Kingdom were subdivided into those with a family history and deaf parents, those with a family history and no deaf parents (FHHP), those with an acquired cause, and those whose aetiology was unknown (12). No significant difference between the four groups in terms of the youngsters' speech intelligibility was found, but those with deaf parents performed significantly better than the other three groups in terms of their reading age and in a speech comprehension ratio of lipreading. In these last two measures, the FHHP group did not differ in performance from those with acquired or unknown aetiologies. Interestingly, in a 20-year follow-up of these young people, it was found that those with an acquired or unknown cause for their hearing impairment were twice as likely to have had psychiatric problems than those with a genetic cause (14).

These findings are compatible with other results in the general literature, which indicate that deaf children of deaf parents

are likely to be better adjusted (15,16), to have a more positive coping framework (17) and less likely to have psychiatric problems (18). It has been strongly argued that many such differences may be attributable to early and effective mother–child communication, leading to the development of a more stable individual (19).

Most of these studies have involved relatively small numbers of subjects, not necessarily controlled for a number of confounding variables. Recently a large-scale study on children with hearing impairments has been conducted in the United Kingdom in which an attempt has been made to control for a range of variables such as hearing level, age of onset of hearing impairment, previous rehabilitative intervention as well as the social class and ethnicity of the parents (20).

The results for 338 children whose parents had some hearing difficulties were compared with those of 2519 children whose parents had no such difficulties. After controlling for gender, age, ethnicity, average unaided hearing level, age of onset of hearing impairment, additional hearing disabilities, parental occupation, and cochlear implantation, they examined any effect of family history. The findings of that study are shown in Table 10.1.

This indicates that, while the auditory receptive communication of those children with hearing-impaired parents was poorer, their sign language skills were better. It also supports the earlier findings of better academic achievement in those children

Table 10.1 Significant findings from main study on UK children (20) in which children with hearing-impaired parents differed from those with hearing parents

Communicative skills	—
Auditory receptive capabilities[a]	Poorer
Use of BSL[a,b]	More likely
Understanding of BSL[a,b]	Better
Use of SSE[a,b]	More likely
Understanding of SSE[a,b]	Better
Academic achievements	—
Academic abilities[a]	Higher
Key stage attainments[a]	Higher
Participation and engagement in education[a]	Better
Quality of life	—
Positive feelings about life[b]	Less
Need for help with social activities, e.g., shopping and inviting friends[b]	Less need

[a]Teacher ratings.
[b]Parent ratings.
Abbreviations: BSL, British sign language; SSE, signed supported English.

with hearing-impaired parents. Finally, in reported quality of life, those children with hearing-impaired parents felt less positive about their lives, but were more independent.

Unfortunately that study considered neither the severity of the parental hearing impairment nor the impact of hearing impairment in siblings, and further analyses were subsequently performed (21). Here children were divided into five groups:

Those with one or more parents "totally deaf";

Those with one or both parents with "some hearing difficulties";

Those with one or more siblings totally deaf, but hearing parents;

Those with one or more siblings with some hearing difficulties, but hearing parents;

Those with neither parents nor siblings with hearing problems.

The first four groups were each compared with group 5 after controlling for the demographic and other variables considered in the earlier analysis.

The results for those children with one or both totally deaf parents are the clearest and account for most of the differences found in Table 10.2. They are also generally in line with the published literature and the broader results of this study (Table 10.1).

Table 10.2 Significant findings from further analyses (21) in which children with one or both "totally deaf" parents differed from those with hearing parents

Communicative skills

Auditory receptive capabilities[b]	Poorer
Use of BSL[a,b]	More likely
Production of BSL[a]	Better
Understanding of BSL[a]	Better
Use of SSE[a,b]	More likely
Production of SSE[a]	Better
Understanding of SSE[a]	Better

Academic achievements

Academic abilities[b]	Higher
Reading age[a]	Older
Engagement in education[a]	Better

Quality of life

Need for help with social activities, e.g., shopping and inviting friends[b]	Less need

[a]Teacher ratings,
[b]Parent ratings.
Abbreviations: BSL, British sign language; SSE, signed supported English.

It may be noted, however, that this group of children do not have the negative feelings about life indicated in the broader study.

The results for the other three subject groups are less clear, although three findings were significant at the ($P < 0.01$) level. These indicate that children with one or both parents with "hearing difficulties" have less positive feeling about their lives. Those with one or more siblings with "total deafness" were reported by their parents to have poorer intelligibility of their British sign language (BSL). Those children with one or more siblings with hearing difficulties were reported by their teachers as achieving better key stage results in their education. The factors responsible for such results are not immediately clear and certainly more research is needed in this field.

Effects of a family history of hearing problems in adults in the community

The results to be considered here are derived from secondary analyses of two large-scale surveys, the UK Medical Research Council's survey of Ear, Nose and Throat problems (MRC-ENT) conducted in 1998 in Wales, Scotland, and England (22,23) and the Australian Blue Mountain Survey conducted in New South Wales between 1997 and 2000 (24). The MRC-ENT study was a household survey administered to 22,000 households and provided data on some 34,000 individuals aged 14 years and older. The Blue Mountain survey combined audiometry and questionnaires and was administered to 2956 participants aged 49 years and older.

Apart from the age and methodological difference between the two surveys, the key question on family history differed markedly between the two, one of the likely consequences of any studies based on secondary analyses. The relevant question in MRC-ENT was "*Did any of your parents, children, brothers or sisters have great difficulty in hearing before the age of 55 years?*" That used in the Blue Mountain Survey was "*Do (or did) any of your close relatives have a hearing loss?*" It is evident that the latter question was more all-encompassing, and this is reflected in the fact that while 11% of the respondents to the MRC-ENT survey answered affirmatively (9.8% of those aged over 60 years), 38% of those in the Blue Mountain survey indicated a family history in response to that question.

Audiometric measures were performed only in the Blue Mountain survey. These indicated that, after controlling for age and sex, those with a parental family history of hearing loss had significantly worse hearing than those without (Fig. 10.1), with a lesser difference found for those with hearing-impaired siblings but hearing parents. This was true for both their better ear (BEHL) and worse ear hearing levels (WEHL), as well as for the mid- and for the high frequencies. However, all differences were relatively small.

The impact of family history on the activity limitation (hearing problems) reported by the subjects was investigated by different general questions in the two surveys. In the MRC-ENT

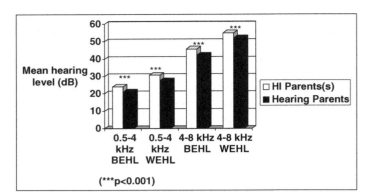

Figure 10.1 Mean better and worse ear hearing levels for respondents with and without a family history of hearing loss (Blue Mountain survey). *Abbreviations*: BEHL, better ear hearing level; WEHL, worse ear hearing level.

survey, the question *"Do you have difficulty with your hearing?"* derived from the Cardiff Health Survey (25) was used. In the Blue Mountain Survey, the question *"Do you feel you have a hearing loss?"* was posed.

In subjects with a family history of hearing loss, a markedly greater proportion of the respondents in the MRC-ENT survey indicated hearing difficulties, irrespective of age-band or gender, compared with respondents with no such family history (Fig. 10.2) (23). In addition in the Blue Mountain survey, again a significantly greater proportion of those respondents with a family history reported hearing difficulties, and these results are compared with the MRC-ENT results for a similar age-band (Fig. 10.2). It may be seen from this figure that the proportions with a family history reporting difficulties were almost identical in the two studies, although the percentage of those without such a family history reporting such problems was lower in the MRC-ENT survey. This could be related to the fact that older subjects, on the whole, complain of hearing problems only when their hearing is poorer, compared with younger subjects (26).

The question then arises as to how much of this family history effect relates to the differences in the hearing thresholds, seen in Figure 10.1, in the Blue Mountain survey. We

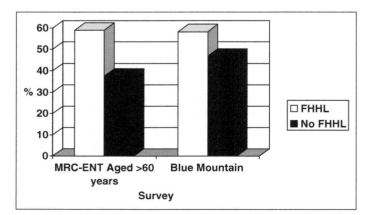

Figure 10.2 Percentages of older respondents with and without an FHHL reporting generic hearing difficulties. *Abbreviation*: FHHL, family history of hearing loss; MRC-ENT, Medical Research Council's survey of Ear, Nose and Throat problems.

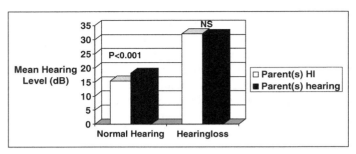

Figure 10.3 Mean hearing levels (500 Hz–4 kHz) by reported hearing loss (Blue Mountain survey).

therefore examined the mean hearing levels as a function of the response to the *"Do you feel you have a hearing loss?"* question and these are shown in Figure 10.3. This shows that while the mean hearing levels for those reporting hearing difficulties are the same in the two groups, the mean hearing level for those reporting no hearing difficulties is lower in the group with parental hearing impairment. This indicates that those with such a parental history are more likely to report hearing difficulties themselves at a better hearing level (i.e., they are more sensitive to milder impairments).

Two quantitative questions about hearing difficulties were used in the MRC-ENT survey (*"Do you have difficulty following TV programmes at a volume others find acceptable without any aid to hearing?"* and *"Do you have any difficulty hearing a conversation with several people in a group?"*). These showed similar results to the results of the generic question with greater difficulties reported by those with a family history. These questions had response options "no difficulty, slight difficulty, moderate difficulty, and severe difficulty" and so provided an indirect estimate of the level of hearing difficulties when we considered other effects of having a family history.

Elsewhere, in a group of patients with tinnitus, the relationship between these "surrogate" measures and the hearing levels has been examined (27). The first of these effects, which was considered was the annoyance caused by the hearing difficulty *"Nowadays how much does any difficulty in hearing worry, annoy or upset you?"* The results of this analysis for those subjects reporting moderate or severe difficulties hearing the television are shown in Figure 10.4. Similarly increased levels of annoyance in the presence of a family history were also found for those with slight difficulties hearing the television and are presented elsewhere (23). Overall, it may be seen that for a given level of hearing difficulty, those with a family history of hearing difficulties find this more annoying than those without such a family history.

The next aspect of hearing difficulties considered in the MRC-ENT survey was that of hypersensitivity to loud sounds as reflected in the question *"Do very loud sounds annoy you?"* Here, in view of the possible complicating factor of "recruitment," the results were examined in terms of the difficulty, which the individuals experienced in hearing the television. Some representative results from this analysis, for those with no difficulties

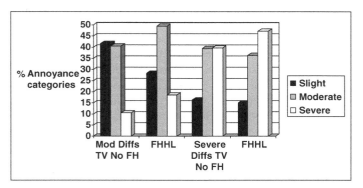

Figure 10.4 Annoyance caused by hearing difficulties for those subjects with moderate or severe difficulties in hearing the TV (Medical Research Council's survey of Ear, Nose and Throat problems). *Abbreviations*: FHHL, family history of hearing loss; FH, family history.

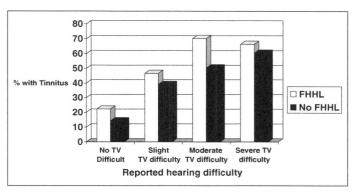

Figure 10.6 Percentage of patients reporting tinnitus by reported hearing difficulty and family history (Medical Research Council's survey of Ear, Nose and Throat problems). *Abbreviation*: FHHL, family history of hearing loss.

and those with moderate difficulties, are shown in Figure 10.5. These show again that, after controlling for the level of reported hearing difficulties, those individuals with a family history of hearing impairment are more annoyed by loud sounds than those without such a family history.

The other aural symptom to be considered in these analyses was tinnitus. The questions were "Nowadays, do you ever get noises in your head or ears (tinnitus), which usually last longer than five minutes" (MRC-ENT) and "Have you experienced any prolonged ringing, buzzing or other sounds in your ears or head within the past year…that is, lasting for five minutes or longer?" (Blue Mountain). While the questions in the two studies regarding tinnitus differed, both indicated that tinnitus was found more commonly in individuals with a family history of hearing impairment than in those without. Thus in the MRC-ENT survey, 34.9% of those with a family history reported tinnitus compared with 21.1% of those without such a family history. The equivalent figures from the Blue Mountain survey were 35.6% and 29.2%.

Hearing level is the best predictor of the occurrence of tinnitus (28) so, to control for this, the reported tinnitus in the MRC-ENT survey for those individuals with different levels of

hearing difficulty was compared. These results are shown in Figure 10.6. This indicates that for all levels of hearing difficulty, those with a family history of hearing loss are more likely to report tinnitus than those without such a family history.

The annoyance caused by the tinnitus and the effects of the tinnitus on the individual's life was also examined in both studies. In the Blue Mountain study, no significant effects were found in this respect. In the MRC-ENT survey, however, some interesting results were found, even after controlling for the frequency of occurrence of the tinnitus and the reported hearing difficulty. The reasons behind this difference in the results from the two studies are not clear and could well be due to the different criteria for the family history, as well as from different wording of the questions in the two studies.

Figure 10.7 shows the levels of annoyance in the MRC-ENT survey (*"Nowadays, how much do these noises worry, annoy or upset you when they are at their worst?"*) caused by the tinnitus as a function of whether the tinnitus is present some or most of the time and the presence or absence of a family history of hearing difficulties. It may be seen that having such a family history results in greater annoyance provoked by the tinnitus.

Finally, the responses to the question *"Nowadays how much do these noises affect your ability to lead a normal life?"* were

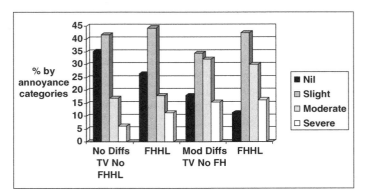

Figure 10.5 Annoyance caused by loud sounds for those with no and moderate difficulties hearing the TV (Medical Research Council's survey of Ear, Nose and Throat problems). *Abbreviations*: FHHL, family history of hearing loss; FH, family history.

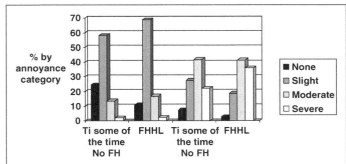

Figure 10.7 Annoyance caused by the tinnitus as a function of tinnitus occurrence and family history (Medical Research Council's survey of Ear, Nose and Throat problems). *Abbreviations*: FHHL, family history of hearing loss; FH, family history.

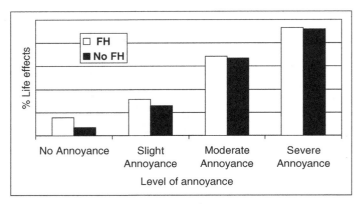

Figure 10.8 Reported life effects of tinnitus of different levels of annoyance by presence of family history (Medical Research Council's survey of Ear, Nose and Throat problems). *Abbreviation*: FH, family history.

examined. Greater effects in the presence of a family history of hearing impairment, even when controlled for hearing level and tinnitus occurrence, were found (23). Most interestingly, even when controlling for the degree of annoyance evoked by the tinnitus, if the subject had a family history of hearing loss, the reported effect on their life was greater (Fig. 10.8). However, this effect was most pronounced at the lower levels of annoyance.

Family history effects in working age adults

In addition to the broad retrospective population studies approached by secondary analysis, two studies have been performed in Sweden on working age adults in which the experimenters returned to a previous experimental group with enquiries about their family history (29,30). The first study involved 50 adults with prelingual or early childhood onset of their hearing impairment seen in a clinic in Karlstad in Sweden and followed up over 15 years. The second comprised 445 respondents with hearing impairment, of onset at a variety of ages, seen in various centres in Sweden, and who were still in the workforce.

In the first of these studies (29), an extensive questionnaire was administered examining a range of psychosocial variables. Of the 50, 14 responded affirmatively to the question "*Do any of your relatives have a hearing impairment?*" and these were compared with those who did not report such a family history. The only significant differences between the two groups were that those with a family history were more likely to have had a university education (36% vs. 11%) and were more likely to report that they wanted to leave their current employment (33% vs. 6%). These responded with yes to the question "*Do you want to leave work because of your hearing impairment?*" The differences occurred despite the fact that the two groups did not differ significantly across a range of demographic variables.

In the second study (30), family history of hearing impairment was defined as onset of hearing problems before the age of 45 years in the respondent's mother and/or father and/or onset before the age of 20 years in the respondent's brother and/or

sister. Twelve percent of the population met this criterion and they were compared with those subjects without any family history. The only significant differences found in the work situation and work experience were that females were more likely to be in work that had required a university education if they had a family history of hearing problems ($\chi^2 = 8.64$; 3df; $p = 0.034$). This is despite having generally poorer hearing levels than those without such a family history. These results are broadly in line with the previous study (29) and a number of the studies discussed earlier in the section of the influence of having such a family history in children.

Reports of the impact of having a family history of hearing impairment

Within this section of the chapter, the results obtained with three different approaches will be described. Firstly, the effects of simply asking patients seen in a clinic, or subjects contacted via the internet, to list the effects on them of having such a family history (31,32) will be described. Secondly, the results obtained using a structured questionnaire based on the results of the first studies (33,34) are presented. Finally, the results of some in-depth interviews of patients with a family history of hearing difficulties (35) will be summarised.

In the first of our open-ended studies (31), patients attending audiological rehabilitation clinics who were found to have a family history of hearing impairment during the clinical interview were administered the following questionnaire:

"*You have mentioned that other members of your family have or have previously had hearing problems. Does this information have any effect on your reaction to your own hearing problems? (please tick the answer that applies most to you) - YES NO*

If YES, please list any ways this knowledge has affected you. Write down as many effects as you can think of."

The study had three specific aims:

- To determine what proportion of such patients saw their family history as having an effect on them
- To determine whether any such perceived effects were positive or negative
- To elucidate the specific nature of any such effects

The questionnaire was administered to 102 consecutive individuals seen in audiological rehabilitation clinics and who had a family history of hearing difficulties. Two-thirds were female and they had a median age of 67 years. Fifty-seven percentage reported that having a family history of hearing problems had influenced their reaction to their own hearing loss. Among these respondents, a total of 150 "effects" were listed. A breakdown of these is shown in Table 10.3. The first category of "general effects" covers those unrelated to the family history, such as nonspecific hearing difficulties (e.g., "having TV volume too loud for others") and will not be considered any further. The "positive" and "negative" categories are self-explanatory and will be considered further below. The "neutral" category comprised those responses, which did not obviously entail

Table 10.3   Nature of responses to the family effects questionnaire

Nature of response	Number of responses
General (nonfamilial) effects	30
Positive effects	68
Negative effects	23
"Neutral" effects	29

either a positive or a negative effect on the respondent (e.g., "*my hearing loss is less of a problem than my sister's, because of treatment in the hearing clinic*").

The nature of the positive responses concerned predominantly early help-seeking and hearing aid fitting as well as a providing a better understanding of their own and others' problems. These, as well as the negative responses will be considered further below. Such negative responses were centred around concerns for their own future or for that of their children and grandchildren.

Within the second part of this study were included the questions on the "Gendeaf," "Hearing Concern," and "Dutch Society of Hard-of-Hearing people" websites. For the last, the questions were translated into Dutch (32). Almost all the responses came from the Dutch website, and only one respondent out of 41 indicated that the family history had no effect. In all, 90 specific responses were obtained, almost equally divided between the "positive," "negative," and "neutral" categories.

In this study, the main aim, apart from a comparison with the clinical population of the previous study, was to define in more detail the specific response categories, following the approach of Graneheim and Lundman (36). This entailed deriving "themes" from the "meaning units" or responses. This

is described in some detail elsewhere (32), and ended with six themes "role modelling," "expectation/anticipation," "acceptance," "help-seeking," "sharing knowledge," and "concern for the future/offspring." Each of these was then considered in terms of "positive," "negative," and "neutral" effects on the individual, and the pattern of results is shown in Figure 10.9. From this it may be seen that role modelling, help-seeking, and sharing knowledge are predominantly characterized by positive reactions. Acceptance and "worry about the future/offspring" evoke predominantly negative reactions, and expectation/anticipation evokes a largely neutral response.

Based on the most commonly found responses from these open-ended questionnaires, which indicated an effect of having a family history (positive, negative, or neutral), we developed a structured questionnaire (33,34). This comprised 20 questions to which the respondent had a response choice of "*definitely true,*" *probably true,*" "*probably not true,*" and "*definitely not true,*" and is shown as Appendix 1. The questionnaire was administered to groups of patients in Cardiff who indicated that they had a family history of hearing impairment, and also to those subjects who had responded by internet to the open-ended questionnaire in the previous study (32). A total of 192 subjects took part in the overall study, with their ages ranging from 17 to 92 years (mean 60.4, SD 13.9 years).

A correlation matrix performed on the responses indicated that 18 of the 20 items related to most of the others, the exceptions being item 4 ("*I didn't realize hearing problems were hereditary*") and item 11 ("*I am not worried about using hearing aids, as I know how much of a problem it is for others without one*"). We therefore excluded these two items from a factor analysis, which subsequently identified five factors, accounting for 58.1% of the total variance. Of these, two factors had acceptable α coefficients and are shown in Table 10.4.

These amounted to "positive effects" of the family history (eight items–factor 1, with an α coefficient of 0.83) and negative effects of the family history (three items – factor 2, with an α coefficient of 0.60). When we related these to demographic and other possible predictor variables, factor 1 was significantly related to the response to question 4—awareness of family history (FH) – ($p = 0.04$), with increased positive feelings related to greater awareness of a family history. Factor 2 was significantly related to overall hearing level ($p = 0.016$) and the study source ($p=0.012$). The former relationship indicates that the more severe the experienced hearing loss, the more negative the respondents consider the impact of a family history to be. The impact of study source is discussed below.

A breakdown of responses showed that, for 12 of the questions, there was no significant difference between the responses from the three groups of subjects (Cardiff clinic patients, Cardiff patients from an age-related hearing impairment study, and Dutch website respondents) (34). A factor analysis on this group of questions revealed three factors accounting for 56.4% of the total variance, with two of the three factors being essentially those shown in Table 10.4. Significant differences between the study groups were found for seven questions

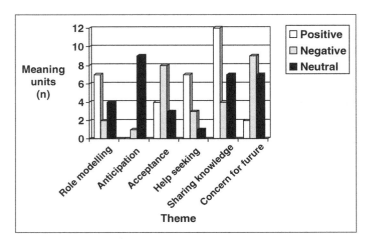

Figure 10.9 Positive, negative, and neutral elements of themes identified.

Table 10.4   Factor structure of the FHHL structured questionnaire with factor loadings, total variance and α coefficients of the two main factors

Item	Factor	% Total variance	α Coefficients	Factor loading
–	*Awareness of family history: positive effects*	*21.8*	*0.83*	–
1	Awareness of danger of social isolation	–	–	0.73
3	Family history made me not ignore the problem	–	–	0.74
7	Open about problems, so that others can help	–	–	0.71
19	Family history prompted me to seek help sooner	–	–	0.70
5	Awareness of other people with hearing problems	–	–	0.67
9	Empathy with people being irritated by me asking for repetition	–	–	0.64
17	Comfort from fact my family had coped in more difficult circumstances	–	–	0.61
13	I try to encourage others who are too proud to seek help	–	–	0.41
–	*Awareness of family history: negative effects*	*10.2*	*0.60*	–
16	Expectancy of problems later in life because of family history	–	–	0.69
15	Knowledge about cause of my problems	–	–	0.68
10	Worry about children's future hearing problems	–	–	0.53

(2,3,4,8,9,12,14 and 20). Within these, the two Cardiff groups generally gave the same response, but differed from the website group who were also younger. Further analyses on all the questions for the Cardiff groups amalgamated indicated again that the two main factors were "positive effects of FH" and "negative effects of FH." Again, "positive effects," accounting for 25% of the total variance, were related to question 4 (awareness of FH), and "negative effects" (12% total variance) were related to severity of hearing loss.

The final study in this series comprised an analysis of in-depth interviews with 11 individuals who had a family history of hearing difficulties (35). Again one of the most important factors to emerge is whether the individual had previously been aware of this family history, with four subjects so aware and seven unaware of the fact that their relatives' hearing losses related to their own. In both groups, there is some effect on transactional communication, but in the aware group, important influences are found also in relational and experiential areas.

A positive experience reported in the transactional domain from one of the individuals aware of the family history was "*knowing there was a system of helping me, that is what encouraged me, knowledge, family encouraging me*". And also the teasing "*you're getting deaf now and that kind of thing, so I was encouraged by the family.*" An example of a less positive, rather neutral, response in a relational context is illustrated by "*My daughter is 44 now in September, I think she is going to be like me, (son) has good hearing, but she is going to follow me, she has to go get her ears syringed quite frequently. So I would imagine she is going to have the same problems as me. She is exactly like I was at that age.*" Finally an example of a positive experiential response is illustrated by the following, concerning the respondent's hearing aid: "*I think aren't I fortunate that I have something that I can wear, whereas my dad had to just put up with it. I would have loved him to have access to something like this.*"

Effects of a family history of hearing loss on reported disabilities, psychological effects, motivation, and rehabilitative outcome

Within this section, three studies, which are in many ways related to each other, will be considered (37–39). They considered adults who were predominantly late middle aged and, in general, only very minor differences were found between those with and without a family history of hearing impairment.

In the first of these studies (37), the 109 subjects were aged between 55 and 65 years of age and had symmetrical sensorineural hearing impairment of adult onset. They were taking part in an aetiological and genetic study on age-related hearing impairment. Fifty-one had no family history of hearing impairment and 58 did. Their mean better ear hearing level was 38.3 dB and the WEHL was 47.0 dB. There were no significant differences in gender, age, or hearing level between the two groups.

Activity limitation and participation restriction were assessed using the quantitative Denver Scale (40), and depression and anxiety were assessed using the Hospital Anxiety and Depression Scale (41). Overall scores for both scales showed no significant difference between the two groups of subjects, although some interesting differences were found with some of the individual questions. Thus on Question 10: *"I tend to be negative about life in general because of my hearing problem,"* a participation restriction question studying the attitude of the patient towards their peers, those with a family history hearing impairment (FHHI) present a more positive attitude about their life despite their hearing impairment ($Z = -2.00; p = 0.04$). Similarly on Question 23: *"I do not like to admit I have a hearing problem,"* another participation restriction question, those with an FHHI are more likely to disagree with the statement that they do not like to admit having a hearing impairment ($Z = -2.15; p = 0.03$).

The other interesting finding to emerge was the association between impairment as measured by the better ear hearing levels or WEHLs averaged over 500 to 4 kHz and the measures of activity limitation and participation restriction. In a range of studies reviewed by Noble (42), impairment has generally been found to have a strong association with activity limitation (formerly disability) and a weaker association with participation restriction (formerly handicap). Table 10.5 shows that in these subjects, those with a family history show a significant relationship between impairment and activity limitation but not with participation restriction. However, those with no family history show significant associations between impairment and both activity limitation and participation restriction. These results suggest that the experience of having a family history of hearing problems may modify the development of participation restrictions from activity limitations.

The second study (38) had two components, a secondary analysis of an earlier study, which had looked the effects of motivation on hearing aid outcome measures (43) and a prospective study on the effects of a family history on motivation for rehabilitative help. In the former, case files on 58 patients, attending a clinic to obtain hearing aids for the first time, were reviewed to obtain details of whether or not they had a family history of hearing problems. Thirty-one had such a family history and 27 did not. These were analysed in terms of whether the individuals' parents were affected. The mean age of this group was 70 years with the mean better ear hearing level 42 dB. Motivation was assessed in terms of duration of reported hearing difficulties prior to attendance, whether or not they came from self-motivation or as a result of family pressures, and a clinician rating of the level of their motivation for hearing aid help. Outcome measures were in terms of satisfaction, reported use of their aid(s), their manipulative skills with the aids, and how they were using the aid. The only significant effects of having a family history were that those with such a history reported a longer duration of hearing problems ($p = 0.024$) and those whose parents had been hearing-impaired were more likely to be self-motivated in their help-seeking ($p = 0.034$). None of the outcome measures showed a significant difference between those with and without such a family history.

In the prospective study, following the introduction of digital signal processing hearing aids in the National Health Service in Wales, 62 first time hearing aid users were seen with a mean age of 67 years and a mean better ear hearing level of 38 dB. The same assessments of motivation were used but, in this case, no significant relationship was found between the measures and whether or not they had a family history of hearing problems. The difference between the two study groups could be related to the fact that the introduction of the new technology (digital signal processing hearing aids) attracted younger patients with milder hearing losses and who had not

Table 10.5   Relationship between impairment and activity limitation and participation restriction in those with and without a family history

Questions (Denver scale)			Better ear		
–	Without FHHI			With FHHI	
–	Kendall's correlation coefficient (τ)	Significance		Kendall's correlation coefficient (τ)	Significance
Activity Limitation	− 0.28	0.006		− 0.341	0.000
Participation Restriction	− 0.23	0.02		− 0.11	0.246

Abbreviation: FHHI, family history of hearing impairment.

been prepared to seek referral when only "old" technology was available.

The final study in this section (39) was a follow-up of patients fitted with hearing aids as part of an investigation on their impact on a range of psychosocial measures (44). They were investigated at 6 and 12 months after being fitted with hearing aids and also questioned about their family history. Of the 171 subjects, 83 reported a family history and 88 did not. The mean age of the group with a family history was younger (68 years vs. 72 years, $\chi^2 = 2.28$; $p = 0.02$). The scores of the two groups on measures of depression, cognitive disorder, anxiety, social isolation, and sensory hyperaesthesia did not differ significantly from each other either at fitting or at 6 or 12 months later. The one difference found concerned hyperacusis on the auditory sensitivity or hyperacusis scale (45), but then only at six months after fitting the hearing aids (Fig. 10.10).

These results indicate that, at that time, hyperacusis was a greater problem in those with a family history of hearing difficulties ($t = 1.99$; $p = 0.05$). These results were mirrored in the emotional response component of the hyperacusis scale ($t = -2.10$; $p = 0.04$), which had further implications in that this was the only measure, which differentiated between those who continued using their hearing aids and those who gave them up. However, after 12 months, there was no significant difference between the groups. Despite this, it is interesting to note some parallelism with one of the epidemiological studies (23), which found higher levels of reported hyperacusis in individuals with a family history of hearing difficulties (Fig. 10.5).

Family history effects on tinnitus

Earlier, epidemiological results were presented indicating that tinnitus was more commonly reported by patients with a family history of hearing loss and also that they found it more annoying and reported that it had a greater effect on their lives (Figs. 10.6–10.8). Two parallel studies (27,46) were subsequently performed to determine whether this applied to members of tinnitus self-help groups and to patients attending a tinnitus clinic. This also provided an opportunity to examine different aspects of any possible family history impact on tinnitus-complaint behaviour.

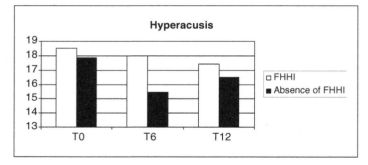

Figure 10.10 Hyperacusis score before and at 6 and 12 months after hearing aid fitting. *Abbreviation*: FHHI, family history hearing impairment.

For both studies, a three-part questionnaire was developed, which comprised a section on general and demographic background including family history of tinnitus and of hearing loss, the International Tinnitus Inventory (ITI) (47), a unidimensional measure covering different aspects of tinnitus impact, and the Tinnitus Reaction Questionnaire (TRQ) (48), which focuses on psychosocial aspect of tinnitus impact. For the purpose of the present chapter, the two studies will be considered together.

The French section of the study comprised 518 subjects (333 males, 185 females) who responded to questionnaires administered at self-help groups or via the website of "France Acouphènes," the French tinnitus association. The mean age of the respondents was 47.1 years (SD 14.1 years) and 88% of the responses came from the website. The Welsh section comprised 102 consecutive patients (56 males and 46 females) seen in the tinnitus clinic of the Welsh Hearing Institute in Cardiff. Their mean age was 57.7 years (SD 14.7 years). The median duration of tinnitus was five years in both samples (interquartile range 3–12 years for the Cardiff subjects and 1.5–10 years for those from Lyon).

The first questions asked whether the individuals had a family history of tinnitus and how it might have influenced them:

"Do or did other members of your family (brothers, sisters, parents, grandparents, etc.) have problems with tinnitus?

If yes, has this influenced your reaction to your own tinnitus?

If yes, please list any ways this knowledge has affected you. Write down as many effects as you can think of."

The related questions asked about a family history of hearing loss and how this might have influenced their reaction to

Table 10.6   Numbers of subjects reporting a family history of tinnitus or hearing loss and its effect on their reaction to their own tinnitus

-	Cardiff participants	Lyon participants
Family history of tinnitus only	3 (2.9%)	41 (8%)
Number indicating an effect	3	12
Family history of hearing difficulty	29 (28.4%)	114 (22%)
Number indicating an effect	11	4
Family history of both together	22 (21.6%)	80 (15.4%)
Number indicating an effect	6	11
Family history of neither	48 (47%)	283 (54.6%)

their tinnitus were *"If yes, has this influenced your reaction to your own tinnitus?"* The responses to the first two questions are summarised in Table 10.6, which indicated that only a minority of those reporting a family history indicated that it influenced their own reaction, and that this proportion was highest in those indicating a family history of tinnitus alone.

The nature of the responses given is shown in Figure 10.11. A number of nonspecific responses from Cardiff such as *"I learned within the past few months that my brother has also suffered with tinnitus for a number of years"* have been excluded. Figure 10.11 indicates that, while overall those with a family history of tinnitus report more positive than negative results and those with a family history of hearing loss more negative than positive results, there is a wide scatter of responses. Thus many with a family history of tinnitus reported a negative impact and a few of those with a family history of hearing problems reported a positive impact.

The specific responses may be analysed using the Graneheim and Lundman (36) technique, used earlier with responses to effects of family history on the individual's reaction to his/her hearing difficulties (e.g., Fig. 10.9). The full list of

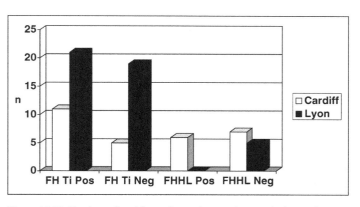

Figure 10.11 Numbers of positive and negative reactions to tinnitus and hearing loss family history. *Abbreviations*: FHHL, family history of hearing loss; FH Ti, family history of tinnitus.

responses may be seen elsewhere (27,46). In terms of the analysis, five themes were developed after analysis of the meaning units. These are shown in Table 10.7, which gives an example of positive and negative meaning units within the different

Table 10.7 "Themes" in responses about the impact of a family history on tinnitus reactions with examples of positive and negative "meaning units"

Meaning unit	Positive/negative	Number of responses	Theme
Made me think of my grandmother's problems and how she coped	Positive	12	Reaction/example of family members
Often saw my father suffering a lot, crying because of his tinnitus, thinking of committing suicide	Negative	4	—
More relaxed about the problems as I can see it's not as debilitating as I may have once thought	Positive	12	Understanding of symptoms
I'm afraid I will become hard-of-hearing because my grandfather's deafness was related to his tinnitus	Negative	8	—
Aware of slight changes in my own hearing	Positive	1	Reaction to symptoms
I'm afraid it will trigger psychological disturbance	Negative	15	—
At first tinnitus got on my nerves, but I did my best to copy her fatalism and serenity	Positive	6	Relieving factors
—	Negative	0	—
I have become more understanding of the suffering of sufferers	Positive	5	Empathy with others
—	Negative	0	—

themes and also the number of such meaning units within each grouping. This indicates a predominance of positive reactions, except for the theme "reaction to symptoms."

Analysis of the impact of family history on responses to the structured questionnaires differed somewhat between the two studies. In terms of the basic measure of tinnitus, the ITI, no significant differences in the total scores between those with and without a family history in either study were found. However, in the Lyon study, the ITI question on sleep ("*Over the past two weeks, how much has your tinnitus affected your sleep?*") showed a significantly better score in those with a family history than in those without ($P < 0.02$). In addition, a number of other significant differences were found in the different family history subgroups (46). In the Cardiff study, significant differences were found in response to three of the individual questions on annoyance ("*Think about your tinnitus over the past two weeks. On an average day, how often have you found it annoying?*"), peace of mind ("*Over the past two weeks, how much has your tinnitus affected your peace of mind?*"), and enjoyment of life ("*Considering everything, how much has your tinnitus changed your enjoyment of life?*"). In all cases, those with a family history were less affected by their tinnitus.

In the TRQ, aimed at tapping particularly the psychosocial aspects of tinnitus, somewhat different family history effects were found, although all pointed towards those with a family history of tinnitus reporting that their own tinnitus had less impact on them. In the Lyon study, the total score for the TRQ showed less impact of tinnitus in the family history group than in those without such a family history ($P < 0.05$). In both populations, examination of the family history subgroups indicated that the significant differences were restricted to those with a family history of tinnitus and did not occur in those with a reported family history of hearing loss alone. The significant differences for the individual questions are shown in Table 10.8. This shows benefits of having a family history of tinnitus in a number of psychosocial domains, but little concordance between the two studies.

Overall it may be concluded that the effects of the role model, of having a member or members of the family with tinnitus, are generally in a positive direction, lessening the impact of tinnitus on the individual. Having family member(s) with only hearing problems has a lesser effect and is sometimes in the direction of increasing the individual's negative reaction.

Otosclerosis

Otosclerosis is interesting in the general context of the psychosocial impact of genetic disorders as it is one of the few genetic disorders resulting in a hearing loss, which may be amenable to surgical intervention. It characteristically causes fixation of the stapes footplate, but can also affect the cochlea. Traditionally it has been regarded as an autosomal-dominant condition with incomplete penetrance, but only some 50% of patients present with a clear family history. Much still needs to be done to identify the detailed genetic background of the condition (see Chapter 8) but, at the time of writing, a number of genes responsible for the condition in different families have been localized (49), although none have been specifically identified.

Previous psychosocial studies of otosclerosis have been very limited (50) and have highlighted some patients' overriding concerns about surgery (51) but have also indicated psychological improvements after successful surgery (52). Two recent studies have examined the attitude of patients with otosclerosis to a range of genetic developments and interventions (53) and to the reported impact in those with a family history of the condition (54).

In the first of these studies (53), 71 patients with the condition were given a structured questionnaire, which had been developed and used in other research involving deaf and hard-of-hearing parents of deaf children (55). The 53% of those with a family history of otosclerosis did not differ significantly in their responses to any of the questions from the 47% who did not have such a family history. In reply to "*If there was a cure or treatment for deafness, would you want to have it?*" 75% indicated that they would like such a treatment. Again some three-quarters of respondents responded with yes to the

Table 10.8 Significant differences in tinnitus reaction questionnaires' individual questions between those with and without a family history of tinnitus

Question	Cardiff	Lyon
3. My tinnitus has made me feel irritable	–	$P < 0.05$
4. My tinnitus has made me feel angry	–	$P < 0.02$
11. My tinnitus has "driven me crazy"	$P < 0.02$	$P < 0.02$
12. My tinnitus has interfered with my enjoyment of life	$P < 0.05$	–
18. My tinnitus has interfered with my ability to work	–	$P < 0.05$
20. My tinnitus has led me to avoid noisy situations	$P < 0.03$	–
21. My tinnitus has led me to avoid social situations	–	$P < 0.05$
23. My tinnitus has interfered with my sleep	–	$P < 0.05$

question about early screening for the condition *"If you could have had a genetic test (blood test) when you were younger that would have predicted whether you were likely to develop a hearing loss when you were older, would you have wanted such a test?"*

Some 89% indicated that they communicated either successfully or very successfully with their partner and only 4% indicated that their condition was a great burden to them and only a quarter of these had difficulty coping. Further elements of the response to this question are shown in Figure 10.12. Seven percent reported feeling either advantaged or both advantaged and disadvantaged by their condition, but 54% felt disadvantaged (Fig. 10.13).

In the second study (54), 22 patients seen in clinics in Belgium and Wales who had a family history of otosclerosis were asked whether this had influenced their reaction to having the condition and, if so, in what way. Seventy percent indicated that it had influenced their reaction and, of these, two-thirds reported that such an effect was positive. When asked to specify ways in which their otosclerosis had affected them, the responses were very similar to those found among other hearing-impaired patients with a family history of hearing impairment (32). The breakdown by themes is shown

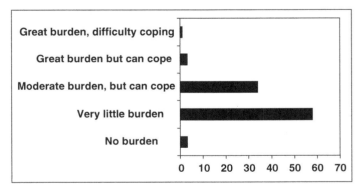

Figure 10.12 Responses to *"Some people with no experience of deafness might assume that this is burdensome for a person who has lost their hearing. Please can you say whether you feel, in reality, an actual burden of having a hearing loss?"*

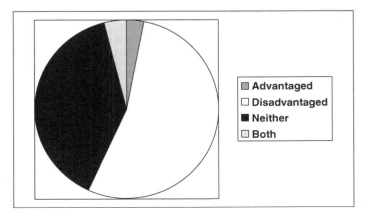

Figure 10.13 Responses to question *"Do you feel you are advantaged/ disadvantaged in any way because of your hearing loss?"*

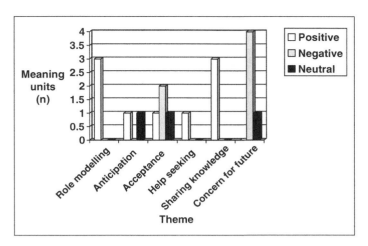

Figure 10.14 Positive, negative, and neutral elements of themes reported in patients with otosclerosis.

in Figure 10.14, which shows again that negative responses are mainly related to "concern about the future and family" and positive responses related to "role models" and "sharing knowledge." Interestingly, none of the responses made any reference to surgery.

In addition, the patients were asked about their attitude towards developments in genetics. In general, these individuals with otosclerosis were more positive about such developments than hard-of-hearing and deaf parents of deaf children investigated by Middleton (see Chapter 11) (55).

Neurofibromatosis 2

This condition is considered here as it is one of the few genetic conditions causing hearing loss, in which premature death may occur. It is a dominantly inherited condition caused by a mutation on chromosome 22. However, only some 50% have a clear family history, with the remainder resulting from new mutations.

Total deafness is likely in most cases as a result of bilateral vestibular Schwannomas or surgery to remove them. In addition, NF2 is associated with meningiomas, gliomas, and ependymomas affecting different parts of the central nervous system, as well as Schwannomas affecting the peripheral nerves. Furthermore, presenile lens abnormalities are common, and some affected individuals experience facial weakness after surgery for removal of the vestibular Schwannomas.

Despite this plethora of consequences of the condition, a recent review (56) was unable to identify any systematic investigations of the psychosocial impact of the condition. This resulted in a pilot open-ended investigation of 20 patients with the condition (57) and 15 of their partners (58).

The first question asked the patients *"What effects has having NF2 had on your life?"* While five of the responses to this question referred to positive effects, the vast majority (43/48) were negative. The most commonly reported areas are shown in

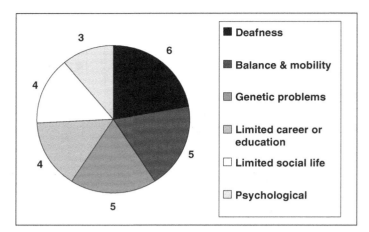

Figure 10.15 Main areas reported in response to *"What effects has having NF2 had on your life?"* in patients with NF2. *Abbreviation*: NF2, neurofibromatosis 2.

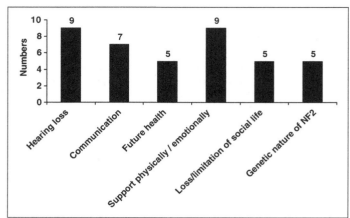

Figure 10.16 The most common responses received from significant others to *"Please could you tell me about the ways in which your partner being diagnosed with NF2 has affected your life?"* *Abbreviation*: NF2, neurofibromatosis 2.

Figure 10.15. In this it may be seen that hearing and balance problems comprise the most common problems for these patients.

They were then asked to specify *"which of the following is the biggest problem: hearing difficulties, facial weakness, mobility problems, visual difficulties or others?"* Of the responses to this question, some individuals specified more than one area. 17 of the 20 specified hearing problems, 10 mobility and seven facial weakness. More detailed results are shown elsewhere (57), as are the results of questions probing further for such effects.

When the question *"Are there any positive effects that the diagnosis has had on your life?"* was posed, 15/20 of the patients listed one or more positive effects. The most commonly reported positive experiences were *"It has made me more considerate, caring and sensitive towards other people,"* specified by five respondents, and *"Has made me more deaf and disability aware,"* specified by three.

Fifteen of the partners of these patients were presented with two questions *"Please could you tell me about the ways in which your partner being diagnosed with NF2 has affected your life?"* and *"Are there any positive effects that the diagnosis of NF2 in your partner has had on your life?"* The commonest areas of response to the first of these questions (16 responses from 14 significant others) comprised hearing difficulties and problems with communication. Fourteen responses from nine significant others specified the need to support the patient physically or emotionally or were concerned with worries about their partner's and children's future health. These and the other most commonly reported areas are shown in Figure 10.16.

Twelve significant others listed one or more positive experiences resulting from their partner's NF2. The most common areas reported are shown in Figure 10.17. The area most commonly specified was increased respect for others with disabilities and increased feeling of closeness to their partner. The genetic component refers to the benefits received from genetic counselling and related advice.

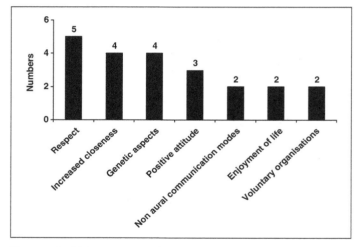

Figure 10.17 Main responses received from significant others to the question *"Are there any positive effects that the diagnosis of neurofibromatosis 2 in your partner has had on your life?"*

Overall, it may be seen that in NF2, the hearing difficulties and their subsequent effects on communication play an important part in terms of the negative impact of the condition on both patients and their partners. However, despite the disabling nature of the condition, both patients and their partners are able to perceive positive consequences of the condition. These are further highlighted in a short autobiographical account by a patient with the condition and his wife (59).

Conclusions

The overall results of the studies described in this chapter indicate a small but significant beneficial effect of having family members with hearing impairment. Provided that the individual with hearing difficulties is aware of the causative relationship between their own hearing problems and those of other family members, such relatives can be taken as role models. This may apply to patients complaining both of hearing difficulties and of tinnitus, although, in the latter case, it seems that having a family history of tinnitus rather than hearing problems is what is important. Indeed, for these people with a family history of hearing loss alone, there may be negative effects on their adjustment to their tinnitus.

An interesting result is that broadly the same positive effects occur with such role models regardless of their specific aural condition (e.g., genetic hearing impairment, tinnitus, otosclerosis, and NF2). In all cases, benefit would seem to come from both the positive experiences of family members and from the affected individual being determined not to make the same mistakes as their relatives.

One of the main limitations of the present studies is that the retrospective studies, based on secondary analyses, used definitions of a family history as well as outcome measures which were far from ideal from the standpoint of research on the impact of genetic hearing impairment. Indeed, even the prospective studies concentrated on aspects of family history rather than directly approaching specific genetic disorder, so do not exclude the possibility of any other impact due to specific genetic disorders or forms of inheritance (e.g., mitochondrial and X-linked). However, given the results currently available, such effects are not likely to be large. In addition, apparent differences between the results of general population-based studies and those based on clinical populations, as well as those between the latter and web-based studies on members of self-help groups, merit further exploration.

Finally, there is a need to explore the way in which these results could be incorporated into the counselling of individuals with hearing difficulties and tinnitus by hearing therapists and audiologists as well as by genetic counsellors. Such counselling will need to cover both generic counselling within the context of the specific genetic disorder and the nonspecific psychosocial impact of hearing impairment, but also will need to take on board the impact of affected family members.

Acknowledgements

This chapter has been published with the support of European Commission, Fifth Framework Programme, Quality of Life and Management of Living Resources programme. The author is solely responsible for this publication. It does not represent the opinion of the community. The community is not responsible for any use that might be made of data appearing therein.

The author is particularly grateful to the contributions by the members of the Psychosocial working group of the GENDEAF project and for their invaluable input to this chapter. He is also grateful to Peter Lewis for his comments on an earlier version of the chapter.

References

1. Stephens D, Jones L, eds. The Impact of Genetic Hearing Impairment. London: Whurr, 2005.
2. Gates GA, Couropmitree NN, Myers RH. Genetic associations in age-related hearing thresholds. Arch Otolaryngol 1999; 125:654–659.
3. Parving A. Epidemiology of genetic hearing impairment. In: Martini A, Read A, Stephens D, eds. Genetics and Hearing Impairment. London: Whurr, 1996:73–81.
4. Kell RL, Pearson JCG, Acton WI, Taylor W. Social effects of hearing loss due to weaving noise. In: Robinson DW, ed. Occupational Hearing Loss. London: Academic Press, 1971:179–191.
5. Groce N. Everyone Here Spoke Sign Language. Cambridge, MA: Harvard University Press, 1985.
6. Woll B, Ladd P. Deaf communities. In: Marschark M, Spencer PA, eds. Deaf Studies, Language, and Education. New York: Oxford University Press, 2003:151–163.
7. Winata S, Arhya IN, Moeljopopawiro S, et al. Congenital non-syndromal autosomal recessive deafness in Bengkala, an isolated Balinese village. J Med Genet 1995; 32:336–343.
8. Friedman TB, Hinnant JT, Ghosh M, et al. DFNB3, spectrum of MYO 15A recessive mutant alleles and an emerging genotype-phenotype correlation. In: Cremers CWR, Smith RJH, eds. Genetic Hearing Impairment. Basel: Karger, 2002:124–130.
9. Branson J, Miller D, Marsaja IG. Everyone here speaks sign language, too: a deaf village in Bali, Indonesia. In: Lucas C, ed. Multicultural Aspects of Sociolinguistics in Deaf Communities. Washington DC: Gallaudet University Press, 1996:39–57.
10. Stephens D, Jones L, eds. The effects of having a family history of hearing impairment. Chichester: Wiley, 2006.
11. Vernon McK, Koh SD. Early manual communication and deaf children's achievement. Am Ann Deaf 1970; 115:527–536.
12. Conrad R. The deaf schoolchild. London: Harper & Row, 1979.
13. Stephens D. The impact of hearing impairment in children. In: Stephens D, Jones L, eds. The Impact of Genetic Hearing Impairment. London: Whurr, 2005:73–105.
14. Griggs M. Deafness and mental health: Perceptions of health within the deaf community. PhD thesis, University of Bristol, 1998.
15. Meadow KP. Deafness and child development. London: Arnold, 1980.
16. Polat F. Factors affecting psychosocial adjustment of deaf students. J Deaf Stud Deaf Educ 2003; 8:325–339.
17. Young A. Family adjustment to a deaf child in a bilingual bicultural environment. PhD thesis, University of Bristol, 1995.
18. Hindley P. Child and adult psychiatry. In: Hindley P, Kitson N, eds. Mental Health and Deafness. London: Whurr, 2000:42–74.
19. Marschark M. Raising and educating a deaf child: a comprehensive guide to the choices, controversies and decisions faced by parents and educators. New York: Oxford University Press, 1997.
20. Stacey PC, Fortnum HM, Barton GR, Summerfield AQ. Hearing Impaired children in the UK I: Auditory performance, communication skills, educational achievements, quality of life and cochlear implantation. Ear Hear 2006; 27:161–186.

21. Fortnum H, Barton G, Stephens D, et al. The impact for children of having a family history of hearing impairment in a UK-wide population study. In: Stephens D, Jones L, eds. The Effects of Having a Family History of Hearing Impairment. Chichester: Wiley, 2006:29–42.

22. Stephens D, Lewis P, Davis A. The influence of a perceived family history of hearing difficulties in an epidemiological study of hearing problems. Audiol Med 2003; 1:228–231.

23. Stephens D, Lewis P, Davis A. The impact of having a family history of hearing loss in elderly people. In: Stephens D, Jones L, eds. The Effects of Having a Family History of Hearing Impairment. Chichester: Wiley, 2006:3–13.

24. Sindhusake D, Stephens D, Newall P, Mitchell P. The impact of a family history of hearing loss in the Blue Mountain Study. In: Stephens D, Jones L, eds. The Effects of Having a Family History of Hearing Impairment. Chichester: Wiley, 2006: 15–27.

25. Stephens SDG, Lewis PA, Charny M. Assessing hearing problems within a community survey. Br J Audiol 1991; 25:337–343.

26. Merluzzi F, Hinchcliffe R. Threshold of subjective auditory handicap. Audiol 1973; 12:65–69.

27. Kennedy V, Stephens D. Tinnitus–the impact of family history. In: Stephens D, Jones L, eds. The Effects of Having a Family History of Hearing Impairment. Chichester: Wiley, 2006:187–205.

28. Coles R, Davis A, Smith P. Tinnitus: its epidemiology and management. In: Jensen JH, ed. "Presbycusis and Other Age Related Aspects." Copenhagen: Jensen, 1990:377–402.

29. Carlsson P-I, Danermark B. Early childhood hearing impairment and family history a long-term perspective. In: Stephens D, Jones L, eds. The Effects of Having a Family History of Hearing Impairment. Chichester: Wiley, 2006:43–54.

30. Gellerstedt L, Danermark B. Effects of a history of hearing problems in the family of origin on the working life. In: Stephens D, Jones L, eds. The Effects of Having a Family History of Hearing Impairment. Chichester: Wiley, 2006:55–68.

31. Stephens D, Kramer SE. The impact of having a family history of hearing problems on those with hearing difficulties themselves: an exploratory study. Int J Audiol 2005; 44:206–212.

32. Kramer SE, Zekveld AA, Stephens D. Effects of a family history on late onset hearing impairment: results of an open-ended questionnaire. In: Stephens D, Jones L, eds. The Effects of Having a Family History of Hearing Impairment. Chichester: Wiley, 2006:71–80.

33. Stephens D, Kramer S, Espeso A. Factors in the effects of a family history on late onset hearing impairment. In: Stephens D, Jones L, eds. The Effects of Having a Family History of Hearing Impairment. Chichester: Wiley, 2006:81–93.

34. Kramer SE, Stephens D, Espeso A. The awareness of having a family history of hearing problems and the impact on those with hearing difficulties themselves: a questionnaire. Audiol Med 2006; 4:179–190.

35. Coulson S. The impact that a family history of late onset hearing impairment has on those with the condition themselves. In: Stephens D, Jones L, eds. The Effects of Having a Family History of Hearing Impairment. Chichester: Wiley, 2006:95–116.

36. Graneheim UH, Lundman B. Qualitative content analysis in nursing research: concepts, procedures and measures to achieve trustworthiness. Nurse Educ Today 2004, 24:105–112.

37. Espeso A, Stephens D. Influence of a family history of hearing impairment on participation restriction, activity limitation, anxiety and depression. In: Stephens D, Jones L, eds. The Effects of Having a Family History of Hearing Impairment. Chichester: Wiley, 2006:117–125.

38. Wilson C, Stephens D. Does a family history of hearing impairment effect help seeking behaviour and attitudes to rehabilitation? In: Stephens D, Jones L, eds. The Effects of Having a Family History of Hearing Impairment. Chichester: Wiley, 2006:127–134.

39. Saglier C, Perez-Diaz F, Collet L, Jouvent R. The impact of a Family History of Hearing Impairment on rehabilitative intervention: a one-year follow-up. In: Stephens D, Jones L, eds. The Effects of Having a Family History of Hearing Impairment. Chichester: Wiley, 2006:135–144.

40. Alpiner JG, Chevrette W, Glascoe E, Metz M, Olsen B. The Denver Scale of Communication Function. Denver: University of Denver, 1971.

41. Zigmond AS, Snaith RP. The hospital anxiety and depression scale. Acta Psychiatr Scand 1983; 67:361–370.

42. Noble W. Self-Assessment of Hearing and Related Functions. London: Whurr, 1998.

43. Wilson C, Stephens D. Reasons for referral and attitudes toward hearing aids: do they affect outcome? Clin Otol 2003; 28:81–84.

44. Saglier C, Perrez-Diaz F, Collet L, Jouvent R. Psychologie, psychopathologie des malentendants et aide auditive. Les cahiers de l'audition 2004; 17:34–40.

45. Khalfa S, Dubal S, Veuillet E, Perrez-Diaz F, Jouvent R, Collet L. Psychometric Normalization of Hyperacusis Questionnaire. ORL 2002; 64:436–442.

46. Chéry-Croze S, Thai-Van H. The influence of a family history of hearing loss and/or of tinnitus on tinnitus annoyance and distress: results of a French study. In: Stephens D, Jones L, eds. The Effects of Having a Family History of Hearing Impairment. Chichester: Wiley, 2006:147–185.

47. Kennedy V, Chéry-Croze S, Stephens D, Kramer S, Thai-Van H, Collet L. Development of the International Tinnitus Inventory (ITI)—a patient-directed problem questionnaire. Audiol Med 2005; 3:228–237.

48. Wilson PH, Henry JL, Bowen M, Haralambous G. Tinnitus Reaction Questionnaire: psychometric properties of a measure of distress associated with tinnitus. J Speech Hear Res 1991; 34:197–201.

49. Van Camp G, Smith R. Hereditary Hearing Loss Homepage http://webhost.ua.ac.be/hhh

50. Lemkens N. The effects of otosclerosis. In: Stephens D, Jones L, eds. The Impact of Genetic Hearing Impairment. London: Whurr, 2005:195–200.

51. Eriksson-Mangold M, Erlandsson SI, Jansson G. The subjective meaning of illness in severe otosclerosis: a descriptive study in three steps based on focus group interviews and written questionnaire. Scand Audiol Suppl 1996; 43:34–44.

52. Gildston H, Gildston P. Personality changes associated with surgically corrected hypoacusis. Audiol 1972; 11:354–367.

53. Middleton A, Moumoulidis I, Crossland G, et al. Attitudes of adults with otosclerosis towards issues surrounding genetics and the impact of hearing loss. In: Stephens D, Jones L, eds. The Effects of Having a Family History of Hearing Impairment. Chichester: Wiley, 2006:237–243.

54. Stephens D, Lemkens N. People's reaction to having a family history of Otosclerosis. In: Stephens D, Jones L, eds. The Effects of Having a Family History of Hearing Impairment. Chichester: Wiley, 2006:245–254.

55. Middleton A. Parents' attitudes towards genetic testing and the impact of deafness in the family. In: Stephens D, Jones L, eds. The Impact of Genetic Hearing Impairment. London: Whurr, 2005:11–53.

56. Neary WJ, Ramsden RT, Evans DGR, Baser ME. Psychosocial aspects of NF2. In: Stephens D, Jones L, eds. The Impact of Genetic Hearing Impairment. London: Whurr, 2005:201–218.

57. Neary W, Stephens D, Ramsden R, Evans G. Psychosocial aspects of Neurofibromatosis type 2 reported by affected individuals. In: Stephens D, Jones L, eds. The Effects of Having a Family History of Hearing Impairment. Chichester: Wiley, 2006:207–226.

58. Neary W, Stephens D, Ramsden R, Evans G. Psychosocial aspects of Neurofibromatosis type 2 reported by relatives/ significant others. In: Stephens D, Jones L, eds. The Effects of Having a Family History of Hearing Impairment. Chichester: Wiley, 2006:227–236.

59. Crawshaw P, Crawshaw C. Living with NF2. In: Stephens D, Jones L, eds. The Effects of Having a Family History of Hearing Impairment. Chichester: Wiley, 2006:319–323.

Appendix 1

1. My family history of hearing loss made me aware of the danger of social isolation.
2. Because of my family history, I didn't think my hearing loss important enough to do anything about my own hearing loss.
3. Having a family history of hearing loss made me determined not to ignore the problem.
4. I didn't realise hearing problems were hereditary.
5. Having a family history of hearing loss made me more aware of other people with hearing problems.
6. Having a family history of hearing loss made me more fatalistic about my hearing problems.
7. A history of hearing loss in the family made me realise the need to be open about my problems so others can help.
8. My hearing problems were a long time being diagnosed so had no effect on me.
9. My experience of a history of hearing loss in the family gave me empathy with people who would possibly find it irritating if I continually asked for repetition or rephrasing.
10. It worries me that my children may develop hearing problems in the future.
11. I am not worried about using a hearing aid as I know how much of a problem it is for others without one.
12. Having a family history of hearing loss has influenced major life decisions [e.g., choice of career, etc.] for me.
13. I try to encourage others who are too proud to seek help.
14. The likelihood of decreasing hearing with age is a depressing prospect.
15. Had I not known of my relatives' deafness, I think I would continually be casting round for the cause of my own problems.
16. I expected problems in later life because of the family history
17. I had some comfort from the fact my family had coped in more difficult circumstances.
18. I am worried that my enjoyment of music will be impaired.
19. My family history of hearing problems made me aware of the problem and prompted me to seek help sooner.
20. Until I came to clinic I thought everyone could hear the same as me.

11 Attitudes of deaf people and their families towards issues surrounding genetics

Anna Middleton

Introduction

Genetic health services in general could be improved with more insight into the particular concerns and fears of patients with different genetic conditions. Previous research has documented the lay understanding of genetics (1,2) and has looked at case-study discussion of the experience of living with a genetic disorder (3). However, more research is needed to fully explore the experience and specific demands that deaf patients and their families have with respect to genetic issues.

This chapter provides an overview of some of the research that has been done to investigate the attitude of deaf people and their families towards genetics and genetic testing. Before this is covered, it is introduced with an overview of the different perspectives of deafness. This is followed by more practical sections on genetic testing services and what happens within genetic counselling. Then, a brief summary is given on the historical context to issues surrounding genetics, eugenics, and deaf people.

Perspectives of deafness

Deafness can develop at any stage of life, the clinical consequences may vary, and this may impact in different ways on the individual's daily functioning. Deaf people may have to alter their use of language and communication in order to function effectively in the hearing world. For a mildly deaf person, this could be through the use of speech with additional lipreading or for a profoundly deaf person this could be through the use of a sign language or its derivatives.

The "pathological" or "medical" model views deafness as a medical defect, which needs treatment or correction. For example, a cochlear implant or hearing aid aims to restore hearing as much as possible, with the view that to be hearing is the preferred option for the patient. However, this perspective is in stark contrast to the way deafness is viewed as part of the "cultural" model. Within this, deafness is not a disability, but rather an experience that is just different, and certainly not defective. Here, the main form of communication is often sign language. People who consider themselves "culturally Deaf" (written with an upper case D) will often not perceive that they have a disability or impairment. They feel positive and empowered by their language and have a strong Deaf identity (4). They also tend to mix and socialize with many other Deaf people (5,6). Deaf identity evolves over time, the process is influenced by the interactions deaf people have with other deaf and hearing peers (7).

Within the United Kingdom, it is thought that there are at least 50,000 deaf people who use British Sign Language (BSL) as their first or preferred language (8), such people may consider themselves culturally Deaf. These people may come from families where there are several relatives who are deaf. Such a "Deaf culture" exists in many countries across the World, e.g., in the United Kingdom, United States, Netherlands, Sweden, Norway, Germany, and Australia.

When there are numerous similarly affected relatives with profound deafness in the same family, there is often a shared use of sign language (e.g., BSL in the United Kingdom). Such individuals may also choose to mix, socialize, and work with other Deaf people and may also choose to have a partner who is Deaf. Approximately 90% of Deaf individuals are thought to marry another Deaf person (not including individuals with late onset deafness) (9).

The audiological level of deafness is not always a direct determinant of membership of the Deaf community (10). Although most people have a congenital or early onset, profound level of deafness, there are many people with this level of deafness who associate themselves more with the hearing world. Conversely, there are people with a mild level of deafness and residual hearing who consider themselves part of the Deaf community.

When a baby is born to deaf parents, there may be an anticipation that it will have inherited its parents' hearing loss. The reaction to this may be mixed. Much depends on the d/Deaf parent's own values and beliefs about their deafness and their experience of being deaf within the wider mainstream society.

Research by the author looking at these issues has shown that deaf parents are much more likely than hearing parents to feel that their deaf children do not place a burden on the family (11). They are also more likely to feel that there are advantages to being deaf within a deaf family; one such deaf parent in the author's research commented: "*I (can) share my skills and knowledge of deafness. I (can) understand her (daughter's) needs better.*" Another deaf parent of deaf children said: "*being deaf myself, the children were advantaged as I knew what the problems were and knew what to do.*" One culturally Deaf parent of deaf children said: "*at home we're all deaf so (the children) never felt left out. It's society without "deaf awareness" that made them feel disadvantaged! Otherwise we are all happy and (a) close-knit family with (the) same rich language (and) culture*" (11).

Preferring to have deaf or hearing children

In 2002, a deaf lesbian couple from the United States chose to have donor insemination from a male deaf friend with the hope that this would increase their chances of having a deaf child (12). Although not actively using genetic intervention, they hoped that genetic inheritance would be favourable for them, as they wanted to increase the chances of passing deafness on. This case caused international debate about the ethics of deliberately creating what some people felt was a "disabled" child (12–17).

The issue of deaf parents preferring to have deaf children is not a new phenomenon; it has been well documented in the past. Passing on deafness to the next generation would keep the Deaf culture alive and would mean that the Deaf community would continue to thrive (18,19). Dolnick (19) comments on this in "Deafness as Culture": "*So strong is the feeling of cultural solidarity that many deaf parents cheer on discovering that their baby is deaf.*"

Deaf people, who do not have ties with the Deaf community, but who nevertheless still prefer to have deaf children, may have this opinion because the thought of having hearing children fills them with worry. This may lead them to asking: "How will I cope?" "How will I teach the child to speak?" "What school will they go to?" The psychological reaction of a deaf parent to having a child of unexpected hearing status (either deaf or hearing) may be very similar to a hearing parent having a deaf child (9). There can be feelings of disbelief, fear, and loss. It is possible that another deaf child would fit better into the family unit if other deaf children were already present, a hearing child may just feel isolated. One hearing individual met by the author indicated that she would actually prefer to have deaf children even though she was personally hearing. This was because her family was all deaf with several generations of deafness and as a hearing person among them, she found it hard to cope with being different from the rest of the family.

Some deaf parents have said that they would choose not to have deaf children, if it could be avoided (11). One participant in the author's research said they "*would not wish deafness on (their) worst enemy.*" This highlighted the negative personal experience they had while growing up with a hearing loss and the struggle they had within a mainstream hearing society. Whereas other d/Deaf parents of deaf children felt the experience was positive—they were lucky to have the opportunity to pass on their language, history, and culture as well as deafness to their children and they were proud of this (11).

Several different pieces of research have shown that deaf parents usually do not mind the hearing status of future children, whereas most hearing parents prefer to have hearing children (11,20,21). This implies that deaf parents may be flexible about coping with either a deaf or a hearing child. They may also have a greater awareness of what deafness in a child would mean and therefore could be more ready to accept this than someone with no such personal experience.

It would be logical to conclude from this that more hearing people than deaf people would be interested to find out whether a baby was likely to be deaf or hearing, via the use of a prenatal genetic test. They may also feel more anxious to learn as soon as possible if their baby is likely to be deaf so that they can have a choice as to whether to continue with the pregnancy or not. Attitudes towards such a use of technology are documented in later sections.

Genes, deafness, and genetic testing services

Deafness can result from different factors, including environmental and genetic causes (22). Out of the 1 in 1000 to 2000 children with severe-profound, congenital, or early onset deafness, between 20% and 60% are thought to be deaf due to genetic causes, 20% to 40% due to environmental causes, and the remaining of unknown cause (23–25). Between 59% and 85% of cases of genetic deafness are thought to be caused by autosomal recessive genes, 15% to 33% by autosomal dominant genes, and up to 5% by X-linked or mitochondrial genes (26–28).

Several hundred genes are known to play a part in inherited deafness (29). Alterations in the *connexin 26* gene are thought to account for up to 50% of childhood genetic deafness, with 1 in 31 people carrying alterations in this gene in certain populations (30,31).

The deafness that results from alterations in the *connexin 26* gene is typically congenital and severe-profound (32), although mild-moderate deafness has also been reported (33). Advances in the molecular genetic research into deafness mean that, for certain families, it is possible to offer a genetic test to define whether a person's deafness is genetic and subsequently, what the chances are of passing this on to children. Such testing and information relating to this is can be obtained via genetic counselling services.

Genetic testing

Genetic testing is a general term that can refer to different types of testing, e.g., diagnostic, carrier, prenatal, and predictive.

- Diagnostic testing is used to diagnose whether a deaf person has a gene alteration(s), which causes his/her deafness.
- Carrier genetic testing tells a hearing individual whether he/she is carrying a gene alteration, which when also carried by their partner, would usually give them as a couple, a one in four chance of having a deaf child.
- Prenatal genetic testing tells a pregnant mother, via an invasive test such as amniocentesis or chorionic villus sampling, whether the foetus has a gene alteration(s) that could cause deafness. The invasive test involves an approximately 0.5% to 1% risk of miscarriage of the pregnancy. Information from a prenatal genetic test could then be used by the parents to decide whether the pregnancy should be continued or not. If not, the mother could have a termination of pregnancy (TOP) from this point on. Prenatal genetic testing is a form of diagnostic testing but it is performed in the prenatal phase, it is also known as prenatal genetic diagnosis (PND).
- Predictive genetic testing could tell a hearing person whether they have a gene alteration(s) that could predispose them to developing deafness later in life.

As more genes linked to deafness are identified and the clinical basis understood, it will become easier to incorporate genetic testing for deafness within routine clinical services. Many clinicians are excited by this prospect (34), but, others may prefer to treat this with some caution. Prenatal testing with selective TOP for deafness raises ethical concerns in relation to whether deafness is a "serious" enough condition to warrant such a course of action. Just because a test is technically possible, does this mean it should necessarily be available? Before such testing becomes routine, it is helpful to consider the longer-term consequences of this procedure.

Genetic counselling for deafness

There is often interest from Deaf individuals to know if and how they have inherited their deafness and what the chances are of passing this on to their children (35). These are issues that can be covered within the clinical service of genetic counselling. Such services are available from genetic counsellors and clinical geneticists working in clinical genetics departments across many parts of the world.

Genetic counselling has been described as "the process by which patients or relatives at risk of a disorder that may be hereditary are (informed) of the consequences of the disorder, (and) the probability of developing or transmitting it" (36). Genetic counselling offers clinical information about different genetic conditions and their heritability within a supportive and nonjudgmental environment.

Some deaf parents worry that they would be told that they should not have children if they came for genetic counselling (37). This would not happen within the present-day genetic counselling services in the United Kingdom as the service is "nondirective," i.e., the genetic counsellor does not tell the client what to do nor give advice. The focus of genetic counselling for deafness is now on the individual needs of the patient and their family and does not have a wider agenda to prevent deafness within larger mainstream society (35). However, aside from this, there is still often the misconception that genetic counselling has an ulterior motive, Das (38) states that: *"The high incidence of genetic causes* (of deafness) *indicates that steps should be taken to facilitate Genetic Counselling and conceivably to reduce the numbers affected"* (38). Therefore, there is an assumption that the process of genetic counselling will inevitably reduce the numbers of deaf children born, which may or may not be the case in reality. Aside from this, the actual focus of genetic counselling is on the provision of information and choice. This means that Deaf parents who prefer to have deaf children would be able to access information about genetics and inheritance in relation to this.

Some patients (deaf and hearing), however, do request genetic counselling because they would rather avoid passing on deafness in their family; others simply want information so that they are better informed of the chances of this happening, just for the sake of information.

Requests for PND for deafness are few and far between. There are limited numbers of people who feel that deafness is a serious enough condition to need to find out about during pregnancy or to opt for a termination if the foetus was likely to be deaf. When asked for their opinion on this subject, the majority of deaf and hearing individuals interested in having a test in pregnancy for deafness said they would only do so just to be prepared (39,40). However, in thinking about having a "nondisabled" child, created outside a natural conception, preimplantation genetic diagnosis could be a viable alternative. Such testing for *connexin 26* deafness has been requested, where two hearing parents wanted to avoid having deaf children, preimplantation genetic diagnosis was requested to select the embryos that did not have the deafness-causing genes with the aim that these would be implanted in the mother (41,42).

Different individuals have different opinions about passing on deafness to the next generation. One deaf couple, known to the author through her work as a genetic counsellor, were so fearful of passing on deafness to their children that they had decided not to have children. The negative personal experience they had in relation to being deaf meant that they felt a heavy responsibility to not "inflict" this on their children. However, the process of diagnostic genetic testing and knowledge of inheritance patterns revealed that their chances of having deaf children were minimal. They were delighted with this news. Another Deaf couple had assumed that because their families were hearing and that their deafness could not be inherited, they were then pleasantly surprised when their two children were born deaf. Genetic testing revealed that they were both deaf due to an alteration in the *connexin 26* gene and consequently all their children would be deaf. They had a strong Deaf identity and were really pleased to pass on their deafness, language, and culture to their children.

Both couples welcomed the opportunity to discuss their concerns about family planning. This in turn meant that they were more fully informed about their genetic heritage and consequently better able to engage in their future. Genetic counselling also offered them the opportunity to confidentially express the burden and responsibility they felt with regards passing (or not) deafness on to their children. This was provided within a sensitive environment away from the perceived "pressure" from their family and community.

Potential outcomes of genetic research

For families who test positive for a specific gene alteration that could cause deafness, it is possible to identify whether hearing parents or siblings are also carriers of such a gene alteration and to offer more specific information about the chances of having deaf children. It could also offer a quick and early diagnosis of deafness in a newborn baby in addition to the audiological testing that they might currently have. Therefore, as more work is done on the molecular genetics of deafness, more accurate information can be offered to families.

Identifying the genetic processes that interplay within the inner ear may lend itself eventually to gene therapies for deafness. This could replace the need for cochlear implants in children, and the obvious pain and risks that major surgery brings. It has also been suggested that, within the next 50 years, hair cell regeneration within the cochlear will be possible (43).

The potential impact of genetic research on families with deafness is summarized by Arnos et al. (35): "*Advances in molecular genetics will eventually bring about new options for prenatal diagnosis of deafness and prenatal or postnatal treatment. Deaf and hard-of-hearing people and parents of deaf children will surely have different feelings and may make different choices regarding the options that will be available to them. Some of the issues that arise may be similar to those that have come up as genetic technology has been applied to the diagnosis and treatment of other hereditary conditions. The sociocultural aspects of deafness will lend additional considerations to these discussions*" (35).

Genetics, eugenics, and deaf people

There have been many attempts throughout history to prevent deaf people from having children so that the numbers of deaf people would be reduced within society. Alexander Graham Bell, inventor of the telephone and also a leader in the eugenics movement, delivered a paper in 1883, called "Memoir Upon the Formation of a Deaf Variety of the Human Race" to the National Academy of Sciences. Here he advocated that deaf people should not be allowed to marry other deaf people, but should marry hearing people so that the chances of passing on deafness to their children would be limited (44). At that time the inheritance of genetic conditions was poorly understood and he mistakenly made the assumption that this would be an effective way of preventing deafness from being passed on. In fact, even if a deaf adult married a hearing partner, if the deafness was due to a dominant gene alteration there would be a 50/50 chance of passing this on to any children. Bell had a great respect for deaf people (his own mother was deaf and so too was his wife), but still felt that deafness was a disability and should be avoided if at all possible. This view, although derived from well-meaning intentions, is seen as insulting by many culturally Deaf people. As such this work has been discussed among British, European, and American deaf studies academics and lay people for over a hundred years since (45).

Another key event in history that involved deaf people related to Hitler's regime in the Second World War. In the Nazi programme, that advocated the eugenic pursuit of the perfect Ayrian Race, Hitler ordered deaf children and adults to be sterilised so that they could not pass on deafness to their children, and this happened to 16,000 to 17,000 deaf people. In addition to this, other deaf people were killed as part of "Operation T4" the Nazi programme designed to "wipe out" disabled citizens (46). Again, the incorrect assumption was made that deafness is always inherited and also another assumption was that deaf people will pass it on to their children. In fact, the majority of deaf children are born to hearing parents.

Given the historical context to the misuse of genetic knowledge, it is not surprising that d/Deaf people are often suspicious of modern day genetics services. The very fact that PND for deafness with selective termination for a deaf foetus is technically possible is sufficient for Deaf people to feel that there is another eugenic agenda being impressed upon them. There is often a sense that genetics services in the past have "devalued" the role of Deaf people in society. With this in mind, it is therefore imperative that genetic counsellors and geneticists are mindful of the historical context within which they practice in the present day.

It is important that a "culturally neutral" genetic counselling service is available to deaf people and their families (47), where Deaf patients are neither judged nor stereotyped. Assumptions should not be made about preferences for having deaf or hearing children and genetic counsellors should be aware of the historical sensitivity of such issues.

General attitudes to the medical model of deafness

As deafness can be viewed from different perspectives, there are often differing beliefs about appropriate medical intervention in relation to this. Deaf people may be sensitive to technology that aims to "cure" deafness and, as such, there has been clear resistance to cochlear implants (48). Here, the view is taken that deaf children should not be put through extensive, painful surgery to try and make them hearing when, to them, being deaf is not insurmountable.

Wheeler, from the Deafness Research Foundation, United States, believes that there is still compatibility between the preservation of the Deaf community and search for a cure/effective treatment for deafness (43). He suggests that by removing communication barriers, so that sign-language users have equal access to *"learning and enjoyment of life,"* a better quality of life will be achieved. At the same time those who wish to use treatments or cures can do so. However, the real argument from many Deaf people is that as most deaf children are born into hearing families, decisions to have treatments or cures will be made by hearing people who probably are not aware of the cultural model of deafness. Such hearing people, with their ignorance of the Deaf World, will make decisions for their deaf child according to their "hearing" perspective. Therefore, such deaf children are "cured" of their deafness before they are old enough to make choices for themselves, so missing the opportunity to be part of a community they could have naturally belonged to.

Having an awareness of what the Deaf community offers is something that many Deaf people aim to educate hearing people about, so that hearing parents are able to make informed decisions about their child's future. However, input from d/Deaf people about the medical or educational management of deafness has largely been ignored in the past (49). This situation is improving but still has a long way to go to create a working partnership between parents of deaf children, the Deaf community, and professionals working in deafness (50).

The British Deaf Association (BDA) or Sign Community is "the U.K.'s largest national organisation run by Deaf people for Deaf people" (51). The BDA has a policy on genetics (updated in May 2003) that stresses concern over the use of PND with selective termination of "deaf" pregnancies. In addition they "demand" that: "*all genetic counsellors should receive Deaf awareness training to ensure a clear understanding of the Deaf community and Deaf culture . . . (and that) . . . parents are not formally or informally pressured to take prenatal tests or to undergo termination where it is discovered that the foetus is deaf*"(52).

Therefore, the BDA believes that d/Deaf and hearing parents attending a genetic counselling clinic in the United Kingdom do not at present receive enough information to enable them to make informed decisions about deafness. The BDA intends to rectify this by implementing more Deaf awareness training among genetics professionals.

The National Deaf Children's Society (NDCS) also has a policy on genetics. In this, they advocate choice and information: "*The Society. . .recognizes the rights of potential parents from families who have a history of deafness to take advantage of genetic testing and antenatal diagnosis and to use the results of such tests in a way that suits the individual family. If asked for advice, the society will ensure that the family receives positive information about deafness in order to enable them to make an informed choice*" (53).

Support groups such as the BDA and NDCS consist of deaf and hearing individuals with an interest in the current clinical, educational, and support services in place for deaf people and their families. These groups are a powerful force that aims to help prevent discrimination and promote acceptance of deafness, whether perceived from the medical or cultural perspective.

Attitudes towards genetics may sometimes be seen as linking in with cultural identity. Those Deaf people who are against the eugenic practices of the past will often have negative views towards modern day genetics services (54). Such attitudes have been well documented over the last ten years, the following gives an overview of some of this work.

Attitudes towards genetics

The views of a collective group of culturally Deaf people attending a conference called "Deaf Nation" at the University of Central Lancashire, United Kingdom in 1997 were studied to ascertain attitudes towards genetics (55,56). Delegates were asked to complete a questionnaire which asked for their views about genetic technology and how they felt about its use with respect to deafness (e.g., for genetic testing in pregnancy for deafness). Of the 87 delegates who completed questionnaires, 55% thought that genetic testing for deafness would "do more harm than good"; 46% thought that its potential use "devalued d/Deaf people," and 49% were concerned about new discoveries in genetics. Some of this group indicated that they felt threatened by the perceived "misuse" of genetic technology, the biggest fear relating to prenatal diagnosis for deafness followed by selective termination if the foetus had the genes for deafness. The worry was that if such actions were utilized to any great extent, then the Deaf community would diminish.

A much larger study ($n = 1314$) has since been completed by the same authors. Here, the attitudes of d/Deaf, hard-of-hearing, and deafened adults as well as hearing parents of deaf children were documented (11,39,40). Participants were collected from medical and educational sources, social services, charities, and support groups for the deaf, i.e., a wider selection of participants were ascertained than gathered in the Deaf Nation study. However, the same findings were replicated among the culturally Deaf participants—involving negative attitudes towards genetic technology. On the other hand, those participants who identified with the wider mainstream hearing society tended to have quite positive views about the use of genetic technology.

Participants were given a list of positive, neutral, and negative words and asked to tick those from the list that described their feelings about new discoveries in genetics. The results showed very different attitudes between groups (Fig. 11.1). Deaf participants were more likely to select negative words ($\chi^2 = 42.2$, df = 6, $P < 0.001$). The most frequently ticked word was "concerned," and just under half of the group ticking this was culturally Deaf. Hearing participants were more likely to select positive words ($\chi^2 = 156.7$, df = 8, $P < 0.001$), the most frequently ticked word being "hopeful." Hard-of-hearing and deafened participants were more likely to tick a mixture of words, the most popular was "cautious."

Participants were given the opportunity to comment on their feelings about new discoveries in genetics. The following are a selection of these.

Some participants felt that new discoveries in genetics would be positive:

"We must go forward in genetics to help us understand causes of deafness and other disabilities caused through genes."
(nonculturally deaf participant)
"I think it is a good idea—to stop the genes passing on into the next generation."
(nonculturally deaf participant)

Some had negative comments about new discoveries in genetics:

"Angry at people trying to mess with nature and interfering with deaf people - leave us alone!"
(culturally Deaf participant)
"My hands is little nerve (I feel nervous). To think it is worst soon (I feel this is the worst situation)"
(culturally Deaf participant, who used BSL as first language, translated their feelings from BSL into written English.)

And some comments were mixed:

"Interested but do not feel involved"
(nonculturally deaf participant)
"Enthusiastic about benefits it can bring—early diagnosis, treatment to improved levels/quality of hearing, BUT concerned it will be used to increase abortion."
(hearing parent of deaf children)

Attitudes towards genetic testing as part of the newborn hearing screening programme

A diagnosis of deafness within a hearing family always has the risk of being delayed, due to neither the parents nor health professionals anticipating or specifically looking out for it. The Newborn Hearing Screening Programme offers the opportunity to obtain a diagnosis as early as possible by screening all newborn babies for audiological deafness (57). The earlier the diagnosis, the sooner that appropriate communication and education tools can be implemented thus giving the d/Deaf child the best possible chance of "normal" development (58). A delayed diagnosis may impact on the acquisition of effective language and this in turn may affect emotional and cognitive development.

Adding genetic testing for the *connexin 26* to the programme and thus making it an automatic part of Newborn Hearing Screening has been discussed (59); this is already in place in some countries. There is some resistance to this, however, due to concern that such testing, although possibly useful for parents to know a genetic cause to their child's deafness, may make it seem implicit that prenatal diagnosis should be utilised in the next pregnancy (60). Therefore, careful consideration of the impact of this should be given before genetic testing services are automatically added onto the audiological testing.

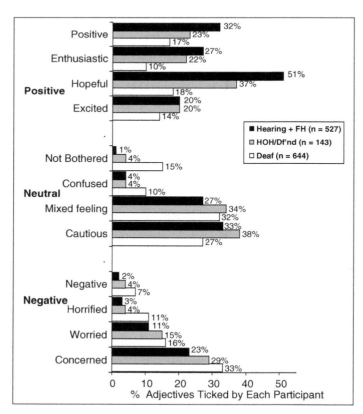

Figure 11.1 Percentage of participants who ticked different adjectives to describe their feelings about new discoveries in genetics. *Abbreviations*: HOH/Df'nd, hard-of-hearing and deafened participants; Hearing + FH, hearing participants who have either a deaf parent or a deaf child. *Source*: From the Journal of Genetic Counseling.

Research looking at the attitudes of deaf adults towards the use of genetic testing as part of the Newborn Hearing Screening Programme has shown that attitudes are generally positive (61) with most deaf participants perceiving the genetic and audiological testing offered as a useful way of diagnosing deafness earlier than has been done in the past. Another study looking at the attitudes of deaf, hard-of-hearing, and hearing participants also showed that most agreed that newborn genetic testing for deafness was appropriate (20). Deaf and hearing people alike appear to agree that the earlier the diagnosis of deafness, the better the outcome for the deaf child.

Attitudes towards genetic testing for deafness from the general public with no knowledge and experience of deafness

Ryan et al. documented the views of 91 pregnant women attending their 12- to 13-week booking scan at a maternity hospital in Scotland towards having a personal carrier test for deafness and subsequent prenatal test should both members of the couple be carriers for a deafness-causing gene (62). The majority had no personal experience of deafness either in themselves or in their relatives. Respondents indicated that the vast majority were interested in carrier and prenatal testing and if found to have a baby that was likely to be deaf, most said they would not have a TOP. This study is interesting as it places a value of what deafness means for people who do not have a family history of it. This study appears to show that people from the general public may perceive it as a condition to know about but not necessarily one to justify the ending of a pregnancy.

Prenatal testing for Cx26 gene alterations is already available to pregnant women having chorionic villus sampling in a pregnancy in Italy (63). Out of more than 5000 such women, with neither experience nor family history of deafness who were offered the testing, 55% chose to go ahead. As yet, only carriers have been identified, however it is only time before foetuses likely to be affected with deafness will be identified. It is not known whether parents would choose to end the pregnancy or not. It is very likely that such a population screening programme for deafness will be rigorously rejected by members of the worldwide Deaf community.

Attitudes towards genetic testing for deafness from deaf people and their families

The author and colleagues documented the views of 87 Deaf participants ascertained from delegates attending a conference on Deaf issues for Deaf people (55,56). This study showed that there was a small group of Deaf participants who said they would be interested in PND for deafness and also preferred to have deaf children. There was the theoretical possibility that they may choose to have a termination for a hearing foetus. The same authors conducted a much larger study documenting the views of 644 deaf individuals, 143 hard-of-hearing individuals and 527 hearing individuals with either a deaf parent or a child (39,40). From this study, 49% hearing participants with a family history of deafness, 39% hard-of-hearing and deafened participants, and 21% deaf participants said they would all be interested in having PND for deafness. From those interested in prenatal testing for deafness, 16% hearing, 11% hard-of-hearing and deafened, and 5% deaf participants said they would do so because they would have a termination if it were to be shown that the foetus was deaf. For the participants who said they would choose this option, it is possible that they may have had such a negative experience of living with a hearing loss in themselves or their family, perhaps observing that deafness created isolation or even discrimination, that they did not want to take the risk of passing on deafness to their children.

Aside from this, the majority of all groups who said they would use PND did so only for preparation for the baby (e.g., so they could learn BSL) rather than because they wanted to have a termination of a deaf foetus. This could be seen as reassuring to members of the Deaf community in that most would not wish to end the pregnancy if the test indicated the baby was likely to be deaf.

Other research has produced similar results; Brunger et al. looked at 96 hearing parents of deaf children ascertained in a hospital setting. There, 96% of the sample had positive views towards genetic testing and 87% said they were interested in having PND for deafness with the intention of using this just for preparation rather than acting on it via a termination (64). Martinez et al. gathered the views of 133 hearing students and 89 deaf and hard-of-hearing students from a U.S. university. They showed that 64% hearing participants and 44% deaf participants said they would be interested in having PND for deafness with no data on opinions about termination (20). Stern et al. used the same study questionnaire and similar groups of participants as the Middleton et al. research described above. They gathered the views of 135 deaf, 166 hard-of-hearing and deafened, and 37 hearing individuals from a number of different sources, including support groups as well as medical and educational settings. The results were classified into those who identified with the Deaf community, those who identified primarily with the Hearing World (including hearing and some deaf participants), and those who identified with both communities. The data showed that 23% participants who identified more with Deaf community were interested in prenatal diagnosis for deafness, compared to 47% of participants who identified more with the hearing world. With regards to attitudes towards termination, approximately 8% of participants who identified with the hearing world said they would consider having this if the foetus was deaf but none of those who identified with the Deaf community said they would (21). Finally, a study by Dagan et al. (65) looked at the views of 139 hearing parents of deaf children from Israeli Jewish families. 49% said they would consider having prenatal diagnosis for deafness with 17% saying they would consider having a termination for deafness (65).

Therefore the results from this selection of studies follow approximately the same patterns, with some participants interested in prenatal diagnosis for deafness, but much less interested in TOP for deafness.

Within work by the author, a very small number of deaf participants, three (2%) did say they would consider having prenatal diagnosis with selective termination of a hearing foetus, since they preferred to have deaf children (39,40). This reaction is somewhat extreme, and it is difficult to say whether, in reality, anyone would choose such a course of action. However, what this does demonstrate is the extent of the feelings of Deaf cultural solidarity that some Deaf people have, and also the fact that deafness is not automatically perceived as a disability. Indeed to be hearing in this instance would be a disadvantage. This fits in with previous literature already documented that shows some deaf parents prefer to have deaf children (14,18,39,40,55,56).

Summary profile of parents interested in prenatal testing for deafness

The author has also documented the attitudes of parents of deaf children towards many different aspects relating to the deafness in the family (11). It is possible from this work to create a profile of the type of person who may choose to have prenatal genetic testing for deafness. In summary, deaf parents of deaf children who were interested in prenatal diagnosis for deafness (because they wanted to avoid passing deafness on) were more likely to prefer to have hearing children, see their deaf children as disadvantaged, feel an actual burden of having a child who is deaf, and want a cure for deafness in their child. Hearing parents interested in prenatal diagnosis for deafness were more likely to consider termination for deafness as acceptable, to find communication with their child less than perfect (ranging from successful to poor), and to find the experience of obtaining education for their child difficult or complicated.

Looking at these collective results, it is possible to infer that many factors influence interest in PND for deafness. If such factors were modified then interest in PND for deafness might decline. For example, if parents were able to see their child as advantaged or less of a burden, or if they felt that communication with their child was easier or there were more straightforward processes to obtaining appropriate education, then they may be less interested in PND for deafness.

Conclusions

This chapter has reviewed some of the literature documenting the attitudes of deaf individuals and their families towards various issues surrounding genetic testing for deafness. This has been considered within the context of Deaf culture and the varying perceptions of the impact of deafness. Deafness does not appear to be a condition that most people (deaf and hearing) feel is "serious" enough to warrant prenatal testing nor selective TOP. However, inevitably there are people who would consider using the technology in this way. Such people tend to perceive deafness as a burden or disadvantage, and one they were inclined to view as a struggle to live with. Despite the negative picture created about deafness, many other people view deafness positively. Culturally Deaf participants are particularly optimistic about their situation and feel that being deaf is not a disability and also not something that genetic technology needs to interfere with. This shows that deafness is not a condition that is clearly detrimental.

If consideration is ever given to large-scale "management" of deafness, for example, by population carrier screening, genetic testing added onto the Newborn Hearing Screening Programme or mass-scale availability of prenatal testing for deafness, involvement in policy decision making surrounding this must include input from deaf, culturally Deaf, hard-of-hearing adults as well as parents of deaf children. All such people are directly affected by such programmes and have valuable insight to offer about the potential impact of this.

Appropriate and effective clinical services for deaf people can be developed as long as health professionals take the time to learn about the diversity of cultural attitudes held by different people affected by deafness (66). Genetic counselling services require a specialist knowledge of deafness, Deaf culture, and the role that genetics has played within history (67). It is also imperative that communication and language differences are embraced. Training in Deaf Awareness would be valuable for any health professional wanting to work in this area.

Acknowledgements

I would like to acknowledge the input of Prof Jenny Hewison and Prof Bob Mueller, my PhD supervisors. Even though it is nearly 10 years since we worked together I am still influenced by their wisdom.

References

1. Chapple A, May C, Campion P. Lay understanding of genetic disease: a British Study of families attending a genetic counseling service. J Genet Counsel 1995; 4:281–301.
2. Richards M. It runs in the family: lay knowledge about inheritance. In: Clarke A, Parsons E, eds. Culture, Kinship and Genes: Towards Cross-Cultural Genetics. Basingstoke: Macmillan 1997:175–197.

3. Marteau T, Richards M, eds. The Troubled Helix: Social and Psychological Implications of the New Human Genetics. Cambridge: Cambridge University Press, 1996.

4. Padden C. The deaf community and the culture of deaf people. In: Wilcox S, ed. American Deaf Culture. Silver Spring, MD: Linstock Press, 1980:1–16.

5. Arnos KS, Israel J, Cunningham M. Genetic Counselling for the deaf: medical and cultural considerations. Ann NY Acad Sci 1991; 630:212–222.

6. Christiansen JB. Sociological implications of hearing loss. Ann NY Acad Sci 1991; 630:230–235.

7. Ohna Stein E. Deaf in my own way: identity, learning and narratives. Deaf Educ Int 2004; 6:20–38.

8. RNID (Royal National Institute for the Deaf) Facts and figures on deafness and tinnitus. In house publication. London, http:/www.rnid.org.uk. Last updated 2003, accessed May 2005.

9. Schein DJ. Family life. In: At Home with Strangers. Washington DC: Gallaudet University Press, 1989:106–134.

10. Woll B, Ladd P. Deaf communities. In: Marschark M, Spencer PE, eds. Oxford Handbook of Deaf Studies, Language and Education. Oxford, Oxford University Press: 2003.

11. Middleton A. Parents' attitudes towards genetic testing and the impact of deafness in the family. In: Stephens D, Jones L, eds. The Impact of Genetic Hearing Impairment. London: Whurr, 2005:11–53.

12. McLellan F. Controversy over deliberate conception of deaf child. Lancet 2002; 359:1315.

13. Levy N. Deafness, culture and choice. J Med Ethics 2002; 28:284–285.

14. Spriggs M. Lesbian couple create a child who is deaf like them. J Med Genet 2002; 28:283.

15. Fletcher JC. Deaf like us: the Duchesneau-McCullough case. L'Observatoire de la genetique - Cadrages. 2002; 5.

16. Anstey KW. Are attempts to have impaired children justifiable? J Med Ethics 2002; 28:286–288.

17. Savulescu J. Deaf lesbians, "designer disability," and the future of medicine. Br Med J 2002; 325:771–773.

18. Jordan IK. Ethical issues in the genetic study of deafness. Ann NY Acad Sci 1991; 630:236–239.

19. Dolnick E. Deafness as culture. Atlantic Monthly 1993; 272(3):37–53.

20. Martinez A, Linden J, Schimmenti LA, Palmer CGS. Attitudes of the broader hearing, deaf, and hard of hearing community toward genetic testing for deafness. Genet Med 2003; 5(2):106–112.

21. Stern SJ, Arnos KS, Murrelle L, et al. Attitudes of deaf and hard of hearing subjects towards genetic testing and prenatal diagnosis of hearing loss. J Med Genet 2002; 39:449–453.

22. Cohen MM, Gorlin RJ. Epidemiology, etiology and genetic patterns. In: Gorlin RJ, Toriello H, Cohen MM, eds. Hereditary Hearing Loss and Its Syndromes. New York: Oxford University Press, 1995:9–21.

23. Newton VE. Aetiology of bilateral sensorineural hearing loss in young children. J Laryngol Otol (suppl) 1985; 10:1–57.

24. Fraser GR. A study of causes of deafness amongst 2355 children in special schools. In: Fisch L, ed. "Research in Deafness in Children". Oxford: Blackwell, 1964:10–13.

25. Parving A. Aetiologic diagnosis in hearing-impaired children - clinical value and application of a modern programme. Int J Pediatr Otorhinolaryngol 1984; 7:29–38.

26. Chung CS, Brown KS. Family studies of early childhood deafness ascertained through the Clarke School for the deaf. Am J Hum Genet 1970; 22:357–366.

27. Fraser GR. The Causes of Profound Deafness in Childhood. Baltimore, MD: John Hopkins University Press, 1976.

28. Marazita ML, Ploughman L, Rawlings B, et al. Genetic epidemiological studies of early-onset deafness in the US school-age population. Am J Med Genet 1993; 46:486–491.

29. Van Camp G, Smith R. Hereditary Hearing Loss Homepage. Antwerpen: University of Antwerpen (cited February 2005). Available from http://webhost.ua.ac.be/dnalab/hhh/

30. Estivill X et al. Connexin-26 mutations in sporadic and inherited sensorineural deafness. Lancet 1998; 351:394–398.

31. Kelley PM, Harris DJ, Comer BC, et al. Novel mutations in the connexin 26 gene (GJB2) that cause autosomal recessive (DFNB1) hearing loss. Am J Hum Genet 1998; 62:792–799.

32. Mueller RF, Nehammer A, Middleton A, et al. Congenital nonsyndromal sensorineural hearing impairment due to connexin 26 gene mutations—molecular and audiological findings. Int J Pediatr Otolaryngol 1999; 50:3–13.

33. Cohn ES, Kelley PM, Fowler TW, et al. Clinical studies of families with hearing loss attributable to mutations in the connexin 26 gene (GJB2/DFNB1). Pediatr 1999; 103:546–550.

34. Reardon W. Connexin 26 gene mutation and autosomal recessive deafness. Lancet 1989; 351:383–384.

35. Arnos KS, Israel J, Devlin L, Wilson MP. Genetic Counselling for the Deaf. Otolaryngol Clin N Am 1992; 25:953–971.

36. Harper P. Practical Genetic Counselling. Oxford: Butterworth-Heinemann, 1993.

37. Israel J. Psychosocial aspects of deafness: perspectives. In: Israel J, ed. An Introduction to Deafness: A Manual for Genetic Counsellors. Washington DC, Genetic Services Center: Gallaudet University, 1995.

38. Das VK. Aetiology of bilateral sensorineural hearing impairment in children: a 10 year study. Arch Dis Childhood 1996; 74:8–12.

39. Middleton A, Hewison J, Mueller RF. Prenatal diagnosis for inherited deafness—what is the potential demand? J Genet Couns 2001; 10:121–131.

40. Middleton A. Deaf and hearing adults' attitudes towards genetic testing for deafness. In: Van Cleve JV, ed. Genetics, Disability, and Deafness. Washington, DC: Gallaudet University Press, 2004:127–147.

41. Kelly J. Designer baby to have perfect hearing. Herald Sun 2002.

42. Australasian Bioethics Information. Designer babies/go ahead to screen out deafness. Australasian Bioethics Information newsletter (serial on the Internet). Accessed Sept 27 2002. Available from: http://www.australasianbioethics.org/Newsletters/047-2002-09-27.html.

43. Wheeler J. The end of all hearing loss is in reach. Editorial. Am J Otol 1998; 19:1–3.

44. Bell AG. Upon the formation of a deaf variety of the human race. Nat Acad Sci Mem 1883; 2:177–262.

45. Murray JJ. "True love and sympathy": The Deaf-Deaf marriages debate in transatlantic perspective. In: Van Cleve JV, ed. Genetics, Disability and Deafness. Washington DC: Gallaudet University Press, 2004:42–71.

46. Primary reference: Biesold H. Crying Hands: Eugenics and Deaf people in Nazi Germany. Washington DC: Gallaudet University Press, 1999. Secondary reference: Schuchman JS. Deafness and eugenics in the Nazi era. In: Van Cleve JV, ed. Genetics, Disability and Deafness. Washington DC: Gallaudet University Press, 2004:72–78.

47. Arnos KS, Pandya A. Genes for deafness and the genetics program at Gallaudet University. In: Van Cleve JV, ed. Genetics, Disability and Deafness. Washington, DC: Gallaudet University Press, 2004:111–127.

48. Gibson WPR. Opposition from deaf groups to the cochlear implant. Med J Aust 1991; 155:212–214.

49. Lane H. When the Mind Hears: a History of the Deaf. New York: Random House 1984.

50. Mohay H. Deafness in children (Letter). Med J Aust 1991; 155:59.

51. SignMatters Website—website for the British Deaf Association. Accessed May 2005. http://www.signmatters.co.uk

52. BDA (British Deaf Association) Genetics policy statement. In house publication, London, also available at http://www.britishdeafassociation.org.uk/ last updated 2003, accessed 2004.

53. NDCS (National Deaf Children's Society) Genetics and deafness—policy statement, London, accessed through http:/www.ndcs.org.uk, last updated 2003, accessed 2005.

54. Middleton A. Genetics and the culturally Deaf. Nature Encyclopaedia of the Human Genome. London, Macmillan Reference, London 2002; 1:1062–1064.

55. Middleton A, Hewison J, Mueller RF. Attitudes of deaf adults towards genetic testing for hereditary deafness. Am J Hum Genet 1998; 63:1175–1180.

56. Middleton A, Hewison J, Mueller R F. Attitudes of deaf adults towards testing in pregnancy for hereditary deafness. Deaf Worlds 1998; 14(3):8.

57. Cone-Wesson B. Screening and assessment of hearing loss in infants. In: Marschark M, Spencer PE, eds. Oxford Handbook of: Deaf Studies, Language and Education. Oxford: Oxford University Press, 2003:420–433.

58. Sass-Lehrer M, Bodner-Johnson B. Early intervention: current approaches to family-centred programming. In: Marschark M, Spencer PE, eds. Oxford Handbook of: Deaf Studies, Language and Education. Oxford: Oxford University Press, 2003:65–81.

59. Arnos KS, Pandya A. Advances in the genetics of deafness. In: Marschark M, Spencer PE, eds. Oxford Handbook of: Deaf Studies, Language and Education. Oxford: Oxford University Press, 2003:392–405.

60. Middleton A. Pre-natal testing for deafness—attitudes and ethics. Department of Health Steering Group Conference on the Newborn Hearing Screening Programme, London, 3rd Sept, 2002.

61. Taneja PR, Pandya A, Foley DL, et al. Attitudes of deaf adults towards genetic testing. Am J Med Genet 2004; 130A:17–21.

62. Ryan M, Miedzybrodzka Z, Fraser L, Hall M. Genetic information but not termination: pregnant women's attitudes and willingness to pay for carrier screening for deafness genes. J Med Genet 2003; 40:e80 (Electronic Letter).

63. Coviello DA, Brambati B, Tului L, et al. First-trimester prenatal screening for the common 35delG GJB2 mutation causing prelingual deafness. Prenat Diag 2004; 24:631–634.

64. Brunger JW, Murray GS, O'Riordan M, et al. Parental attitudes toward genetic testing for pediatric deafness. Am J Hum Genet 2000; 67:1621–1625.

65. Dagan O, Hochner H, Levi H, et al. Genetic testing for hearing loss: different motivations for the same outcome. Am J Med Genet 2002; 113:137–143.

66. Middleton A. Genetic Counselling and the d/Deaf Community. "Delivering genetic information sensitively across culture" Nurs Stand 2005; 20(2):52–56.

67. Middleton A. Genetic Counselling and the d/Deaf Community. In: Stephens D, Jones L, eds. The Effects of Genetic Hearing Impairment in the Family. London: Wiley, 2006:257–284.

12 Genetics of communication disorders

Elisabetta Genovese, Rosalia Galizia,
Rosamaria Santarelli, Edoardo Arslan

Introduction

A communication disorder is an inability to understand and/or use speech and language to relate to others. For the majority of communication disorders, we do not understand the cause. We know that many result from hearing impairment, intellectual disabilities, cerebral palsy, mental retardation, and cleft lip and/or cleft palate.

Over the past 10 years, there has been considerable progress in human genetics, and the mechanisms by which genetic defects can cause speech, language, hearing, cognitive, and behavioral disorders have been described.

Gerber (1) highlighted the fact that, in 1939, Nelson reported that stuttering runs in families. Later, she and her colleagues showed that stuttering is concordant in more than 80% of monozygotic twins but in only 10.5% of dizygotic twins (2). Ingham (3) reported that at least 75% of cases of stuttering are inherited.

Shprintzen (4) considered that virtually all instances of human disability and disease have a genetic component, even if it may not be direct or immediately obvious. He was referring primarily to craniofacial anomalies, but his comment applies generally.

It is well known that clefts of the lip with or without clefts of the palate may be of genetic origin or may be produced by environmental factors or chromosomal anomalies. They are often multifactorial or, as many geneticists believe, caused by a single mutant gene with allelic restriction (5).

Although genetic anomalies resulting in clefting have been known since the early 1970s, research on language disorders has developed only recently. In fact, Rice (6) noted that there is, as yet, no concrete evidence of a connection between genes or some combination of genes and grammatical abilities, but that a genetic contribution of some sort should be expected. More recently, Zoll (7) has suggested that genetic language disorders may be linked to a gene localised at 7q31.

Dyslexia, also a language problem, is known to be inherited (8,9). Phonological language disorders, also, have been shown to be more common among children whose parents had such disorders than among controls (10).

The presence of a genetic component of a disease can be difficult to identify. Evidence supporting a genetic component includes familial clustering of cases, increased incidences of consanguineous mating (i.e., mating between closely related individuals), increased prevalence that exists within genetically segregated communities, increased risk that exists for the children or siblings of affected individuals, and concurrence of identical twins with the disorder. When more than one member in a family is affected by the same rare condition, it is tempting to speculate that there is a genetic contribution to the aetiology.

However, it must be realised that there are several nongenetic reasons why a disease phenotype, causally unrelated to a genetic predisposition, can be seen recurrently in the same family. These nongenetic familial aetiologies should be taken into account when postulating a genetic contribution to a particular disorder.

Members of a family are frequently exposed to the same environmental insults. This may lead to recurrent manifestation of the same condition. A poor or rich educational environment will usually have a marked effect on language outcomes. The combined effects of such factors as age, sex, education, parental education, early intervention, and household income may be appreciable, obscuring the effects of genetic factors.

A shared in utero exposure can lead to familial aggregations of disabilities. Medical conditions such as diabetes, lupus erythematosus, and phenylketonuria can all result in sequelae that can give the appearance of a genetic relationship.

Cultural values and exposures may lead to apparent familial segregation. One example is the language of the home. Dialects and language-related difficulties, despite recurrence in a family, may be due to a shared cultural (rather than genetic) aetiology. Differences in habits and abuse of drugs or alcohol may result in a phenotype that can be misconstrued as being of genetic origin. Foetal alcohol syndrome shows a constellation of features that may include a characteristic facial appearance; cleft lip and palate and hearing loss are examples.

By chance, two members of a family may develop the same condition with no underlying genetic or environmental predisposition. Also, some members of a family may acquire a condition for reasons completely unrelated to other members of the family. A "phenocopy" is an individual with a phenotype similar to other members of a family but with a different aetiology (11). However, some stochastic events may be influenced to some degree by a genetic predisposition (12).

Mendel (13) first delineated the methods by which genetic factors are transmitted and first discovered the basis of heredity in his studies of peas. Although most communicative disorders appear to have a complex inheritance pattern, a select group of communicative disorders has inheritance patterns that directly parallel those observed by Mendel in peas.

Language development

One of the earliest scientific studies to record the language development of a child was that by a German biologist Tiedemann in 1787 (14). He was interested in starting a collection of data about language development in normal children. Interest in language development intensified with the publication of Darwin's theory of evolution, and Darwin (15) himself contributed to the study of language development in children, as did another biologist, Taine (16). When the German physiologist Preyer (17) published a detailed descriptive work carefully recording the first three years of his son's development, the modern descriptive, scientific study of language development had begun, continuing with important work by Shinn (18), Sully (19), Stern (20), and Leopold (21) up to the current "explosion" of literature over the past 20 years.

With regard to the acquisition of human language from the perspective of brain growth and the critical period, we have to consider the following aspects:

- Preconditions to language development (brain development)
- Phonological development
- Critical periods and "feral" children
- Genetically predetermined aspects of language processing

Preconditions for language development

Although children will begin to vocalise and verbalise at different ages and at different rates, most children learn their first language, a highly complex and abstract symbol system, without conscious instruction, from their parents and without any effort. However, before learning can begin, children must be ready to learn; that is, they must be biologically, socially, and psychologically mature enough to undertake the task.

As Kies reported (22), linguists do not agree on exactly how biological factors affect language learning, but most agree with Lenneberg (23) that human beings possess a capacity to learn language that is specific to this species and no other. Lenneberg also suggested that language might be expected from the evolutionary process that humans have undergone, and that the basis for language might be transmitted genetically.

As part of genetically endowed language abilities, Lenneberg (24) hypothesized a "critical period" during which language learning proceeds with unmatched ease. A child's early years are especially crucial for language development because that is the period before the two hemispheres of the human brain become lateralized and specialized in function. As partial proof of this, Lenneberg discussed cases in which children in bilingual communities were able to learn two languages fluently and without obvious signs of effort before the age of about 12. However, learning a second language after the age of 12 becomes enormously difficult for most people.

Similarly, many neurolinguists have argued that children's brains are biologically too immature to comprehend several grammatical concepts commonly used in languages around the world. Concepts such as plurals, auxiliary verbs, inflectional endings, and temporal words will develop in all languages in stages. These stages reflect the biological maturation of the child's brain. The fact that those stages of language development are "identical" and "predictable" in all languages further suggests that there are strong biological preconditions for learning language.

The concept of a sentence is the main guiding principle in a child's attempts to organize and interpret the linguistic evidence that fluent speakers make available to him. These ideas are a part of the "nativist" position discussed later. There is insufficient evidence to conclusively specify the contribution of biology to human language, but all linguists acknowledge that biology does have a role.

The brain will not achieve its final shape for two years, and many interconnections within the brain will not be complete until the child reaches seven years of age. Some neurologists insist, therefore, that the infant who struggles to gurgle and babble is not attempting to articulate speech sounds because the child has not attained sufficient neuromuscular and biological maturity to control the vocal organs before the age of six months.

Before language acquisition can begin, children must be ready to learn. Even before the child has uttered the first word, a long process of growth and language development has already started. The auditory system begins to function some three months before birth. For instance, a newborn baby will recognize his mother's voice at birth and can see with perfect visual acuity his mother's face when nursing him, but no further.

All the neurons are already present at birth. What does increase after birth is the number of dendrites and synapses. In humans, a considerable degree of development continues far

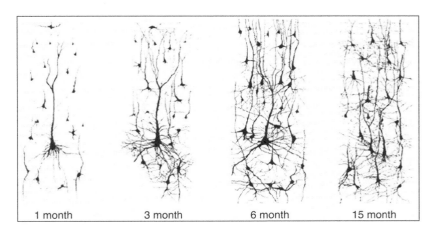

Figure 12.1 The increase in the number of neurones, dendrites, and synapses after birth.

beyond birth: increase in the size of the neurones; increase in the number of connections between neurones (which will allow information transfer); and axon myelinization, which will contribute to increase the speed of neural transmission (Fig. 12.1).

As the baby gets older, myelinization brings increasing numbers of brain areas "on line."

The parietal cortex starts to work fairly early, making babies intuitively aware of the fundamental spatial qualities of the world. The frontal lobes first kick in at about six months, bringing the first glimmering of cognition. The language areas become active about 18 months after birth. The area that confers understanding (Wernicke) matures before the area that produces speech (Broca), so there is a short time when toddlers understand more than they can say.

As may be seen in Figure 12.2, myelinization of the visual system, as expected, reaches maturation earlier than the auditory system and connecting fibers continue to myelinize during the first years of life. Thus, cerebral plasticity that involves language development continues until the age of seven years.

Genes apparently determine the basic pattern of growth and the major lines of connection, the "highways" of the brain and its general architecture, but the details seem to depend on such non-tragenetic factors as the complexity and interest of the environment. The brain overproduces neural connections, establishes the usefulness of certain connections, and then "prunes" the "unwanted" ones (25).

"Establishing the role of genetic influences in diverse aspects of language is only a first step in providing a foundation and a motivation for molecular genetic studies to find the multiple specific genes involved" (26). "Similarly, establishing the relative importance of environmental influences is just a first step towards future research to identify specific environments involved. As specific genes and environments are identified, we can begin to understand the complex mechanisms of development of individual differences in language abilities."

Phonological development

With regard to the steps of phonological development as Kaplan and Kaplan (27) said, babbling serves at least two functions:

First, babbling serves as practice for later speech. This is, of course, the most obvious and intuitive explanation since the

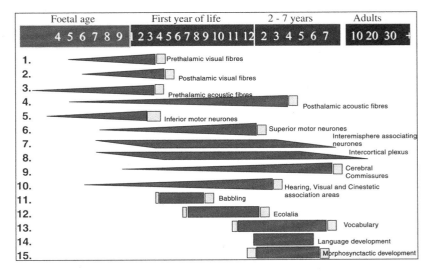

Figure 12.2 Profile of the development of CNS myelinization involved in language development. *Abbreviation*: CNS, central nervous system.

fine neuromuscular control needed later for speech is extensively practiced during the babbling stage. Indeed, the babbling child produces a lot of sound and a greater variety of sounds than is actually needed in the adult language.

Second, babbling provides a social reward. When children babble, their parents attend to them closely and encourage them to continue talking. Cooing and especially babbling are the first experiences a child has of the social rewards of speech. The importance of the social function of babbling is apparent in children who have been severely neglected during this stage. Although they begin to babble at the same age as other children, severely neglected children will stop, unless encouraged by a carer, and their language development is usually irreparably damaged (28).

One of the many unexplained mysteries of child language development is why babbling occurs at more or less the same time in all children, since simple observational evidence shows that children babble to practice their later speech at very different rates. Furthermore, the encouragement children receive for babbling is very variable. If all humans grow at approximately the same rate, then children around the world will begin to babble comparably. In fact, Lenneberg (24) discovered that babies who were prevented from any vocalization by disease or medical procedures would begin to babble spontaneously when they reached six months of age and their medical condition had improved enough to allow vocalization. Lenneberg concluded that previous practice at vocalization was not necessary for the onset of babbling and that biological maturity was a crucial factor. Babbling occurs automatically when the relevant structures in the brain reach a critical level of maturation.

When babbling begins, the nonsense syllables children create develop through a regular progression. Children first produce vowels and later combine consonants and vowels. This quickly involves the production of nonsense syllables: eee, ooo, uuu, ta, di, da, idi, aba, um baba, gigi, tutu, etc. (Table 12.1).

Communication begins before children utter their first words. Children employ the face, body movement, cries, and other preverbal vocalization to communicate their needs, desires, and moods to those around them. According to Meltzoff and Moore (29–31), newborn children not only imitate facial expressions but will also attempt to imitate rudimentary manual gestures.

At the age of six months or so, children in all cultures begin to babble with the production of long sequences of consonants and vowels.

As the child's vocabulary develops, the vocalizations accompanying the gestures become increasingly verbal until the child's language is sufficiently sophisticated to perform speech acts through speech alone. Furthermore, gestures remain an important part of human communication at all stages of development (32,33).

All children pass through this series of fixed "stages" as they develop language. The age at which each stage begins varies considerably from one child to the next, but the relative order of the stages remains constant for all children. The stages are reached in the same order, although the time between stages may be greater for some children than for others. Consequently, it is possible to divide the process of language development into a sequence of phases, remembering always that there is no clear division between stages in real children. The stages always overlap, and the chronological age of the child is only a very rough guide to the stage of language development.

Learning the grammatical structures of language is no less a remarkable achievement than learning the vocabulary. By about 18 to 20 months, the average child is creating his/her first two word utterances, and by 25 months, two word utterances make up the majority of the child's speech. When the child is three years old, on an average, he/she is able to create three- and four-word utterances and, as the child grows, the grammar

Table 12.1　Chronology of the early communicative acts

Age	Vocalisation and communication
Birth	Crying; body movements; facial expressions
12 wk	Reduced crying; smiles and makes vowel-like, pitch-modulated gurgling sound (cooing) when spoken to
16 wk	Responds to human sounds more definitely; turns head; eyes search for speaker; some occasional chuckling sound
20 wk	Vowel-like cooing is interspersed with consonant sounds
6 mo	Cooing changing into babbling, resembling one-syllable utterances; neither vowel nor consonant sound reoccur in any fixed pattern; most common utterances sound like ma, mu, da, and di
8 mo	Reduplication (continuous repetition of a syllable) becomes frequent; intonation patterns become distinct; pitch changes in utterances can signal emotion
10 mo	Vocalisation often mixed with sound play (gurgling, bubble blowing); appears to imitate sounds unsuccessfully; differentiates between words heard
12 mo	More frequent identical repetition of a sequence of sounds; first words (mamma, dadda); understands simple commands (point to your eyes)

Source: From Ref. 24.

grows too, ever increasing in its complexity and variety. Indeed, like vocabulary, the development of grammar need never end, since people can continue to learn new grammatical patterns as they learn new styles of speech and writing and new ways to express themselves with flair and emphasis. Many grammatical structures, particularly those involving coordination and subordination, are not fully mastered until adulthood (34,35).

Critical period and feral children

Focusing on the three essential elements of language, phonology, semantics, and syntax, a time frame for critical/sensitive periods of language development may be presented as a model of central auditory nervous system flexibility. Several studies support the hypothesis that the critical/sensitive period of phonological development is from the sixth month of foetal life to the 12th month of infancy. Data indicate that the critical/sensitive periods for syntax continue until the fourth year of life and for semantics, until the 15th or 16th year of life. The data indicate that there is a time-dependent series of sequential functions that is based on responsive adaptations made by the central nervous system (CNS) to psychophysical and electrophysiological stimuli (36).

Experience has a marked influence on the brain and, therefore, on behavior. When the effect of experience on the brain is particularly strong during a limited period in development, this period is referred to as a sensitive period. Such periods allow experience to instruct neural circuits to process or represent information in a way that is adaptive for the individual. When experience provides information that is essential for normal development and alters performance permanently, such sensitive periods are referred to as critical periods.

Although sensitive periods are reflected in behaviour, they are a property of neural circuits. Mechanisms of plasticity at the circuit level are discussed, which have been shown to operate during sensitive periods. A hypothesis is proposed that experience during a sensitive period modifies the architecture of a circuit in fundamental ways, causing certain patterns of connections to become highly stable and, therefore, preferred. Plasticity, which occurs beyond the end of a sensitive period, alters connection patterns within the architectural constraints established during the sensitive period. By understanding sensitive periods at the circuit level, as well as understanding the relationship between circuit properties and behaviour, we gain a deeper insight into the critical role that experience plays in shaping the development of the brain and the behaviour (37).

Although the critical period hypothesis was hotly debated for some years, there is now compelling supportive evidence. The evidence from feral, confined, and isolated children shows that unless they are exposed to language in the early years of life, humans lose much of their innate ability to learn a language, and especially its grammatical system.

Even if they have missed out on the critical period for language acquisition, feral children can be taught a few words and very simple grammatical constructions. The ability of feral children to learn language on their return to human society is very varied. Some children acquire normal language ability, but only if found before the onset of puberty. In two years, they may cover the stages of learning that usually take six years. Others also learnt to speak normally, but it is assumed that they could speak before their period of isolation.

Genetically predetermined aspects of language processing

Within generative linguistics, it is normally assumed that linguistic universals should be explained by the principles of U(niversal) G(rammar). One of the most remarkable facts about human languages, as traditionally assumed in generative linguistics, is that children learn them in a short period of time. From the input data of the language they hear, children are able to learn the language in a few years. This is taken to be a remarkable fact, because children generally receive very little explicit instruction about how language can and should be used. In order to explain how children can become fluent speakers, they have to be able to form a "model" of their linguistic environment that makes grammaticality judgments not only about sentences they have actually heard but also about those that they never heard before. In the 1950s, Chomsky (38) argued that the behavioural learning theory that was popular at that time, assuming that people start out as a tabula rasa and make use only of simple association and blind induction, could not account for this. Later, this argument was backed up by Gold's (39) results in formal learning theory. Gold proved that learning or identifying an arbitrarily selected language among a collection of languages by "natural" data is impossible in the complete absence of prior information.

Chomsky's argument against the adequacy of simple behavioural language learning and the results of Gold, as well as later results in learning theory, are clear and should be uncontroversial. Chomsky himself, in the 1960s, declared the human ability of language learning despite the limited input to be the central fact that linguistics should explain (40). Chomsky's explanation of children's ability to learn their parents' language is well known. First, humans must have a biological basis for language: Some mental capacities must come as part of the innate endowment of the mind in order for humans to be able to learn language. Chomsky's second claim, however, was that the endowment of language is not for general purpose but rather highly specific for language, a genetically given language acquisition device (LAD).

Hypothesizing the existence of an innate LAD raises the question as to where this acquisition device comes from. Chomsky himself, followed by other linguists such as Bickerton, Newmeyer, and Lightfoot, was not very specific about this question but suggested that it might have evolved through a large mutation or as a by-product of some other evolutionary development. According to Pinker and Bloom (41), the LAD, or what they call the "human language faculty," is a biological adaptation that should be explained by natural selection. A similar view is suggested in various papers of Nowak et al. (42).

Evidence of Chomsky's innatism emerges from neuroscientific theories and against environment-only mechanisms.

However, the proposed language structures cannot be seen. Even if they were visible, it would be impossible to establish that these structures were innate.

Language is creative. We can produce and understand an infinite range of novel grammatical sentences and children do not imitate a fixed number of sentences.

Chomsky argues that creativity is not explicable if language is learnt just from the environment. The grammar of a sentence cannot be deduced from its surface form.

Languages vary greatly, but all are governed by the principles of Universal Grammar. If children do not/cannot learn the rules of grammar from the language in their environment, then these rules must be inborn.

This explains all the difficulties found with environment-only acquisition theories proposed by Skinner (43) and others. In fact, deaf children with normal hearing can learn by imitating adult speech or sign language.

Chomsky states that, "the essential core of grammar is innate."

This means that language (i.e., Universal Grammar) is a separate system in the brain's architecture. It is connected to, but does not interact extensively with, other sorts of thought.

Crucial parts of the human language ability are built into the brain, part of our biology, and programmed into our genes" (40).

Genetics and language disorders

Genetic research has concentrated on two of the main categories of disorders of language, focusing on:

1. Specific language impairment (SLI)
2. Specific reading disability (SRD)

Current quantitative and molecular research in this area has produced many interesting findings that show strong evidence of the presence of a number of genes contributing to these disorders.

Specific language impairment (SLI)

SLI constitutes a complex area of investigation because of the broad interindividual variability that characterizes normal language development and because linguistic competence includes a set of abilities that can be delayed or deficient depending on different lines or dimensions of development. Given the absence of a precise characterization of SLI behavioural profiles, research on the genetic underpinning of such a complex syndrome is still inconclusive. The finding of alterations in various chromosomes and the heterogeneity of SLI from the point of view of the behavioural phenotype suggests that the genetic contribution is complex and that genetic transmission is probably linked to alterations involving more than one gene.

SLI is a heterogeneous set of clinical conditions that presents with a significant delay in language acquisition in the absence of neurological, sensory, cognitive, or emotional impairment. Linguistic deficits can involve both coding (production) and decoding (comprehension) in one or more areas of linguistic competence (phonology, lexicon, morphology, syntax, and pragmatics), giving rise to different behavioural phenotypes.

The impairment includes different subtypes of the disorder that have a variable outcome in relation to factors such as the severity of the initial disorder, the age of the child at the time of diagnosis, and the speech and language therapy. Moreover, the pattern of impairment is not stable over time but tends to change with age.

As regards the genetic hypothesis, Fisher et al. identified (44), for the first time, an alteration of a small segment of chromosome 7 in one KE family, which they called speech-language disorder 1 (SPCH1) or forkhead box P2 (FOXP2). They believed that this alteration was responsible for the family's language disorder. In fact, half of the members of this family had severe speech and grammar impairments. In addition, brain-imaging studies of this family suggested functional abnormalities in the areas of the frontal lobe related to motor activity. They also observed anatomical abnormalities in several brain regions including the neostriatum.

Lai et al. (45) showed a translocation of the same region of the long arm of chromosome 7 (region 7q31) in a patient affected by a severe language disorder and not belonging to this family aggregation. According to these investigators, the gene FOXP2 might disrupt the development of the brain circuitry that underlies language and speech during the fetal stage.

Although rare and severe disorders such as those of the family described by Fisher are often caused by a single gene, common disorders such as language impairment are more likely to be the quantitative extreme of the normal genetic factors responsible for language development throughout the general population.

A recent study (46) showed the essential role of FOXP2 gene in the development of social communication. Disruption of FOXP2 affected the ability of infant rodents to emit ultrasonic vocalizations when separated from their mother and littermates, but it did not appear to influence the structure and neural control of the vocal tract.

Further studies by the same authors on the FOXP2 mice suggest that interference with FOXP2 affects the migration and/or the maturation of neurones in the development of the cerebellum. The gene FOXP2 influences articulation and capacity to control the mouth and influences the individual's capacity to use complex sentences. Chimps do not have the same sequence of amino acids on this gene. This appears to be a genetic impairment that delays language development without affecting nonverbal IQ or cognition.

In recent studies on a large number of cases of SLI with a family history, two additional regions were identified (one on chromosome 16 and one on chromosome 19), which seem to play an important role in determining the genetic risk of SLI (47).

The finding of abnormalities in various chromosomes and the heterogeneity of SLI from the point of view of the behavioral phenotype suggest that the genetic contribution is complex and that genetic transmission is probably linked to an alteration in more than one genetic site. In recent genetic studies of complex traits and disorders, the term "QTL" (quantitative trait loci) has been given to genes contributing to the variance of continuously distributed traits in multiple gene systems (48,49).

Questions about how genetically mediated anomalies in the development of the brain determine SLI are still completely unresolved. One possible hypothesis is that genetic factors can alter the processes of neuronal migration, causing a disruption of cortical cytoarchitectonics at the level of the perisylvian regions. One of the most important structural alterations of the cerebral cortex found at necropsy (50) was symmetry or inverse asymmetry of the plana temporale that was accompanied by cortical ectopias and polymicrogyria in the right and left hemispheres (51). These perisylvian findings were confirmed in morphometric magnetic resonance imaging studies of language-impaired children (52). Atypical asymmetries, characterized by a right temporal planum of the same size as or larger than the left (contrary to what is normally found in control subjects) were also observed by Plante among the family members of affected individuals (53).

Although the clinical and linguistic profiles of children with SLI have been widely described (54–57) and three broad subtypes (mixed receptive–expressive, expressive-only, and phonological disorder) have been identified (58), aetiological studies often treat SLI as a homogeneous condition. As neither a core deficit of SLI nor an alteration of individual processes has been clearly defined, the problem of aetiological interpretation is still open. Given the lack of a precise characterization of behavioural profiles in SLI, research on the genetic underpinning of such a complex syndrome is still inconclusive.

However, the hypothesis that language disorders have a genetic underpinning is supported by various lines of evidence and is based essentially on the following:

- Presence of language disorders in syndromes with known genetic aetiologies
- Epidemiological characteristics of specific language disorders
- Familial aggregation for language disorders and twin studies

Language disorders in pathologies of known genetic aetiologies

Clinical descriptions of the behavioural phenotypes of intellectually retarded children with syndromes of known genetic aetiology (Down, Klinefelter, Prader–Willi, Fragile X, Angelman syndrome, and the syndrome of aneuploidy of sex chromosomes) often document the presence of a selective impairment of verbal abilities. These findings lend support to the hypothesis that alterations of different chromosomes can lead to similar phenotypic expressions (genetic heterogeneity), although the underlying pathophysiological mechanisms remain unknown. One important issue is whether these phenomena are genetically mediated or whether the peculiarity of language function is specifically vulnerable to impairment in a variety of exceptional circumstances that do not necessarily share any common factor (59).

One example of genetic heterogeneity might be represented by the similarities observed between the cognitive language profiles classically described as typical of Williams syndrome (60–63) and of the phenotype of subjects with the syndrome involving deletion of the short arm of chromosome 9 (64).

Epidemiological characteristics of specific language disorders

The incidence of speech and language impairment among children has been difficult to establish. Lindsay and Dockrell (65) estimated that speech and language impairment affects 7% of children, whereas Law et al. (66) arrived at a 10% estimate. The evidence suggests, therefore, that SLI is a significant category of educational need and is not confined to the early years of learning. In fact, the prevalence varies with age and is higher in 24- to 36-month-old children (Fig. 12.3); however, the prevalence of persistent disorders is estimated to be 3% (67,68). SLI constitutes a complex area of investigation because of the broad interindividual variability that characterizes normal language development and because linguistic competence includes a set of abilities that can be delayed or deficient depending on different lines or dimensions of development.

Some children may not be identified as having SLI until they are in the secondary phase of their education (69). If teachers are not aware that a child in their class has a SLI, the student's behavioural response may give rise to perceptions of primary problems such as emotional and behavioural disorders, stubbornness, and noncompliance (70).

Family and twin studies

In the past, most studies of familial effects have focused on single families with multiple cases of language impairment (71–75). Another strategy has been to estimate the frequency of language impairment among the relatives of language-impaired probands (76–80). However, these studies were performed without matched control families unaffected by SLI.

More recently, family studies have included control families in their designs. They have also reported high rates of language impairment in first-degree relatives that ranged between 17% and 43% (6,81–86).

There is also growing evidence in the literature of a hereditary factor in SLI, particularly following from various twin studies, where the prevalence of SLI has been shown to be greater in monozygotic twins than in dizygotic twins (87,88). Additional evidence is accumulating, in the literature, of genetic influence in a family with verbal dyspraxia (the KE family) (44,89) and two sites have been located as being implicated in dyslexia (90).

In a prospective study of language development (16–26 months), Spritz et al. (83) found 50% of children with a

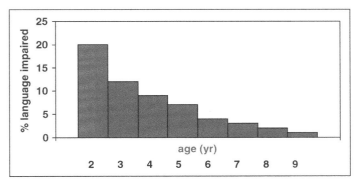

Figure 12.3 The decrease in the prevalence of language impairment with age.

family history demonstrated language delay, whereas none of the children with no family history experienced delay.

The greater prevalence in males (male-to-female ratio approximately 3 to 1) seems explicable on the basis of the complex gene–hormone interactions in the developing brain. Indeed, it is well known that sex hormones influence the expression of many genes responsible for CNS development (91).

- The current investigation has two research questions:
- Firstly, where do genes associated with SLI map?
- Secondly, what is the nature of these genes and their gene products and how do they ultimately lead to SLI.

Stromswold (92) reported that, across seven family studies, the prevalence of SLI in family members of probands ranged from 24% to 78% (mean of 46%) compared with 3% to 46% (mean of 18%) found in the control groups. In addition, twin studies consistently indicated a significant increase in monozygotic concordance rates over those of dizygotic twins, suggesting that much of the reported familial aggregation can be attributed to a genetic influence. However, like many behavioural traits, SLI is assumed to be genetically complex with several loci contributing to the overall risk.

In a recent investigation, the SLI Consortium (47) performed a systematic genome-wide screen using 98 families drawn from epidemiological and clinical populations. All families were selected via a single proband whose standard language scores fall at least 1.5 Standard Deviation (SD) below the mean for their age. Three quantitative measures of language ability were used: the Clinical Evaluation of Language Fundamentals was used to derive scores of receptive and expressive language skills and a Non–Word Repetition test was used as a measure of phonological short-term memory. Separation of the genome screen sample demonstrated independent evidence of linkage on chromosomes 16q and 19q, indicating that these loci may represent universally important loci in SLI and, thus, general risk factors for language impairments.

In summary, SLI appears to be strongly familial, although the rates appear to change with the definition of SLI used. Although family histories suggest a genetic contribution to SLI, it cannot be taken as definitive proof because family similarities can stem from common environmental influences. Clear evidence can come only from other studies that attempt to separate the general influences of genetic and environmental factors. Twin studies are the main example of this type of approach.

Specific reading disability (SRD)

Identifying genes that contribute to the processes underlying the written language may provide important insights into how language is processed. Reading is a complex task that aims to extract meaning from the written word. SRD, or developmental dyslexia, is characterized as a gross difficulty in reading and writing that is not attributable to a general intellectual impairment or to a lack of exposure to an appropriate educational environment. SRD is usually characterized as a deficit of at least

two years in reading age compared to that predicted from the chronological age. However, as with SLI, measures of reading ability differ considerably among studies and, as yet, there are no universal operational definitions of reading disability to allow proper generalization across studies.

A variety of cognitive components have been implicated in the development of SRD. These include deficits of visual processing system (93), deficits in the language processing system (94), and deficits in temporal processing (95). However, most evidence suggests that deficits in phonological processing are central to the development of SRD. The functional unit of phonological processing is the phoneme, the smallest discernible segment of speech. Phonological processing includes phoneme awareness, decoding, storage, and retrieval. Another component of the reading process is the visual appearance of shape (orthographic information) of a written word (96). In addition, the speed at which language-based information is processed may also be of importance (9). Robinson et al. (Robinson L, Morris DW, Turic D, et al. Dimensions of reading disability. Unpublished) have identified three factors that describe severe SRD as comprising phonological, orthographic, and rapid-naming dimensions. Within their population, each factor accounted for a maximum of 18% of the variance.

The genetic background of reading disabilities has not been studied in such depth as that of specific language disorders.

In an early family study of SRD, Rutter et al. (36) observed that 34% of children with specific reading retardation had a parent or sibling with a reading problem compared to 9% of control children. Indeed, four of the major family studies undertaken have consistently reported high sibling recurrence risks of 40.8% (97), 42.5% (98), 43% (99), and 38.5% (48). Although the estimates of population frequency of SRD vary, reasonable estimates range between 5% and 10% (100).

Many early twin studies of SRD that showed significantly greater monozygotic than dizygotic concordance for SRD had methodological flaws, particularly in ascertainment bias and the inconsistent use of operational definitions of SRD (101,102). The first systematic evidence that the high family history of SRD was due to genetic rather than social factors came in the 1980s. At this time, two important twin studies were published: The Colorado Twin Reading Study (103) and The London Twin Study (104). Both provided strong evidence for the role of genetic factors in SRD.

There was also evidence of sex difference in penetrance rates, with females showing lower estimates of penetrance in the autosomal-dominant family. It is possible that this might go some way to explain the slight excess of males observed in SRD (sex ratio of 1.5:1; male:female) (105,106), although the higher ratio of males to females could also be attributed to an artefact of clinical ascertainment (105).

Molecular genetic research on SRD has produced strong evidence of linkage to chromosome 6p (90,106–110), significant evidence of linkage to chromosome 2 (111,112), and suggestive evidence of linkage to chromosome 1 (113). In addition, studies using linkage disequilibrium mapping have fine mapped the region on chromosomes 6 and 15 to areas of approximately 1–6 cM, which show good evidence of containing the putative genes (114).

Grigorenko et al. (90) presented the strongest evidence of linkage to a phenotype characterized as phonemic awareness, although significant linkage was also observed with phonological decoding and single word reading. However, their extended study (110) resulted in a less clear relationship, showing linkage to single word reading, vocabulary, and spelling with phonemic awareness and phonological decoding showing little evidence of a relationship. However, it must be noted that the evidence of relationships with specific reading disabilities phenotypes or dimensions may be influenced by the methods of ascertainment, phenotypic definition, and the frequency of the phenotypes in the sample studied. Furthermore, as most of the phenotypes show significant correlations with each other, which results in many individuals having numerous phenotypes, clear relationships, if they exist, may be difficult to establish.

Conclusions

Although for a long time the ability to speak was considered instinctive and specific to human beings and innate bases were suggested for language acquisition, only quite recently has the genetic role been taken into consideration in language studies.

In the past few decades, language studies and research on the acquisition of a first language have given great importance to the fact that linguistic abilities and their development depend on the existence of innate information. The complex interactions between "nature" and "nurture" have also been underlined; that is the interactions between genes and environment through which the genotype, or the genetic information coded in the DNA of each individual, becomes the phenotype—observable physical and behavioural features. Individual differences in cognitive abilities, primarily verbal, appear to originate at the interface between genetic and environmental aspects, family, school, therapeutic experiences, and so on. On a theoretical basis, finding a genetic influence on individual differences in vocabulary does not contradict the assumption that words are learned. It means that DNA differences between people affect how easily they learn, remember, and use words (49). On the clinical plane, supposing there is a reciprocal interaction between environment and genes in the constitution of a specific behavioural profile means going beyond a diagnosis based on symptoms, in order to try to identify the aetiology of specific cognitive and behavioural phenotypes.

It is known that language acquisition is a phenomenon that occurs naturally and rapidly in most children. However, some children do not show this normal language acquisition. These language-impaired children do not have any type of developmental or neurological delay; they simply have difficulty with language. The children with SLI make more random errors than the group of normal children. This demonstrates the problem, which children with SLI have in learning new vocabulary as well as with grammatical categories.

It was noted earlier that there are several theories as to the origin of SLI. When comparing the brain of a child with SLI to that of a normally developing child, there are no anatomical differences. Research shows that SLI is more prevalent in boys than in girls. Researchers debate the issue of prenatal problems in relation to SLI because low birth weight and socioeconomic factors can be linked to other language impairments. Clinical studies on this matter are contradictory.

Another theory deals with the inability to process sound normally (115). Auditory perceptual deficits could affect the perception of the brief acoustic speech elements.

Limitations in working memory may be an implication for language development according to the study conducted by Adams and Gathercole (116). The study by Marton and Schwartz (117) tested the interaction between working memory and language comprehension in children with SLI. This interaction was tested by studying the effect of sentence length on working memory and syntactic complexity. Working memory is important in language comprehension during language acquisition because it allows the learner to analyze and to determine the structural properties of a language.

The theories discussed above all propose different aetiologies for SLI. The same may be said for intellectual disabilities in which more variables intervene.

Genetics plays a significant role in the development of language disorders as demonstrated by SLI and SRD. The studies reported in this chapter refer to the advances in identifying genes responsible for SLI and SRD. Lewis's work (81) summarizes the latest results on chromosomal regions that show good evidence of containing susceptibility genes (Table 12.2).

As this research increases, there is great optimism that the genes will soon be found and our understanding of the origins of these disorders will truly begin.

Table 12.2   Linkage to chromosomes identified thus far

Chromosome	Phenotype
1	Dyslexia
2	Word recognition; decoding
3	Phonological awareness; rapid auditory naming test; verbal memory
6	Vocabulary; rapid auditory naming test; spelling vocabulary
7	Sequential articulation
13	Reading discrepancy score
15	Word recognition; spelling
16	Non–word repetition
18	Phon and and ortho ortho processing
19	Clinical evaluation of language fundamentals—revised expressive

References

1. Gerber SE. Communication Disorders. In: Gerber SE, ed. Handbook of Genetic Communicative Disorders. Santa Barbara: Academic Press, 2001:12–27.

2. Godai U, Tatarelli R, Bonnani G. Stuttering and tics in twins. Acta Genet Med Gomellologiae 1976; 25:369–375.

3. Ingham RJ. Stuttering: recent trends in research and therapy. In: Winiz H, ed. Human Communication and Its Disorders. Norwood, NJ: Ablex, 1987:1–63.

4. Shprintzen RG. Genetics, Syndromes, and Communication Disorders. San Diego: Singular, 1997.

5. Peterson-Falzone SJ. Basic concepts in congenital craniofacial defects. In: Bzoch KR, ed. Communicative Disorders Related to Cleft Lip and Palate. 3rd ed. Boston: College-Hill, 1989:37–46.

6. Rice ML. Specific language impairments: in search of diagnostic markers and genetic contributions. Mental Retard Develop Disab Res Rev 1997; 3:350–357.

7. Zoll B. Zur genetich der sprachentwicklungsstorungen. Sprach Stimme Gehor 1999; 23:127–180.

8. Regher SM, Kaplan BJ. Reading disability with motor problems may be an inherited subtype. Pediat 1988; 82:204–210.

9. Wolf M, Bowers PG. The double-deficit hypothesis for the developmental dyslexias. J Educ Psychol 1999; 91:415–438.

10. Felsenfeld S, McGue M, Broen PA. Familial aggregation of phonological disorders: result from a 28-year follow-up. J Speech Hear Res 1995; 38:1091–1107.

11. Green GE, Smith RJH. Delineation of genetic components of communicative disorders. In: Gerber SE, ed. The Handbook of Genetic Communicative Disorders. New York: Academic Press, 2001:11–29.

12. Kurnit DM, Layton WM, Matthysse S. Genetics, chance, and morphogenesis. Am J Med Gen 1987; 41:979–995.

13. Mendel G. Versuche über plflanzenhybriden. Verhandlungen des naturforschenden vereines in Brünn, Bd. IV für das Jahr 1865:3–47.

14. Tiedemann D. Beobachtungen ber die entwicklung der seelenfahigkeiten bei kindern. Altenburg 1787.

15. Darwin C. A biographical sketch of an infant. Mind 2 1877:285–294.

16. Taine H. On the acquisition of language by children. Mind 2 1877:252–259.

17. Preyer W. Die seele des kindes. Leipzig, 1882. (Brown HW. The Mind of the Child. Vols. 1 and 2. New York: Appleton, 1888–1890) [English translation].

18. Shinn NW. Notes on the Development of a Child. Berkeley: University of California Press, 1893.

19. Sully J. Studies of Childhood. London: Longmans, 1895.

20. Stern W. Psychology of Early Childhood. London: Allen & Unwin, 1924 [Translated by Barwell A].

21. Leopold WF. Speech Development of a Bilingual Child. Vols. 1–4. Evanston, Ill.: Northwestern University Studies in the Humanities, 1939–1949.

22. Kies D. Language Development in Children. In: Scholes R, ed. The Hyper Text Book. New York: Penguin, 1991:33–37.

23. Lenneberg EH. A biological perspective on language. In: Lenneberg EH, ed. New Directions in the Study of Language. MIT Press, 1964:65–88.

24. Lenneberg EH. Biological Foundations of Language. Wiley J and Sons, eds. New York: MIT Press, 1967.

25. Cowan WM. The development of the brain. Sci Am 1979; 241:106–117.

26. Kovas Y, Hayiou-Thomas ME, Oliver B et al. Genetic influences in different aspects of language development: the etiology of language skills in 4.5-year-old twins. J Child Devel 2005; 76:632–651.

27. Kaplan E, Kaplan G. The Prelinguistic Child. In: Elliot J, ed. Human Development and Cognitive Processes. New York: Holt, Rinehart and Winston, 1971:359–381.

28. Fromkin VA, Krashen S, Curtiss S, et al. The development of language in genie: a case of language acquisition beyond the 'critical period.' Brain Lang 1974; 1:81–107.

29. Meltzoff AN, Moore MK. Imitation of facial and manual gestures by human neonates. Science 1977; 198:75–78.

30. Meltzoff AN, Moore MK. Newborn infants imitate adult facial gestures. Child Development 1983; 54:702–709.

31. Meltzoff AN, Moore MK. The origins of imitation in infancy: paradigm, phenomena, and theories. In: Lipsitt LP, Rovee-Collier CK, eds. Advances in Infant Research. Norwood, NJ: Ablex, 1983:266–276.

32. McNeill D. So you think gestures are nonverbal? Psychol Rev 1985; 92:350–371.

33. Perry M, Breckinridge Church R, Goldin-Meadow S. Transitional knowledge in the acquisition of concepts. Cognit Devel 1988; 3:359–400.

34. Kies D. A functional linguistic view of language development. ERIC Document 1985; 266:462.

35. Kies D. Indeterminacy in sentence structure. Linguistic Edu 1990; 2:231–258.

36. Rutter M, Tizard J, Withmore K. Education, health, and behaviour. ASHA 1970; 27:27–32.

37. Knudsen EI. Sensitive periods in the development of the brain and behavior. J Cognit Neurosci 2004;16:1412–1425.

38. Chomsky N. Syntactic Structures. The Hague: Mouton Humanities Press, 1957.

39. Gold EM. Language identification in the limit. Inform Control 1967; 10:447–474.

40. Chomsky N. Cartesian Linguistics. New York: Harper and Row, 1966.

41. Pinker S, Bloom P. Natural language and natural selection. Behav Brain Sci 1990; 13:707–784.

42. Nowak MA, Komarova N, Niyogi P. Evolution of universal grammar. Sci 2001; 291:114–118.

43. Skinner BF. Verbal Behavior. New York: Appleton-Century-Crofts, 1957.

44. Fisher SE, Vargha-Khadem F, Watkins KE, et al. Localisation of a gene implicated in severe in a severe speech and language disorder. Nature Genet 1998; 18:168–170.

45. Lai C, Fisher S, Hurst J. et al. A forkhead-domain gene is mutated in a severe speech and language disorder. Nature 2001; 413:519–523.

46. Buxbaum JD. Foxp2 gene plays an essential role in the development of social communication. Am J Hum Genet 2005; 68:1514–1520.

47. SLI Consortium. A genomewide scan identifies two novel loci involved in specific language impairment. Am J Hum Genet 2002; 70:384–398.

48. Gilger GW, Pennington BF, DeFries JC. Risk for reading disability as a function of parental history in 3 family studies. Read Writing 1991; 3:205–217.

49. Plomin R, Dale PS. Genetics and early language development: a UK study of twins. In: Bishop DVM, Leonard BE, eds. Speech and Language Impairments in Children: Causes, Characteristics, Intervention and Outcome. Hove, U.K.: Psychology Press, 2000:35–51.

50. Galaburda AM, Sherman GF, Rosen GD, et al. Developmental dyslexia: four consecutive patients with cortical anomalies. Ann Neurol 1985; 18:222–233.

51. Geschwind N, Galaburda AM. Cerebral lateralization. biological mechanisms, associations, and pathology: I. A hypothesis and a program for research. Arch Neurol 1985; 42:428–459.

52. Plante E, Swisher L, Vance R, Rapsack S. MRI findings in boys with specific language impairment. Brain Lang 1991; 41:52–66.

53. Plante E, Boliek C, Binkiewicz A, Erly WK. Elevated androgen, brain development and language/learning disabilities in children with congenital adrenal hyperplasia. Dev Med Child Neurol 1996; 38:423–437.

54. Rapin I, Allen DA. Syndromes in developmental dysphasia and adult aphasia. Res Publ Assoc Res Nerv Ment Dis 1988; 66:57–75.

55. Hayes LA, Watson JS. Neonatal imitation: fact or artefact? Devel Psychol 1981; 17:655–660.

56. Robinson RJ. Causes and associations of severe and persistent specific speech and language disorders in children. Devel Med Child Neurol 1991; 33:943–962.

57. Chilosi AM, Cipriani P. Developmental phenotypes of language specific disorders. In: Riva D, Bellugi U, Denkla M, eds. Neurodevelopmental Disorders: Cognitive Behavioural Phenotypes. London-Paris: Foundation Paediatric Neurology, John Libbey Eurotext Ltd, 2005:1–9.

58. World Health Organization. International classification of diseases. 10th ed. Geneva: WHO, 1992.

59. Mogford K, Bishop D. Language development in unexceptional circumstances. In: Bishop D, Mogford K, eds. Language Development in Exceptional Circumstances. Hove: Lawrence Erlbaum, 1993:10–28.

60. Bellugi U, Lichtenberger L, Mills D, et al. Bridging cognition, the brain, and molecular genetics: evidence from William's syndrome. Trends in Neurosci 1999; 22:197–207.

61. Bellugi U, Lichtenberger L, Jones W, et al. The neurocognitive profile of William's syndrome I: a complex pattern of strengths and weaknesses. J Cogn Neurosci 2000; 12(suppl 1): 7–29.

62. Frangiskakis JM, Ewart AK, Morris CA, et al. LIMkinase1 hemizygosity implicated in impaired visuospatial constructive cognition. Cell 1996; 86:59–69.

63. Reilly J, Klima E, Bellugi U. Once more with feeling: affect and language in atypical populations. Devel Psychopathol 1990; 2:367–391.

64. Chilosi A, Battaglia A, Brizzolara D, et al. The del (9p) syndrome: proposed behavioral phenotype. Am J Med Genet 2001; 100:138.

65. Lindsay, GA, Dockrell JE. The behaviour and self-esteem of children with specific speech and language difficulties. Br J Educ Psychol 2000; 70:583–601.

66. Law J, Boyle J, Harris F, et al. The feasibility of universal screening for primary speech and language delay: findings from a systematic review of the literature. Dev Med Child Neurol 2000; 42:190–200.

67. Silva PA, Williams SM, McGee RA. Longitudinal study of children with developmental language delay at age three: later intelligence, reading and behaviour problems. Dev Med Child Neurol 1987; 29:630–640.

68. Whitehurst GJ, Fischel JE. Practitioner review: early developmental language delay: what, if anything, should the clinician do about it? J Child Psychol Psychiat 1994; 35:613–648.

69. Ripley K, Barrett J, Fleming P. Inclusion for Children With Speech and Language Impairment. London: David Fulton Publishers, 2001.

70. Freeman D. Asking "good" questions: perspectives from qualitative research on practice, knowledge, and understanding in teacher education. TESOL Quart 1995; 29:581–585.

71. Arnold GE. The genetic background of developmental language disorders. Folia Phoniat 1961; 13:246–254.

72. Borges-Osorio MR, Salzano FM. Language disabilities in 3 twin pairs and their relatives. Acta Genet Med et Gemellologiae 1985; 34:95–100.

73. Hurst JA, Baraitser M, Auger E, et al. An extended family with a dominantly inherited speech disorder. Devel Med Child Neurol 1990; 32:352–355.

74. McReady EB. Defects in the zone of language (word-deafness and word-blindness) and their influence in education and behaviour. Am J Psychiat 1926; 6:267–277.

75. Sampless JM, Lane VW. Genetic possibilities in six siblings with specific language learning disorders. Asha 1970; 27:27–32.

76. Bishop DVM, Edmundson A. Is otitis media a major cause of specific developmental language disorders? Br J Dis Communic 1986; 21:321–338.

77. Byrne B, Willerman L, Ashmore L. Severe and moderate language impairment: evidence for distinctive aetiologies. Behav Genet 1974; 4:331–345.

78. Hier DB, Rosenberger PB. Focal left temporal lobe lesions and delayed speech acquisition. J Devel Behav Pediat 1980; 1:54–57.

79. Ingram TTS. Specific developmental disorders of speech in childhood. Brain 1959; 82:450–454.

80. Luchsinger R. In heritance of speech deficits. Folia Phoniat 1970; 22:216–230.

81. Lewis BA. Pedigree analysis of children with phonology disorders. J Learn Disab 1992; 25:586–597.

82. Neils J, Aram D. Family history of children with developmental language disorders. Percept Motor Skills 1986; 63:655–658.

83. Spitz RV, Tallal P, Flax J, Benasich AA. Look who's talking: a prospective study of familial transmission of language impairments. J Speech Hear Res 1997; 40:990–1001.

84. Tallal P, Ross R, Curtiss S. Familial aggregation in specific language impairment. J Speech Hear Dis 1989; 54:287–295.

85. Tomblin JB, Zhang X. Language patterns and aetiology in children with specific language impairment. In: Tager-Flusberg H, ed. Neurodevelopmental Disorders. Cambridge, MA: MIT Press, 1999:361–382.

86. Van der Lely HKJ, Stollwerck L. A grammatical specific language impairment in children: an autosomal dominant inheritance. Brain Lang 1996; 52:484–504.

87. Bishop DVM, North T, Donlan C. Genetic basis of specific language impairment: evidence from a twin study. Devel Med Child Neurol 1995; 37:56–71.

88. Tomblin JB, Buckwalter PR. Heritability of poor language achievement among twins. J Speech Lang Hear Res 1998; 41:188–199.

89. Vargha-Khadem F, Watkins K, Alcock K, et al. Praxic and non-verbal cognitive deficits in a large family with a genetically transmitted speech and language disorder. Proc Nat Acad Sci 1995; 92:930–933.

90. Grigorenko EL, Wood FB, Meyer MS, et al. Susceptibility loci for distinct components of developmental dyslexia on chromosomes 6 and 15. Am J Human Genet 1997; 60:27–39.

91. Geschwind N, Bhean P. Left handedness: association with immune disease, migraine, and developmental learning disorder. Proc Nat Acad Sci USA 1982; 79:5097–5100.

92. Stromswold K. Specific language impairments. In: Feinberg TE, Farah MJ, eds. Behavioral Neurology and Neuropsychology. New York: McGraw Hill 1997:755–772.

93. Stein JF. Visuospatial perception in disabled readers. In: Willows DM, Kruk RS, Corcos E eds. Visual processes in reading and reading disabilities. Hillsdale, NJ: Erlbaum, 1993:331–346.

94. Shankweiler D, Liberman IY, Mark LS, et al. The speech code and learning to read. J Exp Psychol: Hum Learn Mem 1979; 5:531–545.

95. Stein JF, Walsh V. To see but not to read: the magnocellular theory of dyslexia. Trends Neurosci 1997; 20:147–152.

96. Olson RK, Forsberg H, Wise B. Genes, environment, and the development of orthographic skills. In: Berninger VW, ed The Varieties of Orthographic Knowledge. Vol. 1. Theoretical Developmental Issues. Dordrecht: Kluwer, 1994:1–31.

97. Hallgren B. Specific dyslexia: a clinical and genetic study. Acta Psychiat Neurol Scand 1950; (suppl 65).

98. Finucci JM, Guthrie JT, Childs AL, et al. The genetics of specific reading disability. Ann Rev Human Genet 1976; 40:1–23.

99. Vogler GP, DeFries JC, Decker SN. Family history as an indicator of risk for reading disability. J Learn Disab 1985; 18:419–421.

100. Pennington BF. Annotation: the genetics of dyslexia. J Child Psychiat Psychol 1990; 31:193–201.

101. Bakwin H. Reading disability in twins. Develop Med Child Neurol 1973; 15:184–187.

102. Zerbin-Rudin E. Congenital word-blindness. Bull Orton Soc 1967; 17:47–54.

103. DeFries JC, Fulker DW, LaBuda MC. Evidence for a genetic aetiology in reading disability of twins. Nature 1987; 329:537–539.

104. Stevenson J, Graham P, Fredman G, McLoughlin V. A twin study of genetic influences on reading and spelling ability and disability. J Child Psychiat Psychol 1987; 28:229–247.

105. Shaywitz SE, Shaywitz BA, Fletcher JM, Escobar MD. Prevalence of reading disability in boys and girls. J Am Med Assoc 1990; 264:998–1200.

106. Wadsworth SJ, DeFries JC, Stevenson J, et al. Gender ratios among reading-disabled children and their siblings. J Child Psychiat Psychol 1992; 33:1229–1239.

107. Cardon LR, Smith SD, Fulker DW, et al. Quantitative trait locus for reading disability on chromosome 6. Science 1994; 266:276–279.

108. Fisher SE, Marlow AJ, Lamb J, et al. A quantitative trait locus on chromosome 6 p influences aspects of developmental dyslexia. Am J Human Genet 1999; 64:146–156.

109. Gayan J, Smith SD, Cherny SS, et al. Quantitative trait locus for specific language and reading deficits on chromosome 6. Am J Human Genet 1999; 64:157–164.

110. Grigorenko EL, Wood FB, Meyer MS, Pauls DL. Chromosome 6p influences on different dyslexia-related cognitive processes: farther confirmation. Am J Human Genet 2000; 66:715–723.

111. Fagerheim T, Raeymaekers P, Tonnessen FE, et al. A new gene (DYX3) for dyslexia is located on chromosome 2. J Med Genet 1999; 36:664–669.

112. Petryshen TL, Kaplan BJ, Liu MF, Field LL. Absence of significant linkage between phonological decoding dyslexia and chromosome 6p23–21.3, as determined by use of quantitative-trait methods: confirmation of qualitative analyses. Am J Human Genet 2000; 66:708–714.

113. Rabin M, Wen XL, Hepburn M, et al. Suggestive linkage of developmental dyslexia to chromosome 1p34–p36. Lancet 1993; 342:178–180.

114. Morris DW, Robinson L, Turic D, et al. Family-based association mapping provides evidence for a gene for reading disability on chromosome 15q. Human Molec Genet 2000; 9:855–860.

115. Wright BA, Lombardino LJ, King WM, et al. Deficits in auditory temporal and spectral resolution in language-impaired children. Nature 1997; 387:176–178.

116. Adams AM, Gathercole SE. Limitations in working memory: implications for language development. Internat J Lang Communic Dis 2000; 35:95–116.

117. Marton K, Schwartz RG. Working memory capacity and language processes in children with specific language impairment. J Speech Lang Hear Res 2003; 46:1138–1153.

13 Audiometric profiles associated with genetic nonsyndromal hearing impairment: a review and phenotype analysis

Patrick L M Huygen, Robert Jan Pauw, Cor W R J Cremers

Introduction

A useful phenotypic classification of genetic disorders with nonsyndromal hearing impairment comprises the various types of audiometric configurations. Apart from conductive or mixed hearing impairment, Konigsmark and Gorlin (1) and Toriello et al. (2) distinguished several types of nonsyndromal sensorineural hearing impairment (SNHI): (downsloping) high-frequency SNHI, mid-frequency SNHI with a U-shaped audiometric configuration, (upsloping) low-frequency SNHI, and SNHI with a residual-hearing type of audiogram, i.e., measurable thresholds only in the low-frequency range. Additional distinctive features are related to progression (stable and progressive), age of onset (congenital, early, and late onset), and severity (mild, moderate, severe, and profound).

Using such a classification, this review surveys those genetic disorders with nonsyndromal hearing impairment that have already been linked to human chromosomal loci, following the specifications of the Hereditary Hearing Loss Homepage (here called HHH) (3). The autosomal-dominant loci for "deafness"

include DFNA1-5, DFNA6/14/38, DFNA7, DFNA8/12, DFNA9-11, DFNA13, DFNA15-18, DFNA20/26, DFNA21-25, DFNA28, DFNA30-31, DFNA36, DFNA41-44, and DFNA47-50. The autosomal-recessive loci include DFNB1-6, DFNB7/11, DFNB8/10, DFNB9, DFNB12-18, DFNB20-23, DFNB26-27, DFNB29-33, DFNB35-40, DFNB42, DFNB44, DFNB46, and DFNB48-49. The X-linked loci include DFN2-4 and DFN6. In addition, a recently identified Y-linked locus is also included. Otosclerosis is only briefly mentioned, because, on the one hand, the audiometric phenotype of "otosclerosis," which must be a mixed bag of loci yet to be identified, is sufficiently well known, whereas, on the other hand, the phenotypes pertaining to the newly identified loci for otosclerosis, such as OTSC2 and OTSC5, have only just begun to be defined. As regards hereditary auditory neuropathy, the autosomal-recessive type caused by OTOF mutations (DFNB9) is not specifically mentioned here because it fits in with the vast majority of recessive SNHI disorders showing residual hearing. The first locus that has been identified for autosomal-dominant auditory neuropathy (AUNA1s) is included. Furthermore, syndromal hearing impairment is not included in this review. However, Pendred syndrome overlaps with DFNB4, and the differential diagnosis between Pendred syndrome and DFNB4 can be notoriously difficult, with the hearing impairment phenotypes of the two disorders being very similar. This is because the underlying cause is associated with inner ear malformations, i.e., the large endolymphatic duct and sac, which is common to these disorders, so that it is reasonable to include Pendred syndrome.

The purposes of this review are to facilitate (*i*) the differential diagnosis of genetic hearing impairment phenotypes, (*ii*) the consideration of treatment opportunities, (*iii*) the counselling, and (*iv*) the guidance for genotyping efforts of newly defined nonsyndromal hearing impairment traits. Illustrative examples are given as for as possible in figures based on previously reported data, our own original data, or original data communicated to us. In previous review papers, we dealt only with nonsyndromal autosomal-dominant SNHI (4–9). The present review not only updates and extends these reviews regarding autosomal-dominant SNHI disorders (linked to DFNA loci) but also covers autosomal-recessive SNHI (DFNB loci) and X-linked SNHI disorders (DFN loci) as well as a newly identified Y-linked disorder.

Methods

We adopted the classification by Koningsmark and Gorlin (1) with some minor modifications, most of which are in line with the European Union GENDEAF recommendations reported by Mazzoli et al. (10). These include two subcategories of high-frequency configuration: steeply (down)sloping, here designated "high frequency," and flat-to-gently (down)sloping, the latter of which is a combination of the GENDEAF categories "flat" and "gently sloping." The categories of frequency range are the recommended categories: low frequencies, 0.25 to 0.5 kHz; mid-frequencies, 1 to 2 kHz; and high frequencies, 4 to 8 kHz. We invoked previously classified onset categories which, however, appeared to be difficult to apply to many published reports. We therefore preferred to stay as close as possible to the original descriptions and just relay this information about onset age. The recommended categories of severity were applied: mild (20–40 dB HL), moderate (41–70 dB), severe (71–95 dB), and profound (>95 dB), the last of which we considered to be similar to the category of "residual hearing."

The GENDEAF recommendations call hearing impairment progressive if the annual threshold deterioration (ATD) for the pure-tone average (PTA) at 0.5, 1, and 2 kHz, i.e., $PTA_{(0.5,1,2\,kHz)}$, exceeds 1.5 dB. Instead, we specify progression, including the ATD where possible, and then, also specify whether progression is or is not significant. Progression is called significant when the threshold at the appropriate frequencies increases significantly with increasing age. Progression beyond "presbyacusis" is specified if the thresholds are still significantly progressive following correction for median (P50) presbyacusis according to ISO 7029 (11).

What we call "audiometric profile" comprises either a representative audiogram for a "typical" case as a minimum, a "mean audiogram" if hearing impairment does not change appreciably with increasing but not too advanced age, or age-related typical audiograms. These were constructed where possible using the method previously reported (7). The threshold data used to derive such age-related typical audiograms were our own original data, original data obtained from others by personal communication where specified, or data obtained from published papers, using table entries or plotted data points.

Phenotype by audiometric profile

Residual-hearing configuration

DFNA loci

Virtually none of the autosomal-dominant hearing impairment disorders associated with DFNA loci has residual hearing as a key distinctive feature. One exception is the (sub)residual-hearing audiometric configuration shown by a MYO6-based SNHI trait linked to locus DFNA22 (12). However, residual hearing can certainly be the endstage of any progressive autosomal-dominant hearing impairment phenotype. This includes obliterative otosclerosis, where, eventually, the air-bone gap (ABG) can be hardly discernible. Rapid progression to residual hearing is typical of the recently identified autosomal-dominant type of auditory neuropathy linked to the AUNA1 locus (13). Patients with auditory neuropathy have SNHI with intact otoacoustic emissions combined with poor speech recognition even at subresidual-hearing levels and they may not benefit from using hearing aids. However, recent reports suggest there may be a place for cochlear implantation in auditory neuropathy (14–16).

DFNB loci

The autosomal-recessive hearing impairment disorders associated with the DFNB loci generally show residual hearing, i.e., prelingual, severe-to-profound SNHI (17–20). This category includes "rapid progression to residual hearing." This feature has been noticed in a study on a DFNB8/10 trait showing childhood onset with progression to a residual-hearing configuration (21) and a study on a prelingual DFNB13 trait showing progression starting from a flat to a gently downsloping configuration with moderate threshold levels at young ages (22). However, most importantly and most impressively, the feature of early, rapid progression leading to residual hearing is shown (Fig. 13.1) by DFNB4 and/or the (possibly overlapping) Pendred syndrone (23,24) and such progression can be accompanied by substantial threshold fluctuations (25–30). There is no doubt that fluctuations in inner-ear function of this kind that not only include hearing ability but also vestibular function are associated with the features of large endolymphatic duct and sac that can be identified by magnetic resonance imaging or the related feature of a large vestibular aqueduct that was demonstrated when computer tomography was the main imaging

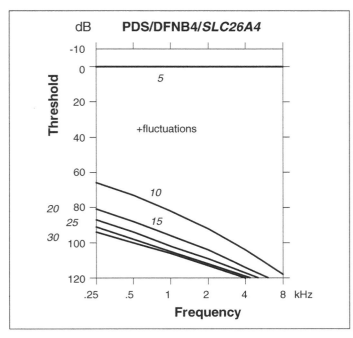

Figure 13.1 Age-related audiograms for Pendred syndrome and/or DFNB4 caused by a mutation in the *SLC26A4* gene showing rapid progression to residual hearing. Age in years is given in italics.

method. Such widening of the bony contours of the endolymphatic duct was identified as a key feature in Pendred syndrome (31) as well as an associated feature in some other syndromal hearing disorders, such as branchio-oto-renal syndrome.

It has been stated in some reports that a minority of patients with DFNB1 and with the 35delG/35delG genotype may show progression (32,33). However, we found no indications of progression in cross-sectional analyses in a recent multicentre study (Snoeckx et al., unpublished data) or in

individual longitudinal analyses (34). One report demonstrates progression in genotypes involving a large deletion in *GJB6* (35). Another report, however, indicates a lack of significant progression in longitudinal analyses of such cases (36). Santos et al. also described the longitudinal analysis of a patient with the *GJB2* H100P/S139 N genotype (H100P is a novel mutation), who showed significant progression in SNHI in both ears, with ATD values of 1 to 2 dB (34).

It should again be emphasised that most of the studies on DFNB1 and other DFNB loci indicate the usual residual-hearing configuration, with few exceptions (see below). The most important exception is that patients with DFNB1 may show variable degrees of SNHI. DFNB1 is a fine example that our genotype–phenotype correlation studies are now becoming more sophisticated at the mutational level. DFNB1 is particularly suitable for such type of studies, because it is, by far, the most prevalent cause of congenital genetic SNHI, which is mainly based on *GJB2* mutations (33). However, refinement of this type of analyses requires large numbers of patients and therefore depends on multicentre research projects. Part of the variability in the SNHI associated with DNFB1 can be explained by recent findings indicating that biallelic compound heterozygous *GJB2* mutation combinations of the type X/Y can show a residual-hearing configuration if both X and Y are some type of truncating mutation, or subresidual or even better hearing levels with a relatively flat audiometric configuration at mild-to-severe threshold levels if X and/or Y are some type of nontruncating mutation (Fig. 13.2) (37). The most important truncating mutations are 35delG (37), 233delC or 235delC (38,39), 167delT (40), W24X (41), as well as a large deletion in the *GJB6* gene [indicated as del(GJB6)] located in the vicinity of the *GJB2* gene responsible for DFNB1 (42). At the moment, the most important *GJB2* mutations in this respect seem to be the nontruncating mutations M34T (43–49), V37I (37,39,44,48,49),

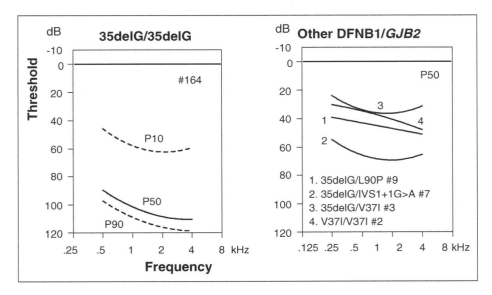

Figure 13.2 The 50th, 10th, and 90th percentiles (P50, P10, and P90, respectively) of the threshold distribution, not related to age, for DFNB1/GJB2 with biallelic, i.e., homozygous, combinations of the truncating 35delG mutation (*left*) and (*right*) biallelic combinations of several different nontruncating mutations, i.e., the missense mutations V37I and L90P, as well as the splice-site mutation IVS1 + 1G > A. Multicentre threshold data underlying the report by Cryns et al. (37); the symbol # indicates the number of patients.

and L90P (37,44,46,48,50), as well as the splice-site mutation IVS1 + 1G > A (Fig. 13.2) (37).

Many authors, especially Cohn and Kelley (19), Murgia et al. (51), Tóth et al. (52), and Cryns et al. (37), have emphasised the wide spectrum of threshold variability shown by 35delG/35delG homozygotes. One possible explanation is that modifying genes are involved. Further research into such a possibility certainly requires additional large-scale efforts.

DFN loci

The majority of the X-linked types of SNHI, i.e., DFN2 (53–55), DFN3 (56,57), and DFN4 (54,55,58–60) have congenital onset and show a residual-hearing type of configuration. In many instances, progression to a residual-hearing type has been specified: for DFN2 (61), as well as for DFN3 (55,62–68). It should be realised that DFN3 patients with a subresidual air-conduction threshold may show a low-frequency audiometric configuration on the basis of their ABG configuration, which,

quite remarkably, is stationary throughout life (Fig. 13.3). DFN3 is also associated with vestibular failure (56,57,63,66,67).

Exceptional X-linked traits linked to DFN2 and DFN6 having different audiometric configurations that are not compatible with residual hearing are specified in the following sections.

High-frequency downsloping audiometric configuration

This category includes stable as well as progressive high-frequency downsloping configurations. Progression is the rule for autosomal-dominant traits (Fig. 13.4) (18). Exceptions are some traits linked to DFNA3 that have been presumed to show stable SNHI and those for which linkage to DFNA23 or DFNA24 was reported. The latter were specified as being nonprogressive. However, threshold data collected by F Häfner (personal communication to P.H. 1999) did show age-related progression in a patient with DFNA24 that may be compatible

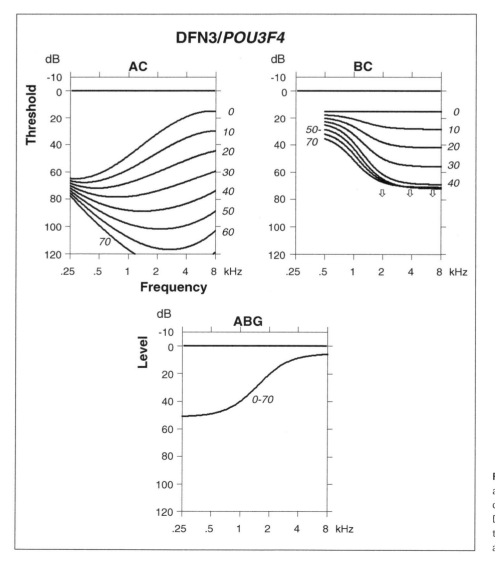

Figure 13.3 Thresholds (i.e., age-related threshold audiograms) for various ages in decade steps for air conduction (AC), bone conduction (BC), and ABG in DFN3 (stapes gusher). Note that ABG is stationary throughout life (0–70 years). *Abbreviation*: ABG, air-bone gap. *Source*: Modified from Ref. 64.

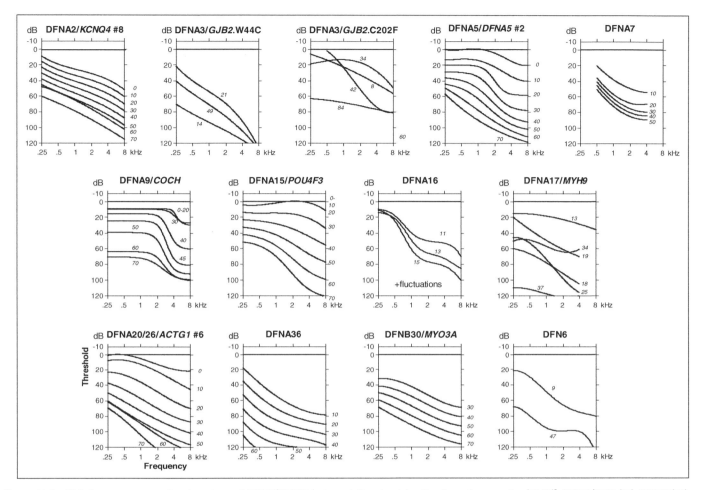

Figure 13.4 High-frequency progressive phenotypes of DFNA2/KCNQ4 (only mutations involving the channel pore region (69,70)], DFNA3/GJB2 (71), DFNA5 (72), DFNA7 (*Source*: Modified from Ref. 8, see that reference and present text for original data sources), DFNA9 (73), DFNA15 (74), DFNA16, and DFNA17 (*Source*: Modified from Ref. 8), DFNA20/26 (sources specified in text), DFNA36 (75), DFNB30 (76), and DFN6 (77). The symbol # followed by a number labels mean age-related typical audiograms covering the specified number of different traits or families.

with "presbyacusis" (data not shown). Stability is the rule for autosomal-recessive traits. Some high-frequency downsloping audiometric configurations can be also interpreted as representing a milder variant of the residual-hearing type.

DFNA2

DFNA2 typically shows a progressive high-frequency audiometric configuration (Fig. 13.4) with, presumably, congenital onset and ATD in the range of 0.7 to 1 dB, regardless of whether it is caused by *KCNQ4* mutations in the channel pore region (4,69,70,78–84), *GJB3* mutations (85), or mutations in as yet unidentified genes at the DFNA2 locus (4,86–88). The traits with genes that have not yet been identified have been reported to have onset ages in the first or second decade of life. A different phenotype was found in a Belgian DFNA2/KCNQ4 trait with a truncating frameshift mutation (Fs71) affecting the first intracellular domain of the *KCNQ4*-related voltage-gated K^{+} channel: only the thresholds for the high frequencies

(>1 kHz) were increased, which produced a much steeper downsloping configuration than in the other DFNA2/KCNQ4 traits (69).

In the present type of progressive SNHI, the lower and the speech frequencies can be relatively spared for many years (Fig. 13.4) and therefore even congenital or early-childhood onset does not necessarily interfere with the normal development of speech and language skills. Bom et al. (89) found remarkably good speech recognition scores in DFNA2 patients, even at advanced ages and levels of hearing impairment.

DFNA3

The report by Grifa et al. (90) only hints at variable audiometric configurations in this *GJB6*-linked SNHI condition. Denoyelle et al. (71,91) indicated a high-frequency to a fairly flat configuration (Fig. 13.4) with stable hearing. Onset was at an age less than four years or in the second decade of life, depending on the *GJB2* mutation (W44C or C202F).

DFNA5

Patients with DFNA5 identified so far show a progressive high-frequency audiometric configuration (Fig. 13.4) with early-childhood to early-adolescent onset and most rapid progression in the first or second decade of life. The review by Kunst et al. (4) reproduces audiometric profiles typical of the original Dutch family (see their refs). Part of this family was reanalysed by De Leenheer et al. (92). Speech recognition remained relatively good (93). A second Dutch family was identified by Bischoff et al. (72). Those authors found that speech recognition in the second family was somewhat better than in the original family, which perhaps related to the slightly more favourable hearing thresholds. A third, Chinese family was recently identified with fairly similar features (94).

DFNA7

This results in a SNHI with a progressive high-frequency configuration (Fig. 13.4) and postlingual (first-decade) onset was described by Fagerheim et al. (95) and Elverland et al. (96) and reviewed by Tranebjærg et al. (97).

DFNA8/12 (1 Trait)

Alloisio et al. (98) described a condition with prelingual onset and a progressive high-frequency configuration at mild-to-moderate threshold levels. The ATD was 0.7 dB at 0.5 to 4 kHz, which, presumably indicates some progression beyond "presbyacusis." A mutation was found in the zonadhesin-like domain of *TECTA*.

DFNA9

All the reported patients show progressive high-frequency SNHI (Fig. 13.4) with midlife onset or, in one American family, onset in the second-to-third decade of life (99,100). Vestibular dysfunction also develops gradually (73) and eventually leads to vestibular areflexia. Hearing deteriorates over a few decades, with maximum ATD values of 2 to 7 dB (101) or even higher in some individual cases, eventually leading to residual-hearing or (sub)residual-hearing threshold levels (102,103). The age-related typical audiograms shown in Figure 13.4 are compatible with an average ATD of 2 to 3 dB. Speech recognition is relatively poor (100), showing features similar to "presbyacusis" that already occur at a younger-than-usual age (89).

DFNA15–17

DFNA15 as described by Frydman et al. (104) showed a progressive high-frequency pattern of hearing impairment (Fig. 13.4) with postlingual onset. Progression beyond "presbyacusis" occurred with ATD values of between 1.1 dB at 0.25 to 1 kHz and 2.1 dB at 2 to 4 kHz (74). The age of onset was estimated at 15 to 25 years using fitting methods in cross-sectional data analysis. Speech recognition continued to be relatively good even at the higher threshold levels (104). Fukushima et al. (105) described a DFNA16 trait with early onset and a high-frequency pattern of hearing impairment with rapid progression (Fig. 13.4) in the first decades of life. A distinctive feature was that large threshold fluctuations occurred that appeared to respond favourably to steroid treatment.

Lalwani et al. (106,107) reported a DFNA17 trait with early onset that showed progressive high-frequency hearing impairment features (Fig. 13.4). Individual longitudinal analyses revealed ATD values of up to about 3 dB. Speech-recognition scores were relatively good, even in members of the family who had substantial SNHI.

DFNA20/26

DFNA20/26 traits show progressive high-frequency audiometric configurations (Fig. 13.4), with postlingual onset varying between childhood and late adolescence (108–112). Teig (113) described a family for whom linkage to the DFNA20/26 locus was recently confirmed and an *ACTG1* mutation was identified (L Tranebjærg, personal communication). Kemperman et al. (112) reported relatively good speech-recognition scores at sound levels of less than 100 dB HL.

Other DFNA loci

SNHI traits with postlingual onset showing progressive high-frequency configurations have been reported with linkage to DFNA30 (114) in which the onset age was relatively late (10–40 years) and to DFNA36. The latter showed SNHI with postlingual onset in the first decade and a high degree of progression (Fig. 13.4), with ATD values in the range of 5 to 8 dB at increasing audio frequencies (75). It should be noted that these high ATD values related to the initial stage of deterioration. Subsequently, the rate of deterioration decreased. The age-related typical audiograms based on threshold data from their last visit (Fig. 13.4) reflect much lower ATD values of around 1 dB. DFNA42 (115), DFNA47 (116), and DFNA48 (117) also showed postlingual onset in the first-to-third decade of life and similar audiometric profiles; progression was fairly slow in patients with DFNA48. Presumably "nonprogressive" types of SNHI, i.e., SNHI that did not appear to show progression beyond "presbyacusis," were reported for DFNA23 (118), which also showed a conductive hearing loss, nor for DFNA24 (119). The last two conditions were of prelingual onset.

DFNB loci

Houseman et al. (45) described two sibs with an M34T/M34T *GJB2* genotype (DFNB1) with a high-frequency audiometric configuration with moderate-to-severe threshold levels. We presume that this type of SNHI is stable. Ahmed et al. (120) described a DFNB8/10 trait with congenital SNHI and a stable high-frequency audiometric configuration. Villamar et al. (121) described a DFNB16 trait with early childhood onset showing a high-frequency configuration with stable thresholds at moderate-to-severe levels. Walsh et al. (76) described a DFNB30 trait (Fig. 13.4) with postlingual (fairly late and variable) onset SNHI showing a progressive, gently to more steeply downsloping audiometric configuration (Fig. 13.4). Substantial progression in SNHI is exceptional for autosomal-recessive hearing impairment disorders. We estimated the ATD to be approximately 1.2 dB at 0.5 to 8 kHz. Progression was certainly beyond "presbyacusis" at the lower frequencies.

DFN6

One reported DFN6 family showed SNHI with postlingual onset in the first decade of life and a progressive high-frequency type of audiometric configuration (Fig. 13.4) (77). We estimated an ATD of about 1 dB from the two audiograms depicted by del Castillo et al. (77).

Flat-to-gently downsloping audiometric configuration

This category includes stable as well as progressive, flat-to-gently downsloping phenotypes (Fig. 13.5). In the following, the majority of the traits show a progressive phenotype. A stable audiometric configuration is shown by the exceptionally mild DFNB1 phenotypes encountered in some patients having DFNB1 with biallelic nontruncating mutations in *GJB2* (see above).

DFNA loci

DFNA4 shows postlingual progressive, flat-to-gently downsloping audiometric configurations as illustrated in Figure 13.5 (122,123). Pusch et al. (124) reported thresholds at moderate-to-severe levels (mean 75 dB) and an ATD of approximately 0.5 dB, which is presumably compatible with normal "presbyacusis" (Fig. 13.5). Although one of the patients described by McGuirt et al. (123)

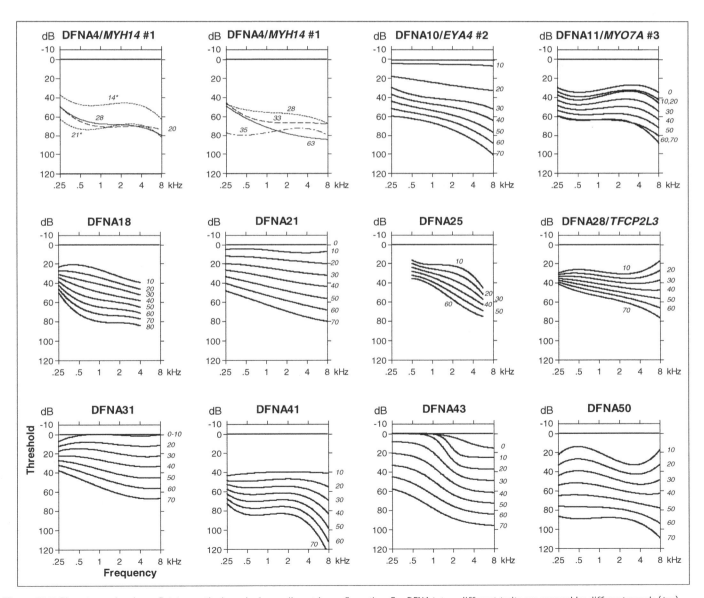

Figure 13.5 Phenotypes showing a flat-to-gently downsloping audiometric configuration. For DFNA4, two different traits are covered by different panels (*top*). *Source*: Trait 1, data from Refs. 122, 123; trait 2, from Ref. 124; asterisks indicate longitudinal data (indicating ATD 3–4dB). Other data or modified figures from: DFNA10, Ref. 9; DFNA11, Refs. 125–127, Bischoff et al. (unpublished data); DFNA18, Ref. 128; DFNA21, Ref. 129; DFNA25, Ref. 130; DFNA28, Ref. 131; DFNA31, Ref. 132; DFNA41, Ref. 133; DFNA43, Ref. 134; and DFNA50, Ref. 135.

was measured twice and the ATD that can be derived from these data is 3 to 4 dB, the ensemble of available threshold data suggests only limited progression given the corresponding ages (Fig. 13.5). The DFNA8/12 trait described by Pfister et al. (136) is exceptional among traits linked to locus DFNA8/12 because it showed a flat-to-gently downsloping hearing impairment rather than a mid-frequency configuration and was progressive with an ATD of about 0.4 dB. The reported DFNA10 patients show postlingual hearing impairments of variable onset within the first four decades of life and a progressive, flat-to-gently downsloping configuration (Fig. 13.5) with an ATD of approximately 0.8 dB (pooled frequencies) (137,138) to 1.1 dB (0.5–4 kHz) (139). McGuirt et al. (123) showed an example of one member of the original DFNA10 family, whose ATD may have been as high as 4 dB in the higher frequency range. Speech recognition was relatively good in the American family according to the phoneme scores analysed by De Leenheer et al. (137).

Fairly similar phenotypes (Fig. 13.5) with postlingual onset in the first two decades of life have been reported for DFNA11 (125–127,140) (Bischoff et al., unpublished data), DFNA18 (128), DFNA21 (129), DFNA25 (130), DFNA28 (131), and DFNA31, which had initially been linked to DFNA13 (Fig. 13.5) (132,141), DFNA41 (133), DFNA43 (134), and DFNA50 (135).

It can be appreciated from Figure 13.5 that some traits, for example, those linked to DFNA25 and DFNA43, showed high-frequency characteristics only at relatively young ages. Other SNHI traits, such as those linked to DFNA10, DFNA18, DFNA28, and DFNA41, tended to develop more high-frequency impairments with increasing age. Progression indicated ATD values of between 0.6 dB for DFNA11 (125,140) and DFNA28 (131) and 1.1 to 1.5 dB for DFNA31 (132) and DFNA50 (135). In DFNA21 (Fig. 13.5), the ATD is 0.7 to 1.1 dB from the low to the high frequencies (129). The subjective age of onset was reported to be in the second decade of life for DFNA41 and DFNA50. For the DFNA21 trait studied by Kunst et al. (129), the subjective age of onset reported by the affected family members varied from childhood to late adolescence and even later. However, the available threshold data allowed for backward extrapolation in linear regression analyses that produced consistent estimates of onset age at about three to five years for all frequencies. Backward extrapolation in cross-sectional linear regression analysis produced estimates of onset ages for the DFNA31 trait of between 5 years (0.25–0.5 kHz) and 12 years (2–8 kHz) (132). Such apparently discrepant findings may be typical of slow postnatal progression of the SNHI. A distinctive feature of DFNA11 is progressive vestibular dysfunction, eventually leading to vestibular areflexia (125,126,140).

OTSC2, 5

At the GENDEAF meeting in Caserta, March 2005, Declau presented a paper specifying a fairly flat audiometric configuration for OTSC2, including the ABG. In a family with OTSC5, which we recently studied, there were fairly similar findings (142). Given the natural history of otosclerosis, the clinical picture must include progression over at least a few years prior to surgery.

DFNB loci

Several of the DFNB1 genotypes with relatively mild SNHI show thresholds at moderate-to-severe levels with a relatively flat audiometric configuration (Fig. 13.2). One study on a DFNB13 trait specified a relatively flat configuration with moderate threshold levels at young ages, probably preceding progression (22).

Y-linked locus

A SNHI trait in a Chinese family showed Y-linked inheritance with onset in childhood to late adolescence and a progressive, flat-to-gently downsloping audiometric configuration. Threshold levels were mild to severe, but there was no profound hearing impairment (143). There was no significant age-related increase in threshold between 9 and 71 years of age. The binaural mean pure tone audiogram averaged over all frequencies was 71 dB. The precise audiometric configuration was not clearly described.

Mid-frequency or U-shaped audiometric configuration

This category includes stable as well as progressive mid-frequency configurations (Fig. 13.6). This phenotype is only encountered among autosomal-dominant traits, although one exceptional

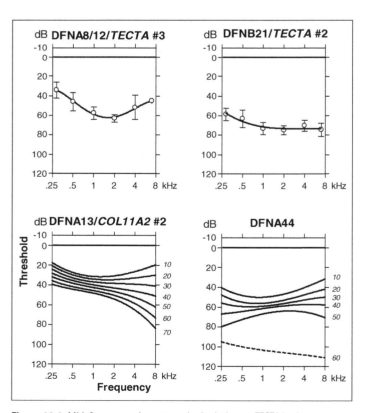

Figure 13.6 Mid-frequency phenotypes. Loci relating to *TECTA* in the top row. The top row panels show the mean ± 1 intertrait SD. The dotted line in the panel for DFNA44 highlights the fact that this threshold line mainly relates to one, possibly exceptional, patient who showed a remarkably unfavourable threshold at an advanced age and therefore should be regarded with reservation. *Source*: Data or modified figures from: DFNA8/12, Refs. 144–146; DFNB21, Ref. 147; DFNA13, Refs. 148–150; and DFNA44, Ref. 151.

X-linked trait has been described as showing mid-frequency–like features. In some of the autosomal-dominant traits, progression may be compatible with "presbyacusis," but there are also traits that show greater progression.

DFNA loci

The majority of the *TECTA*-based traits linked to DFNA8/12 show prelingual onset of SNHI with a stable mid-frequency (sometimes more low-frequency) audiometric configuration (Fig. 13.6) (144–146,152). Almost all of the other autosomal dominant traits with the mid-frequency configuration show progression. This includes the DFNA8/12 trait described by Moreno Pelayo et al. (153) with an ATD of 0.4 dB at 0.5 to 2 kHz, the reported DFNA13 traits (Fig. 13.6) (123,148–150), the DFNA44 trait described by Modamio-Høybjør et al. (Fig. 13.6) (151), and the DFNA49 trait described by Moreno Pelayo et al. (154) that may also have shown some low-frequency characteristics. Some traits showed substantial progression. DFNA44 had an ATD of 1.1 to 1.2 dB and DFNA49 had an ATD of 0.7 dB at all frequencies. However, the DFNA13 trait underlying the report by McGuirt et al. (123) did not show significant progression beyond "presbyacusis." Given the particular threshold configuration and limited degree of SNHI, the normal development of speech and language skills in patients having SNHI linked to DFNA13 does not exclude the possibility of prelingual or congenital onset. One DFNA13 trait studied by De Leenheer et al. (155) using special audiological tests indicated that DFNA13 represents a particular type of intracochlear conductive hearing impairment. Speech recognition was found to be relatively good. The latter finding was also reported for DFNA8/12 by Kirschhofer et al. (144).

DFNB21

The study by Naz et al. (Fig. 13.6) (147) indicates a stable, flat-to-gently downsloping configuration of prelingual SNHI at moderate-to-severe levels for a DFNB21 trait (Fig. 13.6). Although the audiometric configuration could be classified as flat-to-gently downsloping, this SNHI trait is classified here with the mid-frequency traits DFNA8/12 that are also caused by *TECTA* mutations. Minor differences between these

TECTA-based traits seem to relate to the degree of hearing impairment, especially at the high frequencies (Fig. 13.6).

DFN2?

Manolis et al. (Fig. 13.7) (157) described an exceptional trait with presumed linkage to DFN2, which showed congenital SNHI with a progressive low- to mid-frequency audiometric configuration.

Low-frequency audiometric configuration

This category includes stable and progressive low-frequency, i.e., upsloping configurations. This phenotype is almost exclusively encountered among autosomal-dominant traits. Some of the traits have stable hearing and, in those showing progression, in some instances this may be compatible with "presbyacusis."

DFNA loci

The only trait linked to DFNA1 showed early onset of SNHI with a low-frequency configuration with rapid progression (158–160). The age-related typical audiograms shown in Figure 13.7 are compatible with an ATD of 3 to 5 dB. Some of the families linked to the DFNA6/14/38 locus showed an apparently stable low-frequency configuration (4,161), i.e., with progression presumably not beyond "presbyacusis" (18, 162–165). This may also apply to the two traits reported very recently by Gürtler et al. (166). The other DFNA6/14/38 traits (Fig. 13.7), however, showed substantial progression beyond "presbyacusis" (167–170). The traits described by Bom et al. (171) showed ATD values of 0.5 to 1.3 dB at increasing frequencies. Family A described by Bille et al. (167) showed a median ATD of 1.1 dB at 2 to 4 kHz in their individual longitudinal analyses. One of the two families described by Pennings et al. (172) showed no significant progression; the other showed a pooled ATD of 1 dB. The latter study also demonstrated relatively good speech-recognition scores. The onset of hearing impairment in all these traits varied between possibly congenital or somewhere in early childhood and somewhere in the first three decades of life. DFNA54, described by Gürtler et al. (Fig. 13.7) (156), represents the third locus for an autosomal-dominant SNHI that is associated with a low-frequency configuration. It showed relatively late onset (5–40 years) and progression beyond "presbyacusis."

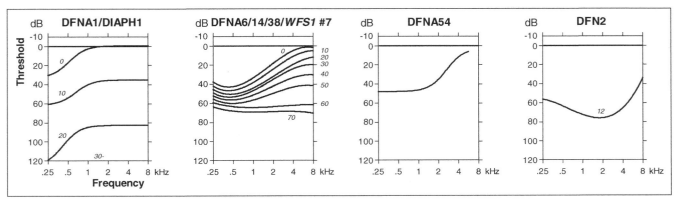

Figure 13.7 Low-frequency progressive phenotypes. *Source*: Data or modified figures from: DFNA1, Ref. 9; DFNA6/14/38, see text; DFNA54, Ref. 156; the subject and age are not specified; and DFN2, Ref. 157.

DFN2?

The exceptional (presumable) DFN2 family reported on by Manolis et al. (Fig. 13.7) (157) can be also mentioned in this category because of its low-frequency–like features.

Discussion

The purposes of this review are several

Facilitating the differential diagnosis, counselling, and guidance for genotyping efforts

As regards the differential diagnosis, it needs to be emphasised that different genotypes may show fairly similar phenotypes. The classification of phenotypes by audiometric configuration seemed to do reasonably well at first sight. From Figures 13.4 to 13.7 it would seem that the differences in audiometric profile between these figures are greater than within these figures. Maximum downward slopes in the audiogram are above 10 dB/octave in high-frequency downsloping configurations (Fig. 13.4) and below 10 dB/octave, with few exceptions in flat-to-gently downsloping configurations (Fig. 13.5). The exceptions in Figure 5 are found in the panels for DFNA41 and DFNA43. Although the average slope in the decade threshold lines is below 10 dB/octave, "local" slopes of $\gg$ 10 dB/octave can be seen in the high frequencies at advanced ages in DFNA41 and in DFNA43 in the mid-frequencies in midlife. Accentuated local slope in the audiogram configuration is also found in high-frequency downsloping configurations (Fig. 13.4). The feature of steepest slope in the mid-frequency range is also found in DFNA5 in late adolescence and in DFNA15 at advanced ages. A midlife-associated steepest slope in the audiogram is found in DFNA9 in the 2 to 4 kHz range. The steepest slopes are found in the low-frequency range in DFNA36 throughout life and in DFNA20/26 at advanced ages (Fig. 13.4).

Despite this type of detailed observations that can be made regarding possibly distinctive features, the differential diagnosis of phenotypes is often quite problematic. We used the threshold features array (TFA) as previously defined (7) in an attempt to find out the apparent similarities or dissimilarities of those traits for which sufficient reliable age-related threshold audiogram data were available in a quantified, objective way. It appeared that regrouping of phenotypes within and between the four main classes pertaining to Figures 13.4 to 13.7 is certainly possible (see sections on TFA below).

The onset age does not generally contribute to the differential diagnosis, apart from the differential diagnosis between DFNA5 (onset in early childhood to early adolescence) and DFNA9 (midlife onset). Early onset with rapid progression may be a useful distinctive feature (see DFNB4/PDS in Fig. 13.1, DFNA1 in Fig. 13.7, and DFNA16, DFNA17, DFNA36, and DFN6 in Fig. 13.4). Progression by itself can be an important item. Extremely rapid deterioration, showing up in the

age-related threshold audiograms as a great distance between consecutive (decade) threshold lines, can be seen in DFNA1 (Fig. 13.7). Rapid initial deterioration with a gradually decreasing rate of deterioration, i.e., nonlinear progression that is associated with nonequidistant (decade) threshold lines in the age-related threshold audiograms, can be noted in traits linked to DFNB4/PDS (Fig. 13.1), DFNA5 and DFNA9 (Fig. 13.4), and DFNA10 (Fig. 13.5).

The occurrence of substantial fluctuations in threshold (DFNB4/PDS and DFNA16) is another distinctive feature of importance. This also holds for vestibular failure (DFNB4/PDS, DFNA9/COCH, DFNA11/MYO7A, and DFN3/POU3F4).

As regards the possible value that careful phenotyping may have for the guidance of genotyping efforts, we and others have already had favourable experiences with some of the more remarkable traits. Congenital residual hearing on a possibly autosomal-recessive basis should be always tested for DFNB1. DFNA2-linked traits are fairly easy to recognise (Fig. 13.4). Although, as stipulated here, there are several traits with fairly similar phenotypes, the relatively high prevalence of DFNA2-linked traits favours guidance in this case (70). This also applies to traits with SNHI caused by WFS1 mutations, whose phenotype is even more easily recognised [DFNA6/14/38, see Fig. 13.7 and the editorial by Smith and Huygen (9)]. The combination of the features of midlife onset and progressive deterioration in hearing and vestibular function is so typical that DFNA9/COCH can be easily recognised (101); in The Netherlands and Belgium (Flanders), the relative prevalence of traits linked to DFNA9 is relatively high. For other traits, especially the less typical or prevalent traits, probably the best strategy for guided phenotyping is to screen all the loci that are associated with possibly similar phenotypes and extend the list of loci to be checked, anyway, if the first search is negative.

Thus, it would seem that, in general, phenotyping does not contribute very much to genotyping efforts in terms of guidance, anyway. Genotyping will always continue to be necessary. Sometimes, however, careful phenotyping does contribute to the guidance of genotyping to the effect that the latter can be limited and considerable time, efforts, and costs can be saved (see the last section below).

Facilitating the consideration of treatment opportunities

It is important to realise in which types of genetic hearing impairment disorder the affected subjects are likely to have only residual hearing. In that case, cochlear implantation is a treatment option. In other types of hearing impairment, i.e., those not associated with residual hearing, fitting a (multiband) hearing aid may be a reasonable option. Given the sometimes remarkably mild types of hearing impairment of DFNB1 phenotypes involving nontruncating GJB2 mutations (Fig. 13.2), it is important to recognise the relatively good opportunities for fitting hearing aids in such cases, where a typical residual-hearing type of SNHI might have been expected to develop. The most important distinctive feature of DFN3 is the ABG and it is important to recognise this phenotype feature because stapes surgery should be avoided because of the risk of perilymphatic gusher. The bone conduction level may allow for effective amplification (Fig. 13.3). An important item for counselling in the slowly progressive types of hearing impairment is that auditory communication will become more difficult from around midlife onward. Although in such cases, the degree of hearing impairment may still be limited at more advanced ages (Fig. 13.5) and aided hearing certainly is a realistic option, the choice of profession made decades before midlife can be critical.

Updating and using the threshold feature array (TFA)

Using the previously described method (7) that bears on the TFA, we updated and extended the previously designed table with TFA data (Table 13.1). We have outlined the purpose of such data and the associated method in the previous paper. Briefly, they can be used to test whether the age-related threshold audiograms and the derived TFA for a given novel trait are similar or dissimilar to previously reported ones (7,70). Testing between complete TFAs derived for the newly established age-related threshold audiograms shown in the present paper was performed as previously outlined using the chi-square test. Table 13.2 shows the result of these tests in the form of S values equalling the P values attached to the corresponding chi-square tests for pairwise comparisons. We replaced the symbol P, for probability, by the symbol S for similarity, because the TFAs do not cover real sampled data. The consecutively sampled values predicted by regression do not pertain directly to the original data points and are unlikely to be stochastically independent. $S = 1$ indicates complete similarity (=identity), whereas $S = 0$

Table 13.1 Threshold feature arrays[a] for suitable loci data that can be used in conventional chi-square tests[b]

Locus, # traits	Cell a	Cell b	Cell c	Cell d	Cell e	Cell f	Cell g	Cell h	Cell i
DFNA2 #8	9	3	1	7	11	8	0	2	7
DFNA5 #2	9	6	3	7	6	5	0	4	8
DFNA6/14/ 38 #7	1	6	10	15	10	6	0	0	0
DFNA9	11	11	8	5	4	2	0	1	6
DFNA10 #2	9	6	6	7	10	7	0	0	3
DFNA11 #3	5	5	4	11	11	10	0	0	2
DFNA13 #2	14	9	7	2	7	8	0	0	1
DFNA15	12	10	8	4	5	4	0	1	4
DFNA18	10	5	–	6	11	–	0	0	–
DFNA20/ 26 #6	7	5	3	8	4	4	1	7	9
DFNA21	12	10	9	4	6	6	0	0	1
DFNA25	–	10	–	–	6	–	–	0	–
DFNA28	12	8	7	4	8	9	0	0	0
DFNA31	15	11	10	1	5	6	0	0	0
DFNA36	5	–	–	4	–	–	7	10	12
DFNA41	3	2	3	12	11	7	1	3	6
DFNA43	12	8	6	4	7	6	0	1	4
DFNA50	7	5	5	7	9	7	2	2	4

[a]Cell count for cells a–i as defined by Huygen et al. (7).
[b]Cells a,b,c pertain to 0–39 dB and 0.25–0.5 kHz, 1–2 kHz, and 4–8 kHz, respectively; cells d,e,f pertain to 40–79 dB and these grouped frequencies; cells g,h,i pertain to 80 dB and over and these grouped frequencies. Averages (**bold**) pertain to norm (*multitrait*) values. It should be noted that a conventional chi-square test can be used for testing across separate arrays (single trait or average), but that a chi-square test for goodness of fit should be used if (average) norm values are applied as representing the expected values for comparison with a single trait. Prior to performing a conventional chi-square test on a given contingency table that can be constructed by combining any arrays, cells should be combined where necessary according to general rules described for chi-square tests in most textbooks on statistics.

Table 13.2 S (similarity) values[a]

Locus	DFNA2	DFNA5	DFNA6/14/38	DFNA9	DFNA10	DFNA11	DFNA13	DFNA15	DFNA20/26	DFNA21	DFNA28	DFNA31	DFNA41	DFNA43
DFNA5	0.48													
DFNA6/14/38	<0.0001	0.0002												
DFNA9	0.0037	0.21	0.0001											
DFNA10	0.21	0.21	0.024	0.11										
DFNA11	0.12	0.031	0.14	0.0016	0.66									
DFNA13	0.0025	0.0071	0.0003	0.055	0.30	0.016								
DFNA15	0.011	0.20	0.0004	0.94	0.37	0.0093	0.39							
DFNA20/26	0.12	0.88	<0.0001	0.054	0.014	0.0023	0.0001	0.0022						
DFNA21	0.0018	0.014	0.0030	0.22	0.43	0.028	0.92	0.67	0.0005					
DFNA28	0.0042	0.0064	0.0055	0.020	0.41	0.070	0.85	0.16	0.0001	0.80				
DFNA31	<0.0001	0.0003	<0.0001	0.029	0.022	0.0003	0.75	0.17	<0.0001	0.65	.49			
DFNA41	0.47	0.19	0.0041	0.0005	0.051	0.18	<0.0001	0.0007	0.11	<0.0001	0.0001	.11		
DFNA43	0.10	0.37	0.0007	0.54	0.78	0.064	0.56	0.94	0.034	0.62	.34	.0060	.42	
DFNA50	0.68	0.84	0.0046	0.12	0.74	0.35	0.034	0.22	0.28	.05+	.043	.34	.0010	.58

[a]For pairwise comparison of the threshold features arrays shown in Table 13.1 resulting from chi-square test between testable traits linked to loci for nonsyndromal hearing impairment. S equals P (probability) for the chi-square test but is no probability measure (see text).

Table 13.3 Decision table indicating which loci should be genetically tested

Locus	DFNA2	DFNA5	DFNA6/14/38	DFNA9	DFNA10	DFNA11	DFNA13	DFNA15	DFNA20/26	DFNA21	DFNA28	DFNA31	DFNA41	DFNA43	DFNA50
DFNA2	test	test													test
DFNA5	test	test							test						test
DFNA6/14/38				test											
DFNA9				test	test		test	test		test				test	
DFNA10	test	test		test	test	Test	test	test		test	test			test	test
DFNA11					test	Test									
DFNA13				test	test		test	test		test	test	test		test	
DFNA15				test	test		test	test		test	test	test		test	
DFNA 20/26		test							test						test
DFNA21				test	test		test	test		test	test	test		test	
DFNA28							test	test		test	test	test		test	
DFNA31							test	test		test	test	test		test	
DFNA41													test		
DFNA43				test	test		test	test		test	test	test		test	test
DFNA50	test	test			test				test					test	test

When a given phenotype (complete age-related threshold audiograms) included in the row title looks like the age-related threshold audiogram for the locus in the column title, initial testing might be limited to the indicated loci.

indicates no similarity at all. All of the present traits whose audiometric profiles are shown in Figures 13.4 to 13.7, for which sufficient testable age-related threshold audiogram data could be obtained are included in this table, with no regard for their tentative classification into the corresponding main phenotypes.

As the S values in Table 13.2 were intended to assist in visual pairwise comparison between the (complete) age-related threshold audiograms of different loci, we performed such a visual comparison for all complete age-related threshold audiograms included in Figures 13.4 to 13.7 in descending order of the corresponding S value. Starting from the highest S value involving a given locus, we looked at the successive other loci. For DFNA11 (age-related threshold audiograms in Fig. 13.5), for example, the highest S value in Table 13.2 is 0.66, which is attached to the comparison with DFNA10 (Fig. 13.5); the next S value involving DFNA11 is 0.35, attached to the comparison with DFNA50 (Fig.13. 5). Looking at the age-related threshold audiograms of the corresponding pairs of loci, we concluded that the age-related threshold audiograms of DFNA11 and DFNA10 might be visually confused, but the age-related threshold audiograms of DFNA11 and DFNA50 would not seem likely to be confused. After having made all the visual comparisons by all the available complete age-related threshold audiograms, we concluded that loci, whose TFAs in pairwise comparison (chi-square test) produce an S value of 0.6 or higher, would seem fairly likely to be visually confused. Remarkably, there are only two loci whose age-related threshold audiograms are unlikely to be visually confused with the age-related threshold audiograms for any other loci: DFNA6/14/38 (Fig. 13.7) and DFNA41 (Fig. 13.5). There are four loci (DFNA2, DFNA9, DFNA11, and DFNA20/26) whose age-related threshold audiograms can be fairly easily confused with the age-related threshold audiograms of one different locus each (Table 13.2). The age-related threshold audiograms of three loci (DFNA5, DFNA28, and DFNA31) can be fairly easily confused with the age-related threshold audiograms of two different loci each, whereas the age-related threshold audiograms of five loci (DFNA10, DFNA13, DFNA15, DFNA43, and DFNA50) could be confused with the age-related threshold audiograms of three loci each. There is one locus, DFNA21 (Fig. 13.5), whose age-related threshold audiograms could be confused with the age-related threshold audiograms of five other loci (DFNA13 in Fig. 13.6, DFNA15 in Fig. 13.4, DFNA28, DFNA31, and DFNA43 in Fig. 13.5). It shows that 8 of the 15 S values above 0.6 in Table 13.2 pertain to pairwise comparisons involving age-related threshold audiograms included in the same figure (Fig. 13.4, 13.5, or 13.6) and 7 S values above 0.6 pertain to comparisons involving age-related threshold audiograms included in different figures (Fig. 13.4, 13.5, or 13.6). This kind of observation demonstrates that our assignment of loci to the main tentative phenotypes for which Figures 13.4 to 13.7 were designed must have been fairly arbitrary. It is indeed possible to group fairly similar age-related threshold audiograms in a number of different clusters that might represent separate phenotypical entities. In order to attempt forming tentative phenotype clusters, we started from the grouped loci specified above and checked whether the attached S value for the group (=P value in simultaneous chi-square test) was 0.6 or higher. This limiting value was chosen because we presume that a value of S = 0.6 attached to simultaneous comparison between TFAs (n > 2) also corresponds to age-related threshold audiograms that might be fairly easily confused on visual inspection. If the tentative cluster had S < 0.6, we searched for the locus or loci that could best be skipped from the cluster in order to obtain S > 0.6. If the tentative cluster had S > 0.6, it was checked whether the cluster could be extended with additional loci while maintaining the condition of S > 0.6. Small tentative clusters were neglected if they were found to form part of any larger tentative cluster(s). The clusters thus obtained were: (A), DFNA6/14/38; (B), DFNA41; (C), DFNA10 and 11; (D), DFNA5, 20/26 and 50; (E), DFNA10, 43 and 50; (F), DFNA13, 21, 28, and 31; (G), DFNA2, 5, 10, and 50; (H), DFNA9, 10, 13, 15, 21, and 43; and (I), DFNA13, 15, 21, 28, 31, and 43. It is of note that DFNA11 initially formed part of a former version of cluster E (with S = 0.47) that is formed by (Table 13.2) starting from DFNA10 but had to be skipped in order to obtain S > 0.6 for the final cluster (S = 0.81). Cluster H was obtained by starting from DFNA15 by combining all the loci whose TFA in pairwise comparison with the TFA for DFNA15 had S > 0.6 (Table 13.2) and then also add the TFAs for DFNA10 and DFNA13 by trial and error to obtain S = 0.62 for the final cluster.

Which loci should be tested for a given new trait?
When complete age-related threshold audiograms have been derived for a newly outlined SNHI trait, Figures 13.4 to 13.7 should be scanned to see what it looks like. If it looks like any of the complete age-related threshold audiograms in these figures, the scheme indicated in Table 13.3 might be followed.

This scheme has been obtained by looking up in which of the above described clusters the look-alike age-related threshold audiograms are included and then specify all the other loci included in these clusters. If newly derived age-related threshold audiograms look most similar to those of the incomplete age-related threshold audiograms included in Figures 13.4 to 13.7, the next most similar complete age-related threshold audiograms should be pinpointed to apply the scheme. Table 13.3 indicates that initial testing of a limited number of loci (n = 1–9) might be sufficient. If all the initial tests are negative, additional loci could be tested, even if the present paper indicates that they seem to be unlikely to be associated with fairly similar phenotypes.

Acknowledgements

We wish to thank Dr. H. Kremer for commenting on the manuscript.

References

1. Konigsmark BW, Gorlin RJ. Genetic and Metabolic Deafness. Philadelphia: Saunders Co., 1976.

2. Toriello HV, Reardon W, Gorlin RJ. Hereditary Hearing Loss and Its Syndromes. Oxford Monographs on Medical Genetics no. 50. Oxford: Oxford University Press, 2004.

3. Van Camp G, Smith RJH. Hereditary Hearing Loss Homepage. http://dnalab-www.uia.ac.be/dnalab/hhh/. Accessed May 2005.

4. Kunst HPM, Marres HAM, Van Camp G, et al. Non-syndromic autosomal dominant sensorineural hearing loss: a new field of research. Clin Otolaryngol 1998; 23:9–17.

5. Bom SJH, Kunst HPM, Huygen PLM, et al. Non-syndromal autosomal dominant hearing impairment: ongoing phenotypical characterization of genotypes. Br J Audiol 1999; 33:335–348.

6. Huygen PLM, Bom SJH, Van Camp G, et al. Clinical presentation of the DFNA loci where causative genes have not yet been cloned. DFNA4, DFNA6/14, DFNA7, DFNA16, DFNA20 and DFNA21. In: Cremers CWRJ, Smith RJH, eds. Genetic Hearing Impairment. Its Clinical Presentations. Adv Otorhinolaryngol Basel: Karger; 2002; 61:98–106.

7. Huygen PLM, Pennings RJE, Cremers CWRJ. Characterizing and distinguishing progressive phenotypes in nonsyndromic autosomal dominant hearing impairment. Audiol Med 2003; 1:37–46.

8. Pennings RJE, Huygen PLM, Van Camp G, et al. A review of progressive phenotypes in nonsyndromic autosomal dominant hearing impairment. Audiol Med 2003; 1:47–55.

9. Smith RJH, Huygen PLM. Making sense of nonsyndromic deafness. Arch Otolaryngol Head Neck Surg 2003; 129:405–406.

10. Mazzoli M, Van Camp G, Newton V, et al. Recommendations for the description of genetic and audiological data for families with nonsyndromic hereditary hearing impairment. Hereditary Hearing Loss Homepage, http://dnalab-www.uia.ac.be/dnalab/hhh/.

11. International Organization for Standardization. ISO 7029. Acoustics: Threshold of Hearing by Air Conduction as a Function of Age and Sex for Otologically Normal Persons. Geneva, Switzerland: International Organization for Standardization, 1984.

12. Melchionda S, Ahituv N, Bisceglia L, et al. MYO6, the human homologue of the gene responsible for deafness in Snell's waltzer mice, is mutated in autosomal dominant nonsyndromic hearing loss. Am J Hum Genet 2001; 69:635–640.

13. Kim TB, Isaacson B, Sivakumaran TA, et al. A gene responsible for autosomal dominant auditory neuropathy (AUNA1) maps to 13q14–21. J Med Genet 2004; 41:872–876.

14. Shallop JK, Peterson A, Facer GW, et al. Cochlear implants in five cases of auditory neuropathy: postoperative findings and progress. Laryngoscope 2001; 111:555–562.

15. Mason JC, De Michele A, Stevens C, et al. Cochlear implantation in patients with auditory neuropathy of varied etiologies. Laryngoscope 2003; 113:45–49.

16. Starr A, Isaacson B, Michalewski HJ, et al. A dominantly inherited progressive deafness affecting distal auditory nerve and hair cells. J Assoc Res Otolaryngol 2004; 5:411–426.

17. Van Camp G, Willems PJ, Smith RJH. Nonsyndromic hearing impairment: unparalleled heterogeneity. Am J Hum Genet 1997; 60:758–764.

18. Van Camp G, Kunst H, Flothmann K, et al. A gene for autosomal dominant hearing impairment (DFNA14) maps to a region on chromosome 4p16.3 that does not overlap the DFNA6 locus. J Med Genet 1999; 36:532–536.

19. Cohn ES, Kelley PM. Clinical phenotype and mutations in connexin 26 (DFNB1/GJB2), the most common cause of childhood hearing loss. Am J Med Genet 1999; 89:130–136.

20. Cremers CWRJ, Smith RJH, eds. Genetic Hearing Impairment. Its Clinical Presentations. Adv Otorhinolaryngol; Basel: Karger, 2002:61.

21. Veske A, Oehlmann R, Younus F, et al. Autosomal recessive non-syndromic deafness locus (DFNB8) maps on chromosome 21q22 in a large consanguineous kindred from Pakistan. Hum Mol Genet 1996; 5:165–168.

22. Mustapha M, Chardenoux S, Nieder A, et al. A sensorineural progressive autosomal recessive form of isolated deafness, DFNB13, maps to chromosome 7q34-q36. Eur J Hum Genet 1998; 6:245–250.

23. Campbell C, Cucci RA, Prasad S, et al. Pendred syndrome, DFNB4, and PDS/SLC26A4 identification of eight novel mutations and possible genotype-phenotype correlations. Hum Mutat 2001; 17:403–411.

24. Napiontek U, Borck G, Müller-Forell W, et al. Intrafamilial variability of the deafness and goiter phenotype in Pendred syndrome caused by a T416P mutation in the SLC26A4 gene. J Clin Endocrinol Metab 2004; 89:5347–5351.

25. Cremers CWRJ, Admiraal RJC, Huygen PLM, et al. Progressive hearing loss, hypoplasia of the cochlea and widened vestibular aqueducts are very common features in Pendred's syndrome. Int J Pediatr Otorhinolaryngol 1998; 45:113–123.

26. Kitamura K, Takahashi K, Noguchi Y, et al. Mutations of the Pendred syndrome gene (PDS) in patients with large vestibular aqueduct. Acta Otolaryngol 2000; 120:137–141.

27. Stinckens C, Huygen PLM, Joosten FBM, et al. Fluctuant, progressive hearing loss associated with Meniere like vertigo in three patients with the Pendred syndrome. Int J Pediatr Otorhinolaryngol 2001; 61:207–215.

28. Stinckens C, Huygen PLM, Van Camp G, et al. Pendred syndrome redefined. Report of a new family with fluctuating and progressive hearing loss. In: Cremers CWRJ, Smith RJH, eds. Genetic Hearing Impairment. Its Clinical Presentations. Adv Otorhinolaryngol Basel: Karger; 2002;61:131–141.

29. Tsukamoto K, Suzuki H, Harada D, et al. Distribution and frequencies of PDS (SLC26A4) mutations in Pendred syndrome and nonsyndromic hearing loss associated with enlarged vestibular aqueduct: a unique spectrum of mutations in Japanese. Eur J Hum Genet 2003; 11:916–922.

30. Blons H, Feldmann D, Duval V, et al. Screening of SLC26A4 (PDS) gene in Pendred's syndrome: a large spectrum of mutations in France and phenotypic heterogeneity. Clin Genet 2004; 66:333–340.

31. Cremers CWRJ, Bolder C, Admiraal RJC, et al. Progressive sensorineural hearing loss and a widened vestibular aqueduct in

Pendred syndrome. Arch Otolaryngol Head Neck Surg 1998; 124:501–505.

32. Cohn ES, Kelley PM, Fowler TW, et al. Clinical studies of families with hearing loss attributable to mutations in the connexin 26 gene (GJB2/DFNB1). Pediatrics 1999; 103:546–550.

33. Denoyelle F, Marlin S, Weil D, et al. Clinical features of the prevalent form of childhood deafness, DFNB1, due to a connexin-26 gene defect: implications for genetic counselling. Lancet 1999; 353:1298–1303.

34. Santos RLP, Aulchenko YS, Huygen PLM, et al. Hearing impairment in Dutch patients with connexin 26 (GJB2) and connexin 30 (GJB6) mutations. Int J Pediatr Otorhinolaryngol 2005; 69:165–174.

35. Feldmann D, Denoyelle F, Chauvin P, et al. Large deletion of the GJB6 gene in deaf patients heterozygous for the GJB2 gene mutation: genotypic and phenotypic analysis. Am J Med Genet A 2004; 127A:263–267.

36. Stinckens C, Kremer H, van Wijk E, et al. Longitudinal phenotypic analysis in patients with connexin 26 (GJB2) (DFNB1) and connexin 30 (GJB6) mutations. Ann Otol Rhinol Laryngol 2004; 113:587–593.

37. Cryns K, Orzan E, Murgia A, et al. A genotype-phenotype correlation for GJB2 (connexin 26) deafness. J Med Genet 2004; 41:147–154.

38. Matsushiro N, Doi K, Fuse Y, et al. Successful cochlear implantation in prelingual profound deafness resulting from the common 233delC mutation of the GJB2 gene in the Japanese. Laryngoscope 2002; 112:255–261.

39. Oguchi T, Ohtsuka A, Hashimoto S, et al. Clinical features of patients with GJB2 (connexin 26) mutations: severity of hearing loss is correlated with genotypes and protein expression patterns. J Hum Genet 2005; 50:76–83.

40. Sobe T, Vreugde S, Shahin H, et al. The prevalence and expression of inherited connexin 26 mutations associated with nonsyndromic hearing loss in the Israeli population. Hum Genet 2000; 106:50–57.

41. RamShankar M, Girirajan S, Dagan O, et al. Contribution of connexin26 (GJB2) mutations and founder effect to non-syndromic hearing loss in India. J Med Genet 2003; 40:e68.

42. del Castillo I, Villamar M, Moreno Pelayo MA, et al. A deletion involving the connexin 30 gene in nonsyndromic hearing impairment. N Engl J Med 2002; 346:243–249.

43. Griffith AJ, Chowdhry AA, Kurima K, et al. Autosomal recessive nonsyndromic neurosensory deafness at DFNB1 not associated with the compound-heterozygous GJB2 (connexin 26) genotype M34T/167delT. Am J Hum Genet 2000; 67:745–749.

44. Wilcox SA, Saunders K, Osborn AH, et al. High frequency hearing loss correlated with mutations in the GJB2 gene. Hum Genet 2000; 106:399–405.

45. Houseman MJ, Ellis LA, Pagnamenta A, et al. Genetic analysis of the connexin-26 M34T variant: identification of genotype M34T/M34T segregating with mild-moderate non-syndromic sensorineural hearing loss. J Med Genet 2001; 38:20–25.

46. Janecke AR, Hirst-Stadlmann A, Günther B, et al. Progressive hearing loss, and recurrent sudden sensorineural hearing loss

associated with GJB2 mutations-phenotypic spectrum and frequencies of GJB2 mutations in Austria. Hum Genet 2002; 111:145–153.

47. Engel-Yeger B, Zaaroura S, Zlotogora J, et al. Otoacoustic emissions and brainstem evoked potentials in compound carriers of connexin 26 mutations. Hear Res 2003; 175:140–151.

48. Lim LHY, Bradshaw JK, Guo Y, et al. Genotypic and phenotypic correlations of DFNB1-related hearing impairment in the Midwestern United States. Arch Otolaryngol Head Neck Surg 2003; 129:836–840.

49. Roux AF, Pallares Ruiz N, Vielle A, et al. Molecular epidemiology of DFNB1 deafness in France. BMC Med Genet 2004; 5:5.

50. Gualandi F, Ravani A, Berto A, et al. Exploring the clinical and epidemiological complexity of GJB2-linked deafness. Am J Med Genet 2002; 112:38–45.

51. Murgia A, Orzan E, Polli R, et al. Cx26 deafness: mutation analysis and clinical variability. J Med Genet 1999; 36:829–832.

52. Tóth T, Kupka S, Sziklai I, et al. Phänotypische Charakterisierung schwerhöriger Patienten mit homozygoter 35delG-Mutation im Connexin-26-Gen. HNO 2003; 51:400–404.

53. Tyson J, Bellman S, Newton V, et al. Mapping of DFN2 to Xq22. Hum Mol Genet 1996; 5:2055–2060.

54. Pfister MHF, Lalwani AK. Clinical phenotype of DFN2, DFN4 and DFN6. In: Cremers CWRJ, Smith RJH, eds. Genetic Hearing Impairment. Its Clinical Presentations. Adv Otorhinolaryngol Basel: Karger; 2002; 61:168–171.

55. Pfister MHF, Lalwani AK. X-linked hereditary hearing impairment. Audiol Med 2003; 1:29–32.

56. Phelps PD, Reardon W, Pembrey M, et al. X-linked deafness, stapes gushers and a distinctive defect of the inner ear. Neuroradiology 1991; 33:326–330.

57. Hagiwara H, Tamagawa Y, Kitamura K, et al. A new mutation in the POU3F4 gene in a Japanese family with X-linked mixed deafness (DFN3). Laryngoscope 1998; 108:1544–1547.

58. Lalwani AK, Brister JR, Fex J, et al. A new nonsyndromic X-linked sensorineural hearing impairment linked to Xp21.2. Am J Hum Genet 1994; 55:685–694.

59. Pfister MHF, Apaydin F, Turan O, et al. A second family with nonsyndromic sensorineural hearing loss linked to Xp21.2: refinement of the DFN4 locus within DMD. Genomics 1998; 53:377–382.

60. Pfister MHF, Apaydin F, Turan O, et al. Clinical evidence for dystrophin dysfunction as a cause of hearing loss in locus DFN4. Laryngoscope 1999; 109:730–735.

61. Cui B, Zhang H, Lu Y, et al. Refinement of the locus for non-syndromic sensorineural deafness (DFN2). J Genet 2004; 83: 35–38.

62. Nance WE, Setleff R, McLeod A, et al. X-linked mixed deafness with congenital fixation of the stapedial footplate and perilymphatic gusher. Birth Defects Orig Artic Ser 1971; 7:64–69.

63. Cremers CWRJ, Hombergen GCHJ, Scaf JJ, et al. X-linked progressive mixed deafness with perilymphatic gusher during stapes surgery. Arch Otolaryngol 1985; 111:249–254.

64. Cremers CWRJ, Snik AFM, Huygen PLM, et al. X-linked mixed deafness syndrome with congenital fixation of the stapedial

footplate and perilymphatic gusher (DFN3). In: Cremers CWRJ, Smith RJH, eds. Genetic Hearing Impairment. Its Clinical Presentations. Adv Otorhinolaryngol Basel: Karger; 2002; 61:161–167.

65. Carlson DL, Reeh HL. X-linked mixed hearing loss with stapes fixation: case reports. J Am Acad Audiol 1993; 4:420–425.

66. Reardon W, Bellman S, Phelps P, et al. Neuro-otological function in X-linked hearing loss: a multipedigree assessment and correlation with other clinical parameters. Acta Otolaryngol 1993; 113:706–714.

67. Arellano B, Ramirez Camacho R, Garcia Berrocal JR, et al. Sensorineural hearing loss and Mondini dysplasia caused by a deletion at locus DFN3. Arch Otolaryngol Head Neck Surg 2000; 126:1065–1069.

68. Oh N, Kupka S, Mirghomizadeh F, et al. Klinische und molekulargenetische Analyse monozygoter Zwillinge mit Stapes-Gusher-Syndrom (DFN3). HNO 2003; 51:629–633.

69. De Leenheer EMR, Ensink RJH, Kunst HPM, et al. DFNA2/KCNQ4 and its manifestations. Genetic Hearing Impairment. Its Clinical Presentations. Adv Otorhinolaryngol Basel: Karger; 2002; 61:41–46.

70. Topsakal V, Pennings RJE, te Brinke H, et al. Phenotype determination guides swift genotyping of a DFNA2/KCNQ4 family with a hot spot mutation (W276S). Otol Neurotol 2005; 26:52–58.

71. Denoyelle F, Lina Granade G, Petit C. DFNA3. In: Cremers CWRJ, Smith RJH, eds. Genetic Hearing Impairment. Its Clinical Presentations. Adv Otorhinolaryngol Basel: Karger; 2002; 61:47–52.

72. Bischoff AMLC, Luijendijk MWJ, Huygen PLM, et al. A novel mutation identified in the DFNA5 gene in a Dutch family: a clinical and genetic evaluation. Audiol Neurootol 2004; 9:34–46.

73. Bom SJH, Kemperman MH, Huygen PLM, et al. Cross-sectional analysis of hearing threshold in relation to age in a large family with cochleovestibular impairment thoroughly genotyped for DFNA9/COCH. Ann Otol Rhinol Laryngol 2003; 112:280–286.

74. Gottfried I, Huygen PLM, Avraham KB. The clinical presentation of DFNA15/POU4F3. In: Cremers CWRJ, Smith RJH, eds. Genetic Hearing Impairment. Its Clinical Presentations. Adv Otorhinolaryngol Basel: Karger; 2002; 61:92–97.

75. Makishima T, Kurima K, Brewer CC, et al. Early onset and rapid progression of dominant nonsyndromic DFNA36 hearing loss. Otol Neurotol 2004; 25:714–719.

76. Walsh T, Walsh V, Vreugde S, et al. From flies' eyes to our ears: mutations in a human class III myosin cause progressive nonsyndromic hearing loss DFNB30. Proc Natl Acad Sci USA 2002; 99:7518–7523.

77. del Castillo I, Villamar M, Sarduy M, et al. A novel locus for non-syndromic sensorineural deafness (DFN6) maps to chromosome Xp22. Hum Mol Genet 1996; 5:1383–1387.

78. Marres HAM, van Ewijk M, Huygen PLM, et al. Inherited nonsyndromic hearing loss. An audiovestibular study in a large family with autosomal dominant progressive hearing loss related to DFNA2. Arch Otolaryngol Head Neck Surg 1997; 123:573–577.

79. Kunst H, Marres H, Huygen P, et al. Nonsyndromic autosomal dominant progressive sensorineural hearing loss: audiologic analysis of a pedigree linked to DFNA2. Laryngoscope 1998; 108: 74–80.

80. Coucke PJ, Van Hauwe P, Kelley PM, et al. Mutations in the KCNQ4 gene are responsible for autosomal dominant deafness in four DFNA2 families. Hum Mol Genet 1999; 8:1321–1328.

81. Talebizadeh Z, Kelley PM, Askew JW, et al. Novel mutation in the KCNQ4 gene in a large kindred with dominant progressive hearing loss. Hum Mutat 1999; 14:493–501.

82. Ensink RJH, Huygen PLM, Van Hauwe P, et al. A Dutch family with progressive sensorineural hearing impairment linked to the DFNA2 region. Eur Arch Otorhinolaryngol 2000; 257:62–67.

83. Akita J, Abe S, Shinkawa H, et al. Clinical and genetic features of nonsyndromic autosomal dominant sensorineural hearing loss: KCNQ4 is a gene responsible in Japanese. J Hum Genet 2001; 46:355–361.

84. De Leenheer EMR, Huygen PLM, Coucke PJ, et al. Longitudinal and cross-sectional phenotype analysis in a new, large Dutch DFNA2/KCNQ4 family. Ann Otol Rhinol Laryngol 2002; 111:267–274.

85. Liu XZ, Xia XJ, Xu LR, et al. Mutations in connexin31 underlie recessive as well as dominant non-syndromic hearing loss. Hum Mol Genet 2000; 9:63–67.

86. Djelantik B. Progressive Autosomal Dominant Hearing Loss. [PhD Thesis] University of Antwerp, 1996.

87. Goldstein JA, Lalwani AK. Further evidence for a third deafness gene within the DFNA2 locus. Am J Med Genet 2002; 108: 304–309.

88. Stern RE, Lalwani AK. Audiologic evidence for further genetic heterogeneity at DFNA2. Acta Otolaryngol 2002; 122:730–735.

89. Bom SJH, De Leenheer EMR, Lemaire FX, et al. Speech recognition scores related to age and degree of hearing impairment in DFNA2/KCNQ4 and DFNA9/COCH. Arch Otolaryngol Head Neck Surg 2001; 127:1045–1048.

90. Grifa A, Wagner CA, D'Ambrosio L, et al. Mutations in GJB6 cause nonsyndromic autosomal dominant deafness at DFNA3 locus. Nat Genet 1999; 23:16–18.

91. Denoyelle F, Weil D, Levilliers J, et al. DFNA3. In: Kitamura K, Steel KP, eds. Genetics in Otorhinolaryngology. Adv Otorhinolaryngol Basel: Karger; 2000; 56:78–83.

92. De Leenheer EMR, van Zuijlen DA, Van Laer L, et al. Clinical features of DFNA5. In: Cremers CWRJ, Smith RJH, eds. Genetic Hearing Impairment. Its Clinical Presentations. Adv Otorhinolaryngol Basel: Karger; 2002; 61:53–59.

93. De Leenheer EMR, van Zuijlen DA, Van Laer L, et al. Further delineation of the DFNA5 phenotype: results of speech recognition tests. Ann Otol Rhinol Laryngol 2002; 111:639–641.

94. Yu C, Meng X, Zhang S, et al. A 3-nucleotide deletion in the polypyrimidine tract of intron 7 of the DFNA5 gene causes nonsyndromic hearing impairment in a Chinese family. Genomics 2003; 82:575–579.

95. Fagerheim T, Nilssen Ø, Raeymaekers P, et al. Identification of a new locus for autosomal dominant non-syndromic hearing impairment (DFNA7) in a large Norwegian family. Hum Mol Genet 1996; 5:1187–1191.

96. Elverland HH, Hansen PW, Fagerheim T, et al. Audiological variation in a family with autosomal dominant non-syndromic hearing impairment linked to the DFNA7 locus—a need for reclassificiation of deafness. J Audiol Med 1998; 7:109–119.

97. Tranebjærg L, Elverland HH, Fagerheim T. DFNA7. In: Kitamura K, Steel KP, eds. Genetics in Otorhinolaryngology. Adv Otorhinolaryngol Basel: Karger; 2000; 56:97–100.

98. Alloisio N, Morlé L, Bozon M, et al. Mutation in the zonadhesin-like domain of a-tectorin associated with autosomal dominant non-syndromic hearing loss. Eur J Hum Genet 1999; 7:255–258.

99. Manolis EN, Yandavi N, Nadol JB Jr, et al. A gene for non-syndromic autosomal dominant progressive postlingual sensorineural hearing loss maps to chromosome 14q12–13. Hum Mol Genet 1996; 5:1047–1050.

100. Halpin C, Khetarpal U, McKenna M. Autosomal-dominant progressive sensorineural hearing loss in a large North American family. Am J Audiol 1996; 5:105–111.

101. Verhagen WIM, Bom SJH, Fransen E, et al. Hereditary cochleovestibular dysfunction due to a COCH gene mutation (DFNA9): a follow-up study of a family. Clin Otolaryngol 2001; 26:477–483.

102. Kemperman MH, Bom SJH, Lemaire FX, et al. DFNA9/COCH and its phenotype. In: Cremers CWRJ, Smith RJH, eds. Genetic Hearing Impairment. Its Clinical Presentations. Adv Otorhinolaryngol Basel: Karger; 2002; 61:66–72.

103. Lemaire FX, Feenstra L, Huygen PLM, et al. Progressive late-onset sensorineural hearing loss and vestibular impairment with vertigo (DFNA9/COCH): longitudinal analyses in a Belgian family. Otol Neurotol 2003; 24:743–748.

104. Frydman M, Vreugde S, Nageris BI, et al. Clinical characterization of genetic hearing loss caused by a mutation in the POU4F3 transcription factor. Arch Otolaryngol Head Neck Surg 2000; 126:633–637.

105. Fukushima K, Kasai N, Ueki Y, et al. A gene for fluctuating, progressive autosomal dominant nonsyndromic hearing loss, DFNA16, maps to chromosome 2q23–24.3. Am J Hum Genet 1999; 65:141–150.

106. Lalwani AK, Goldstein JA, Mhatre AN. Auditory phenotype of DFNA17. In: Cremers CWRJ, Smith RJH, eds. Genetic Hearing Impairment. Its Clinical Presentations. Adv Otorhinolaryngol Basel: Karger; 2002; 61:107–112.

107. Lalwani AK, Linthicum FH, Wilcox ER, et al. A five-generation family with late-onset progressive hereditary hearing impairment due to cochleosaccular degeneration. Audiol Neurootol 1997; 2: 139–154.

108. Morell RJ, Friderici KH, Wei S, et al. A new locus for late-onset, progressive, hereditary hearing loss DFNA20 maps to 17q25. Genomics 2000; 63:1–6.

109. Elfenbein JL, Fisher RA, Wei S, et al. Audiologic aspects of the search for DFNA20: a gene causing late-onset, progressive, sensorineural hearing loss. Ear Hear 2001; 22:279–288.

110. DeWan AT, Parrado AR, Leal SM. A second kindred linked to DFNA20 (17q25.3) reduces the genetic interval. Clin Genet 2003; 63:39–45.

111. Zhu M, Yang T, Wei S, et al. Mutations in the γ-actin gene (ACTG1) are associated with dominant progressive deafness (DFNA20/26). Am J Hum Genet 2003; 73:1082–1091.

112. Kemperman MH, De Leenheer EMR, Huygen PLM, et al. A Dutch family with hearing loss linked to the DFNA20/26 locus: longitudinal analysis of hearing impairment. Arch Otolaryngol Head Neck Surg 2004; 130:281–288.

113. Teig E. Hereditary progressive perceptive deafness in a family of 72 patients. Acta Otolaryngol 1968; 65:365–372.

114. Mangino M, Flex E, Capon F, et al. Mapping of a new autosomal dominant nonsyndromic hearing loss locus (DFNA30) to chromosome 15q25–26. Eur J Hum Genet 2001; 9:667–671.

115. Xia J, Deng H, Feng Y, et al. A novel locus for autosomal dominant nonsyndromic hearing loss identified at 5q31.1–32 in a Chinese pedigree. J Hum Genet 2002; 47:635–640.

116. D'Adamo P, Donaudy F, D'Eustacchio A, et al. A new locus (DFNA47) for autosomal dominant non-syndromic inherited hearing loss maps to 9p21–22 in a large Italian family. Eur J Hum Genet 2002; 11:121–124.

117. D'Adamo P, Pinna M, Capobianco S, et al. A novel autosomal dominant non-syndromic deafness locus (DFNA48) maps to 12q13-q14 in a large Italian family. Hum Genet 2003; 112: 319–320.

118. Salam AA, Häfner FM, Linder TE, et al. A novel locus (DFNA23) for prelingual autosomal dominant nonsyndromic hearing loss maps to 14q21-q22 in a Swiss German kindred. Am J Hum Genet 2000; 66:1984–1988.

119. Häfner FM, Salam AA, Linder TE, et al. A novel locus (DFNA24) for prelingual nonprogressive autosomal dominant nonsyndromic hearing loss maps to 4q35-qter in a large Swiss German kindred. Am J Hum Genet 2000; 66:1437–1442.

120. Ahmed ZM, Li XC, Powell SD, et al. Characterization of a new full length TMPRSS3 isoform and identification of mutant alleles responsible for nonsyndromic recessive deafness in Newfoundland and Pakistan. BMC Med Genet 2004; 5:24.

121. Villamar M, del Castillo I, Valle N, et al. Deafness locus DFNB16 is located on chromosome 15q13-q21 within a 5-cM interval flanked by markers D15S994 and D15S132. Am J Hum Genet 1999; 64:1238–1241.

122. Chen AH, Ni L, Fukushima K, et al. Linkage of a gene for dominant non-syndromic deafness to chromosome 19. Hum Mol Genet 1995; 4:1073–1076.

123. McGuirt WT, Lesperance MM, Wilcox ER, et al. Characterization of autosomal dominant non-syndromic hearing loss loci: DFNA 4, 6, 10 and 13. In: Kitamura K, Steel KP, eds. Genetics in Otorhinolaryngology. Adv Otorhinolaryngol Basel: Karger; 2000; 56:84–96.

124. Pusch CM, Meyer B, Kupka S, et al. Refinement of the DFNA4 locus to a 1.44 Mb region in 19q13.33. J Mol Med 2004; 82:398–402.

125. Tamagawa Y, Ishikawa K, Ishikawa K, et al. Phenotype of DFNA11: a nonsyndromic hearing loss caused by a myosin VIIA mutation. Laryngoscope 2002; 112:292–297.

126. Luijendijk MWJ, van Wijk E, Bischoff AMLC, et al. Identification and molecular modelling of a mutation in the motor head domain of myosin VIIA in a family with autosomal dominant

hearing impairment (DFNA11). Hum Genet 2004; 115:149–156.

127. Street VA, Kallman JC, Kiemele KL. Modifier controls severity of a novel dominant low-frequency MyosinVIIA (MYO7A) auditory mutation. J Med Genet 2004; 41:e62.

128. Bönsch D, Scheer P, Neumann C, et al. A novel locus for autosomal dominant, non-syndromic hearing impairment (DFNA18) maps to chromosome 3q22 immediately adjacent to the DM2 locus. Eur J Hum Genet 2001; 9:165–170.

129. Kunst HPM, Marres HAM, Huygen PLM, et al. Non-syndromic autosomal dominant progressive non-specific mid-frequency sensorineural hearing impairment with childhood to late adolescence onset (DFNA21). Clin Otolaryngol 2000; 25:45–54.

130. Thirlwall AS, Brown DJ, McMillan PM, et al. Phenotypic characterization of hereditary hearing impairment linked to DFNA25. Arch Otolaryngol Head Neck Surg 2003; 129:830–835.

131. Peters LM, Anderson DW, Griffith AJ, et al. Mutation of a transcription factor, TFCP2L3, causes progressive autosomal dominant hearing loss, DFNA28. Hum Mol Genet 2002; 11:2877–2885.

132. Ensink RJH, Huygen PLM, Snoeckx RL, et al. A Dutch family with progressive autosomal dominant non-syndromic sensorineural hearing impairment linked to DFNA13. Clin Otolaryngol 2001; 26:310–316.

133. Blanton SH, Liang CY, Cai MW, et al. A novel locus for autosomal dominant non-syndromic deafness (DFNA41) maps to chromosome 12q24-qter. J Med Genet 2002; 39:567–570.

134. Flex E, Mangino M, Mazzoli M, et al. Mapping of a new autosomal dominant non-syndromic hearing loss locus (DFNA43) to chromosome 2p12. J Med Genet 2003; 40:278–281.

135. Modamio Høybjør S, Moreno Pelayo MA, Mencia A, et al. A novel locus for autosomal dominant nonsyndromic hearing loss, DFNA50, maps to chromosome 7q32 between the DFNB17 and DFNB13 deafness loci. J Med Genet 2004; 41:e14.

136. Pfister MHF, Thiele H, Van Camp G, et al. A genotype-phenotype correlation with gender-effect for hearing impairment caused by TECTA mutations. Cell Physiol Biochem 2004; 14:369–376.

137. De Leenheer EMR, Huygen PLM, Wayne S, et al. The DFNA10 phenotype. Ann Otol Rhinol Laryngol 2001; 110:861–866.

138. De Leenheer EMR, Huygen PLM, Wayne S, et al. DFNA10/EYA4—the clinical picture. In: Cremers CWRJ, Smith RJH, eds. Genetic Hearing Impairment. Its Clinical Presentations. Adv Otorhinolaryngol Basel: Karger; 2002; 61:73–78.

139. Verstreken M, Declau F, Schatteman I, et al. Audiometric analysis of a Belgian family linked to the DFNA10 locus. Am J Otol 2000; 21:675–681.

140. Tamagawa Y, Ishikawa K, Ishikawa K, et al. Clinical presentation of DFNA11 (MYO7A). In: Cremers CWRJ, Smith RJH, eds. Genetic Hearing Impairment. Its Clinical Presentations. Adv Otorhinolaryngol Basel: Karger; 2002; 61:79–84.

141. Snoeckx RL, Kremer H, Ensink RJH, et al. A novel locus for autosomal dominant non-syndromic hearing loss, DFNA31, maps to chromosome 6p21.3. J Med Genet 2004; 41:11–13.

142. Pauw RJ, De Leenheer EMR, Van den Boogaerd K et al. The phenotype of the first otosclerosis family linked to OTSCS. OTOL Neurotol 2006; 27:308–315.

143. Wang QJ, Lu CY, Li N, et al. Y-linked inheritance of non-syndromic hearing impairment in a large Chinese family. J Med Genet 2004; 41:e80.

144. Kirschhofer K, Kenyon JB, Hoover DM, et al. Autosomal-dominant, prelingual, nonprogressive sensorineural hearing loss: localization of the gene (DFNA8) to chromosome 11q by linkage in an Austrian family. Cytogenet Cell Genet 1998; 82: 126–130.

145. Govaerts PJ, De Ceulaer G, Daemers K, et al. A new autosomal-dominant locus (DFNA12) is responsible for a nonsyndromic, midfrequency, prelingual and nonprogressive sensorineural hearing loss. Am J Otol 1998; 19:718–723.

146. Iwasaki S, Harada D, Usami S, et al. Association of clinical features with mutation of TECTA in a family with autosomal dominant hearing loss. Arch Otolaryngol Head Neck Surg 2002; 128: 913–917.

147. Naz S, Alasti F, Mowjoodi A, et al. Distinctive audiometric profile associated with DFNB21 alleles of TECTA. J Med Genet 2003; 40:360–363.

148. Kunst HPM, Huybrechts C, Marres HAM, et al. The phenotype of DFNA13/COL11A2: nonsyndromic autosomal dominant mid-frequency and high-frequency sensorineural hearing impairment. Am J Otol 2000; 21:181–187.

149. De Leenheer EMR, Kunst HPM, McGuirt WT, et al. Autosomal dominant inherited hearing impairment caused by a missense mutation in COL11A2 (DFNA13). Arch Otolaryngol Head Neck Surg 2001; 127:13–17.

150. De Leenheer EMR, McGuirt WT, Kunst HPM, et al. The phenotype of DFNA13/COL11A2. In: Cremers CWRJ, Smith RJH, eds. Genetic Hearing Impairment. Its Clinical Presentations. Adv Otorhinolaryngol Basel: Karger; 2002; 61: 85–91.

151. Modamio Høybjør S, Moreno Pelayo MA, Mencía A, et al. A novel locus for autosomal dominant nonsyndromic hearing loss (DFNA44) maps to chromosome 3q28–29. Hum Genet 2003; 112:24–28.

152. Govaerts PJ, De Ceulaer G, Daemers K, et al. Clinical presentation of DFNA8-DFNA12. In: Cremers CWRJ, Smith RJH, eds. Genetic Hearing Impairment. Its Clinical Presentations. Adv Otorhinolaryngol Basel: Karger; 2002; 61:60–65.

153. Moreno Pelayo MA, del Castillo I, Villamar M, et al. A cysteine substitution in the zona pellucida domain of α-tectorin results in autosomal dominant, postlingual, progressive, mid frequency hearing loss in a Spanish family. J Med Genet 2001; 38:E13.

154. Moreno Pelayo MA, Modamio Høybjør S, Mencía A, et al. DFNA49, a novel locus for autosomal dominant non-syndromic hearing loss, maps proximal to DFNA7/DFNM1 region on chromosome 1q21-q23. J Med Genet 2003; 40:832–836.

155. De Leenheer EMR, Bosman AJ, Kunst HPM, et al. Audiological characteristics of some affected members of a Dutch DFNA13/COL11A2 family. Ann Otol Rhinol Laryngol 2004; 113:922–929.

156. Gürtler N, Kim Y, Mhatre A, et al. DFNA54, a third locus for low-frequency hearing loss. J Mol Med 2004; 82:775–780.

157. Manolis EN, Eavey RD, Sangwatanaroj S, et al. Hereditary postlingual sensorineural hearing loss mapping to chromosome Xq21. Am J Otol 1999; 20:621–626.

158. León PE, Bonilla JA, Sánchez JR, et al. Low frequency hereditary deafness in man with childhood onset. Am J Hum Genet 1981; 33:209–214.

159. Lalwani AK, Jackler RK, Sweetow RW, et al. Further characterization of the DFNA1 audiovestibular phenotype. Arch Otolaryngol Head Neck Surg 1998; 124:699–702.

160. Leon PE, Lalwani AK. Auditory phenotype of DFNA1. In: Cremers CWRJ, Smith RJH, eds. Genetic Hearing Impairment. Its Clinical Presentations. Adv Otorhinolaryngol Basel: Karger; 2002; 61:34–40.

161. The Vanderbilt University Hereditary Deafness Study Group. Domintantly inherited low-frequency hearing loss. Arch Otolaryngol 1968; 88:242–250.

162. Kunst HPM, Marres HAM, Huygen PLM, et al. Autosomal dominant non-syndromal low-frequency sensorineural hearing impairment linked to chromosome 4p16 (DFNA14): statistical analysis of hearing threshold in relation to age and evaluation of vestibulo-ocular functions. Audiology 1999; 38: 165–173.

163. Bespalova IN, Van Camp G, Bom SJH, et al. Mutations in the Wolfram syndrome 1 gene (WFS1) are a common cause of low frequency sensorineural hearing loss. Hum Mol Genet 2001; 10:2501–2508.

164. Komatsu K, Nakamura N, Ghadami M, et al. Confirmation of genetic homogeneity of nonsyndromic low-frequency sensorineural hearing loss by linkage analysis and a DFNA6/14 mutation in a Japanese family. J Hum Genet 2002; 47:395–399.

165. Tóth T, Kupka S, Nürnberg P, et al. Phänotypische Charakterisierung einer DFNA6-Familie mit Tieftonschwerhörigkeit. HNO 2004; 52:132–136.

166. Gürtler N, Kim Y, Mhatre A, et al. Two families with nonsyndromic low-frequency hearing loss harbor novel mutations in Wolfram syndrome gene 1. J Mol Med 2005; 83:553–560.

167. Bille M, Munk Nielsen L, Tranebjærg L, et al. Two families with phenotypically different hereditary low frequency hearing impairment: longitudinal data and linkage analysis. Scand Audiol 2001; 30:246–254.

168. Brodwolf S, Böddeker IR, Ziegler A, et al. Further evidence for linkage of low-mid frequency hearing impairment to the candidate region on chromosome 4p16.3. Clin Genet 2001; 60: 155–160.

169. Young TL, Ives E, Lynch E, et al. Non-syndromic progressive hearing loss DFNA38 is caused by heterozygous missense mutation in the Wolfram syndrome gene WFS1. Hum Mol Genet 2001; 10:2509–2514.

170. Lesperance MM, Hall JW III, San Agustin TB, et al. Mutations in the Wolfram syndrome type 1 gene (WFS1) define a clinical entity of dominant low-frequency sensorineural hearing loss. Arch Otolaryngol Head Neck Surg 2003; 129:411–420.

171. Bom SJH, Van Camp G, Cryns K, et al. Autosomal dominant low-frequency hearing impairment (DFNA6/14): a clinical and genetic family study. Otol Neurotol 2002; 23:876–884.

172. Pennings RJE, Bom SJH, Cryns K, et al. Progression of low-frequency sensorineural hearing loss (DFNA6/14-WFS1). Arch Otolaryngol Head Neck Surg 2003; 129:421–426.

14 Early detection and assessment of genetic childhood hearing impairment

Agnete Parving

Introduction

Throughout life, the hearing organ, with its different anatomical areas, i.e., outer ear and ear canal, middle ear, inner ear and auditory pathways, may be affected by numerous damaging factors, resulting in a hearing disorder. The loss of auditory sensitivity—which in clinical terms is hearing impairment (HI)—may, in children, result in reduced or delayed acquisition of language and development of communication, which in turn can lead to poor educational achievements and reduced quality of life, self-esteem, and employment opportunities.

HI, in children, caused by genetic factors is permanent, irrespective of the site of lesion in the auditory organ and may be conductive or sensorineural and progressive or stable, with early or late onset. Thus, it may be congenital, acquired early (i.e., in the neonatal period), or acquired through childhood although it is currently impossible to distinguish between genetic HI present at birth and HI acquired in the neonatal period, which is thus termed congenital. Because genetic HI may develop before or after language acquisition, some prefer to use the terms prelingual and postlingual HI. Because language and speech development is essential for communication, the impact and adverse effects of a prelingual HI can be devastating if not treated (1–3).

This contribution will concentrate on the detection of congenital HI with some reference to hereditary HI (HHI) and the assessment of genetic factors causing HI in infancy and childhood, with their potential for primary and secondary prevention of HI.

Detection of congenital HI

It has been documented and long recognised that infants with congenital permanent HI are detected and identified with a severe delay and thus have a high risk of speech and language deficits (1–3).

Most HHI is caused by genes resulting in only HI (i.e., non-syndromal) and 90% of the parents have normal hearing so a difference in age at identification between genetic and nongenetic HI has, to the author's knowledge, not been documented. However, it may be anticipated that problems in children with parents affected by HI and infants with hearing-impaired older siblings may be detected earlier when compared to other children. Thus, based on an ongoing paediatric audiological register (4,5), a comparative analysis was performed of the age at identification of congenital HI caused by genetic and nongenetic factors in the case of children born between 1985 and 2000. The 289 diagnosed as having hereditary congenital HI were diagnosed at a median age of 78 months, whereas the 334 with nongenetic factors causing congenital HI were diagnosed at a median age of 66 months. The difference is not significant and complies with the major proportion of sporadic and inherited autosomal recessive HI among children, and thus the early detection of hearing-impaired children is described without specific relationship to HHI.

The early detection of hearing impaired infants/children has been emphasized since the late 1960s, which resulted in implementation of hearing screening programmes in the 1970s either as universal hearing screening or as targeted groups.

However the screening tests had poor sensitivity/specificity (6) and the behavioural hearing-screening tests were performed at an age far too late for optimal intervention, which, on current evidence, is considered to be no later than six months of age (7–9). A list of risk indicators has represented a screening method (10), although, even if 100% effective, the indicators would only detect about 40% to 50% of children with congenital HI.

Throughout the 1990s, Universal Neonatal Hearing-Screening programmes (UNHS) have been implemented—predominantly in the United States—but within the last five years, several European countries have also introduced and implemented UNHS on a national level. In many European regions and health authority districts, UNHS is performed with a high compliance. In addition, the challenges imposed upon the diagnostic and intervention process by the early detection of hearing-impaired infants have resulted in early-detection and hearing-intervention (EDHI) programs of benefit to the entire paediatric audiological services.

Neonatal hearing screening is most often performed as a two-stage screening procedure using otoacoustic emissions (OAEs) or automated brainstem audiometry (ABR) or a combination of the two methods (11). Mass hearing screening in children, irrespective of age, is based on the concept of secondary prevention and it is a requirement for the implementation of all screening programmes that the condition represents an important health problem with serious consequences if the condition is undetected and thus untreated. Some prevalence estimates of congenital and acquired childhood HI will be briefly reported.

Prevalence estimates

The estimated prevalence of permanent childhood HI varies according to the definition and severity of the HI, the classification into conductive/sensorineural/mixed HI, the time of onset, whether progressive or stable, whether unilateral or bilateral, and, in addition, the estimated prevalence rate may also vary as a function of country or local area (12,13). Prevalence estimates of congenital HI (40 dB or greater for the average of 0.5–4 kHz) of 1 to 2 per 1000 live births are usually quoted based on clinical series of children included in hearing health–surveillance programs, which has been confirmed by UNHS (Table 14.1) (13,17).

The hearing level is graded according to a scale such as mild, moderate, severe, and profound. However, other descriptors may be used and should be defined because no uniform internationally accepted criteria for description of the degree of hearing level exist. A comprehensive national study from the United Kingdom has been conducted, including 17,160 hearing-impaired children with permanent HI above 40 dB for the averaged frequencies of 0.5 to 4 kHz in the better hearing ear and born between 1980 and 1995. The hearing loss was moderate (41–70 dB) in 52.9%; severe (71–95 dB) in 21.0%; and profound (>95 dB) in 24.8%. (In 1.3%, the hearing loss was unspecified.) Among those with permanent childhood HI, a varying proportion of 7.7% to 25.2% with acquired or late-onset HI has been reported (18).

Audiological assessment of children

The hearing level in infants can be determined in the clinic by behavioural observation audiometry (BOA), conditioned orientation reflex (COR), and by visual reinforcement audiometry (VRA). The BOA includes stimulation with different sound sources with a more or less well-defined frequency content and a relatively well-defined stimulus intensity, which may be varied by distance and force applied to provide the sound. In cooperative infants tested by experienced testers, the hearing level may be determined fairly reliably. However, in infants suffering from mental retardation, autistic behaviour or other additional handicaps, BOA is highly unreliable. The COR and VRA are

Table 14.1 Prevalence of HI based on the outcome of universal neonatal hearing-screening programs using a two-stage screening procedure with transient oto-acoustic emissions (TEOAE) and/or auditory brainstem response testing (ABR)

	Screened	Confirmed HI	Incidence (confidence interval)	Screening tests
	N	N	N = 1/1000	
Prieve et al. (14)	43311	85	1.96 (1.74–2.19)	TEOAE
Messner et al. (15)	7771	9	1.56 (0.54–2.58).	ABR
Mehl and Thomson (16)	148240	291	1.96 (1.74–2.19)	ABR/TEOAE

Note: 95% confidence intervals are indicated in brackets.
Abbreviations: ABR, automated brain-stem audiometry, HI; hearing impairment; TEOAE, transient oto-acoustic emissions.

important test procedures, and it has been shown that both reliable air- and bone-conduction hearing thresholds can be determined in infants using VRA (19,20).

Several studies have shown that there is a difference between infant thresholds and those of older children over the frequency range of 500 to 4000 Hz, the difference being greater at the lower frequencies than in the higher frequencies, a consistent finding in free-field testing and under earphone testing (21). The poorer auditory sensitivity in infants compared to that in older children may have many explanations such as difficulties in concentrating, inadequate motivation, poor fitting of earphones and, not the least, lack of developmental maturation and changes with age. However, it can be stated that behavioural hearing testing of infants performed by experienced testers—irrespective of the measurement procedure—can provide reliable information on the hearing sensitivity of infants/children unable to cooperate in formal pure-tone audiometric testing (22).

From the age of three to four years, at least three pure-tone hearing thresholds can be obtained by motivational games ranging from peep shows to finger raising techniques, and at an age of six years, most normally developed children can perform formal audiometry as used in adults.

In uncooperative children, and thus in most infants, various electrophysiological methods are used for hearing-threshold determination (23). In the clinic, ABR is used mostly due to its noninvasive nature and its high diagnostic sensitivity/specificity. In recent years, the auditory steady-state response technique has also been implemented in order to reliably predict pure-tone thresholds in infants. By using a combination of OAEs and ABR, auditory neuropathy—that may be related to genetic HI—can be diagnosed (24).

Apart from the assessment of hearing thresholds, the measurement of speech recognition is important. Procedures independent of speech and language production have been developed, whereby the perception of specific speech features can be discriminated (21,25). Some tests or modification of tests use target words or objects to measure speech recognition in two- to four-year-old children and, in older children, word recognition scores can be used as part of a play situation. In general, the older the child, the better the opportunity to perform speech recognition tasks, thus giving important information on their hearing capacity. These also have the potential to distinguish between peripheral and central auditory disorders.

Most HHI is sensorineural and to classify a HI as sensorineural, coherent air- and bone-conduction thresholds are essential. In addition, to classify HI in general, admittance audiometry including recording of stapedial reflex thresholds—often elicited by contralateral stimulation—should be part of the test procedure. The interpretation and diagnostic validity of stapedial-reflex-threshold testing in children are similar to the testing of adults, but the test may be difficult to perform in young children. Valuable information on site-of-lesion testing can also be obtained by electrophysiological methods, e.g.,

electrocochleography may differentiate between a conductive/sensorineural HI and a presynaptic or postsynaptic lesion.

In general, age-appropriate procedures including a whole battery of tests should be used for both hearing-sensitivity determination and classification of HI into conductive/sensorineural/mixed hearing loss. The testing is dependent only on the degree of cooperation of the child and the experience of the tester. The progress made in the early detection of HI in infants by neonatal hearing screening over the past few years will force clinicians to provide accurate, reliable, and comprehensive audiological assessment of infants and young children. To avoid pitfalls and misdiagnosis, it is recommended that the testing be based on a firm protocol using cross-checks of procedures (26).

Aetiological assessment of HI in children

Although an audiological assessment may offer some information on the factor(s) causing HI in children—information often provided by thorough history taking and clinical examination including otoscopy—a systematic evaluation protocol based on an interdisciplinary approach should be offered to each child and their family. An example of such a protocol is outlined in Table 14.2 and evidence that such a protocol improves the aetiological evaluation has been provided (27,28).

Table 14.2   Protocol for routine aetiological evaluation

1) Thorough clinical evaluation

2) Hearing-threshold determination (including that of parents, siblings, and other family members)

3) Classification of the hearing impairment (i.e., site of lesion)

4) Vestibular testing

5) Ophthalmological assessment

6) Computed tomography/magnetic resonance scanning

7) Blood testing: e.g.,

   Viral antibodies (rubella, cytomegalovirus, HIV, and others)

   Bacterial antibodies (syphilis, toxoplasmosis, and others)

   Thyroid function (thyroid-stimulating hormone, triiodothyronine, thyroxine, and others)

   Cytogenetic testing (chromosomal abnormalities)

8) Urine analysis

9) Electrocardiogram

10) Mutation analysis in Connexins (*GBJ2* and *GBJ6*) and other relevant genes such as *WFS1* and *SLC26A4*

11) Specific, e.g., perchlorate test

Table 14.3   Proportion of genetic factors causing permanent hearing impairment in children and "unknown cause" reported in various studies

Studies (Ref.)	Genetic factors (%)	Unknown cause (%)
Parving (29)	46	20
France and Stephens (27)	50	31
Maki-Torkko (30)	46	38
Billings and Kenna (31)	25	25
Fortnum (14)	30	49

Table 14.3 shows the proportion of some factors causing permanent HI in children reported in various studies, but consideration here will be given to genetic factors.

It has been estimated that more than 50% of permanent HI in children can be ascribed to genetic factors. However, as a proportion of 20% to 50% of hearing impaired children are categorized as "unknown" (Table 14.3), genetic factors are assumed to account for a much higher proportion. Traditionally, genetic HI has been described according to the mode of transmission of the mutant gene in terms of autosomal dominant (accounting for approximately 10–25%), autosomal recessive (accounting for approximately 80%), and X-linked recessive (accounting for 1–2%). However, developments in audiological genetics since 1994 (32,33) and the initial sequencing and analysis of the human genome (34,35) has resulted in the localization of more than 100 genes related to both nonsyndromal and syndromal HI (i.e., with other organ manifestations in addition to HI caused by the mutant gene in question); the previous proportions of subcategories according to the classical Mendelian mode of transmission may change in the future. Thus, it has been shown, for example, that mutations in the mitochondrial DNA can result in both syndromal and nonsyndromal HI (36).

Although more than 100 gene mutations causing autosomal-dominant (DFNA) and autosomal-recessive (DFNB) nonsyndromal HI have been localised, only about 40 genes have so far been identified. There is, however, limited knowledge of the function of the genes relating to the mechanism of hearing such as the hair-cell transduction, the hair-cell synaptic activity, the outer hair cell motor, the role of the tectorial membrane, the ionic environment of hair cells, and the molecules involved in the homeostasis of the endolymph and the perilymph (37). In addition, a potential phenotype/genotype correlation may be difficult to establish due to inadequate descriptions of either phenotypes or genotypes in journals related to audiology and genetics, respectively, which has led to guidelines for the description of genetic HI being proposed (38). In a recent sample of more than 1500 hearing-impaired individuals with biallelic GBJ2 mutations, with identification of 83 different mutations, a phenotype/genotype correlation

was confirmed, showing that truncating mutations cause more severe HI than nontruncating mutations and that homozygous 35delG mutations were the most frequent (39,40). Although a phenotype can be predicted from various GBJ2 genotypes with some degree of probability, it is still not possible—in the individual hearing-impaired child—to assess the genetic factor(s) causing the HI from the phenotype, unless the child appears with special features characteristic of a syndrome (41).

It should be mentioned that, for nonsyndromal HI, mutant mouse models have provided useful insights into some of the functions of genes related to the inner ear (42) and much can be learned by studying shared developmental pathways in other organisms such as flies, worms, and yeast (43).

Paediatric audiological services should offer children with sensorineural HI—irrespective of the degree of HI—testing for mutations in Connexin proteins because mutations in at least three Connexins have been implicated in nonsyndromal HI (GBJ2, GBJ3, and GBJ6). As mentioned above, the most frequent mutation is found in Connexin 26 encoded by the GBJ2 gene, resulting in DFNB1 but has also been found responsible for DFNA3, thus resulting in both a recessive and a dominant mode of transmission of the mutant gene. As also mentioned, numerous mutations in Connexin 26 have been described, the most frequent being the 35delG mutation (44). Mutations in Connexin 26 result in sporadic and familial severe/profound prelingual HI (45,46) and account for about 50% of recessive and 10% to 25% of sporadic nonsyndromal HI in Southern European children. An evaluation from United States has shown that nearly 30% have Connexin 26–related HI with all degrees of HI (44) and thus it can be stated that mutations in Connexin 26 may result in all degrees of HI (39).

Thus, it is recommended that all children under 18 years of age with bilateral, permanent, nonsyndromal sensorineural or mixed HI—irrespective of the level of impairment—for which there is no other explanation, should be offered testing. The initial testing should check for 35delG and/or the other most frequent mutations in the background population. Unless the first screening identifies mutations on both alleles, testing should go on to screening of the entire coding region and splice sites for mutations. In addition, the presence of GBJ6/Cx30 deletions should be sought (47).

As part of the protocol for diagnostic evaluation (Table 14.2), imaging techniques should be used in order to detect aplasia/hypoplasia and/or malformations such as enlarged vestibular aqueduct (EVA) and Mondini malformation (48,49). EVA and Mondini defects are often found in subjects with Pendred syndrome, a diagnosis previously depending on an abnormal perchlorate test. The syndrome is a recessive genetic hearing disorder. However, the clinical picture differs in many cases from the original description (50) of two sisters with congenital deafness and goitre developing during puberty. The gene responsible for Pendred syndrome has been located to chromosome 7q31 and designated PDS. The gene product, pendrin, is a transmembrane chloride-iodide cotransporter protein, probably essential for endolymphatic homeostasis. The sensorineural HI may be fluctuant or progressive, ranging from mild to profound, and an EVA may be found by radiological examination, with the perchlorate test being negative. The diagnosis of Pendred syndrome (or DFNB4) in such cases depends on analysis of mutations in the *PDS* gene, where the most frequent mutation is the *SLC26A4* (51).

Ophthalmological examination is of utmost importance in order to assess visual acuity and to examine for involvement of structures in the eyes such as, e.g., retinitis pigmentosa found in Usher syndrome and differences in eye color as in, e.g., Waardenburg type I syndrome. In addition, many other impairments of hearing are associated with eye manifestations (52).

Systematic testing for mutations in known genes causing nonsyndromal HI as part of a diagnostic evaluation has not been performed in clinical series, but developments within molecular biology and genetic testing may, in the future, lead to screening for numerous mutations related to HI by means of DNA chips. However, many other factors, apart from the diagnostic evaluation, should be taken into account—factors such as the possibility for genetic counseling and the attitudes towards genetic testing for HI and deafness (53). This will result in improved diagnostic evaluation, improved counseling, and, ultimately, in prevention of genetic HI.

In order to be updated on genetic HI as part of the diagnostic evaluation, the reader is recommended to consult the hereditary hearing loss home page: http://webhost.ua.ac.be/hhh (54).

Some future aspects

Concurrent with the implementation of EDHI programmes, genetic testing may be of benefit to both the parents and the infant, because the genetic testing may reveal the cause of the HI and thus avoid numerous other aetiological investigations in the child. As previously mentioned, it is recommended that all children identified with sensorineural HI be tested for Connexin 26 mutations (47), but genetic testing may be part of screening in combination with screening for other diseases such as congenital hypothyroidism and various other inborn errors of metabolism using the blood spots obtained in the Guthrie cards (55). Thus, when confirming reduced hearing sensitivity of the child, the aetiological diagnosis may already be known. However, as part of the general screening in the neonatal period, there are disadvantages to this procedure, the costs and also problems arising from the identification of potential carriers and how to share this information with parents of unaffected infants being not the least of them (56,57). Thus, at present, it seems most appropriate to perform the diagnostic evaluation after the identification of the HI, although this may change in the future. Testing after the identification of HI should also take the attitudes of many deaf and hard-of-hearing people into account because especially the deaf community welcomes deafness not as a disease or handicap but as an integral part of their identity (58). Cause finding, offered as a postidentification procedure, can then be a choice for the parents, meeting the historically negative perception of the medical community among the Deaf who consider the medical community as trying to "treat" an "inability." Some recent surveys have shown that members of the Deaf community have a predominantly negative attitude toward genetic testing for deafness (59,60), but it should also be mentioned that about 90% of parents of hearing-impaired children with normal hearing, who understand the problem of HI/deafness, consider genetic testing as an improvement and support it (61). To further clarify these problems, additional surveys need to be performed including Deaf communities and parents of hearing-impaired children from many different countries, reflecting different social and cultural backgrounds.

Conclusions

For the identification and audiological assessment—and as part of surveillance and support programs offered to children with HI, hereditary or not—it is recommended that age-appropriate and reliable hearing tests be used, and when the HI has been documented, a systematic evaluation of the aetiological factors causing the HI be performed. This evaluation should be considered as a process in which every due caution should be taken with the individual child.

As a result of future diagnostic procedures, factors causing HI will be detected and recognised and, with the implementation of early detection programmes, including genetic testing for known mutations related to HI, HHI will also be diagnosed. This will ultimately render possible primary and secondary prevention of HHI in children. To meet this challenge, a formal collaboration between geneticists and audiologists must be established.

References

1. Yoshinaga-Itano C, Sedey AL, Coulter DK, Mehl AL. Language of early- and later-identified children with hearing loss. Pediatrics 1998; 102:1161–71.
2. Yoshinaga-Itano C. Universal newborn hearing screening programs and developmental outcomes. Audiol Med 2003; 1:199–206.
3. Moeller MP. Early intervention and language development in children who are deaf and hard of hearing. Pediatrics 2000; 106:E43.
4. Parving A. Paediatric audiological medicine—a survey from a regional department. J Audiol Med 1992; 1:99–111.
5. Parving A, Hauch A-M. Permanent childhood hearing impairment—some cross-sectional characteristics from a surveillance program. Int Pediatrics 2001; 16:33–37.
6. Davis A, Bamford J, Wilson I, et al. A critical review of the role of neonatal hearing screening in the detection of congenital hearing impairment. Health Techn Assess 1997; 1.

7. NIH Consensus Statement. Early identification of hearing impairment in infants and young children. Bethesda: United States Dept. Health & Human Services Publications, 1993.

8. Joint Committee on Infant Hearing. Position statement: principles and guidelines for early hearing detection and intervention program. Am J Audiol 2000; 9:9–29.

9. Grandori F, Collet L, Kemp D, et al. Universal screening for infant hearing impairment. European Concerted Action on Otoacoustic Emissions. Pediatrics 1994; 94:956–963.

10. Joint Committee on Infant Hearing. Position statement. ASHA 1994; 36:3841.

11. Watkin PM. Neonatal hearing screening—methods and outcome. Audiol Med 2003; 1:165–174.

12. Fortnum H. Epidemiology of permanent childhood hearing impairment: implications for neonatal hearing screening. Audiol Med 2003; 1:155–164.

13. Parving A. Looking for the hearing-impaired child: past, present and future. In: Seewald RC, Gravel J, eds. A Sound Foundation Through Early Amplification. Proceedings of the 2nd Int. Conference 2001. Great Britain: St. Edmundsbury Press, 2002: 251–259.

14. Prieve B, Dalzell L, Berg A, et al. The New York State universal newborn hearing screening project: outpatient outcome measures. Ear Hear 2000; 21:92–103.

15. Messner AH, Price M, Kwast K, et al. Volunteer-based universal newborn hearing screening program. Int J Ped Otorhinolaryngol 2001; 60:123–130.

16. Mehl AL, Thomson V. The Colorado newborn hearing screening project, 1992–1999: on the threshold of effective population-based universal newborn hearing screening. Pediatrics 2002; 109:1–8.

17. Fortnum HM, Marshall DH, Summerfield AQ. Epidemiology of the UK population of hearing-impaired children, including characteristics of those with and without cochlear implants—audiology, aetiology, comorbidity and affluence. Int J Audiol 2002; 41:170–179.

18. Fortnum HM, Summerfield AQ, Marshall DH, et al. Prevalence of permanent childhood hearing impairment in the UK and implications for universal hearing screening. Questionnaire-based ascertainment study. Br Med J 2001; 323:536–539.

19. Gravel JS, Traquina DN. Experience with the audiologic assessment of infants and toddlers. Int J Ped Otorhinolaryngol 1992; 23:59–71.

20. Widen JE, Folsom RC, Cone-Wesson B, et al. Identification of neonatal hearing impairment: hearing status at 8 to 12 months corrected age using a visual reinforcement audiometry protocol. Ear Hear 2000; 21:471–485.

21. Nozza RJ. Development psychoacoustics: science to practice. In: Seewald RC, Gravel J, eds. A Sound Foundation Through Early Amplification. Proceedings of the 2nd Int. Conference, 2001. Great Britain: St. Edmundsbury Press, 2002:37–46.

22. Hickson F. Behavioural tests of hearing. In: Newton VE, ed. Pediatric Audiological Medicine. London & Philadelphia: Wurr Publishers, 2002:91–112.

23. Cone-Wesson B. Paediatric audiology. A review of assessment methods for infants. Audiol Med 2003; 1:25–45.

24. Hall J, Penn T. Neurodiagnostic paediatric audiology. In: Newton VE, ed. Pediatric Audiological Medicine. London & Philadelphia: Wurr Publishers, 2002:113–145.

25. Kuhl PK, Williams KA, Lacerda F, et al. Linguistic experience alters phonetic perception in infants by six months of age. Science 1992; 255:606–608.

26. Gravel J. Potential pitfalls in the audiological assessment of infants and young children. In: Seewald RC, Gravel J, eds. A Sound Foundation Through Early Amplification. Proceedings of the 2nd Int. Conference, 2001. Great Britain: St. Edmundsbury Press, 2002:85–102.

27. France EA, Stephens SDG. All Wales audiology and genetic service for hearing impaired young adults. J Audiol Med 1995; 4:67–84.

28. Parving A. Aetiological diagnosis in hearing-impaired children—clinical value and application of a modern examination programme. Int J Ped Otorhinolaryngol 1984; 7:29–38.

29. Parving A. Factors causing hearing impairment: some perspectives from Europe. J Am Acad Audiol 1995; 6:387–395.

30. Mäki-Torkko EM, Lindholm PK, Väyrynen MRH, et al. Epidemiology of moderate to profound childhood hearing impairments in Northern Finland. Any changes in ten years? Scand Audiol 1998; 27:95–103.

31. Billings KR, Kenna MA. Causes of pediatric sensorineural hearing loss. Arch Otolaryngol Head Neck Surg 1999; 125:517–521.

32. Hutchin T, Telford E, Mueller R. Autosomal recessive nonsyndromic hearing impairment: an overview. Audiol Med 2003; 1:12–20.

33. Van Laer L, Van Camp G. Autosomal dominant nonsyndromic hearing impairment: an overview. Audiol Med 2003; 1:21–28.

34. Lander E, Linton LM, Birren B, et al. Initial sequencing and analysis of the human genome. Nature 2001; 409:860–921.

35. Venter JC, Adams MD, Meyers EW, et al. The sequence of the human genome. Science 2001; 291:1304–1351.

36. Fischel-Ghodsian N. Mitochondrial hearing impairment. Audiol Med 2003; 1:56–66.

37. Petit C, Llevilliers J, Hardelin JP. Molecular genetics of hearing loss. Ann Rev Genet 2001; 35:589–646.

38. Mazzoli M, Van Camp G, Newton V, et al. Recommendations for the description of genetic and audiological data for families with nonsyndromic hereditary hearing impairment. Audiol Med 2003; 1:148–150.

39. Snoeckx R, Huygen P, Feldmen D, et al. The predictability of Connexin 26 hearing loss, the most prevalent form of childhood deafness. AM J Human Genet 2005; 77:945–957.

40. Green GE, Mueller R, Cohn SE, et al. Audiological manifestations and features of Connexin 26 deafness. Audiol Med 2003; 1:5–11.

41. Mazzoli M, Parving A. Genotype-phenotype correlations—can we expect to find them? Audiol Med 2004; 2:255–258.

42. Steel KP. Using mouse mutants to understand the genetics of deafness. In: Tranebjaerg L, Christen-Dalgaard J, Andesen T, Poulsen T. ed. Genetics and the function of the Audiory System. 19th Dauavox Symposium, Holmens, Trykkeri-Denmark, 2002:109–129.

43. Read AP. Lessons about syndromic hearing impairment from shared developmental pathways in other organisms. In: Tranebjaerg L, Christen-Dalgaard J, Andesen T, Paulsen T. ed. Genetics and

the function of the Audiory System. 19th Dauavox Symposium, Holmens, Trykkeri-Denmark, 2002:99–107.

44. McGuirt W, Prasad SD, Gucci RA, et al. Clinical presentation of DFNB1. In: Cremers CWRJ, Smith RJH, eds. Genetic Hearing Impairment—Advances in Oto-Rhino Laryngology. Basel: Karger, 2002:113–119.

45. Denoyelle F, Lina-Granade G, Plauchu H, et al. Connexin 26 gene linked to a dominant deafness. Nature 1998; 393:319–320.

46. Estivill X, Fortina P, Surrey S, et al. Connexin-26 mutations in sporadic and inherited sensorineural deafness. Lancet 1998; 351: 394–398.

47. Mazzoli M, Newton V, Murgia A, et al. Guidelines and recommendations for testing of CX26 mutations and interpretation of results. Int J Ped Otorhinolaryngol 2004; 68:1397–1398.

48. Ludman CN. Recent advances in magnetic resonance imaging of the inner ear. Audiol Med 2000; 9:191–204.

49. Phelps P. Radiological abnormalities of the ear. In: Newton VE, ed. Pediatric Audiological Medicine. London & Philadelphia: Wurr Publishers, 2002:36–64.

50. Pendred V. Deaf mutism and goitre. Lancet 1896; 532:ii.

51. Stinckens C, Huygen P, Van-Camp G, Cremers CWRJ. Pendred syndrome redefined. Report of a new family with fluctuating and progressive hearing loss. In: Cremers CWRJ, Smith RJH, eds Genetic Hearing Impairment—Advances in Oto-Rhino Laryngology. Basel: Karger, 2002:131–141.

52. Toriello HV, Reardon W, Gorlin RJ. Hereditary hearing loss and its syndromes. 2nd ed. Oxford University Press Inc., 2004.

53. Robin NH, Smith RJH, Matthews AL. Genetic testing for deafness in clinical practice. Audiol Med 2003; 1:89–93.

54. http://webhost.ua.ac.be/hhh.

55. ACMG statement. Genetics evaluation guidelines for the etiologic diagnosis of congenital hearing loss. Genet Med 2002; 4: 162–171.

56. Schimmenti LA, Martinez A, Fox MS, et al. Genetic testing as part of the early hearing detection and intervention (EHDI) process. Genet Med 2004; 6:521–525.

57. Robin NH. Genetic testing for deafness is here, but how do we do it? Genet Med 2004; 6:463–464.

58. Jones L. Future perfect: social aspects of genetics and deafness. In: Stephens D, Jones L, ed. The Impact of Genetic Hearing Impairment. London: Whurr Publisher, 2005:1–10.

59. Middleton A, Hewison J Mueller R. Prenatal diagnosis for inherited deafness-what is the potential demand? J Genet Counseling 2001; 10:121–131.

60. Middleton A. Parents' attitudes towards genetic testing and the impact of deafness in the family. In: Stephens D, Jones L, eds. The Impact of Genetic Hearing Impairment. London: Whurr Publisher, 2005:11–53.

61. Brunger JW, Murray GS, O'Riordan MA, et al. Parental attitudes toward genetic testing for pediatric deafness. Am J Hum Genetics 2000; 67:1621–1625.

15 What genetic testing can offer

Paolo Gasparini, Andrew P Read

Why perform genetic testing in hearing impairment?

Genetic testing in both children and adults with hearing loss can be very helpful to patients and their families. DNA analysis can make it possible to identify the molecular basis of nonsyndromal hearing impairment (NSHI), for which an accurate genetic diagnosis is impossible on the basis of clinical features alone. Moreover, syndromal forms that lack the typical clinical features in childhood or present atypically can also be identified through molecular testing. Even when the test result does not lead to specific decisions on management or reproductive options, much clinical genetic experience underlines the benefit to families of knowing the cause of a condition. A clear genetic diagnosis puts an end to the searching and questioning over what went wrong and whether somebody is to blame and allows the family to move on. It is clear that with the widespread implementation of newborn hearing screening, the demand for genetic testing will increase significantly (1). Considering the current lack of guidelines for follow-up testing and the variability of implementation, for the next few years, a decision on whether or not to perform genetic testing will depend mainly on the audiological physician or ENT clinician. This will require familiarity with the molecular diagnostic options available and the probability of each individual assay being able to find causative mutations.

Molecular genetic testing is minimally invasive. It can often be performed on a very small amount of blood obtained through venepuncture or from a neonatal blood spot card or on a cheek brush sample or even saliva. With each passing year, DNA testing becomes more comprehensive and relevant through the implementation of new diagnostic technologies and increasing knowledge about the genes involved and their spectra of mutations (2). Finally, as genetic testing for hearing loss becomes more widely accepted and available, genotype–phenotype correlations can be made more reliably and the physical effect of individual mutations, or combinations of mutations, can be predicted with greater confidence.

Once the cause of hearing loss has been identified, genetic counselling can be more specific. Matters covered may include the chance of recurrence in a future pregnancy, the expected course (progressive vs. nonprogressive, possible eventual involvement of other organs or systems), and an evaluation of the pedigree to assess which other family members may potentially benefit from the same test. In some cases, the DNA diagnosis may affect the type and timing of treatment, with potentially major benefits to the patient.

Thus, summarising, molecular diagnostic testing has revolutionised the ability of clinicians to provide insight into the aetiology of hearing impairments. State-of-the-art molecular testing is now available for the most common causes of hereditary hearing impairment. In addition, family studies can be performed for less common causes of hearing impairment. The benefits of genetic testing include the following:

- Providing an accurate diagnosis of the aetiology of the hearing impairment
- Avoiding the need for more expensive and invasive testing
- Providing the basis for prognostic information about future hearing
- Giving direction and improving genetic counselling
- Defining new guidelines for treatment

What is genetic testing?

Genetic testing is the process by which our unique genetic code (the sequence of A, G, C, and T nucleotides that make up our DNA) is examined to discover the cause of a particular genetic disorder. It is estimated that humans have about 24,000 genes, and several thousand of these may be involved in enabling the sense of hearing to function. Most will also have other functions, but some will function specifically in the hearing mechanism. Mutations in genes required exclusively for hearing are likely to cause NSHI, while those that are also performing other functions may cause syndromal hearing loss when mutated. Evidence from family studies suggests that at least 100 genes may, when mutated, cause NSHI. To date, mutations in some 50 different genes have been identified as causes of some cases of NSHI.

Any one genetic test focuses on one particular small segment of DNA and asks if it has any sequence variant that might be pathogenic. The central problem in genetic testing is seeing this one small piece of DNA of interest—typically a few hundred base pairs—against a background of the huge amount (6×10^9 base pairs) of irrelevant DNA in every cell. There are two general solutions to this:

- Selectively amplify the sequence of interest to such an extent that the sample consists largely of copies of that sequence.
- Pick out the sequence of interest by hybridising it to a matching sequence that is labelled, e.g., with a fluorescent dye.

In the past, selective amplification was achieved by cloning the sequence into a bacterium, but nowadays, the "polymerase chain reaction" (PCR) is universally used. For details of this technique, see S&R2 Section 6.1 (Basic features of PCR; see Bibliography); for present purposes, it suffices to know that PCR allows the investigator to amplify any chosen sequence of up to a few kilobases (1000 base pairs) to any desired degree in a few hours. All that is necessary is to know a few details of the actual nucleotide sequence that is to be amplified and to order some specific reagents (PCR primers) from one of the firms that custom-produce these. Almost all genetic testing involves PCR, although some companies make kits based on alternative methods, mainly to avoid the royalty payments required of users of the patented PCR process. The major limitation of PCR is that it can only be used to amplify sequences of, at most, a few kilobases. It is not possible to PCR-amplify a whole gene (average size 27 kb), still less a whole chromosome (average size 100,000 kb).

"Hybridisation" depends on the fact that the two strands of the DNA double helix can be separated ("denatured") by brief boiling, and when the resulting single-stranded DNA solution is cooled, each Watson strand will try to find a matching Crick strand. If a dye-labelled single strand corresponding to the sequence of interest (a "probe") is added, some of the test DNA will stick to the probe, and by using the label, it can be isolated, followed, or characterised. Hybridisation was important in the now largely obsolete technique of Southern blotting and has regained importance as the principle behind microarrays ("gene chips").

Various applications of PCR and/or hybridisation make it relatively straightforward to check any predetermined short stretch of a person's DNA—but the key word is "short." As described in Chapter 1, the coding sequence of almost all genes is divided into short segments called exons, which are spaced out along the DNA of a chromosome. Genes can have any number of exons, from 1 to over 100. In general, each exon of a gene must be the subject of a separate PCR amplification and check on its sequence. When DNA is sequenced, a maximum of around 500 to 700 bp can be sequenced in a single test. Details of how these methods work are given in S&R2 Sections 6.3 (DNA sequencing) and 17.1 (Direct testing is like any other pathology laboratory investigation a sample from the patient is tested to see if it is normal or abnormal) but the key point to appreciate is that our ability to answer questions about a

person's DNA depends crucially on the precision with which the question is posed.

DNA technology is developing very fast. Sequencing and genotyping become cheaper every year and new technologies allow both to be done on scales that were unthinkable a few years ago. Some companies claim to be developing methods that would allow a person's entire genome to be sequenced in a few days for a few thousand dollars. Optimists and pessimists alike dream of the day when everybody's complete genome sequence will be stored in vast databases—they differ only in their reaction to this prospect. Among all this heady talk, it is important to remember that DNA analysis can reveal only those things about us that are genetically determined.

When should genetic testing be performed?

It would be tempting to ask the laboratory to determine whether a patient has any genetic cause for his/her hearing loss, and whether this can be tested at a molecular level. But such a general question is unanswerable in any diagnostic setting—it might well be too challenging even for a PhD project. The problem is the great heterogeneity of genetic hearing loss. Genetic heterogeneity takes two forms:

- "*Locus heterogeneity*" is where the same clinical condition can be caused by mutations in any one of a number of genes. NSHI is a prime example.
- "*Allelic heterogeneity*" is when a condition is caused by mutations in one particular gene, but different unrelated patients have different sequence variants in that gene. Some forms of syndromal hearing impairment fall into this category.

All too often, both forms of heterogeneity are present. As mentioned above, our ability to answer questions about a person's DNA depends crucially on the precision with which the question is posed, and genetic heterogeneity is the major factor limiting the applications of genetic testing in hearing impairment.

Ideally, the laboratory should be asked to check for the presence or absence of a specific mutation (sequence variant) in a specific gene. Any one of a variety of PCR-based methods allows such a question to be answered efficiently and cheaply in a few hours. The main circumstance in which it is possible to ask such a specific question is if somebody is being tested to see if they have inherited a mutation that has already been defined by the study of other family members. Additionally, there are some diseases that depend on such a specific pathogenic mechanism that they can only be caused by one specific DNA sequence change. Sickle-cell disease and Huntington disease are examples. The nearest approximation to this in hearing impairment is a specific mutation (g.1555A > G) in the DNA of the mitochondria that leads to extreme sensitivity to the ototoxic effects of aminoglycoside antibiotics.

Although NSHI shows extreme genetic heterogeneity, many patients with autosomal recessive NSHI carry mutations in the GJB2 gene, which encodes the protein Connexin 26 (DFNB1 locus). The actual percentages vary markedly, on the basis of the ethnic origin of the tested individuals, but in southern Europe, in particular, more than half of all affected individuals have mutations in this gene. Moreover, specific GJB2 mutations are common in different populations. In Caucasians, the c.35delG mutation is the most prevalent, with a high carrier frequency demonstrated in Estonia and in all Mediterranean countries; in Ashkenazi Jews, the most prevalent mutation is c.167delT while most East Asian cases carry the c.235delC mutation. Gypsies are another population group with their own common mutation in GJB2.

A large variety of molecular diagnostic assays are available to test the GJB2 gene. Many of these are tests for specific mutations, but multiplexed so that a number of different mutations are checked in a single operation. Allele-specific assays such as PCR followed by restriction enzyme digestion, allele-specific PCR, primer extension, or real-time PCR are all relatively fast, cost effective, highly sensitive, and specific. The mutation panel needs to be appropriate for the population being tested. Although these allele-specific methods are widely used and can be appropriate, testing that checks only for the most common GJB2 mutations is often too limiting to find the full complement of mutations in the majority of patients. The GJB2 gene is fairly simple to analyse exhaustively because it is small and has only two exons. Direct DNA sequencing allows the detection of almost all point mutations, small deletions, and insertions and is ideal for this small gene. Due to recessive inheritance, two pathogenic mutations are expected in order to make the molecular diagnosis with certainty (3). GJB2 plays a prominent role in the aetiology of NSHI and its analysis should be the first step in molecular diagnostic testing.

It is important to note that when only one GJB2 mutation can be identified, despite sequencing both copies of the whole gene, the hearing loss may be due to other causes and the individual may be a coincidental carrier of a GJB2 sequence variant. This is not a rare occurrence, especially for the common mutations, which have a high carrier frequency in the general population. Before reaching this uncertain conclusion, however, it is preferable to investigate whether a large deletion in the adjacent GJB6 gene (which encodes the protein Connexin 30) is present. This has been shown to be quite a common cause of NSHI, in conjunction with a single GJB2 mutation or occasionally in homozygous form (4). The high carrier rate in the general population also explains the occasional examples of "pseudo-dominant" inheritance, where autosomal recessive NSHI occurs in two or more generations of a family—such a pedigree pattern is a strong indication for testing the GJB2 and GJB6 genes. Finally, we should note that extensive phenotype–genotype studies have shown that it is possible to broadly predict the hearing impairment associated with GJB2 mutations on the basis of the specific genotype (5). In conclusion, genetic testing of the GJB2 gene and the GJB6 gene should be considered in the evaluation of all individuals with congenital NSHI.

Locus heterogeneity poses a major problem for current testing technologies. With syndromal hearing impairment, it is often possible to define a single candidate gene: EYA1 for branchio-oto-renal syndrome, PAX3 for type 1 Waardenburg syndrome, TCOF1 for Treacher Collins syndrome, and so on. Nevertheless, even for well-defined syndromes, there is often some degree of locus heterogeneity; for example, type 1 Usher syndrome can be caused by mutations in any one of at least eight genes. For NSHI, either dominant or recessive, locus heterogeneity is a serious obstacle. Family studies of dominant NSHI have confirmed that, as with recessive loss, heterogeneity is high, but unlike in autosomal recessive NSHI, no single gene has been identified that is responsible for a high proportion of cases.

Occasionally, careful examination can provide a pointer to a candidate gene:

- Mutations in WFS1 are found in 75% of families in which autosomal dominant NSHI initially affects low frequencies while sparing high frequencies.
- Mutations in SLC26A4 are associated with inner-ear defects (enlarged/dilated vestibular aqueduct and Mondini dysplasia).

Detection of these temporal bone anomalies by computed tomography examination should prompt consideration of molecular genetic testing. SLC26A4 mutations cause Pendred syndrome but can also cause nonsyndromal recessive hearing impairment (DFNB4 locus). SLC26A4-related hearing impairment is likely to be underdiagnosed at present. Molecular testing of this gene should be considered in unresolved cases, especially in conjunction with imaging studies.

Allelic heterogeneity, creating the need to scan an entire gene for mutations that might be anywhere, is more or less of a problem depending on the size and complexity of the gene. For mutation scanning, direct DNA sequencing is considered the gold standard, but it has the disadvantage of potentially missing deletions of entire exons or genes; also the cost is significant, and the interpretation is complex and relatively labour intensive. Other screening methods such as, for example, denaturing high performance liquid chromatography can be used to provide a quick initial screen and reduce the sequencing load. Sometimes a two-stage protocol can be used: the majority of SLC26A4 mutations are clustered in 4 of the 20 coding exons, so costs can be contained by first analysing the commonly affected exons and analysing the remaining part of the gene only when necessary.

Many other genes, when mutated, cause hearing impairment and a similar approach can be used: allele-specific tests for a limited panel of mutations, if the epidemiology justifies this, or systematic sequencing of the gene to search for any mutation. Inherited diseases, in general, including genetic hearing impairment, belong to two different groups according to the number of mutations present in the causative gene/s: those characterised by high allelic heterogeneity and those for which one or few common alleles have been detected (due to founder effect or mutational hot-spot). In the first case, it is necessary to screen each patient for a large number of mutations, while in the latter case, it could be more useful to have a testing technology able to analyse a large number of individuals for the same mutation.

Although molecular genetic testing is available for a number of other genes implicated in hearing impairment, the large size of many genes (*MYO7A*, *MYO15*, *MYO6*, *MYH14*, etc.) and their low relative contribution to hearing impairment (*OTOF*, *HDIA1*, *TECTA*, *COCH*, *POU4F3*, etc.) make it impractical to offer such testing on a clinical basis at this time. Updated information on tests available can be obtained through the Gene Tests website (http://www.genetests.org/) (6).

New approaches for genetic testing

Genetics and molecular medicine have an expanding need for technologies that allow rapid genotyping, mutation analysis, and DNA sequencing. The keys to high throughput screening lie in miniaturisation, parallelisation and automation. Conventional methods for mutation detection, such as direct sequencing, single strand conformation polymorphism, denaturing gradient gel electrophoresis, or chemical cleavage are labour intensive (7) and handle only one or a few samples at a time. A promising alternative technology uses oligonucleotide microarrays. Microarray assays are based on nucleic acid hybridisation (8–10) or hybridisation coupled with an enzyme-mediated reaction (11–13). One of the most currently successful and widely used variants of this technology is arrayed primer extension (APEX) (14). An array of oligonucleotides is immobilised on a glass surface. DNA from individuals to be investigated is amplified by PCR, digested enzymatically, and annealed to the immobilised primers. A DNA polymerase is then used to extend each primer by adding a single modified nucleotide. The modified nucleotides are dideoxynucleotides, ensuring that the polymerase reaction can add only a single nucleotide to each primer, and the four dideoxynucleotides each carry a different fluorescent label. After the primer extension reaction, a mutation is detected by a change in the colour code of the primer sites. APEX arrays have been developed for detection of mutations in several genes such as β-globin and the *TP53* tumour suppressor (15,16). It is also possible to invert the target and probe configuration by arraying aminomodified PCR products on slides, so as to check for the same mutation in a large number of samples. Very recently, Asper Biotech Ltd. (Tartu, Estonia) has developed a highly sensitive and specific assay that addresses multiple mutations in multiple genes causative for hearing impairment. It evaluates a panel of hundreds of mutations underlying sensorineural (largely nonsyndromal) hearing impairment in a series of genes including *GJB2*, *GJB6*, *GJB3*, *GJA1*, *SLC26A4*, *SLC26A5*, and the mitochondrial genome. Because the spectrum of mutations checked is much larger than most laboratories currently offer, the APEX microarray could possibly double the current mutation detection rate. The assay is robust, relatively inexpensive, and easily modifiable.

The APEX technique belongs to the category of passive methodologies, which have an intrinsic limit to the degree to which hybridisation speed and selectivity can be improved. Recently, "active" microelectronic chip devices that use electric fields have been developed (Nanochip from Nanogen). They facilitate (*i*) the rapid transport and selective addressing of DNA probes to any position or test site on the array surface; (*ii*) acceleration of the basic hybridisation process; and (*iii*) the ability to rapidly discriminate single base mismatches in target DNA sequences. These new "active" devices will further improve the use of micro devices in diagnostics and help in screening large numbers of individuals at a low cost and with great accuracy. An example of Nanochip results is given in Figure 15.1, in which the detection of a common polymorphism (M34T mutation) within the Connexin 26 gene is reported.

Finally, another example of an array-based hearing impairment assay is a gene chip capable of holding 28,000 anchored oligonucleotide probes. This array allows rapid screening of nine genes and is being developed on the Affymetrix platform (Affymetrix Corp.) A validation study of this approach is ongoing at Cincinatti Children's Hospital Medical Center in collaboration with Harvard Partners Group in Boston (17). Although it is hard to predict exactly which technologies will emerge as dominant over the next decade, we can be fairly confident that the extensive locus and allelic heterogeneity of NSHI will steadily become less of an obstacle and will allow the benefits of genetic testing to be much more widely disseminated.

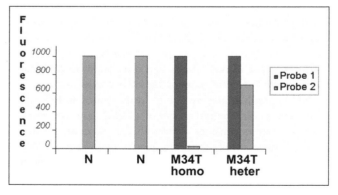

Figure 15.1

References

1. Baroch KA. Universal newborn hearing screening: fine-tuning the process. Curr Opin Otolaryngol Head Neck Surg 2003; 11: 424–427.

2. Schrijver I. Hereditary non-syndromic sensorineural hearing loss: transforming silence to sound. J Mol Diagn 2004; 6:275–284.

3. Del Castillo I, Moreno-Pelayo MA, Del Castillo FJ, et al. Prevalence and evolutionary origins of the del(*GJB6–D13S1830*) mutation in the DFNB1 locus in hearing-impaired subjects: a multicenter study. Am J Hum Genet 2003; 73:1452–1458.

4. Pandya A, Arnos KS, Xia XJ, et al. Frequency and distribution of *GJB2* (Connexin 26) and *GJB6* (Connexin 30) mutations in a large North American repository of deaf probands. Genet Med 2003; 5:295–303.

5. Snoeckx RL, Huygen PL, Feldmann D et al. *GJB2* mutations and degree of hearing loss: a multicenter study. Am J Hum Genet 2005; 77:945–57.

6. http://www.genetests.org/

7. Mutation Detection: A Practical Approach. Cotton RGD, Edkins E, Forrest S, eds. New York: Oxford University Press, 1998.

8. Chee M, Yang R, Hubbell E, et al. Accessing genetic information with high-density DNA arrays. Science 1996:274:610–614.

9. Cronin MT, Fucini RV, Kim SM, Masino RS, Wespi RM, Miyada CG. Cystic fibrosis mutation detection by hybridization to light-generated DNA probe arrays. Hum Mutat 1996; 7:244–255.

10. Hacia JG, Brody LC, Chee MS, Fodor SP, Collins FS. Detection of heterozygous mutations in BRCA1 using high-density oligonucleotide arrays and two-colour fluorescence analysis. Nat Genet 1996; 14:441–447.

11. Shumaker JM, Metspalu A, Caskey CT. Mutation detection by solid phase primer extension. Hum Mutat 1996; 7:346–354.

12. Head SR, Rogers YH, Parikh K, et al. Nested genetic bit analysis (N-GBA) for mutation detection in the p53 tumor suppressor gene. Nucleic Acids Res 1997; 25:5065–5071.

13. Pastinen T, Kurg A, Metspalu A, Peltonen L, Syvanen AC. Minisequencing: a specific tool for DNA analysis and diagnostics on oligonucleotide arrays. Genome Res 1997; 7:606–614.

14. Kurg A, Tonisson N, Georgiou I, Shumaker J, Tollett J, Metspalu A. Arrayed primer extension: solid-phase four-color DNA resequencing and mutation detection technology. Genet Test 2000; 4:1–7.

15. Tonisson N, Zernant J, Kurg A, et al. Evaluating the arrayed primer extension resequencing assay of TP53 tumor suppressor gene. Proc Natl Acad Sci USA 2002; 99:5503–5508.

16. Shumaker JM, Tollet JJ, Filbin KJ, Montague-Smith MP, Pirrung MC. APEX disease gene resequencing: mutations in exon 7 of the p53 tumor suppressor gene. Bioorg Med Chem 2001; 9:2269–2278.

17. Shafer DN. Genetic hearing test moves ahead: goal is to identify sensorineural hearing loss earlier. ASHA 2005; 5:27.

Bibliography

S&R: Strachan T, Read AP. Human Molecular Genetics. 3rd ed. Garland, 2004. The 2nd ed. ("S&R2"; Bios Scientific Publishers, 2000) is freely available as full searchable text at http://www.ncbi.nlm.nih.gov/entrez/query.fcgi?db = Books. Because of this ready availability, in this chapter references are given to this edition.

16 Pharmacotherapy of the inner ear

Ilmari Pyykkö, Esko Toppila, Jing Zou, Erna Kentala

Introduction

The auditory system seems better equipped to deal with injuries in lower species than in mammals. In fish and amphibians, the inner ear will produce new sensory cells (hair cells) throughout their life and, consequently, injured cells can be replaced continuously. Birds lose this ability during embryonic development, but possess the capacity to replace the injured sensory cells by regeneration and thus maintain hearing function. In contrast, mammalian hair cell loss has always been considered irreversible.

The mechanism of cell death in the cochlea is produced in two ways: through "necrotic cell death" mediated by very loud noise, or "apoptosis," mediated by the activation of cysteine protease family within the cells, the caspases [very loud noise can also induce immediate apoptosis (1)]. Originally these mechanisms, necrosis versus apoptosis, were thought to operate with different initiators (as an extrinsic cellular pathway and an intrinsic cellular pathway, respectively), but it may be assumed that these mechanisms are more or less under statistical control in that dependent on the characteristics of the stimulus the extent of cell death and damages is brought about by one of these two major mechanisms. Each of these mechanisms provides the possibility to reduce and, in some cases, to prevent cochlear cell death through active intervention with pharmacotherapy.

Recently, many researchers have investigated the role of antioxidant agents in different models of peripheral hearing disorders. It has been found that antioxidants protect the cochlea from noise-induced trauma, as well as cisplatin and aminoglycoside exposure (2–4). Van De Water et al. recently suggested that protection of auditory sensory cells from cisplatin is carried out at the molecular level by three mechanisms: prevention of reactive oxygen species (ROS) formation; neutralisation of toxic products, and blockage of apoptotic pathways (5).

Several genes regulate the differentiation of cochlear hair cells and supporting cells from their common precursor cells during mammalian embryogenesis. Recent experiments have provided new and exciting information about the processes related to inner ear damage. For example, in the mammalian vestibular system, hair cell regeneration has been shown to occur under certain circumstances (6). The situation in the auditory system is less clear. There is evidence of hair cell regeneration in newborn mice given explants of cochlear duct (7) and in replacing the damaged hair cells by converting the supporting cells (8). A key gene is Atoh1 (also known as Math1). This is the mouse homologue of the drosophila gene atonal that encodes a basic helix-loop-helix transcription factor (9). Overexpression of Atoh1 in nonsensory cells of the normal cochlea generates new hair cells, both in vitro and in vivo. Atoh1 has been shown to act as a "prohair cell gene" and is required for the differentiation of hair cells from multipotent progenitors. Recently, Izumikawa et al. (2005) demonstrated that in mammals by using gene therapy, the lost hair cells will regenerate and that hearing may be returned to the profoundly deaf mammalian ear (10). This finding opens new perspectives for the treatment of hearing loss and justifies the efforts to encapsulate nucleotides encoding the Math1 gene within the nanostructures for the treatment of deafness.

In addition, a moderate degree of spontaneous recovery of hearing after noise trauma has been observed in humans, implying that humans may also have the capacity to regain hearing function (11). However, the mechanisms behind the recovery have not yet been fully delineated. There is, however, substantial evidence that cochlear damage induced by noise can be prevented by the application of different pharmacologically active substances (12). Thus, there are grounds to expect that hearing disorders in mammals may, under certain circumstances, be successfully treated.

Drugs can reach the inner ear by systemic application (orally, intravenously, or via the cerebrospinal fluid) or locally [from the middle ear over the round window membrane (RWM) through permeation, direct injection through the RWM or the oval window, and also with an osmotic pump by passing through the lateral wall of the cochlea]. However, not all of these approaches are clinically possible.

Mechanisms of noise-induced hearing loss

Normal auditory stimulation elicits pressure differences across the cochlear partition causing a number of mechanical events within the organ of Corti: vibrations, shearing motion, and deflection of the stereocilia (13). The end result is excitation of the outer and inner hair cells and, following release of transmitter substances, increased activity in the cochlear nerve. The outer hair cells are activated and react in a linear manner to sinusoidal sound stimulation with one impulse to one sinusoid up to 1000 Hz. At higher frequencies, other mechanisms are involved in coding the amplification of the signal. These are not known in detail.

Assisting the tight coupling between the tectorial membrane and the basilar membrane, the tips of the stereocilia of the outer hair cells are buried within the tegmentum. The contractions of the outer hair cell bodies amplify the basilar membrane vibration and transduce the vibration to shear forces that will activate the inner hair cells. The perceived and actively enhanced basilar membrane vibration is transmitted into the central auditory system and is perceived as sound. The role of the supporting cells is not clear yet but they may serve as a supporting organ to provide stability and damping of excessive vibration. Damage to the cochlea may also lead to hyperacusis and we hypothesise that this symptom may be linked to supporting cell damage (Fig. 16.1).

Obviously, noise or excessive auditory stimulation will elicit shear forces in the cochlea but at much larger amplitudes. There are two fundamentally different ways by which overstimulation may lead to cochlear injury: mechanical or metabolic (14). Intense noise exceeding 125 dB sound pressure level (SPL) in animal experiments leads to large amplitude vibration that may mechanically alter or disrupt cochlear structures causing mechanical damage to cell membranes and nerve endings and disturb the blood circulation. Cellular distortion, disorganisation of the stereocilia, and possible rupture of cell membranes

disable the cochlear fluid barriers and will cause immediate reduction of auditory sensitivity (15).

At SPLs of less than 125 dB, sound-induced overstimulation and overactivity of the cochlea can result in disturbed cochlear homeostasis and subsequent functional impairment in the absence of direct and immediate mechanical damage. Experimental evidence suggests a critical level about 125 dB SPL, at which the cause of damage changes from predominantly metabolic to mechanical (16). Thus, at moderate SPLs, damage would mainly be caused by metabolic mechanisms while at higher levels, mechanical mechanisms would predominate. As changes in homeostasis may also occur in mechanical trauma and the effects of metabolic stress are also likely to be expressed as mechanical damage, it is not meaningful to make a strict separation between metabolic and mechanical causes of noise-induced hearing loss.

When the metabolic and/or mechanical stress is too large, the cells will die and a permanent hearing loss results. Cell death is a result of either apoptosis or necrosis. Apoptosis is a strictly controlled process to eliminate dysfunctional cells without affecting the surrounding tissue. It can be viewed as a counterbalance to cell division, and a disturbance may, for example, result in degenerative disorders or tumour growth. Necrosis on the other hand is a more passive type of cell death, involving a rapid and disorganised breakdown of a cell, often as a consequence of acute trauma (toxic substances, ischaemia, etc.). As the cell contents are released directly into the surrounding tissue and an inflammatory reaction usually follows. Thus, for the organism, apoptosis is the preferred method when it is necessary to eliminate cells. In the auditory system, there is no conclusive evidence that apoptosis does play a significant role. Structural observations of DNA fragmentation may suggest the involvement of either apoptotic or necrotic mechanisms during peri- and postnatal development of the inner ear (17). A recent study on autopsy materials from subjects with no history of acoustic trauma suggests that apoptosis does not contribute significantly to the regulation of the cell population in the normal adult inner ear (18). Nevertheless, apoptosis may be involved during noise-induced trauma, although there is to date no direct evidence in humans.

Changes in cochlear blood flow have generally been suggested as contributing to noise-induced hearing loss (19). Recent findings have clearly demonstrated noise-induced alterations in the cochlear microcirculation causing local ischaemia (20). The effect varies with the intensity and duration of the exposure, but when vascular insufficiency is manifest, the reduced oxygen and energy supply to the cochlea and the accumulation of metabolites will be accompanied by severe functional alterations. It has been shown experimentally that applying drugs blocking vasoconstriction prevents a noise-induced microcirculatory disorder and maintains normal hearing (21). However, the exact role of local blood flow alterations is unclear and it should be noted that it has been observed that hearing loss and cochlear hypoxia may actually precede changes in cochlear blood flow (22).

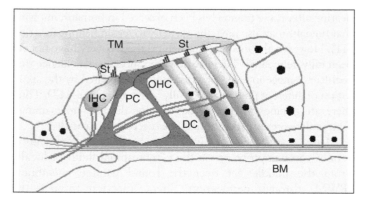

Figure 16.1 Schematic drawing of organ of Corti. *Abbreviations*: BM, basilar membrane, DC, dieters cells; IHC, inner hair cells; OHC, outer hair cells; PC, pillar cell; ST, stereocilia; TM, tectorial membrane.

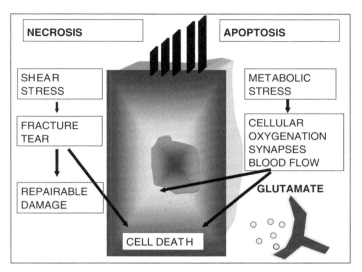

Figure 16.2 Schematic drawing representing the necrotic and apoptotic cell death mechanisms, as excitotoxicity caused by glutamate.

Table 16.1 Comparison between apoptosis and necrosis

Apoptosis	Necrosis
May happen under both physiological and pathological conditions	Only happens under pathological conditions
A gene-directed process	Not a gene-directed process
An energy-dependent process	Not an energy-dependent process
Protein synthesis is increased	Protein synthesis is decreased
ATP content is normal	ATP content is decreased
Single cell involved	Several cells involved
A delayed degeneration process	An immediate degeneration process
Cellular shrinkage	Cellular oedema
Organelles are intact	Organelles are destroyed
Chromatin condensation	Chromatin destruction
Late membrane damage	Early membrane damage
Does not cause inflammation	Causes inflammation

Abbreviation: ATP, adenosine triphosphate.

There are several mechanisms leading to cellular damage after acoustical overstimulation (Fig. 16.2). The damage can be repaired or can be irreversible leading to cell death. Some of the mechanisms are mainly related to metabolic changes, e.g., oxidative stress, synaptic hyperactivity, and altered cochlear blood flow, while others are predominantly mechanical. It is likely, however, that the resulting damage to the auditory system is partly mediated by similar mechanisms irrespective of the cause. Although definite evidence of a common final pathway is missing, experimental data suggest that free radicals and other highly reactive endogenous substances play a significant role in noise-induced hearing loss.

The mechanisms causing cell death through necrosis are fundamentally different from those in apoptosis. Table 16.1 summarises the differences. The apoptotic mechanism is, in the developmental stage and in some disease stages, such as in cancer or granulomatous infection (for example in tuberculosis), a normal and vital part of life. With these mechanisms, the body shelters from infection, eliminates small tumours, and controls the growth of larger tumours.

Apoptotic mechanisms and free radicals

It is well known, from other biological systems, that reactive oxygen metabolites (ROMs) are important mediators of cell injury. ROMs are free radicals or other molecules, which have a chemical structure, making them extremely reactive. As they react very easily with cellular components such as lipids, proteins, and DNA, they are potentially cytotoxic. ROMs are produced continuously as part of normally occurring reactions, e.g., in the mitochondria. However, protection is offered by several endogenous antioxidants. These are either enzymes

catalysing reactions to neutralise the ROM, or scavengers binding them. When there is an imbalance between the production of ROMs and the endogenous protective mechanisms, the tissue is under oxidative stress. Increased ROM production can cause cell death, whereas overactive protective mechanisms may lead to tumour growth. In the auditory system, there are several reports demonstrating both elevated levels of either ROMs or antioxidants following noise exposure (23), and reduced hearing loss by treatments increasing the antioxidant level (24).

The key element in apoptosis is the caspase-induced cell death pathway. Caspases consist of a family of cysteine proteases that are present in the cells in an inactive form. In short, when the cell is damaged, a lethal chain reaction occurs that is triggered by activation of *Bax* gene. In the reaction, apaf-1 interacts with cytochrome C that is located on the mitochondrial surface, the complex interacts with procaspase-9 (a complex called to apoptosome) that cleaves and results in the caspase-9 that finally activates the caspase-3 through cleavage of some other procaspases. The "killer" caspase-3 reacts with the mitochondrial membrane and causes membrane lysis by liberating the lysosome enzymes from the cell leading to degradation of DNA and the proteins and disintegration of the cell (Fig. 16.3).

There are today 14 members of caspase family, but not all members of caspase family participate in the apoptosis, as caspase-1 and -11 function in the regulation of cytokines. The initiator includes caspase-9 and -8 and the effector includes

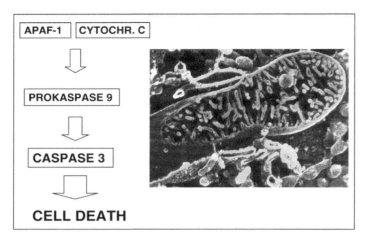

Figure 16.3 A diagram showing activation of caspase pathway in the final apoptotic pathway leading to disintegration of the cell.

caspase-3, -6, and -7. The initiation of the caspase reaction can be regulated by the external cell death receptor pathway through the Fas ligand—receptor activation or through the intrinsic cell death pathway [the mitogen-activated protein kinase (MAPK)/Jun N-terminal kinases (JNK) pathway]. Both these pathways trigger responses that lead to final stage activation of caspase-3 that acts as the executioner molecule for the cell. Nevertheless, caspase-3 appears to participate in the normal development and maturation of the membranous labyrinth and its cochleovestibular ganglion, so that a loss of function mutation of the gene for caspase-3 could result in maldevelopment of the inner ear and a hearing deficit.

ROS and the caspase-induced cell death pathway

Oxidative stress is a key factor in apoptosis with the creation of ROS and other free radicals (e.g., hydroxyl radical), which activate the apoptotic pathway through cellular mechanisms that are linked to caspase activation (5). These ROS and other radicals damage the affected cell's organelles and internal membranes resulting in mitochondrial membrane damage and a loss of the membrane potential. This loss of mitochondrial membrane integrity results in a release of cytochrome C from the damaged mitochondria into the cytoplasm. Once cytochrome C enters the cytoplasm, it combines with a facilitating molecule termed apoptotic protease-activating factor-1, dATP (an energy-supplying molecule), and procaspase-9 to form the apoptosome (also known as the aposome), which cleaves procaspase-9 and generates activated caspase-9 (25). A small mitochondrial "proapoptosis molecule" facilitates apoptosis of an affected cell by inhibiting some of the damaged cell's naturally occurring caspase-inhibitory molecules (e.g., NIAP-neuronal inhibitor of apoptosis protein). Once procaspase-9 has been activated, its downstream targets are effector caspases, e.g.,

caspase-3, -6, and -7 (26). The naturally occurring cellular apoptosis-inhibitory proteins are thought to target activated effector caspases such as caspases-3 and -7 for deactivation (27).

The activated effector caspases can interact with a large number of targets within an affected cell to bring about its destruction by apoptosis. Some of the cellular molecules targeted by the caspases are summarised by van de Water et al. (5) as: poly (ADP-ribose) polymerase (PARP-1); DNA within the nucleus and a DNA repair enzyme; nuclear lamin molecule A, B, and C; DNA fragmentation factor 45; inhibitor of caspase-activated DNase; receptor-interacting protein; DNA topoisomerase; signal transducer and activator of transcription-1; Rb; X-linked inhibitor of apoptosis; U1 small nucleoprotein; fodrin; vimentin; and procaspase-2, -6, and -10. Caspase-3 has been suggested as being the primary executioner in most cellular apoptosis during both normal developmental cell death and the removal of damaged cells after injury (i.e., apoptosis) (25).

Hu et al. examined noise trauma–initiated apoptosis of cochlear outer hair cells in the chinchilla (28). In a double-labelled study, the authors localised the activated caspase-3 to the cell bodies of damaged hair cells undergoing apoptosis. The results show a relationship between post–noise exposure progression of hair cell loss, apoptosis of damaged hair cells, and activation of caspase-3. The study also demonstrated that activation of caspase-3 persists for at least two days after the initial noise trauma exposure. There was a correlation between post–exposure loss of noise-damaged outer hair cells, apoptotic changes in the outer hair cell nuclei, and the presence of activated caspase-3, -8, and -9 in the cell bodies of damaged sensory cells. The finding also indicates that the treatment window for noise-induced apoptosis of cochlea lasts at least two days.

The MAPK/JNK-induced cell death pathway

The extrinsic cell pathway involves the binding of cell death receptors that are members of tumour necrosis factors (TNF)-α pathway. In this, there are two receptors in the cell that are both activated in the shear stress injury by TNF-α, the type 1 (p55 receptor pathway) and type 2 (p75 receptor pathway). As in most instances in upregulation of cellular function, one leads to cell death and the other tries to rescue the cell. The TNF-α type 1 receptor pathway is the apoptotic pathway. TNF, through its two types of receptors, activates two signalling pathways within cells (29). One, linked to receptor type 1 leads to programmed cell death (apoptosis), whereas the other, linked to receptor 2, counters the death signal and leads to survival. When both receptors are expressed, the type 2 receptor of the TNF-α may enhance the receptor 1–mediated death pathway. The final consequence may depend on the level of type 1 expression. The survival pathway activates a transcription factor, nuclear factor (NF)-B, which works by turning on a set of antiapoptotic genes.

NF-B is normally composed of two subunits, p50 and p65. It is usually held captive in the cytoplasm of a cell because it associates with an inhibitor protein called inhibitory protein-B (IB), which stops NF-B from entering the nucleus. After cells are treated with TNF-α, the IB protein becomes labelled with phosphate groups, which marks it out for degradation. With its jailer destroyed, NF-B is free to move into the nucleus, where it binds to relevant sites in its target genes and activates a new programme of gene expression, ensuring that the cell survives. The IB kinase complex mediates the key phosphorylation of IB in this chain of events.

In Mongolian gerbils, it was found that changes in the levels of apoptosis-related proteins correlated with decreases in cochlear function as measured by distortion product otoacoustic emissions (DPOAEs) (30). The apoptosis-related proteins that correlated with a decrease in DPOAEs were (i) an antiapoptotic fast response gene Bcl, bcl-2, which was decreased in the tissues of the aged cochlea and (ii) activated caspase-3 molecules, which increased in the tissues of the aged cochlea when these tissues were compared with the same tissue types obtained from the cochleae of the young animals. The level of Bax (a proapoptosis protein caused by cell death gene Bax) did not show any ageing-related increase or decrease. Both bcl-2 and activated caspase-3 are involved in the control and execution of the MAPK/JKN-mediated cell death pathway, which is thought to be the primary mediator of oxidative stress-induced apoptosis of inner ear sensory cells. Thus the reported higher shear stress vulnerability of older animals may be linked to differences in regulation of the components in the apoptotic pathway (31).

During intense sound exposure, the inner hair cells are overstimulated resulting in synaptic hyperactivity and an excessive release of transmitter substance. The afferent neurotransmitter is most likely to be glutamate, which, like other excitatory amino acids, has toxic effects when released in large amounts. The resulting overstimulation of the glutamate receptors elicits an inflow of calcium ions, which, in combination with other ions, brings about the entry of water and subsequent swelling of the nerve endings. The result may be a total disruption of the synapses between the inner hair cells and the afferent nerve fibres in the cochlear nerve (32). A dorsal root acid sensing ion channel has been detected in the spiral ganglion cells (SGCs) and the organ of Corti including the nerve fibres innervating the organ of Corti (33). It is known that opening of the acid sensing ion channel may flux Ca^{2+} and induce cell death (34). This mechanism may also be involved in noise-induced hearing loss and ischaemia-induced hearing loss because both shear stress and ischaemia can result in a low pH extracellular homeostasis.

In addition to the accumulation of ROMs seen following metabolic and/or mechanical stress, it has been demonstrated that acoustical overstimulation leads to a significant rise in intracellular calcium levels in the outer hair cells (35). A sustained increase in the intracellular calcium concentration is known to result in severe cell injuries such us cytoskeletal breakdown, membrane defects, and DNA damage (36). One probable consequence of the increased calcium concentration

in the outer hair cells is the loss of cell body stiffness observed after intense acoustical stimulation (37). Moreover, a structural reorganisation of the organ of Corti has recently been demonstrated following acoustical overstimulation (15). The noise-induced changes in cellular stiffness and structure of the hearing organ seem to be, at least partly, reversible and the results may thus contribute to knowledge of the mechanisms involved (Fig. 16.4).

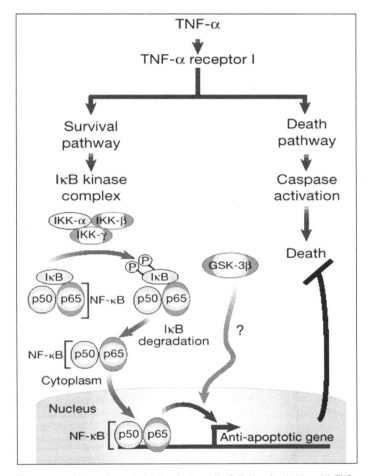

Figure 16.4 Life-and-death decision in the cells. Cellular stimulation with TNF-α (*top*) simultaneously activates survival (*left*) and death (*right*) signalling pathways. The survival pathway leads to the activation of NF-κB, which induces the expression of antiapoptotic genes in the nucleus. NF-κB (subunits p50 and p65) is normally held captive in the cytoplasm by the IkB protein. Cellular stimulation with TNF-α leads to activation of the IKK complex, which phosphorylates IkB. The phosphate tag (*circled* "p") singles out IkB for destruction. NF-κB is then free to move into the nucleus and activate its target genes. Hoeflich et al. have revealed an unexpected requirement for GSK-3b in the NF-κB–mediated activation of genes needed for survival (39). It is not yet clear how GSK-3b works in this pathway, but it probably involves a critical step following the movement of NF-κB to the nucleus. Targeted disruption in mice of any of the molecules coloured red leads to death of the embryo, accompanied by TNF-α–induced apoptosis of hepatocytes. *Abbreviations*: GSK, glycogen synthase kinase; IKB, inhibitory kinase-B; IKK, IkB kinase; NF, nuclear factor; TNF, tumour necrosis factor. *Source*: From Ref. 38.

Necrosis induced by sound stimulation

Very loud sound leads to mechanical damage of the organ of Corti with fractures of the cellular membrane, liberation of lysosome content, and, exposure of the cell content to extracellular fluids. In necrosis, there is abundance of proinflammatory cytokines such as interleukin (IL)-1β, IL-6, and TNF-α, and migration of inflammatory cells (40).

TNF-α is involved in cellular survival/damage mechanism especially through the TNF receptor 1 (p55). The survival pathway can induce activation of c-Jun NH2-terminal kinases and NF-κB (41). There is also another TNF-α–mediated pathway that acts through receptor 2 (p75), the necrosis stimulating pathway. This pathway is also self-feeding; as the receptor 2 pathway is activated, it enhances production of TNF-α. The upregulation of receptor type 2 leads to inflammation and cytotoxic effects.

Upregulation of growth factors in noise trauma

The role of upregulation of growth factors is not yet well known. One of the nerve growth factors (NFG), the NFG1, is expressed in the cochlea during traumatizing noise leading to permanent threshold shift (PTS) but not during nontraumatic noise leading to temporary threshold shift (TTS) (41). One of the immediate responses by *NFG1* gene production is activation of c-fos. Loud noise at a damaging level also upregulates genes producing glial cell line–derived neurotrophic factor (GDNF) in rats. The upregulation starts after four hours, peaks after 12 hours, and levels out after 12 hours from cessation of the noise exposure (42). GDNF has a protective effect on noise-induced cellular damage but the exact mechanism has not yet been delineated. It has been hypothesised that GDNF is involved in the consolidation of recovery function from noise damage. It is also possible that GDNF has a function that is related to protection from additional noise-induced stress, rather than recovery from the first stress. GDNF upregulation may be related to the training effect, toughening, or conditioning of the organ of Corti (42).

Vascular endothelial growth factor (VEGF) is also upregulated during shear stress that leads to traumatic changes (43). The expression of VEGF is limited to the hair bundles and SGCs after traumatic vibration. VEGF receptor 1 (VEGF R1) is not detected in the vibrated cochlea, whereas VEGF R2 expression is present in the lower part of the outer hair cells, Dieters' cells, Hensen's cells, Claudius cells, the basal membrane of the organ of Corti, the internal sulcus cells, nucleus of the SGCs, the lateral wall of scala tympani, and the spiral ligament (Fig. 16.6). No expression of VEGF R2 was observed in the stria vascularis.

It is well accepted that shear movement exists in the organ of Corti, but there is no documentation of shear stress within

the SGCs. Shear forces within the bone matrix stimulate bone cells and mechanically transform them causing upregulation of genes in the cells (44). The SGCs are surrounded by perilymph and bone matrix. The shear force produced by the transcranial vibration is conducted to the SGCs and is able to cause shear stress. In our study, *VEGF* and *VEGF R2* gene expression in the SGCs supports this hypothesis (Fig. 16.5).

Vibration induces *VEGF* and *VEGF R2* expression in the cochlea, but not *VEGF R1*. Our results confirm the biological significance of a previous in vitro study, which indicated that in vascular endothelial cells, high shear stress induced an increase in VEGF R2 expression. This upregulation reached its maximum and was in a linear relationship to the stress strength within a range of 2 to 40 dyne/cm^2 (45). The authors interpreted this as showing that an increase in the shear stress in the vasculature by postischaemic reperfusion stimulates VEGF R2 expression, resulting in an increase in vascular permeability and leading to neovascularisation. After myocardial infarction, the newly formed myofibroblasts express VEGF and VEGF R2 that seem to play a significant role in tissue repair/remodelling (46). When the cochlea is exposed to mechanical vibration, a shear stress presented in the various cell types of the cochlea with concomitant increase of expression of VEGF and VEGF R2. Thus, VEGF may contribute to tissue remodelling and angiogenesis at the site of damage in an autocrine manner and may be important in preventing further damage to the cochlea. The most enhanced expression was located in the SGCs, stereocilia, supporting cells, the internal sulcus cells, and epithelial cells of the lateral wall of the scala tympani. No obvious expression was found in the hair cells. This means that the hair cells are rather stable and not affected by the VEGF-induced reaction and seem not to be able to be remodelled/repaired by VEGF when they are damaged. Conversely, the spiral ganglion may be repaired with the assistance of VEGF because both VEGF and VEGF R2 are expressed there.

Shear stress–induced VEGF expression seems to be time-dependent. After acute shear stress within six hours of the

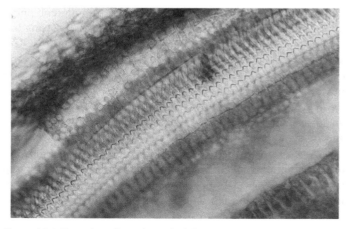

Figure 16.5 Expression of vascular endothelial growth factor in the hair bundles of the outer and inner hair cells after shear stress–induced cochlear trauma in a guinea pig. It is quite possible that this staining covers the tip links.

exposure, it is not expressed (47); whereas after longer shear stress, its expression is increased up to 14 days (48). In the cochlea, we observed expression of VEGF and VEGF R2 one to three days after vibration. This is in accordance with time limit of previous reports. In pathological states, especially at the acute phase of brain ischaemia and myocardial infarction, VEGF was expressed and could induce oedema, which is deleterious. This happened within six hours (49). The naturally occurring upregulation of VEGF at a later phase (six hours later) means that VEGF and VEGF R2 responses are protective responses in the individual. There is no evidence to show whether VEGF and VEGF R2 are expressed in the spiral ganglion within six hours of cochlea shear stress. It is worth investigating this response to provide reference data for clinical treatment.

Pharmacotherapy of the inner ear

Free radical scavengers

At least three important ROS are generated in the reduction of O_2 to H_2O: superoxide anion (O_2^-), hydrogen peroxide (H_2O_2), and hydroxyl radical (OH^-). It has been demonstrated that ROSs are involved in noise trauma (50–52), cisplatin ototoxicity (53–55), and aminoglycoside ototoxicity (56). Direct evidence of ROS ototoxicity has been demonstrated using isolated outer hair cells and by intraperilymphatic infusion (57). ROS ototoxicity is believed to be mediated by deleterious effects at multiple sites including lipid peroxidation, DNA strand breaks, and alterations in carbohydrate and protein structures.

Increased knowledge of the processes leading to cellular injuries is of fundamental importance in order to develop clinical means for protection and repair. Many recent reports on the protection against noise-induced hearing loss offered by drugs such as antioxidants and neurotrophins (NTs) are promising. Table 16.2 shows the antioxidants for which this has been experimentally demonstrated, and some are currently in use.

In addition to these agents, there are several other compounds that have been tried and some may be useful, but there are insufficient data on their efficacy in preventing or healing cochlear injury.

There are several different pharmacologically active agents that have been tried or are in use to treat sudden acoustic trauma. In general, few experiments have been prospective with relevant control material. The experiments carried out in military camps with the use of Mg^{2+} are effective and usable, but the limitation in their use is that Mg^{2+} should be administered before exposure to inner ear trauma. The efficacy seems to be limited to preventative action by alleviating the accumulation of excessive Ca^{2+} in the cochlea.

An iron chelator and free radical scavengers have been shown to attenuate cochlear damage caused by noise (58). Also the antioxidant D-methionine has proved to be useful in preventing gentamicin-induced ototoxicity (4). N-acetylcysteine (NAC) is metabolised to cysteine (among other molecules) and may provide cellular needs for glutathione (GSH) in the presence of ROS. Several recent articles demonstrate that L-NAC or related drugs could reduce noise-induced hearing loss (59). ROS-induced damage may occur in vibration-induced hearing loss, and ROS scavengers such as NAC may prevent vibration-induced hearing loss. In an animal model, NAC could not prevent vibration-induced hearing loss, although different

Table 16.2   Possible reactive oxygen species scavengers

1. Glutathione is a nucleophilic scavenger and an electron donor via the SH group of it business residue, cysteine

2. N-acetylcysteine, the acetylated variant of the amino acid L-cysteine, is an excellent source of SH groups and is converted in the body into metabolites capable of stimulating glutathione synthesis, promoting detoxification and acting directly as free radical scavengers

3. Ascorbic acid and its sodium, potassium, and calcium salts are commonly used as antioxidant food additives. These compounds are water soluble and thus cannot protect fat from oxidants: For this purpose, the fat soluble esters of ascorbic acid with long-chain fatty acids (ascorbyl palmitate or ascorbyl stearate) can be used as food antioxidants

4. Salicylic acid is able to absorb hydroxyl ions and thus impede a main step in the process of membrane lipid peroxidation

5. Melatonin, once oxidised, cannot be reduced to its former state because it forms several stable end products upon reacting with free radicals. Therefore, it has been referred to as a terminal (or suicidal) antioxidant

6. Tocopherols are the most abundant and efficient scavengers of hydroperoxyl radicals in biological membranes

7. The iron chelator (desferrioxamine) forms a stable complex with ferric iron, decreasing its availability for the production of reactive oxygen species. Desferrioxamine is a powerful inhibitor of iron-dependent lipid peroxidation and hydroxyl radical formation

8. Mannitol is free radical scavenger of the hydroxyl radical to which the aldehyde moiety of mannitol reacts and binds. This forms a mannitol radical that undergoes disproportionation or dimerises, and thus becomes less cytotoxic than the former hydroxyl radical, causing less damage to the cellular ultrastructure

Abbreviation: SH, sulfhydryl.

administration approaches have been tested (60). Figure 16.6 shows the results of NAC on vibration-induced hearing loss. In fact, NAC appears to have synergistic neurotoxic effects in combination with glutamate, which may be the primary afferent neurotransmitter of the cochlea (61,62).

Several compounds have been tried in the prevention or treatment of noise-induced hearing loss in humans (Table 16.3).

Few of these experiments have control group or are randomised and prospective. So far, based on evidence in humans, only Mg^{2+} seems to be effective in prevention of noise-induced hearing loss. The study of Attias was carried out in Israeli army forces and included controls, indicating that replacement of Ca^{2+} ions in body led to protection from noise damage (63).

In animal studies, the control of noise dose and environmental factors can be minimised. There has been much research conducted in animals with several pharmacological compounds. In general, all seem to work in animal experiments that have been tried for prevention, but their clinical value needs to be documented. For treatment of sudden deafness, there are several substances suggested for use. These are listed in Table 16.4.

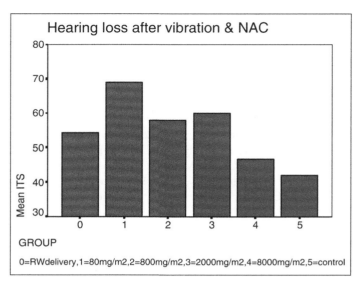

Figure 16.6 Mean hearing threshold change after exposure of the guinea pigs on traumatizing vibration causing shear stress, which was administered with NAC before vibration. *Note*: 0—round window delivery; 1—80 mg/m²; 2—800 mg/m²; 3—2000 mg/m²; 4—8000 mg/m²; 5—control. *Abbreviation*: NAC, *N*-acetylcysteine.

Table 16.3   Clinical trial of drug treatment of acute acoustic trauma

Drugs	Sample number	Method	Efficacy	Authors
Vitamin A		Re	No	Ward and Glorig, (64)
Dextran	72	Re,Co	Yes	Martin and Jakobs, (65)
	209	Re,Co	No	Eibach and Borger, (66)
Dextran; + pentoxifylline	147	Pr,Ra	No	Probst et al., (67)
	50	Pr,Co	No	Eibach and Borger, (68)
Bencyclan	85	Re,Co	No	Eibach and Borger, (68)
Xantinol nicotinate	85	Re,Co	No	Eibach and Borger, (68)
ATP	136	Re,Co	No	Eibach and Borger, (68)
Vitamin A, B, E	85	Re,Co	No	Eibach and Borger, (68)
Methionine	85	Re,Co	No	Eibach and Borger, (68)
Cinnarizine	57	Re,Co	No	Eibach and Borger, (68)
Betahistine	122	Pr,Ra	No	Pilgramm and Schumann, (69)
Magnesium	320	Pr,Ra	Yes	Joachim et al., (70)
4 g, drink	80		No	Pilgram et al., (71)
10 mg/kg, infusion	300	Pr,Co	Yes	Attias et al., (63)
167 mg, drink	100	Pr,Ra	No	Maurer et al., (72)
Diltiazem				

Abbreviations: Co, control group; Pr, prospective study; Ra, randomised study; Re, retrospective study.
Source: From Refs. 63–72.

Table 16.4   Animal studies of drug treatment of acute acoustic trauma

Drugs	Animal species	Efficacy	Parameters	Authors
NAC	Guinea pig	++	ROS, ABR, hair cell loss	Ohinata et al., (73)
NAC; + acetyl-salicylic acid	Chinchilla	+++	ABR, cytocochleogram	Kopke et al., (59)
HES70, ES200, pentoxifylline, *ginkgo biloba*, betahistidine	Guinea pigs	HES +++; betahistidine +; others	pO2, CAP, ABR, CM	Lamm and Arnold, (21)
Allopurinol	Guinea pigs	+	ROS, ABR	Attanasio et al., (74)
Allopurinol, SOD-PEG	Rat	+	ABR, CAP	Seidman et al., (75)
Dipyridamol, allopurinol	Guinea pigs	+	CAP	Bergmann, (76)
DFO, mannitol, GDNF	Guinea pigs	++	Cytocochleogram, ABR	Yamasoba et al., (58)

Abbreviations: ABR, brainstem evoked response; CAP, compound action potential; CM, cochelar microphonics; DFO, desferroxamine; GDNF, glial cell line–derived neurotrophic factor; HES, hydroxyethyl starch; NAC, *N*-acetylcysteine; PEG, polyethylene glycol; ROS, reactive oxygen species; SOD, superoxide dismutase.
Source: From Refs. 21, 58, 59, 73–76.

TNF-α and its antagonists

After shear stress of the cochlea, Zou et al. demonstrated a weak TNF receptor 1 staining mainly in Hensen's cells, Claudius cells, the internal sulcus cells, and the capillaries of the spiral ganglion (Fig. 16.7) (43). Much stronger expression of TNF receptor 2 was found mainly in the SGCs, Henson's cells, Claudius cells, the internal sulcus cells, Dieters' cells, the basal membrane of the organ of Corti, the spiral ligament, the spiral vascular prominence, with weaker staining in the lower part of the out hair cells (43). No TNF receptor expression was detected in the normal cochlea.

Although TNF-α, TNF receptor 1, and receptor 2 were observed in the vibrated cochlea, the expression of TNF receptor 2 was more prominent in the cochlea. The combination of TNF-α with TNF receptor 2 is capable of activating JNK and NF-κB (41). The activation of JNK and NF-κB has the function of an antiapoptotic agent (41). On the other hand, the activation of TNF receptor 1 induces apoptosis (77). When both receptors are expressed, the activation of TNF receptor 2 enhances the effects

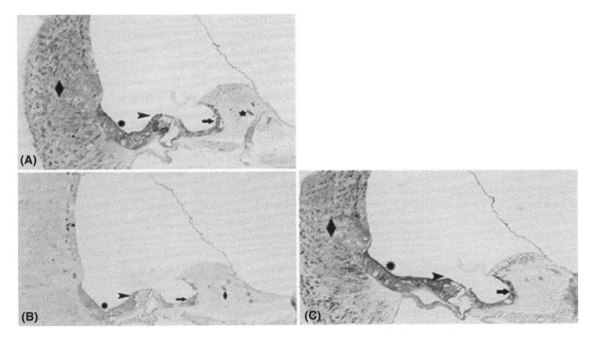

Figure 16.7 Expression of TNF-α and receptor upregulation in guinea pig cochlea after induction of powerful shear stress. TNF-α (**A**) and receptor 2 (**C**) are markedly expressed in the vibrated cochlea. Receptor 1 (**B**) only showed slight expression in the vibrated cochlea. *Abbreviation*: TNF, tumour necrosis factor.

of receptor 1 activation. The final fate of the cells should be related to the expression ratio of both receptors. Shear stress inhibits TNF-α–induced apoptosis by activating phosphatidylinositol 3-kinase and inhibiting caspase-3 (Fig. 16.7) (78).

Recently anticytokine therapies have become a common treatment in diseases of autoimmune origin such as rheumatoid arthritis and Crohn's disease (79). Treatment with monoclonal antibodies against TNF-α suppresses inflammation and improves patient well being (79). TNF-α is a proinflammatory cytokine released during infection or inflammation, which calls the immune system to action (38). Anti–TNF-α antibody administration in vivo results in the rapid downregulation of a spectrum of cytokines, cytokine inhibitors, and acute-phase proteins (79).

Etanecerp and infliximab are drugs that potently and selectively bind TNF-α in the cellular microenvironment, thereby preventing TNF-α from interacting with membrane-bound TNF receptors on target cells. Etanecerp is a recombinant fusion protein of the soluble type 2 TNF receptor on a human IgG1 backbone, whereas infliximab is a chimeric anti–TNF-α monoclonal antibody containing a murine TNF-α–binding region and human IgG1 backbone.

Both etanecerp and infliximab are reported to have a positive effect on hearing loss or hearing fluctuation in Menière's disease and idiopathic sensorineural hearing loss (80). In the animal model in which keyhole limpet hemocyanin (KLH) was used to induce autoimmune hearing loss in guinea pigs, etanecerp could effectively alleviate the hearing loss and cochlear damage in the animal model (81). The findings were confirmed in later study in the same animal model (82). However, a multicentre study on immunomediated cochleovestibular disorders by Matteson et al. could not demonstrate that etanecerp was effective in alleviating vertigo and tinnitus or improving hearing in these patients (83). Zou et al. studied the effect of infliximab on the prevention of hearing loss after shear stress–induced cochlear trauma (unpublished data). In this trauma, TNF-α and its receptor 1 and 2 are upregulated in the cochlea. Infliximab was administered through different approaches in the experiments, intravenously, intraperitoneally, and transtympanically. None of the administration methods could prevent the animals from developing hearing loss. In a subsequent trial, four patients with vertigo and bilateral severe sensorineural hearing loss were followed up for three months and infliximab with azathioprine were administered intravenously according to protocol used for treatment of severe rheumatoid arthritis. In none of the patients was hearing improved or preserved. It is noteworthy was that one of the subjects responded to corticosteroids with an improvement of hearing of 50 dB, but did not show a similar responsiveness to infliximab.

Infliximab may cause severe adverse effects, the main being hypersensitivity reactions, development of antinuclear antibodies, possibly lymphoproliferative disorders, and reactivation of latent tuberculosis. Also a case has been reported with severe neutropaenia and thrombocytopaenia associated with infliximab (84). Infliximab infusions are accompanied by acute reactions in approximately 5% of infusions (85).

To summarise the findings of TNF-α, it seems well documented that in a damaged cochlea, there is upregulation of TNF type 1 and 2 receptors but the efficacy of the blocking agents have not yet been demonstrated, so that neither etanecerp nor infliximab can be recommended for treatment of hearing loss in humans.

Neuroprotection: calpain, nitric oxide, and glutamate receptors

The accumulation of free radicals severely damages the inner ear and other tissues. Through a complex chain of events, this damage can then cause a release and accumulation of glutamate and calpains. Nitric oxide (NO) plays a role in a great range of important functions in the organism, such as vasodilatation, relaxation of muscles, neurotransmission, and neuromediation. NO has been found to cause ototoxicity. Ruan et al. demonstrated that sodium nitroprusside, a NO donor, produced both outer hair cell and inner hair cell damage when it was applied at the cochlear round window (86). NO synthase (NOS) has been shown to play an active role in the initiation of degeneration of the SGCs of the rat cochlea (87). It has been suggested that noise-induced hearing loss is partly due to excessive release of the excitatory amino acids such as glutamate and consequently exciting the postsynaptic receptors leading to swelling of the nerve endings (88). It has also been suggested that the ototoxicity of noise trauma and aminoglycosides may result from the same excitatory process at the glutamate receptor (89). NO mediates the effects of excitatory amino acids in the central nervous system and may play a similar role in the peripheral auditory system, since glutamate is considered to be the afferent neurotransmitter at the inner hair cell synapses. NO plays an important role in kainic acid–induced ototoxicity (90). A study demonstrated that 7-nitroindazole, a competitive inhibitor of neuronal NOS, could attenuate the compound action potential (CAP) threshold shift caused by kainic acid, suggesting that NO is coupled to a glutamate receptor (91). Indeed, Amaee et al. suggested that NO might be involved in sensorineural hearing loss–induced by bacterial meningitis (92).

Recently Barkdull et al. used cochlear microperfusion to treat sensorineural hearing loss caused by inflammation in a guinea pig model (93). The microperfusion was effective in the acute phase that is associated with elevations in cytokines, NO, and cellular infiltrates and the breakdown of the blood–labyrinthine barrier. The chronic phase leads to irreversible ossification of the labyrinth demanding other kinds of treatment to facilitate removal of inflammatory cells and their byproducts. The benefit of microperfusion may be sustained when combined with local delivery of immunosuppressive agents to the inner ear.

Studies have shown that excessive glutamate may play a role in the production of tinnitus. They also show that glutamate antagonists can have a protective effect on the inner ear and possibly be a treatment for peripheral tinnitus, which is generated by the inner ear. Several such drugs are currently under investigation for hearing loss and tinnitus as, for example, memantine, caroverine and magnesium. Caroverine has been shown to restrict the activity of glutamate receptors and protect the hearing of guinea pigs. Its safety and tolerance have been demonstrated in some clinical studies. In one study, 63% of patients treated with intravenous caroverine reported a significant improvement in their tinnitus immediately after intravenous infusion (94). Over 48% of patients remained stable after one week. No severe adverse effects were identified for the majority of patient. However, a few patients experienced mild transient side effects. There is, however, conflicting data that suggest that the placebo effect may have been responsible for the reduction in tinnitus. More clinical studies need to be conducted to resolve the controversy.

Glutamate receptor antagonists have been found to protect the cochlea from noise trauma and aminoglycoside ototoxicity. Excitotoxicity can be prevented by a non-NMDA (NMDA, N-methyl-D-aspartic acid) receptor antagonist (95). Swelling of the dendrites under the inner hair cells induced by the glutamate agonist alpha-amino-3-hydroxy-5-methyl-4-isoxazolepropionic acid (AMPA) can be partly prevented by the non-NMDA receptor antagonist dinitroquinoxaline-2,3-dione (DNQX). Noise-induced swelling of the dendrites under the inner hair cells has been found to be prevented by either dizocilpine (MK) 801, an NMDA receptor antagonist, or kynurenic acid, a wide glutamate receptor antagonist for both NMDA and non-NMDA receptors (96). Aminoglycoside-induced hearing disorders could be prevented by the NMDA receptor antagonist MK 801 (97). This suggests that the glutamate receptor plays an important role in noise and drug-induced hearing loss.

Puel et al. observed total disruption of all synapses between the inner hair cells and spiral ganglion neurone dendrites, together with the disappearance of cochlear potentials after applying AMPA, a glutamate agonist, to the cochlea (98). In addition, recovery of both the normal pattern of inner hair cell innervation and the physiological responses has been observed within five days.

Treatment of cochlea trauma with nerve growth factors

NTs, including nerve growth factor (NGF), brain-derived NGF (BDNF), NT-3, and GDNF, are known to play a role in the survival of injured cochlear neurones both in vitro and in vivo. Schindler et al. found that NGF significantly prevented damage to spiral ganglion neurones from neomycin in vivo (99). BDNF and NT-3 have been shown to protect spiral ganglion neurones from ototoxicity of cisplatin and aminoglycoside both in vitro and in vivo (100). BDNF and GDNF have also been found to protect the cochlea from noise-induced damage (101). In addition, Pirvola et al. found that fibroblast growth factor (FGF) receptor (FGFR)-3 mRNA was present in the organ of Corti following acoustic overstimulation and suggested that FGFR-3 could be involved in protecting the cochlea from noise-induced damage (102).

Recent findings that GDNF, BDNF, NT-3, and transforming growth factor-α can protect the auditory hair cells from

acoustic trauma or aminoglycoside ototoxicity in vivo raise the question of whether other neurotrophic factors can also protect the hair cells in vivo (103–106). FGF-2 can protect hair cells from neomycin ototoxicity in vitro, and an in vivo study has shown upregulation of FGFR-3 in the cochlea following noise exposure, suggesting that some FGF family members might play a role in protection or repair of the cochlea from damage (107). However, no significant difference in threshold shifts was observed between the treated and untreated ears in any of the groups (108). The extent of hair cell damage was also comparable among the different treatment groups. These findings indicate that exogenous FGF-1 or FGF-2 does not influence noise-induced hair cell damage under the experimental conditions used in this study, suggesting that these FGFs are not good candidates as auditory hair cell protectors in vivo.

Zou et al. demonstrated, in the guinea pig, that after damage under shear stress in cochlea, the hearing loss could be alleviated by combining BDNF and Connective Tissue Nitrient Formula (CTNF) (60). Because BDNF + Ciliary Neuro Trophic Factor (CNTF) can improve the survival of SGCs while affording no protection to hair cells from noise, protection from hearing loss with BDNF + CNTF suggests that ganglion cell damage may be important in vibration-induced hearing loss (109). Apparently we need to protect the hair cells, ganglion cells, and possibly other structures such as supporting cells and strial cells from vibration-induced hearing loss. Because of severe side effects from BDNF + CNTF, it is still too risky to give NTs systemically but, in the future, local application may be useful in preventing inner ear trauma.

The development, within the mammalian cochlea, of neurite sprouting and integrity of SGCs is influenced by members of several growth factor families. Among these NGF, BDNF, NT-3, and NT-4/5 are important (110). NGF, BDNF, NT-3, and NT-4/5 can promote the survival of postnatal mammalian SGCs in culture (111). Delivery of exogenous BDNF, NT-3, and NGF to the mammalian inner ear can prevent loss of SGCs following administration of ototoxic drugs (100). NTs have been associated with regenerating neurones in avian cochleae (112). CNTF and leukaemia-inhibitory factor are members of the neuropoietic cytokine family and can also promote the survival of SGCs (113). These cytokines and NTs act in concert upon mammalian SGCs. For example, the combination of CNTF and NT-3 is more effective in promoting the survival of dissociated SGCs in vitro than either factor alone (113).

In recent years, studies on antioxidants and/or NTs show promise in protecting the inner ear (hair cells and SGCs) from trauma such as noise (58). The next question, of clinical relevance, is to assess such pharmacological treatment in the prevention of surgically induced trauma to the human inner ear. In a previous experimental study, we showed that vibration resulted in significant hearing loss (31). Therefore, experimental studies mimicking the clinical situation are required to provide information on the mechanism underlying this kind of damage.

Based on the evidence of animal experiments on the neurotrophic factors, it is possible in the future, when targeted drug therapy will become feasible, that the NTs may be the key molecules used in hearing preservation.

Treatment of cochlear trauma with corticosteroids

The inner ear contains both glucocorticoid and mineralocorticoid receptors providing substrate for the biological action of corticosteroids. The normal cortisol production in human plasma is 14 to 70 μmol/day (5–25 mg/day) and peaks in the early morning. Injuries, infections, cold, and pain result in a 10-fold and a greater increase in the rate of production of cortisol. Dexamethasone has a biological half-life in plasma of about two to five hours [baxter dexamethasone data sheet, (114)]. For cortisol, this is about 80 minutes. The anti-inflammatory effect lasts longer than the half time in the plasma.

Bachmann et al. evaluated the prednisolone level in perilymph after round window application (115). They applied 0.1 mL of 50 mg/mL prednisolone solution directly to the round window niche. Samples were taken from the apex of the cochlea. The steroid concentration in the scala tympani reaches a peak of 1 mg/mL after one hour, which is equal to 2% of the steroid concentration of the solution applied to the RWM.

The dexamethasone concentration found by Parnes in the cochlea was about 10 times higher than that found by Chandrasekhar et al., although Parnes used a lower dexamethasone concentration applied on the RWM (4.4 mg/mL) than Chandrasekhar (10 mg/mL), who completely filled the bulla (116,117). Parnes used a much slower perilymph sampling technique. Since both Parnes and Chandrasekhar et al. took 10 μL samples from the cochlea base and Bachmann from the apex, the latter data are the most reliable. Also, Bachmann put the steroid solution directly onto the round window niche (the others just filled the bulla) and left the animal under anaesthesia for a longer time. In addition, his periods of sampling cover a longer total period. The other authors rinsed the bulla with saline 30 minutes after the steroid injection.

Ikeda and Morizono studied possible adverse effects of triamcinolone in the middle ear of chinchillas (118). Triamcinolone did not influence the CAP when compared with the saline-treated control animals. Jinn et al. investigated the length changes in outer hair cells from the chinchilla in vitro (119). Tobradex diluted 1:40 resulted in an in vitro dexamethasone concentration of 25 μg/mL. Dexamethasone at this concentration had the least effect on the outer hair cell length when compared with the others. Kroin et al. perfused the subarachnoid space of the spinal cord in rats (intrathecal) with dexamethasone, via an osmotic minipump (0.5 μL/hr) over 14 days (120). The objective was to evaluate stability, bioavailability, and safety of long-term drug delivery. They concluded that a dose of 300 ng/day (=12.5 ng/hr) is safe. Higher doses resulted in morphological changes. However, the dose without information on the volume of the spinal cord fluid does not give the correct value of drug concentration. In order to transfer this figure into humans, the relevant volume of the spinal cord fluid of the rat should be compared with the scala tympani volume in humans. The rat spinal cord fluid volume could be in the range of 10 μL, as the guinea pig perilymph respecting the human perilymph volume. Nordang et al. investigated morphological changes of the RWM in rats, after the instillation of either dexamethasone (1 μg in 20 μL) or hydrocortisone (2%, 20 μL) every second day for either 5 or 10 days, through the tympanic membrane into the middle ear cavity (121). Control groups received 20 μL of saline. In the group treated with dexamethasone, no morphological differences were found between the steroid group and the control group. However, epithelial thickening and inflammatory cells were found in the RWMs of the hydrocortisone groups as compared to the controls. The authors suggest that every instillation of fluid into the middle ear causes some swelling, but dexamethasone reduces the symptoms because it is the most potent drug. Unfortunately, hearing was not monitored.

Spandow et al. observed that hydrocortisone instilled into the middle ear cavity of rats caused irreversible threshold shift in the brainstem evoked response (ABR) (122). No morphological changes in the inner ear were observed. The hydrocortisone was dissolved in distilled water. Distilled water served as control in the other ear. It has been suggested that the threshold shift was due to distilled water rather than hydrocortisone (118).

It has been suggested that acute noise trauma can also be treated with corticosteroids or other treatments aimed at improving the microcirculation of the cochlea (123). The efficacy of corticosteroids has been evaluated in idiopathic progressive sensorineural hearing loss, sudden deafness, and Menière's disease. Nevertheless, no conclusive evidence on their efficacy on treatment in any of these diseases has been achieved (Tables 16.5–16.7).

Novel substances still at an experimental stage

Peptide inhibitor AM-111 (D-JNKI-1)

D-c-jun N-terminal kinase peptide inhibitor (D-JNKI-1) is a cell permeable peptide that selectively blocks MAPK/JNK-mediated apoptosis of stress injured hair cells and neurones in the cochlea to protect against permanent hearing loss. When administered within a therapeutic window after the incident, D-JNKI-1 can effectively protect cochlear hair cells and neurones that would otherwise undergo apoptosis and be lost (139). D-JNKI-1 is an efficient inhibitor of the action of all three JNK isoforms produced by linking the 20 amino acid terminal JNK-inhibitory sequence (JNK-binding domain) of JIP-1/IB1 to a 10 amino acid HIV transactivating regulatory protein (TAT) transporter sequence (140). The otoprotective properties of D-JNKI-1 have been tested and confirmed in various animal models so far, including acute acoustic trauma, surgically induced acoustic trauma (cochlear implant electrode insertion), and aminoglycoside ototoxicity. After acute acoustic trauma in guinea pigs, D-JNK-1 was shown to protect against permanent sensorineural hearing loss even if administered only "after" noise exposure (6 kHz pure tone, 120 dB for 30 minutes) and in just one single dose. The therapeutic window was 12 hours.

Table 16.5 Animal studies of drug treatment of acute acoustic trauma

Drugs	Anti-inflammatory efficacy	Biological $t_{1/2}$ (hours)	Human plasma $t_{1/2}$ (hours)
Hydrocortisone	1	8–12	1–1.5
Prednisolone	4	12–36	2–3
Triamcinolone (Volon A, Kenacort A)	5	12–36	2–3
Dexamethasone	25–30	36–72	3
Methyl-prednisolone	5	12–36	1.5–3

Table 16.6 Clinical studies on the efficacy of corticosteroids in Menière's disease

Drugs	Number of subjects participating in the study (n)	Administration of the drug	Dose of administration	Positive effect the drug	Authors
Dexamethasone	15	Intratymp	8 mg in hyaluron solution	5/15	Arriaga and Goldman, (124)
Dexamethasone	21	Intratymp	4 mg/mL, 1/wk, 4 wk	11/21; 9/21	Barrs et al., (125)
Dexamethasone	17	Intratymp	16 mg/mL; 3 × 0.2–0.4 mL, 1 wk	0/17	Hirvonen et al., (126)
Prednisone + Dexamethasone	12	ES	P: 20 mg, into ES; D: 32 mg/mL, outside ES	0/12	Kitahara et al., (127)
Dexamethasone	21	Intratymp	1 × 4 mg/mL solution	21/21	Sakata et al., (128)
Dexamethasone	24	Intratymp	0.25 mg/0.25 mL, ventilation tube	Vertigo 17/24; hearing 0/24	Sennaroglu et al., (129,130)
Dexamethasone	28	Intratymp; + IV; + oral	RWM: 3 × 0.2 mg; IV: 16 mg; oral: 0.25 mg, daily, 1 mo	Hearing 19/28; tinnitus 23/28; dizziness 27/28	Shea et al., (131)
Dexamethasone	22	Intratymp	Intratymp 1 mg/ml intravenous 4 mg/mL	Tinnitus 10/22; hearing 9/22	Silverstein et al., (132)
Dexamethasone	17	Intratymp	8 mg/mL	0/17	Silverstein et al., (133)

Abbreviations: ES, electrolyte solution; IV, intravenous; RWM, round window membrane.
Source: From Refs. 124–133.

This pathway appears to be different from that of [cephalic sensilla (1346 vai 11004) (CEP-1346)]. The inhibitory action of AM-111 is thought to be fundamentally different from the action of small chemical inhibitors such as CEP-1347 (141,142). AM-111 does not interfere with intrinsic JNK activity that might be involved in such physiological activities as cellular differentiation and neuritic outgrowth, but rather it targets access of MAPK/JNK to substrates within a cell nucleus by a competitive mechanism (143–146).

CEP-1346

Increased JNK activity and c-Jun induction is observed in stressed cells during various conditions, including degeneration and regeneration. Combined with data from tissue culture experiments dissecting the JNK pathway, this suggests that activation of the JNK pathway via c-Jun induction or other mechanisms is important in cell death processes involved in hearing loss and potentially other neurodegenerative disorders.

Table 16.7 Efficacy of treatment with corticosteroids on tinnitus and sensorineural hearing loss

Diseases (number of subjects participating in the study)	Drugs	Administration of the drug	Dose of administration	Positive effect of drugs	Authors
Tinnitus (1214)	Dexamethasone	Intratymp	4 mg/mL	862/1214	Sakata et al., (128)
Tinnitus (56)	Dexamethasone	Intratymp	2 mg, 4 mg, 4/wk	40/56	Sakata et al., (134)
Tinnitus (3041)	Dexamethasone	Intratymp	4–8 wk, 1 mg/mL	2068/3041	Sakata et al., (135)
Tinnitus (24)	Dexamethasone	Intratymp	1/2 days, 3 mo; Dexamethasone, 4 mg/mL	2/24	Sennaroglu et al., (129,130)
SNHL and various (37)	Dexamethasone (20); methyl-prednisolone (17)	Intratymp	Methyl-prednisolone, 40 mg/mL	SNHL, 13/37	Parnes et al., (116)
Sudden SNHL (6)	Methyl-prednisolone	Microcath on RWM	62.5 mg/mL, 14 days	AIED, 7/13	Kopke et al., (136)
Sudden SNHL (12)	Methyl-prednisolone	Microcath on RWM	62.5 mg/mL, 10 days	5/6	Lefebvre and Staecker, (137)
Labyrinthine fistula (12)	Prednisolone	IV single dose	500 mg	12/12 Prevent HL	Milewski et al., (138)

Abbreviations: AIED, autoimmuno inner ear disease; HL, hearing loss; IV, intravenous; RWM, round window membrane; SNHL, sensory neural hearing loss.
Source: From Refs. 116, 128–130, 134–138.

The development of the neurotrophic molecule CEP-1347 is based on the observations of the survival-promoting and neurotrophic effects of the naturally occurring small molecule K252a (147). K252a possesses two activities in neurones. At high concentration, K252a inhibits the survival-promoting and neurotrophic effects of NTs, whereas at low concentrations, K252a, by itself, promotes survival and differentiation similar to the effects of the NTs. Compounds based on the K252a structure were synthesised to enhance the neurotrophic effects of K252a while decreasing its ability to inhibit tyrosin kinase (Trk) phosphorylation. The conjugation of alkyloxy- or alkylthio–side chains to the outer benzene rings of the indolocarbazole structure increases choline acetyltransferase mRNA (ChAT) activity in both the rat spinal cord and basal forebrain cultures. Compared to other bulkier alkylthio-derivatives, the 3,9-*bis*-[ethylthio(methyl)]-substituted K252a has the most potent neurotrophic effects. The 3,9-*bis*-[ethylthio(methyl)]-substituted K252a was named CEP-1347 or KT-7515. Compared to K252a, CEP-1347 is not cytotoxic above 200 nM, as is K252a, and does not possess the nonselective serine/threonine kinase inhibitor property of K252a, having binding affinities three orders of magnitude lower than K252a to protein kinase A (PKA) and protein kinase C (PKC) and myosin light chain kinase. Thus, the semisynthetic derivative of K252a, CEP-1347, has the desired neurotrophic effects while greatly reducing the nonselective-inhibitory profile of K252a.

Recent studies in disparate species demonstrate that hair cell loss in response to noise or exposure to aminoglycoside antibiotics is associated with activation of the JNK pathway and subsequent apoptosis (148). CEP-1347 (1 mg/kg) administered to guinea pigs a few hours before and daily for two weeks after six hours of 120 dB, 4 kHz noise exposure significantly reduces hair-cell death and hearing loss observed 14 days post–noise exposure (149).

Latanoprost

Endogenous production of prostaglandins has been demonstrated in the cochlea, but no information is available on the distribution of the cyclo-oxygenase (COX) or prostanoid receptors in the cochlea. Stjernschantz et al. investigated the localisation of the FP, prostaglandin E receptor 1 (EP1), and EP3 prostanoid receptors as well as the COX-1 and COX-2 in the cochlea of guinea pigs and human (149). In both the guinea pig and human, the FP prostanoid receptor was abundantly distributed in the cochlea, e.g., in the stria vascularis, spiral ligament, spiral ganglion, and organ of Corti. The immunohistochemical staining of the EP1 and EP3 receptors in the same structure was significantly weaker and sometimes lacking altogether (e.g., EP3 receptor in human cochlea). Weak, but mostly consistent immunostaining of COX-1 was found in the cochlear structures. At the same time, COX-2 was absent. The abundant distribution of the FP receptor in several important cochlear structures in both the guinea pig and human suggests a physiological function for (prostaglandin F, PGF) PGF2a in the cochlea. COX-1 seems to be expressed in cochlea in contrast to COX-2.

Latanoprost is a selective agonist for the FP prostanoid receptor (receptor for PGF2α). Many prostaglandins, including PGF2α, are produced in the inner ear (150). Rask-Andersen et al. administered latanoprost by intratympanic injection once daily for three days (151). Before the first injection (day 1) and on day 5 and 15, hearing capacity and tinnitus were determined. The patients' vertigo was assessed on a visual analogue scale on days 1 to 15. The study was randomised, double-blind, and placebo-controlled. Latanoprost reduced vertigo/disequilibrium by about 30% and improved speech recognition by about 15%. Tinnitus loudness was not reduced by latanoprost. There were few side effects. It is likely that latanoprost may be a useful agent for acute hearing loss and also environmental noise-induced hearing loss.

Targeted drug delivery—future treatment

The specific cell targeting treatment of the inner ear disease represents another challenge. The possibility of nanocarrier-based drug targeting is under development. In this nanocarrier, it can be a nanoparticle (NP) of size less than 200 nm in diameter (Fig. 16.8). The NPs can be produced by different techniques including interfacial deposition, emulsion, micellular structures, or sonication. Poly (lactic-co-glycolic acid) (PLGA) and poly (E-capro-lactone) (PCL) are biodegradable approved polymers, but typically suffer from low drug incorporation and rapid drug release rates for low-molecular-weight organic drug molecules. Other materials such as chitosan, silica-based materials, demonstrate better incorporation and slower release rates, but suffer from poorer biodegradability and biocompatibility. Additionally, physicochemical properties of drugs affect loading and release, thus choice of drugs and compatible polymers will be important for development and clinical therapy.

NPs should be appropriately surface modified to reduce toxicity and immunogenicity. Obviously both of these features represent a challenge. Circumventing the immune response may be solved by (*i*) using peptide ligands to avoid protein tags on the NP surfaces and (*ii*) coating the surface of nanostructures with polyethylene glycol (PEGylating) to avoid nonspecific reactions with inner ear proteins and opsonisation or false targeting of the nanostuctures. Coating can be created either by the addition of a PEG-containing surfactant at NP production or after NP manufacture. NP coating must also inhibit aggregation and reduce uptake by nontargeted cells. Unless particles demonstrate significant charge stabilisation, they will tend to aggregate due to their hydrophobic action. Proteins and buffering salts may increase aggregation or may adsorb to the particle surface, resulting in nontargeted cell uptake. Hydrophobic particles and positively charged complexes (as in uncoated polyplexes) will also tend to bind to cell surfaces, which will lead to a nonspecific uptake by macrophages into cells.

A peptide-based targeting ligand can be attached with covalent bonds to the outer surface of the NP. The NP will bind with this ligand to specific receptors present, for example, in hair cells, supporting cells and cells in stria vascularis. In hair cells, there are several possibilities of targets, including prestin, cadherin, claudin, anion exchanger 2, and myosin IVa. On the cochlear nerve, the SGCs have TrkB and TrkC receptors that can be targeted. Metalloprotein matrix proteins (MMP), MMP2 and MMP9, can be expressed in the stria vascularis after lesions. Conjugation of ligands may be achieved via PEG-like linkers to ensure that the uptake is specific. Ligands will be identified with a phage display technique. In this technique, 10^9 different DNA sequences coding for a peptide library are cloned to the coat protein gene of the virus and are displayed in the phage plasmid after protein synthesis. Using immobilised receptors in vitro, it is possible to select and isolate peptides with different binding specificities. This procedure of ligand screening is called biopanning and results in highly selective peptides binding to specified receptors, thus allowing accurate targeting.

Several genes regulate the differentiation of cochlear hair cells and supporting cells, during mammalian embryogenesis, from their common precursor cells. A key gene is known to be *Atoh1* (also known as *Math1*). This is the mouse homologue of the Drosophila gene *atonal* that encodes a basic helix-loop-helix transcription factor. Overexpression of *Atoh1* in nonsensory cells of the normal cochlea generates new hair cells, both in vitro and in vivo. *Atoh1* has been shown to act as a "prohair cell gene" and is required for the differentiation of hair cells from multipotent progenitors. Recently our adjunct research institute demonstrated that, in mammals, by using gene therapy the lost hair cells will regenerate and also return hearing to the profoundly deaf mammalian ear. This finding opens new perspectives for the treatment of hearing loss and justifies the efforts to incapsulate nucleotides encoding the *Math1* gene within the nanostructures.

Another approach for the inner ear-targeted treatment is to selectively open the passage from blood to perilymph without interference with endolymph because perilymph is essential for the surviving of cochlear hair cells and other cells. When VEGF is delivered to the RWM, it could significantly enhance the transport of gadolinium (111) complexed with

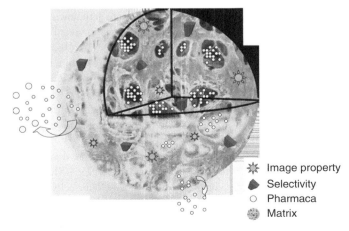

Figure 16.8 Multifunctional, biocompatible, biodegradable, nontoxic polymer matrix nanoparticle with a matrix integrated "tracer" for magnetic resonance imaging and selective drug delivery.

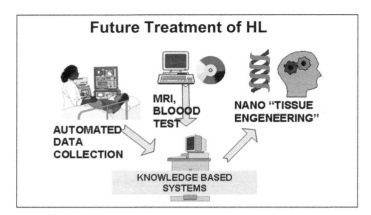

Figure 16.9 Future aspects of inner ear treatment are based on integrated action with internet-based data collection interface, genotyping with proteomics, data mining and evaluation with artificial intelligence-based systems, and robotic tissue engineering.

diethylentriamine pentaacetic acid bis-methylamide (Gd DTPA-BMA) from blood to perilymph without disturbing the blood–labyrinth barrier (152). This site-specific response might be explained by the different structure of the blood–labyrinth barrier located in the stria vascularis and the blood–perilymph barrier, which is located in the spiral ligament and cochlear glomeruli. This response might be used to accelerate the penetration of intravenously administered drugs to the cochlea (Fig. 16.9).

References

1. Hu BH, Henderson D, Nicotera TM. Extremely rapid induction of outer hair cell apoptosis in the chinchilla cochlea following exposure to impulse noise. Hear Res 2006; 211(1–2):16–25.

2. Lynch ED, Kil J. Compounds for the prevention and treatment of noise-induced hearing loss. Drug Discov Today 2005; 10(19): 1291–1298.

3. Kalkanis JG, Whitworth C, Rybak LP. Vitamin E reduces cisplatin ototoxicity. Laryngoscope 2004; 114(3):538–542.

4. Sha SH, Schacht J. Antioxidants attenuate gentamicin-induced free radical formation in vitro and ototoxicity in vivo: D-methionine is a potential protectant. Hear Res 2000; 142(1–2):34–40.

5. Van De Water TR et al. Caspases, the enemy within, and their role in oxidative stress-induced apoptosis of inner ear sensory cells. Otol Neurotol 2004; 25(4):627–632.

6. Sage C, Huang M, Karimi K, et al. Proliferation of functional hair cells in vivo in the absence of the retinoblastoma protein. Science 2005; 307(5712): 1114–1118.

7. Sobkowicz HM, Bereman B, Rose JE. Organotypic development of the organ of Corti in culture. J Neurocytol 1975; 4(5):543–572.

8. Fekete DM, Muthukumar S, Karagogeos D. Hair cells and supporting cells share a common progenitor in the avian inner ear. J Neurosci 1998; 18(19):7811–7821.

9. Gopfert MC, Stocker H, Robert D. Atonal is required for exoskeletal joint formation in the Drosophila auditory system. Dev Dyn 2002; 225(1):106–109.

10. Izumikawa M et al. Auditory hair cell replacement and hearing improvement by Atoh1 gene therapy in deaf mammals. Nat Med 2005; 11(3):271–276.

11. Cacace AT, Silver SM, Farber M. Rapid recovery from acoustic trauma: chicken soup, potato knish, or drug interaction? Am J Otolaryngol 2003; 24(3):198–203.

12. Henderson D et al. The role of antioxidants in protection from impulse noise. Ann N Y Acad Sci 1999; 884:368–380.

13. Ulfendahl M, Khanna SM, Heneghan C. Shearing motion in the hearing organ measured by confocal laser heterodyne interferometry. Neuroreport 1995; 6(8):1157–1160.

14. Ulehlova L. Stria vascularis in acoustic trauma. Arch Otorhinolaryngol 1983; 237(2):133–138.

15. Tsuprun V et al. Structure of the stereocilia side links and morphology of auditory hair bundle in relation to noise exposure in the chinchilla. J Neurocytol 2003; 32(9):1117–1128.

16. Scheibe F, Haupt H, Ludwig C. Intensity-dependent changes in oxygenation of cochlear perilymph during acoustic exposure. Hear Res 1992; 63(1–2):19–25.

17. Leon Y, Sanchez-Galiano S, Gorospe I. Programmed cell death in the development of the vertebrate inner ear. Apoptosis 2004; 9(3):255–264.

18. Jokay I et al. Apoptosis in the human inner ear. Detection by in situ end-labeling of fragmented DNA and correlation with other markers. Hear Res 1998; 117(1–2):131–139.

19. Nakashima T et al. Disorders of cochlear blood flow. Brain Res Brain Res Rev 2003; 43(1):17–28.

20. Lamm K, Arnold W. Successful treatment of noise-induced cochlear ischemia, hypoxia, and hearing loss. Ann N Y Acad Sci 1999; 884:233–248.

21. Lamm K, Arnold W. The effect of blood flow promoting drugs on cochlear blood flow, perilymphatic pO(2) and auditory function in the normal and noise-damaged hypoxic and ischemic guinea pig inner ear. Hear Res 2000; 141(1–2):199–219.

22. Lamm K, Arnold W. Noise-induced cochlear hypoxia is intensity dependent, correlates with hearing loss and precedes reduction of cochlear blood flow. Audiol Neurootol 1996; 1(3):148–160.

23. Banfi B et al. NOX3, a superoxide-generating NADPH oxidase of the inner ear. J Biol Chem 2004; 279(44):46065–46072.

24. Yamashita D et al. Post-exposure treatment attenuates noise-induced hearing loss. Neuroscience 2005; 134(2):633–642.

25. Budihardjo I et al. Biochemical pathways of caspase activation during apoptosis. Annu Rev Cell Dev Biol 1999; 15:269–290.

26. Slee EA, Adrain C, Martin SJ. Executioner caspase-3, -6, and -7 perform distinct, non-redundant roles during the demolition phase of apoptosis. J Biol Chem 2001; 276(10):7320–7326.

27. Maier JK et al. The neuronal apoptosis inhibitory protein is a direct inhibitor of caspases 3 and 7. J Neurosci 2002; 22(6): 2035–2043.

28. Hu BH, Henderson D, Nicotera TM. F-actin cleavage in apoptotic outer hair cells in chinchilla cochleas exposed to intense noise. Hear Res 2002; 172(1–2):1–9.

29. Pomerantz JL, Baltimore D. NF-kappaB activation by a signaling complex containing TRAF2, TANK and TBK1, a novel IKK-related kinase. Embo J 1999; 18(23):6694–6704.

30. Alam SA et al. The expression of apoptosis-related proteins in the aged cochlea of Mongolian gerbils. Laryngoscope 2001; 111(3):528–534.

31. Zou J et al. Sensorineural hearing loss after vibration: an animal model for evaluating prevention and treatment of inner ear hearing loss. Acta Otolaryngol 2001; 121(2):143–148.

32. Puel JL et al. Excitotoxicity and repair of cochlear synapses after noise-trauma induced hearing loss. Neuroreport 1998; 9(9): 2109–2114.

33. Hildebrand MS et al. Characterisation of DRASIC in the mouse inner ear. Hear Res 2004; 190(1–2):149–160.

34. Waldmann R et al. A proton-gated cation channel involved in acid-sensing. Nature 1997; 386(6621):173–177.

35. Fridberger A, Ulfendahl M. Acute mechanical overstimulation of isolated outer hair cells causes changes in intracellular calcium levels without shape changes. Acta Otolaryngol 1996; 116(1):17–24.

36. Maurer J, Heinrich UR, Mann W. Morphologic damage and changes of intracellular calcium-binding sites after acute noise trauma in the organ of Corti of the guinea pig. ORL J Otorhinolaryngol Relat Spec 1993; 55(1):7–12.

37. Fridberger A, van Maarseveen JT, Ulfendahl M. An in vitro model for acoustic overstimulation. Acta Otolaryngol 1998; 118(3):352–361.

38. Pomerantz JL, Baltimore D. Signal transduction. A cellular rescue team. Nature 2000; 406(6791):26–27, 29.

39. Hoeflich KP et al. Requirement for glycogen synthase kinase-3beta in cell survival and NF-kappaB activation. Nature 2000; 406(6791):86–90.

40. Satoh H et al. Proinflammatory cytokine expression in the endolymphatic sac during inner ear inflammation. J Assoc Res Otolaryngol 2003; 4(2):139–147.

41. Goeddel DV. Signal transduction by tumor necrosis factor: the Parker B. Francis Lectureship. Chest 1999; 116(1 suppl): 69S–73S.

42. Nam YJ et al. Upregulation of glial cell line-derived neurotrophic factor (GDNF) in the rat cochlea following noise. Hear Res 2000; 146(1–2):1–6.

43. Zou J et al. Vibration induced hearing loss in guinea pig cochlea: expression of TNF-alpha and VEGF. Hear Res 2005; 202(1–2): 13–20.

44. Turner CH, Forwood MR, Otter MW. Mechanotransduction in bone: do bone cells act as sensors of fluid flow? Faseb J 1994; 8(11):875–878.

45. Abumiya T et al. Shear stress induces expression of vascular endothelial growth factor receptor Flk-1/KDR through the CT-rich Sp1 binding site. Arterioscler Thromb Vasc Biol 2002; 22(6):907–913.

46. Chintalgattu V, Nair DM, Katwa LC. Cardiac myofibroblasts: a novel source of vascular endothelial growth factor (VEGF) and its receptors Flt-1 and KDR. J Mol Cell Cardiol 2003; 35(3):277–286.

47. Gan L et al. Distinct regulation of vascular endothelial growth factor in intact human conduit vessels exposed to laminar fluid shear stress and pressure. Biochem Biophys Res Commun 2000; 272(2):490–496.

48. Milkiewicz M et al. Association between shear stress, angiogenesis, and VEGF in skeletal muscles in vivo. Microcirculation 2001; 8(4):229–241.

49. Weis SM, Cheresh DA. Pathophysiological consequences of VEGF-induced vascular permeability. Nature 2005; 437(7058): 497–504.

50. Van Campen LE et al. Oxidative DNA damage is associated with intense noise exposure in the rat. Hear Res 2002; 164(1–2): 29–38.

51. Yamane H et al. Appearance of free radicals in the guinea pig inner ear after noise-induced acoustic trauma. Eur Arch Otorhinolaryngol 1995; 252(8):504–508.

52. Ohlemiller KK, Wright JS, Dugan LL. Early elevation of cochlear reactive oxygen species following noise exposure. Audiol Neurootol 1999; 4(5):229–236.

53. Ravi R, Somani SM, Rybak LP. Mechanism of cisplatin ototoxicity: antioxidant system. Pharmacol Toxicol 1995; 76(6):386–394.

54. Lautermann J et al. Glutathione-dependent antioxidant systems in the mammalian inner ear: effects of aging, ototoxic drugs and noise. Hear Res 1997; 114(1–2):75–82.

55. Rybak LP, Somani S. Ototoxicity amelioration by protective agents. Ann N Y Acad Sci 1999; 884:143–151.

56. Wu WJ, Sha SH, Schacht J. Recent advances in understanding aminoglycoside ototoxicity and its prevention. Audiol Neurootol 2002; 7(3):171–174.

57. Clerici WJ, Yang L. Direct effects of intraperilymphatic reactive oxygen species generation on cochlear function. Hear Res 1996; 101(1–2):14–22.

58. Yamasoba T et al. Attenuation of cochlear damage from noise trauma by an iron chelator, a free radical scavenger and glial cell line-derived neurotrophic factor in vivo. Brain Res 1999; 815(2):317–325.

59. Kopke RD et al. Reduction of noise-induced hearing loss using L-NAC and salicylate in the chinchilla. Hear Res 2000; 149(1–2): 138–146.

60. Zou J et al. Comparison of the protective efficacy of neurotrophins and antioxidants for vibration-induced trauma. ORL J Otorhinolaryngol Relat Spec 2003; 65(3):155–161.

61. Puka-Sundvall M, Eriksson P, Nilsson M, Sandberg M, Lehmann A. Neurotoxicity of cysteine: intraction with glutamate. Brain Res 1995; 705(1–2):65–70.

62. Nordang L, Cestreicher E, Arnold W, Anniko M. Glutamate is the afferent neurotransmitter in the human cochlea. Acta otalaryngol 2000; 120(3):359–362.

63. Attias J et al. Oral magnesium intake reduces permanent hearing loss induced by noise exposure. Am J Otolaryngol 1994; 15(1): 26–32.

64. Ward WD, Glorig A. The relation between vitamin A and temporary threshold shift. Acta Otolaryngol 1960; 52:72–78.

65. Martin JG. The treatment of acute acoustic trauma (blast injury) with dextran 40 [author's transl.]. HNO 1977; 25(10):349–352.

66. Eibach H. Borger U. Therapeutic results in acute acoustic trauma [author's transl.]. Arch Otorhinolaryngol 1980; 226(3):177–186.

67. Probst R et al. A randomized, double-blind, placebo-controlled study of dextran/pentoxifylline medication in acute acoustic trauma and sudden hearing loss. Acta Otolaryngol 1992; 112(3): 435–443.

68. Eibach H, Borger U. Acute acoustic trauma. The therapeutic effect of bencyclan in a controlled clinical trial [author's transl.]. HNO 1979; 27(5):170–175.

69. Pilgramm M, Schumann K. Hyperbaric oxygen therapy for acute acoustic trauma. Arch Otorhinolaryngol 1985; 241(3):247–257.

70. Joachims Z et al. Oral magnesium supplementation as prophylaxis for noise-induced hearing loss: results of a double blind field study. Schriftenr Ver Wasser Boden Lufthyg 1993; 88:503–516.

71. Pilgramm M et al. Do magnesium infusions protect the inner ear during middle ear surgery? A randomized double blind study. Schriftenr Ver Wasser Boden Lufthyg 1993; 88:517–528.

72. Maurer J et al. Diltiazem for prevention of acoustical trauma during otologic surgery. ORL J Otorhinolaryngol Relat Spec 1995; 57(6):319–324.

73. Ohinata Y, Miller JM, Schacht J. Protection from noise-induced lipid peroxidation and hair cell loss in the cochlea. Brain Res 2003; 966(2):265–273.

74. Attanasio G et al. Protective effect of allopurinol in the exposure to noise pulses. Acta Otorhinolaryngol Ital 1999;19(1):6–11.

75. Seidman MD, Shivapuja BG, Quirk WS. The protective effects ofallopurinol and superoxide dismutase on noise-induced cochlear damage. Otolaryngol Head Neck Surg 1993; 109(6): 1052–1056.

76. Bergmann K. Experiments on the medicamental treatment of the noise-induced cochlear damage. Part I. The effect of dipyridamol and allopurinol on the RMP of the cochlea (guinea pig) after noise [author's transl.]. Arch Otorhinolaryngol 1976; 212(3): 171–177.

77. Ashkenazi A, Dixit VM. Death receptors: signaling and modulation. Science 1998; 281(5381):1305–1308.

78. Pavalko FM et al. Fluid shear stress inhibits TNF-alpha-induced apoptosis in osteoblasts: a role for fluid shear stress-induced activation of PI3-kinase and inhibition of caspase-3. J Cell Physiol 2003; 194(2):194–205.

79. Charles P et al. Regulation of cytokines, cytokine inhibitors, and acute-phase proteins following anti-TNF-alpha therapy in rheumatoid arthritis. J Immunol 1999; 163(3):1521–1528.

80. Rahman MU, Poe DS, Choi HK. Etanercept therapy for immune-mediated cochleovestibular disorders: preliminary results in a pilot study. Otol Neurotol 2001; 22(5):619–624.

81. Satoh H et al. Tumor necrosis factor-alpha, an initiator, and etanercept, an inhibitor of cochlear inflammation. Laryngoscope 2002; 112(9):1627–1634.

82. Wang M, Bregenholt S, Petersen JS. The cholera toxin B subunit directly costimulates antigen-primed CD4 + T cells ex vivo. Scand J Immunol 2003; 58(3):342–349.

83. Matteson EL et al. Etanercept therapy for immune-mediated cochleovestibular disorders: a multi-center, open-label, pilot study. Arthritis Rheum 2005; 53(3):337–342.

84. Vidal F, Fontova R, Richart C. Severe neutropenia and thrombocytopenia associated with infliximab. Ann Intern Med 2003; 139(3):235.

85. Cheifetz A et al. The incidence and management of infusion reactions to infliximab: a large center experience. Am J Gastroenterol 2003; 98(6):1315–1324.

86. Ruan RS, Leong SK, Yeoh KH. Ototoxicity of sodium nitroprusside is not due to nitric oxide. Exp Neurol 1999; 158(1):192–201.

87. Zdanski CJ et al. Nitric oxide synthase is an active enzyme in the spiral ganglion cells of the rat cochlea. Hear Res 1994; 79(1–2):39–47.

88. Pujol R et al. Pathophysiology of the glutamatergic synapses in the cochlea. Acta Otolaryngol 1993; 113(3):330–334.

89. Matsuda K et al. A role of glutamate in drug-induced ototoxicity: in vivo microdialysis study combined with on-line enzyme fluorometric detection of glutamate in the guinea pig cochlea. Brain Res 2000; 852(2):492–495.

90. Johnson KL et al. Role of nitric oxide in kainic acid-induced elevation of cochlear compound action potential thresholds. Acta Otolaryngol 1998; 118(5):660–665.

91. Irons-Brown SR, Jones TA. Effects of selected pharmacological agents on avian auditory and vestibular compound action potentials. Hear Res 2004; 195(1–2):54–66.

92. Amaee FR et al. Possible involvement of nitric oxide in the sensorineural hearing loss of bacterial meningitis. Acta Otolaryngol 1997; 117(3):329–336.

93. Barkdull GC et al. Cochlear microperfusion: experimental evaluation of a potential new therapy for severe hearing loss caused by inflammation. Otol Neurotol 2005; 26(1):19–26.

94. Denk DM et al. Caroverine in tinnitus treatment. A placebo-controlled blind study. Acta Otolaryngol 1997; 117(6):825–830.

95. Kopke RD et al. Candidate's thesis: enhancing intrinsic cochlear stress defenses to reduce noise-induced hearing loss. Laryngoscope 2002; 112(9):1515–1532.

96. Jager W et al. Noise-induced aspartate and glutamate efflux in the guinea pig cochlea and hearing loss. Exp Brain Res 2000; 134(4):426–434.

97. Bienkowski P et al. Ototoxic mechanism of aminoglycoside antibiotics–role of glutaminergic NMDA receptors. Pol Merkuriusz Lek 2000; 9(52):713–715.

98. Puel JL et al. Alpha-amino-3-hydroxy-5-methyl-4-isoxazole propionic acid electrophysiological and neurotoxic effects in the guinea-pig cochlea. Neuroscience 1991; 45(1):63–72.

99. Schindler RA et al. Enhanced preservation of the auditory nerve following cochlear perfusion with nerve growth factors. Am J Otol 1995; 16(3):304–309.

100. Staecker H et al. NT-3 and/or BDNF therapy prevents loss of auditory neurons following loss of hair cells. Neuroreport 1996; 7(4):889–894.

101. Altschuler RA et al. Rescue and regrowth of sensory nerves following deafferentation by neurotrophic factors. Ann N Y Acad Sci 1999; 884:305–311.

102. Pirvola U et al. The site of action of neuronal acidic fibroblast growth factor is the organ of Corti of the rat cochlea. Proc Natl Acad Sci U S A 1995; 92(20):9269–9273.

103. Keithley EM et al. GDNF protects the cochlea against noise damage. Neuroreport 1998; 9(10):2183–2187.

104. Ylikoski J et al. Guinea pig auditory neurons are protected by glial cell line-derived growth factor from degeneration after noise trauma. Hear Res 1998; 124(1–2):17–26.

105. Shoji F et al. Differential protective effects of neurotrophins in the attenuation of noise-induced hair cell loss. Hear Res 2000; 146(1–2):134–142.

106. Kawamoto K et al. Hearing and hair cells are protected by adenoviral gene therapy with TGF-beta1 and GDNF. Mol Ther 2003; 7(4):484–492.

107. Low W et al. Basic fibroblast growth factor (FGF-2) protects rat cochlear hair cells in organotypical culture from aminoglycoside injury. J Cell Physiol 1996; 167(3):443–450.

108. Yamasoba T et al. Absence of hair cell protection by exogenous FGF-1 and FGF-2 delivered to guinea pig cochlea in vivo. Noise Health 2001; 3(11):65–78.

109. Yamagata T et al. Delayed neurotrophic treatment preserves nerve survival and electrophysiological responsiveness in neomycin-deafened guinea pigs. J Neurosci Res 2004; 78(1):75–86.

110. Wheeler EF et al. Expression of BDNF and NT-3 mRNA in hair cells of the organ of Corti: quantitative analysis in developing rats. Hear Res 1994; 73(1):46–56.

111. Zheng JL, Stewart RR, Gao WQ. Neurotrophin-4/5 enhances survival of cultured spiral ganglion neurons and protects them from cisplatin neurotoxicity. J Neurosci 1995; 15(7 Pt 2):5079–5087.

112. Pirvola U et al. Expression of neurotrophins and Trk receptors in the developing, adult, and regenerating avian cochlea. J Neurobiol 1997; 33(7):1019–1033.

113. Staecker H et al. NT-3 combined with CNTF promotes survival of neurons in modiolus-spiral ganglion explants. Neuroreport 1995; 6(11):1533–1537.

114. Conroy PJ. New quinolone/steroid combination for topical treatment of acute otitis: early- and late-phase study results. Ear Nose Throat J 2003; 82(8 suppl 2):2–4.

115. Bachmann G et al. Permeability of the round window membrane for prednisolone-21-hydrogen succinate. Prednisolone content of the perilymph after local administration vs. systemic injection. Hno 2001; 49(7):538–542.

116. Parnes LS, Sun AH, Freeman DJ. Corticosteroid pharmacokinetics in the inner ear fluids: an animal study followed by clinical application. Laryngoscope 1999; 109(7 Pt 2):1–17.

117. Chandrasekhar SS et al. Dexamethasone pharmacokinetics in the inner ear: comparison of route of administration and use of facilitating agents. Otolaryngol Head Neck Surg 2000; 122(4):521–528.

118. Ikeda K, Morizono T. Effect of ototopic application of a corticosteroid preparation on cochlear function. Am J Otolaryngol 1991; 12(3):150–153.

119. Jinn TH et al. Determination of ototoxicity of common otic drops using isolated cochlear outer hair cells. Laryngoscope 2001; 111(12):2105–2108.

120. Kroin JS, Schaefer RB, Penn RD. Chronic intrathecal administration of dexamethasone sodium phosphate: pharmacokinetics and neurotoxicity in an animal model. Neurosurgery 2000; 46(1):178–182; discussion 182–183.

121. Nordang L, Linder B, Anniko M. Morphologic changes in round window membrane after topical hydrocortisone and dexamethasone treatment. Otol Neurotol 2003; 24(2):339–343.

122. Spandow O, Anniko M, Hellstrom S. Hydrocortisone applied into the round window niche causes electrophysiological dysfunction of the inner ear. ORL J Otorhinolaryngol Relat Spec 1989; 51(2):94–102.

123. Lamm K, Arnold W. The effect of prednisolone and non-steroidal anti-inflammatory agents on the normal and noise-damaged guinea pig inner ear. Hear Res 1998; 115(1–2):149–161.

124. Arriaga MA, Goldman S. Hearing results of intratympanic steroid treatment of endolymphatic hydrops. Laryngoscope 1998; 108(11 Pt 1):1682–1685.

125. Barrs DM et al. Intratympanic steroid injections for intractable Meniere's disease. Laryngoscope 2001; 111(12):2100–2104.

126. Hirvonen TP, Peltomaa M, Ylikoski J. Intratympanic and systemic dexamethasone for Meniere's disease. ORL J Otorhinolaryngol Relat Spec 2000; 62(3):117–120.

127. Kitahara T et al. Effects of exposing the opened endolymphatic sac to large doses of steroids to treat intractable Meniere's disease. Ann Otol Rhinol Laryngol 2001; 110(2):109–112.

128. Sakata E et al. Treatment of Meniere's disease. Middle ear infusion with lidocaine and steroid solution. Auris Nasus Larynx 1986; 13(2):79–89.

129. Sennaroglu L et al. Transtympanic dexamethasone application in Meniere's disease: an alternative treatment for intractable vertigo. J Laryngol Otol 1999; 113(3):217–221.

130. Sennaroglu L et al. Intratympanic dexamethasone, intratympanic gentamicin, and endolymphatic sac surgery for intractable vertigo in Meniere's disease. Otolaryngol Head Neck Surg 2001; 125(5): 537–543.

131. Shea JJ Jr, Ge X. Dexamethasone perfusion of the labyrinth plus intravenous dexamethasone for Meniere's disease. Otolaryngol Clin North Am 1996; 29(2):353–358.

132. Silverstein H et al. Intratympanic steroid treatment of inner ear disease and tinnitus (preliminary report). Ear Nose Throat J 1996; 75(8):468–471, 474, 476 passim.

133. Silverstein H et al. Dexamethasone inner ear perfusion for the treatment of Meniere's disease: a prospective, randomized, double-blind, crossover trial. Am J Otol 1998; 19(2):196–201.

134. Sakata E, Itoh A, Itoh Y. Treatment of cochlear-tinnitus with dexamethasone infusion into the tympanic cavity. Int Tinnitus J 1996; 2:129–135.

135. Sakata E, Ito Y, Itoh A. Clinical experiences of steroid targeting therapy to inner ear for control of tinnitus. Int Tinnitus J 1997; 3(2):117–121.

136. Kopke RD et al. Targeted topical steroid therapy in sudden sensorineural hearing loss. Otol Neurotol 2001; 22(4):475–479.

137. Lefebvre PP, Staecker H. Steroid perfusion of the inner ear for sudden sensorineural hearing loss after failure of conventional therapy: a pilot study. Acta Otolaryngol 2002; 122(7):698–702.

138. Milewski C, Dornhoffer J, DeMeester C. Possibilities for preserving hearing in labyrinth fistulas of different degrees of severity. Laryngorhinootologie 1995; 74(7):408–412.

139. Wang J et al. A peptide inhibitor of c-Jun N-terminal kinase protects against both aminoglycoside and acoustic trauma-induced auditory hair cell death and hearing loss. J Neurosci 2003; 23(24):8596–8607.

140. Vives E, Brodin P, Lebleu B. A truncated HIV-1 Tat protein basic domain rapidly translocates through the plasma membrane and

accumulates in the cell nucleus. J Biol Chem 1997; 272(25): 16010–16017.

141. Maroney AC et al. Cep-1347 (KT7515), a semisynthetic inhibitor of the mixed lineage kinase family. J Biol Chem 2001; 276(27):25302–25308.

142. Harris C, Maroney AC, Johnson EM Jr. Identification of JNK-dependent and -independent components of cerebellar granule neuron apoptosis. J Neurochem 2002; 83(4): 992–1001.

143. Ip YT, Davis RJ. Signal transduction by the c-Jun N-terminal kinase (JNK)—from inflammation to development. Curr Opin Cell Biol 1998; 10(2):205–219.

144. Bodner A et al. Mixed lineage kinase 3 mediates gp120IIIB-induced neurotoxicity. J Neurochem 2002; 82(6): 1424–1434.

145. Bonny C et al. Cell-permeable peptide inhibitors of JNK: novel blockers of beta-cell death. Diabetes 2001; 50(1):77–82.

146. Barr RK, Kendrick TS, Bogoyevitch MA. Identification of the critical features of a small peptide inhibitor of JNK activity. J Biol Chem 2002; 277(13):10987–10997.

147. Wang LH, Besirli CG, Johnson EM Jr. Mixed-lineage kinases: a target for the prevention of neurodegeneration. Annu Rev Pharmacol Toxicol 2004; 44:451–474.

148. Ylikoski J et al. Blockade of c-Jun N-terminal kinase pathway attenuates gentamicin-induced cochlear and vestibular hair cell death. Hear Res 2002; 166(1–2):33–43.

149. Stjernschantz J, Wentzel P, Rask-Andersen H. Localization of prostanoid receptors and cyclo-oxygenase enzymes in guinea pig and human cochlea. Hear Res 2004; 197(1–2):65–73.

150. Escoubet B et al. Prostaglandin synthesis by the cochlea of the guinea pig. Influence of aspirin, gentamicin, and acoustic stimulation. Prostaglandins 1985; 29(4):589–599.

151. Rask-Andersen H et al. Effects of intratympanic injection of latanoprost in Meniere's disease: a randomized, placebo-controlled, double-blind, pilot study. Otolaryngol Head Neck Surg 2005; 133(3):441–443.

152. Zou J et al. MRI evidence of exogenous vascular endothelial growth factor-enhanced transport across inner ear barriers in guinea pigs. Zhonghua Er Bi Yan Hou Tou Jing Wai Ke Za Zhi 2005; 40(4):266–270.

17 Diagnosis and management strategies in congenital middle and external ear anomalies

Frank Declau, Paul Van De Heyning

Introduction

Congenital middle ear abnormalities can be divided into major and minor anomalies. The major malformations represent the congenital atresias of the external auditory canal; the minor ones relate to the congenital defects of the ossicular chain. The term "congenital atresia of the ear" is generally used to describe a series of malformations of the external and middle ear. Although atresia anatomically implies an absence of an external auditory canal, clinically it is usually applied in a broader sense, varying from a mild abnormality with only narrowing to a complete absence of the external ear canal. Abnormalities of the external auditory canal are usually associated with a deformity or an absence of the pinna as well as middle-ear abnormalities. The inner-ear structures are only rarely involved. There is a considerable divergence of opinion as to the necessity and advisability of treatment for congenital atresia. Furthermore, there is much disagreement as to the procedure of choice and which criterion should be used to determine a surgical success.

Epidemiology

In Europe, a prevalence of 1.07 per 10,000 births for microtia-anotia (M-A) was found in the period 1980–2003 (1). Health Department statistics of the City of New York for a 10-year period (1952–1962) showed that there was a rate of 1 in 5800 births (2). According to the Swedish Board of Welfare statistics, the frequency of isolated external-ear and external-ear-canal malformations in 1980 amounted to 0.92 per 10,000 live births (3). Variable prevalence rates can be due to variable registration. A lack of standardisation of definition and diagnosis was previously described (1). Also, substantial variations in the incidence between different years have been found (4).

Mastroiacovo et al. (5) studied the epidemiology and genetics of M-A, using data collected from the Italian Multicentre Birth Defects Registry (IPIMC) from 1983 to 1992. Among 1,173,794 births, they identified 172 with M-A, a rate of 1.46/10,000; 38 of the 172 infants (22.1%) had anotia. Of the 172 infants, 114 (66.2%) had an isolated defect, 48 (27.9%) were multimalformed infants (MMI) with M-A, and 10 (5.8%) had a well-defined syndrome. The frequency of bilateral defects among nonsyndromal cases was 12% compared to 50% of syndromal cases. Among the MMI, only holoprosencephaly was preferentially associated with M-A; four cases were observed as against the 0.7 expected ($P = 0.005$). Neither was geographical variation in the prevalence of nonsyndromic cases observed nor was there evidence of time trends. Mothers with parity 1 had a higher risk of giving birth to an MMI with M-A. Mothers with insulin-dependent diabetes were at a significantly higher risk of having a child with M-A. Mastroiacovo et al. (5) suggested autosomal dominant inheritance with variable expression and incomplete penetrance "in a proportion of cases" or multifactorial aetiology. Three cases had consanguineous parents, but there were no other affected siblings to support recessive inheritance.

M-A can occur as an isolated defect or in association with other defects. A genetic or environmental cause has been found in only a minority of the cases. In such cases, M-A is usually part of a specific pattern of multiple congenital anomalies. For instance, M-A is an essential component of isotretinoin embryopathy, is an important manifestation of thalidomide embryopathy, and can be a part of the prenatal alcohol syndrome and maternal diabetes embryopathy. M-A occurs with a number of single-gene disorders such as Treacher Collins syndrome or chromosomal syndromes such as trisomy 18. M-A also occurs as a part of seemingly nonrandom patterns of multiple defects such as Goldenhar syndrome.

Congenital aural atresia (CAA) has been reported in patients with chromosomal anomalies, especially terminal deletions starting at chromosome 18q23. Veltman et al. (6) stated that CAA occurs in approximately 66% of all patients who have a terminal deletion of 18q. They reported a series of 20 patients with CAA, of whom 18 had microscopically visible 18q deletions. The extent and nature of the chromosome 18 deletions were studied in detail by array-based comparative genomic hybridisation. A critical region of 5 Mb on chromosome 18q22.3–q23 was deleted in all patients. Veltman et al. (6) concluded that this region could be considered a candidate region for aural atresia.

Aural atresia is usually (70–85%) unilateral (7–9). The deformity on each side can vary in complexity. For unknown reasons, males outnumber females and the right ear is more commonly involved (10). There are no reliable data on the prevalence or incidence of minor anomalies. The latter are syndromal in 25% of the cases.

Patient evaluation

These congenital anomalies cause moderate-to-severe hearing loss and require determination of the hearing level within three months of birth, using evoked potentials. In bilateral anomalies, amplification by air- or bone-conduction hearing aids within six months of birth is essential to avoid delays in speech or language development. According to current international opinion, infants whose permanent hearing impairment is diagnosed before the age of three months and who receive appropriate and consistent early intervention at an average of two to three months after identification of hearing loss have significantly higher levels of receptive and expressive language, personal–social development, expressive and receptive vocabulary, general development, situation comprehension, and vowel production (11,12). Speech development is progressively impaired by increased age at the diagnosis of hearing loss (13). Impairment is measurable as early as the age of three years and has consequences throughout life, leading to lower reading abilities, poorer school performance, and under- or unemployment. Linguistic experience already alters phonetic perception in infants by six months of age (14). Experimental data suggest nonregressive modifications of brain organisation due to absence of or inappropriate cochlear stimulation during the first half year of life (15).

Genetic counselling is also required not only to establish the hereditary pattern but also to rule out associated anomalies in other organ systems.

During early childhood, it is important to monitor both ears for the presence of otitis media. Especially in cases with unilateral atresia, the normal ear should be regularly followed up to exclude otitis media with effusion. If otitis media with effusion is present, prompt medical and/or surgical therapy is needed. Also, the atretic ear may be involved and may exhibit signs of acute otitis media. If the atretic ear is suspected of having acute otitis media, prompt antibiotic treatment should be initiated to minimise the risk of complications such as coalescent mastoiditis or subdural abscess.

History and physical examination

Middle and external ear anomalies may be isolated or associated with other malformations. To determine a syndromal aetiology, a systematic physical examination and history are needed not only of the craniofacial region but also of other organ systems. The examiner should include questions on drug utilisation or toxic exposure during pregnancy and any family history of hearing impairment as well as auricular or other developmental craniofacial abnormalities. In addition to these, information regarding low birth weight, maternal intrauterine infections, or trauma should be sought. If the patient is a young child, achievement of neurological milestones such as speech and ambulation are assessed through history and direct observation.

According to Schuknecht (9), 45% of patients with aural atresia had concomitant abnormalities. In particular, the spine and genitourinary tract systems require careful evaluation (16). The calibre of the external auditory canal should be graded as normal, stenotic, blindly ending, or atretic. Patients with a stenotic or blindly-ending external canal may escape diagnosis for years if the auricle is normal or only slightly deformed. There is no general agreement as to whether the degree of differentiation of the external ear correlates with the degree of malformation of the middle ear. Because the external ear develops embryologically earlier than the middle ear, one would be unlikely to find a normal middle ear with microtia, whereas a malformed middle ear can occur with a normal pinna (2). The face of the patient should be carefully examined to reveal any muscle weakness. It is rare to encounter a facial paresis or paralysis involving the entire hemiface, although occasionally there is involvement of the lower face or lip area. The most common anomaly of facial function is a congenital absence of the depressor anguli oris muscle (17).

Audiometric evaluation

According to the high-risk register (18), CAA can be identified as a high-risk factor. The child's usable residual hearing and the need for amplification should be determined as soon as possible after birth. When congenital atresia is diagnosed in a newborn baby, the paediatrician must rapidly refer the child to the ear surgeon or the audiological physician for further audiological evaluation. Delay in testing or a wait-and-see strategy is not in the infant's best interest. In the vast majority of cases, sensorineural function is normal and the atresia of the external ear canal causes a 45 to 60 dB conductive hearing loss. If both ears are affected, early hearing-aid fitting is called for. If it seems that the atresia is unilateral, then the status of normal hearing in the opposite ear must be clearly established. Pure-tone audiometry, speech-reception thresholds, or accurate behavioural testing cannot be performed on these young infants. Auditory-evoked brainstem response (and steady state evoked potentials) derived technology can be used as a test of the hearing status. This test will establish presence of cochlear function and overall degree of hearing loss, thus aiding the determination of the type of auditory rehabilitation needed.

According to Bellucci (19) and to Kaga and Suzuki (20), adequacy of inner-ear balance function can also be assessed using a rotational vestibular test.

Radiology

Axial and coronal computed tomography (CT) scans of the temporal bone are necessary in all patients with atresia as well as those with severe stenosis of the external auditory canal. In the latter group, radiographic studies are important in examining for possible cholesteatoma formation. High-resolution, thin-cut (1.5 mm) imaging modalities form the standard for evaluation of congenital atresia. CT scans provide information on the position of the facial nerve. Special attention is focused on its relationship with the oval window (i.e., normally positioned or overhanging) and the position of its vertical segment. Anterior displacement of the vertical segment of the nerve restricts access to the middle-ear space, reducing the chance for a successful hearing result from surgery and increasing the risk of facial nerve injury. In addition, the extent and type of the atretic plate as well as ossicular and inner ear development, and the pneumatisation of the middle ear and mastoid can be examined. Rarely, an abnormality of the horizontal semicircular canal or vestibule is seen. This finding may suggest an abnormal communication between the perilymph and the cerebrospinal fluid (CSF). In such cases, manipulation of the stapes should be minimised to avoid the potential complication of a CSF gusher. Three-dimensional CT may aid in their visualisation and can be used to view the radiographic reconstruction from the surgical position (21,22). Also, stereolithographic model reconstruction from CT has been used for the assessment and the surgical planning in CAA (23).

The CT scan may be obtained after birth or at the time of surgical repair. Although studies at an early age are rarely applicable to immediate rehabilitative plans, they may be important to establish the syndromal aetiology. Periodic CT scans are not necessary in patients with completely atretic ear canals, given the rarity of cholesteatoma in that setting (24).

Classification

The classification of the minor middle-ear anomalies shown has been modified from that of Teunissen and Cremers (25) (Table 17.1) and was approved by the HEAR consensus group of the European Workgroup on Genetics of Hearing Impairment (26). This classification is based on the preoperative findings and has direct impact on the reconstruction technique applied.

This classification is not based on the degree of abnormality but depends on the degree of fixation of the stapedial footplate or the presence or absence of accompanying anomalies of the other ossicles. Preoperative inclusion criteria are (i) age older than 10 years; (ii) no existence of intermittent periods of secretory otitis media; (iii) performance of tonal and speech audiogram as well as tympanometry with contralateral stapedial reflexes completed; and (iv) performance of high-resolution CT scan completed.

The further rehabilitation of patients with atresia is performed either with a surgical correction or with a bone-anchored hearing aid (BAHA). Atresia repair surgery should be performed only in carefully selected patients after a thorough investigation of all parameters involved. A proper selection based on stringent audiological and radiological criteria is obligatory. Preoperatively, a complete audiometric survey is performed as well as a high-resolution CT scan of the temporal bones.

The atresias are classified according a modification of the classification of Altmann (Table 17.2) (27).

This classification is based on the degree of malformation present. Altmann (27) was the first to propose a histopathological classification according to the severity of the atresia. He divided his cases into three categories: mildly-, moderately-, and severely-malformed types.

Table 17.1 HEAR-classification for ossicular malformations

I: Isolated congenital stapes ankylosis

   Footplate fixation

   Stapes suprastructure fixation

II: Idem + another ossicular chain anomaly

   Discontinuity of the chain

   Epitympanic fixation

   Tympanic fixation

III: Congenital anomaly of the ossicular chain but a mobile stapes footplate

   Discontinuity of the chain

   Epitympanic fixation

   Tympanic fixation

IV: Congenital aplasia or severe dysplasia of the oval or round window: a- or dysplasia; crossing N VII; persistent stapedial artery

Table 17.2 HEAR-classification of congenital atresia of the external ear canal

Type I: mild: tympanic membrane is hypoplastic; various kinds of ossicular malformations exist

Type II: moderate: atretic plate exists; tympanic cavity is within normal limits

Type IIa: tympanic bone is hypoplastic; course of the facial nerve is usually normal

Type IIb: tympanic bone is absent; course of the facial nerve is abnormal

Type III: severe: atretic plate is with a severely hypoplastic tympanic cavity

In mild cases (type I), the tympanic membrane is still present but hypoplastic. The tympanic bone is normal or hypoplastic. Various kinds of ossicular malformations have been described.

In moderate cases (type II), an atretic plate is present. The tympanic bone may be hypoplastic or absent. The course of the facial nerve may be abnormal; the tympanic cavity is within normal limits.

In severe cases (type III), the above-mentioned abnormalities can be found in association with a severely hypoplastic tympanic cavity.

Marquet et al. (17,28,29) as well as Cremers et al. (30–32) further subclassified the grade II patients based on the surgical and functional outcome.

Marquet et al. (17) based their subclassification of the moderate cases (type II) on Altmann's classification scheme on the course of the facial canal in its third segment, the morphology of the atretic plate, the presence or absence of a tympanic bone, and the distance between the glenoid cavity and the anterior surface of the mastoid. The surgical outcome was highly related to the proposed subclassification (33).

In type IIa, the course of the facial nerve is normal in its third segment. The tympanic bone is present but is hypoplastic or dysmorphic. The morphology of the atretic plate demonstrates the presence of an upper part formed by the squamous bone and an inferior one formed by the malformed tympanic bone. This inferior bony ledge extends laterally off the scutum of the squamous bone. The distance between the glenoid cavity and the mastoid is within normal limits.

In type IIb, the course of the facial nerve is more anteriorly situated in its third segment. The tympanic bone is virtually absent. The atretic plate constitutes an upper part formed by the squamous bone and an inferior one formed by a bony ledge, extending from the otic capsule. This bony lamella is very thin and never extends lateral to the scutum of the squamous bone. In between, there is often a fibrous ledge containing the facial nerve. Also, a hyperplastic Reichert's cartilage may be present here. The distance between the glenoid cavity and the mastoid is significantly diminished.

Cremers et al. (30) also reported an additional classification of type II cases in Altmann's classification scheme, depending on the thickness of the atretic plate. This subclassification proved to be useful in predicting the postoperative hearing level. In type IIa, there is total bony atresia over only a part of the length of the canal or the canal is partially aplastic and ends blindly with a fistula tract, sometimes leading to a rudimentary tympanic membrane (30).

For radiological criteria, the scoring system defined by Jahrsdoerfer et al. (34) is recommended.

Results

The surgical results of ossicular malformations without atresia are quite good (25). With the exception of severe dysplasia or aplasia of the oval and/or round window, (group IV), a postoperative air-bone gap of 20 dB or below was found in 72% of the operated cases.

A meta-analysis of the surgical results on atresia surgery showed a mean hearing gain of 20 to 25 dB in atretic type II and 30 to 35 dB in atresia type I cases (35). Surgical correction is recommended only if postoperative hearing better than 25 to 30 dB can be achieved. The long-term results remain almost unchanged (30). Most frequently, the anterior approach is used to open the atretic plate. This type of surgery can be performed from the age of five to six years. In the literature, no agreement can be found for the surgery of unilateral cases: Some surgeons will not operate on these cases, whereas others wait until the age of 18, so that the patient himself/herself can decide.

Less-favoured patients should be helped by BAHA. The results of BAHAs show not only a hearing gain in 89% but also better comfort when compared to classical bone-conduction hearing aids (36). Also, the speech recognition scores are much better (37,38). Owing to the requirements concerning the thickness of the cortical bone and its composition, the age limit for implantation has been set around two to three years in most centres (38). In children, this comprises a two-stage procedure performed under general anaesthesia: In the first stage, the titanium fixtures are placed in the bone at the mastoid (usually two), and at least three months later after osseointegration has taken place, the fixtures are liberated. The implant can be loaded two weeks after.

Medical management

The otological surgeon is usually alerted to the possibility of an atresia by the obstetrician or paediatrician shortly after birth. Quite often, the parents have some guilt about a particular incident or practice, and it is important to ascertain if this is the case so that these fears can be alleviated (39). During early infancy, the child should be evaluated in a complete and thorough fashion to determine the need for amplification. Genetic counselling is equally important to establish the aetiology and to rule out associated anomalies in other organ systems. During early childhood, it is important to monitor both ears for the presence of otitis media. Especially in cases with unilateral atresia, the normal ear should be regularly followed up to exclude otitis media with effusion. If this is present, prompt medical and/or surgical therapy is needed. Also, the atretic ear may be involved and may exhibit signs of acute otitis media. If the atretic ear is suspected of having acute otitis media, prompt antibiotic treatment should be initiated to minimise the risk of complications such as coalescent mastoiditis or subdural abscess (40).

Unilateral atresia

Medical intervention is not necessary in the infant discovered to have unilateral atresia. Paediatric audiometry should be performed to confirm that the child has normal hearing in the other ear. The parents are then reassured that speech, language, and intellectual development will proceed normally. As the child enters school, preferential seating is advised, but rarely is a hearing aid recommended because of poor acceptance by most children. In classrooms with unavoidable background noise, an auditory trainer can be helpful. Teenagers and adults often find the consequences of unilateral hearing loss from atresia to be a significant problem in social settings and at work, and they may more readily accept a hearing aid. However, a bone-conduction hearing aid is rarely helpful. If the canal is only stenotic, an air-conduction aid is preferred because of cosmetic considerations, better sound localisation, broader frequency response, and less sound distortion. Also, a contralateral routing of signal (CROS) system, possibly mounted in a spectacle frame, can be proposed in selected cases.

Bilateral atresia

In infants with bilateral atresia, amplification as early as the third month of life is essential. Auditory training should begin at six months of age (2). The initial medical and audiometric evaluations can be completed within the first few months of life, and a bone-conduction hearing aid fitted soon after. In children, a conventional bone-conduction hearing aid consisting of an electromagnetic vibrator pressed against the mastoid process on one side of the head by a steel spring or headband is the sole option. With the latest addition to the BAHA system, the BAHA Softband, even the youngest children who need amplification by bone conduction can be helped (41). The Softband is an elastic band with a BAHA sound processor connected to a plastic snap connector disk sewn into the band. The band has a Velcro fastening that enables it to be easily adjusted to fit the size of the baby's head. The results of this transcutaneous transmission are comparable with those of conventional bone conductors. In this application, the more powerful BAHA Classic is more appropriate than the BAHA Compact.

Scientific research shows that bilateral bone-conduction hearing aids mounted on spectacles are not feasible in young children, especially if the pinnas are malformed: Often there is insufficient support for the frame due to anotia or microtia. The conventional bone-conduction hearing aid may have a number of disadvantages. To function properly, the transducer of the bone conductor must be pressed very firmly against the skull. This can lead to skin irritation and ulceration. The body-level receiver, which is usually worn under the clothes, may provoke unwanted background noise. These children will remain deprived of bilateral speech "cues." However, there is experimental evidence that the auditory system is able to adapt in some way to binaural inputs even after childhood (42–44).

Surgical management

Since 1843, when Thomson published the first attempt of an operative treatment for CAA (45), much work has been done to improve the surgical technique and many authors have published their techniques. The surgical management is aimed at obtaining functional hearing gain and establishing an appropriate auditory canal eventually for the application of hearing aids. Surgical correction of hearing is a one-stage procedure. However, revision surgery is often needed (25–50%) (2,39).

Atresia repair surgery

Selection criteria

Accurate preoperative assessment is essential in determining surgical candidacy, because only 50% of patients with aural atresia are candidates for repair (34).

Jahrsdoerfer et al. (34) have developed a grading system (Table 17.3) based on preoperative temporal bone CT and auricular appearance to aid in patient selection for surgical correction.

Table 17.3 Selection criteria

Parameter	Points
Stapes present	2
Oval window open	1
Middle ear space	1
Facial nerve	1
Malleus/incus complex	1
Mastoid pneumatisation	1
Incus-stapes connection	1
Round window	1
Appearance of external ear	1
Total available points	*10*

In their system, there is a maximum score of 10 points. The total score aids in determining whether the patient will benefit from surgery to correct the hearing mechanism. A patient with a score of 5 or less is not a suitable candidate. This grading system correlated well with the degree of hearing improvement achieved, because 80% of patients with scores of 8 or higher had a postoperative speech-reception threshold of 25 dB or greater (46). Patients with syndromes involving craniofacial maldevelopment (Treacher Collins or hemifacial microsomia) are considered poor surgical candidates. In these and other familial syndromes, the middle ear is usually poorly developed and the surgical grade is often 5/10 (poor or marginal candidate) or worse.

Unilateral vs. bilateral atresia repair

Although most otological surgeons would consider atresia repair in bilateral cases, many are reluctant to operate on unilateral atresias. This reluctance is based on expectations of hearing recovery and the potential morbidity of the surgery (Fig. 17.1).

In patients with unilateral aural atresia, the operated ear should compete against the good hearing threshold in the other, normal ear. A patient with a unilateral congenital ear defect will only benefit materially from middle-ear surgery if the hearing is sufficiently improved to provide binaural hearing. The patient with a unilateral conductive loss must be made to understand what he or she can expect from successful surgery. He or she will be able to hear stereo music, tell the direction of

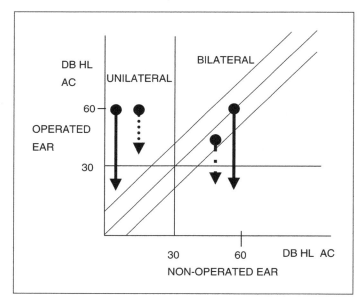

Figure 17.1 Glasgow benefit plot for unilateral and bilateral aural atresias. In this plot, surgical success for aural atresia has been defined as a postoperative hearing level better than 30 dB HL. If the preoperative hearing level is about 60 dB HL, the surgical procedure will be successful only if the hearing gain is more than 30 dB. However, as pointed out in Table 17.5, a hearing gain of only 20 to 25 dB is more realistic. The dashed arrow at the left represents a unilateral case with a functionally unsuccessful operation, whereas the dashed arrow at the right demonstrates a favourable bilateral case with an acceptable postoperative hearing gain. *Source*: From Ref. 35.

sound, and will hear more readily in a situation where there is background noise; in a quiet room, on a one-to-one basis, no appreciable difference would be noted.

Evidence indicates that children with unilateral hearing loss from any cause may be at the risk of delayed language development, attention deficit, and poor school performance (47). Speech recognition in patients after successful surgery for unilateral ear anomalies seems to be satisfactory although poorer than that of the normal ears (44). Dichotic listening tests have revealed a nonatretic ear advantage in postoperative unilateral atresia patients, suggesting a sensitive and critical period for aural development before the age of five years (48).

Patients with bilateral atresia present less of a surgical dilemma. The surgeon has to compare the expected hearing improvement following surgery with the rehabilitation using a bone-conduction hearing aid (conventional or bone-anchored). The goal in these individuals is to restore sufficient hearing so that amplification is no longer needed. Therefore, the "better" (as determined on CT scan evaluation) ear is selected for the initial surgical procedure.

Timing of surgery

Timing of surgical repair depends on whether unilateral or bilateral aural atresia is present.

The vast majority of authors agree that surgery for bilateral atresia of the external meatus should not be carried out before the age of five-to-six years and they point out that surgical treatment of younger patients is justified only if complications such as cholesteatoma are present. By this time, accurate audiometric tests can be obtained, pneumatisation of the temporal bone is well advanced, and the children are capable of cooperating with postoperative care. Although most surgeons are comfortable operating on the first ear of a child with bilateral atresia as he or she approaches school age, some are reluctant to recommend surgery at that age in unilateral cases. Delay until adulthood, when the patient can make his or her own decision, is then recommended.

Timing of microtia repair

According to Jahrsdoerfer (2), what really matters is the cooperation and dialogue between plastic and otological surgeons, and the willingness to integrate their ideas and surgical needs for the good of the patient.

Bellucci (19) and Marquet (28) believed that atresia repair should precede microtia repair. It was their belief that the opening in the mastoid could only be made precisely when the original position of the auricular remnant and the temporomandibular joint was known. Furthermore, it was believed that there would be less manoeuvrability of the skin and access to the middle ear would be limited. However, Aguilar and Jahrsdoerfer (49) demonstrated that the auricular framework could be sufficiently manoeuvred to align the meatus and the new canal. Auricular reconstruction should be performed first in order to preserve the integrity of the blood supply.

Cholesteatoma

A patient with CAA and chronic otorrhea or cholesteatoma requires surgery for eradication of the disease to prevent further complications, regardless of the potential for hearing improvement. Should there be a draining fistula or trapped cholesteatoma, surgical intervention is warranted immediately. Congenital aural stenosis (canal opening of 4 mm or less), as compared to CAA, carries a much greater risk of cholesteatoma.

According to Cole and Jahrsdoerfer (50), a bony ear-canal opening of 2 mm or less puts the patient at a risk of cholesteatoma formation. In their study, 91% of the ears with a stenosis of 2 mm or less had developed a cholesteatoma at 12 years of age. Surgery is recommended for patients with stenosis of the external ear canal measuring 2 mm or less. The appropriate time is late childhood or early adolescence, before irreversible damage has occurred.

Surgical techniques

There are three surgical approaches to the creation of a new external auditory canal:

Anterior approach: This method requires the removal of the atretic plate before the middle ear is reached. Dissection begins along the linea temporalis immediately posterior to the temporomandibular joint. The mastoid cells are not opened and the posterior wall of the external auditory canal is preserved. The dura mater at the tegmen tympani superiorly and the glenoid fossa anteriorly are the key landmarks in this approach. These are followed medially through the atresia plate into the epitympanum, allowing the identification of the ossicles. This approach avoids injury to the variably located vertical portion of the facial nerve, as long as the dissection is carried out in an anterosuperior manner, with entrance into the epitympanum prior to the exposure of the mesotympanum. The atretic plate is delicately removed with diamond burrs and curettes to avoid acoustic trauma to the inner ear from drill vibration. The abnormally located facial nerve is most commonly found in the inferoposterior portion of the atretic plate, lateral to the middle-ear space.

Transmastoid approach: This method employs a posterior approach to the middle ear and atretic plate. Dissection begins along the linea temporalis over the region of the mastoid cavity. The dura mater of the middle fossa, the sigmoid sinus, and the sinodural angle are used as landmarks. Following these medially, the mastoid antrum is entered, allowing identification of the horizontal semicircular canal and atretic plate. If possible, the facial nerve should be identified. The atretic plate is removed, exposing the mesotympanum. The facial ridge is lowered, creating an open mastoid cavity. The cavity must be centred either on the lateral semicircular canal or on the stapes: The hypotympanum is usually never revealed (17).

Modified anterior approach: Marquet et al. (17) and also Molony and De la Cruz (51) used a combined method. First, the mastoid at the antrum was opened to identify the short process of the incus. Then the bone immediately anterior to the mastoid was drilled away to obtain a new external auditory canal, preserving an intact bony wall between the mastoid cavity and the newly formed canal. The approach can be compared with an intact canal wall-like procedure.

Surgical results

Surgical results are difficult to compare because the selection criteria for surgery are quite divergent, leading to considerable differences between patient populations.

Moreover, every surgeon uses his own audiological criteria to define their operation as a surgical success (Table 17.4).

Although the kind of approach is readily defined, the surgical details differ considerably between different surgeons. To make meaningful comparisons of outcome, a consensus should be reached on the criteria for audiological success. A successful operation can reasonably be defined as one that obviates the need for a hearing aid. Even for such a criterion, differences of interpretation can be found: average hearing threshold level better than 30 to 35 dB (32) or than 20 dB (9).

The reported surgical successes are summarised in Table 17.5.

Although these results are not really comparable, it seems obvious that the audiological results are not very encouraging in the ears with more severe atresia. The variability of hearing improvement depends on the severity of the malformation. Whether the aura atresia is unilateral or bilateral does not influence the results (67).

However, even in the hands of the best surgeons, a mean hearing gain of about 20 to 25 dB is attained in atresia type II (Altmann classification) and 30 to 35 dB in type I. The mean hearing gain with atresia repair surgery seems to be somewhat better in less severely malformed ears. The more favourable cases usually have better preoperative hearing. As demonstrated on a Glasgow benefit plot (Fig. 17.1) (68), the combination of these factors leads to the conclusion that atresia repair surgery should be done only in very selected patients after a thorough investigation of all parameters involved (age, anatomy, uni-/bilateral, hearing status, etc.): Only the most favourable cases may sufficiently benefit from that kind of surgery.

Although some authors argue that the surgical results are only temporary and decline after some years, long-term results of Cremers and Teunissen (67), Marquet et al. (17), and Jahrsdoerfer and Hall (69) clearly demonstrate the stability of the postsurgical hearing results.

Table 17.4 Methods of assessing surgical success

Closure of air-bone gap	Surgical success of the procedure
Hearing gain	Lessening of monaural disability
Socially acceptable hearing (HL < 30 dB)	Lessening of bilateral aural disability
Glasgow benefit plot	Degree of benefit for the patient

Table 17.5 Surgical results in congenital atresia surgery

Author	Reference	Publication year	Classification	Success criterion	Atresia type	Patient number	Success rate (% or dB)	Follow-up (yr)
Gill	52	1969	Gill	HG > 30 dB	I	11	70	
					II	50	38	
					III	16	0	
Ombrédanne	53	1970	Ombrédanne	HG > 35%		600 Ears	69	
Wigand	54	1975	Altmann	Mean HG = 25 dB	II + III	26	50	
Jahrsdoerfer	2	1978	Jahrsdoerfer	< 30 dB HL		17	65	2–8
Pulec and Freedman	55	1978	Pulec	AB-gap < 30 dB		35 Ears	49	
Nager and Levin	56	1980	Nager	< 30 dB HL		23	70	
Belluci	19	1981	Altmann	< 30 dB HL		71	55	> 2
Portmann and Le Grignou	57	1982	Ombrédanne	Mean HG		100 Ears	22 dB	
de la Cruz	58	1985	de la Cruz	< 30 dB HL		56	73	0.5
Chiossone	59	1985	Chiossone	AB-gap < 30 dB	I–III	12 Ears	75	1–6
Mattox and Fisch	60	1986		HG > 30 dB		11	45	> 2
Lund	61	1987	Altmann	AB-gap < 20 dB		35 Ears	11	0.5–10
Manach	8	1987	Ombrédanne	< 25 dB HL		92	10	> 5
Cremers	31	1987	Cremers	< 35 dB HL	IIa + b	36 Ears	47	
Marquet	17	1988	Marquet	Mean HG	I	78 Ears	30 dB	
					II	126 Ears	15 dB	
Lambert	62	1988	Altmann			15	53	
Cremers	32	1988	Cremers	Mean HG	IIa	33 Ears	21 dB	
				Mean HG	IIb	20 Ears	20 dB	
Jahnke and Schrader	63	1988	Altmann	AB-gap < 20 dB	I + II + III	168	65	
Minatogawa	64	1989	Altmann	HG > 20 dB	I + II + III	9 Ears	58	> 2
Schuknecht	9	1989	Schuknecht	< 20 dB HL	II–IV	55	20	3
Molony and de la Cruz	51	1990	Jahrsdoerfer	< 30 dB HL		24 Ears	71	0.5–4
Federspil	65	1992	Cremers	< 30 dB HL	I	6	83	
					IIa	6	65	
					IIb	13	77	
					III	6	0	
Jahrsdoerfer	34	1992	Jahrsdoerfer	< 25 dB HL	8/10	112	82	
Helms[a]		1998	Jahrsdoerfer	Mean HG		125 Ears	13 dB	0.8
Tjellström[b]		1998	Cremers	Mean HG		37 Ears	20	15
Zhao	66	2005		HG > 30 dB		635	35	7.9

[a]Helms, 1998, personal communication.
[b]Tjellström, 1998, personal communication.
Note: HG, hearing gain.

Complications

The most common anatomical complications are chronic infection of the newly formed external auditory canal, lateral displacement of the tympanic graft or canal, and/or meatal stenosis. Anatomical complication rates of 20% to 60% are reported (9,40,70).

Functional complications are related to labyrinthine injury and facial-nerve injury. High-frequency sensorineural hearing loss due to noise trauma is quite common, whereas accidental labyrinthine fenestration is rare. Despite anomalous positions of the facial nerve, injury to the nerve is rare, with most series reporting no injury or an infrequent transient paralysis. Facial-nerve monitoring in surgery for CAA is obligatory (71).

Bone-conduction implant surgery

Based on the experience with dental implants, the idea of inserting titanium implants into the temporal bone for fixation of a hearing aid by bone conduction was raised. The concept of direct bone conduction was introduced by Tjellström et al. (72) and is achieved by using a skin-penetrating coupling from an osseointegrated titanium implant in the mastoid bone to an impedance-matched transducer that the patients can apply and remove at will. Long-term results have been published from centres in Göteborg (73), Nijmegen (74), and Birmingham (75).

Another clinical application of these implants in the temporal bone is the fixation of an auricular prosthesis. Four different systems are now in the market: Divino, Classic 300, Compact, and Cordelle II.

Selection criteria

Otological criteria

Patients with congenital malformations of the middle/external ear or microtia are good candidates for implant surgery, especially those with a good cochlear function. In particular, it is a valuable alternative in those patients for whom reconstructive surgery for ear canal atresia cannot be performed. Chronically draining ears, which do not allow the use of an air-conduction hearing aid, can be helped with a BAHA. Patients with a single-sided deafness combined with contralateral conductive hearing loss due to ossicular disease are also candidates for a BAHA.

Audiological criteria

The average bone-conduction thresholds (0.5–4 kHz) should be better than 45 dB HL for an ear-level or better than 60 dB HL for a body-worn hearing device. The speech recognition score should be better than 60%.

The Divino is suitable for people with bone-conduction thresholds of the indicated ear better than or equal to 45 dB HL (measured at 0.5, 1, 2, and 3 kHz). Additionally, patients with unilateral, profound sensorineural hearing loss in the indicated ear with normal contralateral hearing (as defined by 20 dB HL air-conduction pure-tone average) may also benefit from the Divino sound processor.

The Classic 300 is suitable for patients with a pure-tone average bone-conduction threshold in the indicated ear better than or equal to 45 dB HL (measured at 0.5, 1, 2, and 3 kHz.) This enables patients with air thresholds down to 105 dB HL to be successfully treated (60 dB air bone gap+45 dB bone thresholds).

The Compact is suitable for patients with a pure-tone average bone-conduction threshold in the indicated ear better than or equal to 45 dB HL (measured at 0.5, 1, 2, and 3 kHz.) This enables patients with air thresholds down to 105 dB HL to be successfully treated (60 dB air-bone gap+45 dB bone thresholds).

The Cordelle II is recommended for patients who have the same indications as those described for the other BAHA devices but when they are "too weak." The output from the Cordelle II is on an average 13 dB stronger than the Classic 300 (measured at 0.5, 1, 2, and 3 kHz).

Age criteria

BAHAs have been implanted in children as young as two years of age (37). At Nijmegen, only children older than 10 years were initially implanted, although recently the age limit also was decreased to five years. Also, Hamann et al. (76) start with implantation at five years.

Psychosocial criteria

The patient needs to have realistic expectations and a reasonable social support. Patients should be able to maintain the abutment/skin interface of the BAHA.

Anatomical and biological criteria

Diseases that might jeopardise osseointegration are a formal contraindication for implant surgery.

Surgical technique

Initially, it was described as a two-stage procedure with an interval of three to four months, allowing for osseointegration to start before a load was applied. The single-stage technique was first suggested by Tjellström et al. (77,78) shortly after the Nijmegen group (79) developed their own single-stage technique. Simultaneously, a single-stage technique has evolved in Birmingham (80). The two-stage procedure is still in use for children under the age of 10 years and older individuals with poor cognitive skills (39,81). The surgical procedure is well tolerated under local anaesthesia with minor sedation except in children who undergo the procedure under general anaesthesia. For the placement of the fixtures, surgical equipment specially designed by Brånemark is needed. After healing (about three months), the external hearing aid may then be attached to the bone-anchored implant.

Results

The application of BAHAs in patients with congenital atresia resulted in, marginally, the best free-field thresholds and speech discrimination as compared to other BAHA users (74,81–83). All studies report that the audiometric benefit from BAHAs is clearly greater than that from conventional bone-conduction hearing aids.

In a 10-year follow-up study by Håkansson et al. (36) on 114 patients, 89% of the patients reported improved hearing and 95% reported improved comfort when compared to their old device. For the patients, improved sound quality, aesthetic appearance (no steel spring), physical comfort (no constant pressure against the skin), and practical handling (single-housing construction and stable position) as compared to a bone-conduction hearing aid seemed to be equally important. Also, in relation to feedback, the BAHA was more popular (84). This improvement is due to less distortion, particularly in the low frequency range and/or due to the direct coupling to the bone. Håkansson et al. (36) found an improvement of 10 to 20 dB in thresholds, in Békésy audiometry, when skin penetration was performed (in the frequency range 600–6000 Hz). The BAHA was also evaluated in 65 patients by Snik et al. (38). These authors found an improvement in hearing threshold (pure tones) of 15 to 20 dB. Also, Powell et al. (37) found better free-field warble-tone thresholds in children.

In the majority of patients who previously used a conventional bone conductor, significantly improved speech recognition scores were found (38). The speech recognition score in noise improved from 50% to 75%. Also, Powell et al. (37) found an improvement in speech recognition tests in 50% of children with congenital hearing loss.

Mylanus et al. (84) concluded in their study that the BAHA is also a highly acceptable alternative for air-conduction hearing aids. However, when comparing BAHA with air-conduction hearing aids, a break-even point occurs at an air-bone gap of 25 to 30 dB: Patients with a lesser air-bone gap may feel a possible deterioration in speech recognition. If the air-bone gap was larger than 30 dB, better speech reception was obtained with a BAHA in the majority of patients. Further, Browning and Gatehouse (85) found ambiguous results when comparing BAHA with air-conduction devices. Håkansson et al. (36) reported on the subjects' assessment of BAHA as compared to their previous air-conduction aid and found no significant difference in sound quality, aesthetic appearance, practical handling, or physical comfort.

In children with previous air-conduction aids, the speech recognition was better in 71% whereas 29% had the same results as with their BAHA (37). Also, a majority of children felt BAHA to be more effective for hearing in noisy as well as in quiet conditions.

Van der Pouw et al. (44) examined the effect of bilateral fitting of BAHAs. Compared to unilateral fitting, speech recognition with bilateral BAHAs showed a significant improvement in quiet and, to a lesser extent, in noise. With bilateral fitting, the improvement of the speech-reception threshold in quiet was 5.4 dB (86). In addition, sound localisation improved (44). In patients with bilateral inoperable CAA, application of bilateral BAHAs is the only means for them to receive binaural cues because fitting a conventional bone conductor mounted in spectacles is often troublesome in children and adults if the pinnas are malformed. According to Thomas (87), postoperative training improves auditory speech recognition and needs to be followed by speech training.

Complications

Intraoperative complications are the inadvertent penetration of the lateral venous sinus or the inadequate thickness of bone. The most serious complication is loss of the osseointegrated fixture from its placement at the skull. Loss of fixture is reported in 3% to 10% of the cases (45,65,78,79,81).

Conclusions

Aural atresia surgery is mostly performed to alleviate a patient's hearing disability and seldom to manage pathology. Surgical management is usually aimed at obtaining functional hearing gain. Assessing the real benefit from surgery is, unfortunately, much more complicated than we usually realise. Owing to the fact that aural atresia surgery is considered one of the most difficult forms of ear surgery, it is very tempting to the less-experienced surgeon to consider a BAHA to be the best and most accessible solution for patients with aural atresia. This dilemma also reflects the differences between surgical teams, regarding selection criteria and the criteria for surgical success. Review of the literature demonstrated large differences in the interpretation of this term. However, even in the hands of the best surgeons, a mean hearing gain of only 20 to 25 dB is attained in atresia type II and 30 to 35 dB in type I. The more favourable cases usually also have better preoperative hearing. Therefore, atresia repair surgery is worthwhile if proper patient selection is done using stringent audiolometric and radiographic criteria. A postoperative air-bone gap of less than 25 to 30 dB should be pursued. The combination of these factors leads to the conclusion that atresia repair surgery should only be done in very selected patients after a thorough investigation of all parameters involved (age, anatomy, uni-/bilateral, hearing status, etc.). Only the most favourable cases may benefit sufficiently from this kind of surgery. Less-suitable patients should be helped with BAHAs because this type of surgery does not interfere with the future use of new techniques.

References

1. Eurocat. European Registration of Congenital Anomalies, 2003 (http://www.eurocat.ulst.ac.uk/).
2. Jahrsdoerfer RA. Congenital atresia of the ear. Laryngoscope 1978; 88(suppl 13):1–48.
3. Tjellström A, Jacobsson M, Albrektsson T, Jansson K. Use of tissue integrated implants in congenital aural malformations. Adv Otorhinolaryngol 1988; 40:24–32.
4. Lidén G, Kankkunen A, Tjellström A. Multiple handicaps and ear malformations in hearing impaired preschool children. In:

Mencher G, Gerber S, eds. The Multiply Handicapped Hearing Impaired Child. New York: Grune and Stratton, 1983:67.

5. Mastroiacovo P, Corchia C, Botto LD, Lanni R, Zampino G, Fusco D. Epidemiology and genetics of microtia-anotia: a registry based study on over one million births. J Med Genet 1995; 32:453–457.

6. Veltman JA, Jonkers Y, Nuijten I, et al. Definition of a critical region on chromosome 18 for congenital aural atresia by array CGH. Am J Hum Genet 2003; 72:1578–1584.

7. Cremers CW, Teunissen E. When to choose reconstructive ear surgery and when to choose a BAHA for major and minor congenital ear anomalies. In: Ars B, ed. Congenital External and Middle Ear Malformations. Amsterdam: Kugler, 1992:33–36.

8. Manach Y. La prise en charge des aplasies majeures de l'oreille. Acta Otorhinolaryngol Belg 1987; 41:564–573.

9. Schuknecht HF. Congenital aural atresia. Laryngoscope 1989; 99:908–917.

10. Okajima H, Takeichi Y, Umeda K, Baba S. Clinical analysis of 592 patients with microtia. Acta Otolaryngol (Stockh) 1996; (suppl 525):18–24.

11. Yoshinaga-Itano C, Sedey A, Coulter D, Mehl AL. Language of early- and later identified children with hearing loss. Pediatrics 1998; 102:1161–1171.

12. Moeller M. Early intervention and language development in children ho are deaf and hard of hearing. Pediatrics 2000; 106:43.

13. Gabbard SA, Schryer J. Early amplification options. Ment Retard Dev Disabil Res Rev 2003; 9:236–242.

14. Kuhl P, Williams K. Linguistic experience alters phonetic perception in infants by six months of age. Science 1992; 225:606–608.

15. Lustig LR, Leake PA, Snyder RL, Rebscher SJ. Changes in the cat cochlear nucleus following neonatal deafening and chronic intracochlear electrical stimulation. Hear Res 1994; 74:29–37.

16. Cressman WR, Pensak ML. Surgical aspects of congenital aural atresia. Otolaryngol Clin North Am 1994; 27:621–633.

17. Marquet J, Declau F, De Cock M, et al. Congenital middle ear malformations. Acta Otorhinolaryngol Belg 1988; 42:123–302.

18. American Academy of Pediatrics. Joint Committee on Infant hearing: position statement 1982. Pediatrics 1982; 70:496–497.

19. Bellucci RJ. Congenital aural malformation: diagnosis and treatment. Otolaryngol Clin North Am 1981; 14:95–124.

20. Kaga K, Suzuki JI. Bilateral congenital atresia. Auditory and vestibular testing and surgical approach. Acta Otorhinolaryngol Belg 1991; 45:51–57.

21. Jahrsdoerfer RA, Garcia ET, Yeakley JW, Jacobson JT. Surface contour three-dimensional imaging in congenital aural atresia. Arch Otolaryngol Head Neck Surg 1993; 119:95–99.

22. Andrews JC, Anzai Y, Mankovich NJ, Favilli M, Lufkin RB, Jabour B. Three-dimensional CT scan reconstruction for the assessment of congenital aural atresia. Am J Otol 1992; 13:236–240.

23. Andrews JC, Mankovich NJ, Anzai Y, Lufkin RB. Stereolithographic model construction from CT for assessment and surgical planning in congenital aural atresia. Am J Otol 1994; 15:335–339.

24. Lambert PR, Dodson EE. Congenital malformations of the external auditory canal. Otolaryngol Clin North Am 1996; 29:741–760.

25. Teunissen E, Cremers CW. Classification of congenital middle ear anomalies. Report on 144 ears. Ann Otol Rhinol Laryngol 1993; 102:606–612.

26. Van de Heyning P, Declau F, Martini A, Cremers C. The European congenital ear anomaly inventory. In: Martini A, Mazzoli M, Stephens D, Read A, eds. Definitions, Protocols & Guidelines in Genetic Hearing Impairment. London: Whurr, 2001:44–49.

27. Altmann F. Congenital aural atresia of the ear in man and animals. Ann Otol Rhinol Laryngol 1955; 64:824–858.

28. Marquet J. Homogreffes tympano-ossiculaires dans le traitement de l' agenesie de l'oreille. Acta Otorhinolaryngol Belg 1971; 25:885.

29. Marquet J, Declau F. Considerations on the surgical treatment of congenital ear atresia. In: Ars B, Van Cauwenberghe P, eds. Middle ear structure, Organogenesis, and Congenital Defects. Amsterdam: Kugler, 1991:85–98.

30. Cremers CW, Oudenhoven J, Marres EH. Congenital aural atresia. A new subclassification and surgical management. Clin Otolaryngol 1984; 9:119–127.

31. Cremers CW, Marres EH. An additional classification for congenital aural atresia. Acta Otorhinolaryngol Belg 1987; 41:56–601.

32. Cremers CW, Teunissen E, Marres EH. Classification of congenital aural atresia and results of reconstructive surgery. Adv Otorhinolaryngol 1988; 40:9–14.

33. Declau F, Offeciers F, Van de Heyning P. Classification of the non-syndromal type of meatal atresia. In: Devranoglu I, ed. The Proceedings of the XVth World Congress of ORL & Head and Neck Surgery: Panel Discussions, 1997:135–137.

34. Jahrsdoerfer RA, Yeakley JW, Aguilar EA, Cole RR, Gray LC. Grading system for the selection of patients with congenital aural atresia. Am J Otol 1992; 13:6–12.

35. Declau F, Cremers C, Van de Heyning P. Diagnosis and management strategies in congenital atresia of the external ear canal. Brit J Audiol 1999; 33:313–327.

36. Håkansson B, Liden G, Tjellström A, et al. Ten years of experience with the Swedish bone-anchored hearing system. Ann Otol Rhinol Laryngol 1990; 99(suppl 151):1–16.

37. Powell RH, Burrell SP, Cooper HR, Proops DW. The Birmingham bone anchored hearing aid programme: paediatric experience and results. J Laryngol Otol 1996; (suppl 21):21–29.

38. Snik AF, Mylanus EA, Cremers CW. The bone-anchored hearing aid compared with conventional hearing aids. Audiological results and the patients' opinions. Otolaryngol Clin North Am 1995; 28:73–83.

39. Glasscock ME, Schwaber MK, Nissen AJ, Jackson CG. Management of congenital ear malformations. Ann Otol Rhinol Laryngol 1983; 92:504–509.

40. Close LG, Scholl PD. Coalescent mastoiditis in a case of congenital aural atresia. Int J Ped Otorhinolaryngol 1982; 4:69–76.

41. Hol MK, Cremers CW, Coppens-Schellekens W, Snik AF. The BAHA Softband. A new treatment for young children with bilateral congenital aural atresia. Int J Pediatr Otorhinolaryngol 2005; 69:973–980. [Epub 2005 Mar 24].

42. Wilmington D, Gray L, Jahrsdoerfer R. Binaural processing after corrected congenital unilateral conductive hearing loss. Hear Res 1994; 74:99–114.

43. Snik FM, Teunissen B, Cremers CW. Speech recognition in patients after successful surgery for unilateral congenital ear anomalies. Laryngoscope 1994; 104:1029–1034.

44. van der Pouw KT, Snik AF, Cremers CW. Audiometric results of bilateral bone-anchored hearing aid application in patients with bilateral congenital aural atresia. Laryngoscope 1998; 108:548–553.

45. Thomson A. Description of congenital malformation of the auricle and external meatus of both sides in three persons. Proc R Soc Edinb 1843; 1:443–446.

46. Yeakley JW, Jahrsdoerfer RA. CT evaluation of congenital aural atresia: what the radiologist and surgeon need to know. J Comput Assist Tomogr 1996; 20:724–731.

47. Linstrom CJ, Aziz MH, Romo T. 3rd Unilateral aural atresia in childhood: case selection and rehabilitation. Am J Med Genet 1989; 34:574–578.

48. Breier JI, Hiscock M, Jahrsdoerfer RA, Gray L. Ear advantage in dichotic listening after correction for early congenital hearing loss. Neuropsychologia 1998; 36:209–216.

49. Aguilar EA, Jahrsdoerfer RA. The surgical repair of congenital microtia and atresia. Otolaryngol Head Neck Surg 1988; 98: 600–606.

50. Cole RR, Jahrsdoerfer RA. The risk of cholesteatoma in congenital aural stenosis. Laryngoscope 1990; 100:576–578.

51. Molony TB, de la Cruz A. Surgical approaches to congenital atresia of the external auditory canal. Otolaryngol Head Neck Surg 1990; 103:991–1001.

52. Gill NW. Congenital atresia of the ear. A review of the surgical findings in 83 ears. J Laryngol Otol 1969; 83:551–587.

53. Ombrédanne M. Malformations du conduit auditif externe et de l'oreille moyenne. Encyclopédie Médico-Chirurgicale. Paris, 1970:20182D10:1–8.

54. Wigand ME. Tympano-méatoplastie endaurale pour les atrésies congénitales sévères de l'oreille. Rev Laryngol 1978; 99:15–28.

55. Pulec JL, Freedman HM. Management of congenital ear abnormalities. Laryngoscope 1978; 88:420–434.

56. Nager GT, Levin LS. Congenital aural atresia: embryology, pathology, classification, genetics and surgical management. In: Paparella M, Schumrick D, eds. Otolaryngology. Vol. 2. The Ear. Philadelphia: Saunders, 1980:1303–1344.

57. Portmann M, Le Grignou P. Chirurgie des agénésies majeures de l'oreille. Rev Laryngol 1982; 103:347–352.

58. De la Cruz A, Linthicum F, Luxford W. Congenital atresia of the external auditory canal. Laryngoscope 1985; 95:421–427.

59. Chiossone E. Surgical management of major congenital malformations of the ear. Am J Otol 1985; 6:237–242.

60. Mattox DE, Fisch U. Surgical correction of congenital atresia of the ear. Otolaryngol Head Neck Surg 1986; 94:574–577.

61. Lund WS. The surgery of congenital deafness: the Oxford, England. Series of 235 ears. Acta Otorhinolaryngol Belg 1987; 42:5–11.

62. Lambert PR. Major congenital ear malformations: surgical management and results. Ann Otol Rhinol Laryngol 1988; 97:641–649.

63. Jahnke K, Schrader M. Surgery for congenital aural atresia. The Tübingen study. Adv Otorhinolaryngol 1988; 40:1–8.

64. Minatogawa T, Nishimura Y, Inamori T, Kumoi T. Result of tympanoplasty for congenital aural atresia and stenosis, with special reference to fascia and homograft as the graft material of the tympanic membrane. Laryngoscope 1989; 99:632–637.

65. Federspil P, Delb W. Treatment of congenital malformations of the external and middle ear. In: Ars B, ed. Congenital External and Middle Ear Malformations: Management. Amsterdam: Kugler, 1992:47–70.

66. Zhao SQ, Dai HJ, Han DM, et al. Long-term surgical results for congenital aural atresia and hearing reconstruction. Zhongua Er B, Yan Hou Tou Jing Wai Ke Za Zhi, 2005; 40(5):327–330.

67. Cremers CW, Teunissen E. Long-term results of surgery for unilateral and bilateral congenital aural atresia. In: Charachon R, Garcia-Ibanez E, eds. Proceedings of the Politzer Society conferences in Ibiza 1989 and Courchevel 1990. Amsterdam: Kugler, 1991: 13–15.

68. Browning GG, Gatehouse S, Swan I. The Glasgow benefit plot: a new method for reporting benefits from middle ear surgery. Laryngoscope 1991; 101:180–185.

69. Jahrsdoerfer RA, Hall JW. Congenital malformations of the ear. Am J Otol 1986; 7:267–269.

70. Chang SO, Min Y, Kim CS, Koh T. Surgical management of congenital aural atresia. Laryngoscope 1994; 104:606–611.

71. Linstrom CJ, Meiteles LZ. Facial nerve monitoring in surgery for congenital auricular atresia. Laryngoscope 1993; 103:406–415.

72. Tjellström A, Hakannson B, Ludstrom J. Analysis of the mechanical impedance of bone anchored hearing aids. Acta Otolaryngol (Stockh) 1980; 89:85–92.

73. Tjellström A, Granström G. Long-term follow-up with the bone anchored hearing aid: a review of the first 100 patients between 1977 and 1985. Ear Nose Throat J 1994; 73:112–114.

74. Cremers CW, Snik AF, Beynon AJ. Hearing with the bone-anchored hearing aid (BAHA, HC200) compared to a conventional bone conduction hearing aid. Clinical Otolaryngol 1992; 17:275–279.

75. Cooper H, Burell S, Powell R, et al. The Birmingham bone anchored hearing aid programme: referrals, selection, rehabilitation, philosophy and adult results. J Otol Laryngol 1996; 110(suppl 21):13–20.

76. Hamann C, Manach Y, Roulleau P. La prothèse auditive à ancrage osseux BAHA- résultats applications bilatérales. Revue de Laryngol 1991; 112:297–300.

77. Tjellström A, Jacobsson M, Norvell B, Albrektsson T. Patient's attitudes to the bone-anchored hearing aid. Results of a questionnaire study. Scand Audiol 1989; 18:119–123.

78. Tjellström A, Granström G. The one stage procedure for implant in the mastoid. 3rd International Winter Seminar on Implants in Craniofacial Rehabilitation and Audiology. Selva Val Gardena, 1993.

79. Mylanus EA, Cremers CW. A one stage procedure for placement of percutaeous implants for the bone anchored hearing aid. J Laryngol Otol 1994; 108:1020–1033.

80. Proops DW, Wake MJC. A single stage technique for the BAHA. 3rd International Winter Seminar on Implants in Craniofacial Rehabilitation and Audiology. Selva Val Gardena, 1993.

81. Proops DW . The Birmingham bone anchored hearing aid programme: surgical methods and complications. J Laryngol Otol 1996; (suppl 21):7–12.

82. Tjellström A, Rosenhall U, Lindstrom J, et al. Five-years experience with skin-penetrating bone-anchored implants in the temporal bone. Acta Otolaryngol (Stockh) 1983; 95:568–575.

83. Mylanus EA, Snik AF, Jorritsma FF, Cremers CW. Audiological results of the bone anchored hearing aid HC200. Ear Hear 1994; 15:87–92.

84. Mylanus EAM, van der Pouw KC, Snik AF, Cremers CW. Intraindividual comparison of the bone-anchored hearing aid and air-conduction hearing aids. Arch Otolaryngol Head Neck Surg 1998; 124:271–276.

85. Browning GG, Gatehouse S. Estimation of the benefit of bone-anchored hearing aids. Ann Otol Rhinol Laryngol 1994; 103:872–878.

86. Priwin C, Stenfelt S, Granstrom G, et al. Bilateral bone-anchored hearing aids (BAHAs): an audiometric evaluation. Laryngoscope 2004; 114:77–84.

87. Thomas J. Speech and voice rehabilitation in selected patients fitted with a bone anchored hearing aid (BAHA). J Laryngol Otol 1996; (suppl 21):47–51.

18 Cochlear implantation in genetic deafness

Richard Ramsden, Shakeel Saeed, Rohini Aggarwal

Introduction

In this chapter, we will discuss cochlear implantation (CI), which is now widely employed in the rehabilitation of many forms of genetically determined deafness. We will point out the difficulties that may be encountered in implanting various inner ear dysplasias, the risks that might be encountered, and results that might be expected. We also look at the outcomes that one might reasonably hope for in the largest group of implanted children, those with recessively inherited connexin 26 mutation. The genetic causes of deafness are many and the numbers of individuals with the less common syndromes who have received CI are small; so information about outcomes in specific conditions is still scanty, if it exists at all. With the current state of our knowledge, therefore, this chapter must of necessity be somewhat rudimentary. Nevertheless, generalisations can be made about the pattern of phenotype that is likely to predict good or bad outcomes. The risks associated with comorbidity in certain deafness syndromes are touched upon. Finally the indications for the auditory brainstem implant (ABI) are discussed for that small group of patients who are not suitable for CI.

Background to CI

CI has evolved over the last two decades as a remarkably successful component of the rehabilitation of certain individuals with a severe-to-profound bilateral cochlear hearing loss. Such hearing loss is usually the result of hair cell loss in the organ of Corti and the causes are many. In the normal inner ear, the organ of Corti acts a transducer that converts the travelling wave in the inner ear fluids to electrical activity in the cochlear nerve; this then progresses through the brainstem centres of the auditory pathways to the higher centres, the primary auditory cortex and the association areas. The process of transduction is performed by the hair cells. Shearing forces on the stereocilia cause alteration in the properties of the hair cell membranes and synaptic transmission to the dendrites of the first-order neurone, the cell bodies of which constitute the spiral ganglion. The ganglion is situated in the modiolus of the cochlea. Its central axons pass through the lamina cribrosa to form the cochlear nerve, which passes through the internal auditory meatus (IAM), traverses the cerebellopontine angle, and joins the brainstem, where its fibres synapse with the second-order neurones in the dorsal and ventral cochlear nuclei.

The cochlea has a very elegant tonotopic arrangement by means of which sounds of a progressively lower frequency are perceived as one passes along the cochlea from the oval window toward the helicotrema. The main determinant of pitch in the normal inner ear, therefore, is the point along the cochlear partition where maximum depolarisation of the hair cells occurs. This in turn is defined by the peak of the travelling wave. In addition, some frequency information is conveyed by alteration in the rate of stimulation of the cochlear nerve, especially at low frequencies. The cochlear nucleus on the other hand does not have such a clearly defined tonotopic map, and this has some significance when we consider the use of the ABI in the rehabilitation of certain cases of total hearing loss.

Until the development of the cochlear implant, the treatment of severe-to-profound sensorineural deafness was based on the use of high-powered hearing aids, lipreading, and signing. Adults deafened in adult life have acquired and retained language, although there might with time be some degradation in their speech. Children born deaf or deafened in the first years of life, however, have had no access to sound and have usually acquired very little in the way of spoken language; they may have faced a life of social, educational, and professional isolation and often economic hardship. The cochlear implant has changed things in a quite spectacular manner and has transformed the lives of many thousand deaf people since its introduction about 20 years ago.

The cochlear implant, in effect, takes the place of the deficient organ of Corti by introducing electrical stimuli into the auditory system where they can be interpreted by the brain as sound. A multichannel electrode array is inserted into the cochlea, usually into the scala tympani, and coils round in the cochlea for a distance of 25 mm. The array in most frequent use worldwide has a series of 22 electrodes mounted on a silastic carrier. The stimulation strategy takes advantage of the tonotopic arrangement of the cochlea. The most distal electrodes deliver low-frequency information and those in the basal turn deliver high frequencies. It is probable that the electrodes stimulate the spiral ganglion cells or possibly surviving distal dendrites and performance with the implant is related to the ganglion cell population. The implanted component of the system also comprises a receiver coil that picks up the incoming signal from the external transmitter and a stimulator containing a microchip that directs electrical stimuli to the appropriate electrode at a rate that may be as high as 90,000 times per second.

The internal component is inserted during an operation that usually takes about one to two hours. The middle ear is entered through a transmastoid facial recess approach and a small cochleostomy is drilled in the promontory just in front of the round window to allow access to the scala tympani of the basal turn. The electrode is threaded in and the receiver stimulator is located in a shallow bony well in the skull just above and behind the pinna. The external component comprises a microphone, a signal processor, and a transmitter that sends the processed signal through the skin to the internal component encoded on to a radiofrequency carrier wave.

CI in adults

The first patients to receive implants were adults who had lost their hearing after childhood and had already acquired normal speech and language. Cochlear deafness in this group is the result of acquired pathology such as ototoxicity, otosclerosis (OTSC), Menière's disorder (MD), meningitis, head injury, chronic middle ear disease, autoimmune inner ear disease, and surgery. In some cases, the cause is not readily identifiable and some of these represent a genetically determined progressive pathology. Assuming good patient selection, the majority of these recipients acquire good open set speech recognition and are able to use the telephone to a greater or lesser extent. They rapidly become socially integrated, get back their independence, and progress professionally. So good have been the results that the candidacy criteria are constantly changing and now include subjects with quite reasonable aided speech recognition.

Some of the conditions leading to deafness in adults may have a clear genetic basis or a genetic predisposition notably OTSC, aminoglycoside ototoxicity, some of the autoimmune disorders, and probably some cases of MD.

Otosclerosis

OTSC is an osseous dyscrasia of the temporal bone. Familial OTSC usually exhibits autosomal-dominant inheritance with reduced penetrance and variable expression (1). Linkage analysis has identified seven loci (OTSC1–OTSC7) of which four are published and three are reserved (2,3). The specific genes within these loci have not as yet been identified or cloned. In addition, there is emerging evidence that postnatal exposure to paramyxoviruses, particularly measles, in sporadic or genetically predisposed individuals is part of the process leading to clinical OTSC (4–6). Most cases present with a conductive hearing loss that may be managed by stapes surgery, but, in severe retrofenestral disease, there may be a profound cochlear loss, and this group may be candidates for CI. There are surgical issues that are specific to OTSC. There may be partial obliteration of the scala tympani by otosclerotic bone necessitating a drill-out, but usually the extent of new bone formation is confined to the first few millimetres of the basal turn and the problem is easily solved and insertion of the electrode array is not difficult. More of an issue is the spread of current from the array through the otospongiotic bone of the otic capsule to the facial nerve causing twitching of the face. This is most likely to be caused by electrodes close to the first genu of the nerve. It is managed by removing the rogue electrodes from the map but, as time goes by, it is not uncommon for more and more electrodes to have to be deactivated, as demineralisation of the otic capsule proceeds, so that eventually the device may become unusable (7). The other problem that can occur is result of osteolysis and cavitation in the petrous bone; the electrode may become displaced out of the cochlea into a cavity or into the internal auditorycanal (8).

Susceptibility to aminoglycoside deafness

Susceptibility to aminoglycoside deafness is associated with mutations in mitochondrial DNA. Mutations in the *12SrRNA* gene account for the majority of cases, usually the A1555G mutation. These mutations are most commonly encountered in familial cases in China and South East Asia when compared to sporadic cases (9). These cases are usually associated with severe hair cell loss but usually with good preservation of the spiral ganglion population and do very well with CI.

The other nonsyndromal mitochondrial deafness gene identified is *MT RNR1* (3). As expected, both types are characterised by maternal inheritance.

Mitochondrial syndromes

Mitochondrial syndromes associated with sensorineural hearing loss include the following:

- Mitochondrial encephalopathy, lactic acidosis, and stroke-like episodes syndrome
- Maternally inherited diabetes and deafness MT-CO3 syndrome

■ Kearns–Sayre (KSS syndrome)
■ Chronic progressive external ophthalmoplegia (MT-NDS)

The inner ear changes in these syndromes appear to be initially confined to the outer hair cells in the basal turn, but hair cell loss is progressive and it is possible that changes occur in the spiral ganglion cells at a later stage although the histological evidence is scanty. Only a small number of patients with syndromal mitochondrial deafness have received cochlear implants, so information is relatively scanty, but the majority have good open set speech recognition (10).

MD is an inner ear disorder with a proposed genetic and autoimmune aetiopathogenesis. Studies by Morrison et al. suggest that many human leukocyte antigen-A, -B, -C, and -DR alleles are either associated with the condition or confer protection against it (11). End-stage MD may be characterised by a profound bilateral hearing loss, and of course certain surgical procedures for the condition may produce a total loss of hearing as either a predictable (labyrinthectomy) or an unintended (vestibular neurectomy and saccus drainage) consequence. Ganglion cell survival is usually good, however, and these patients, who feature in any large adult cochlear implant program, usually do well with cochlear implants.

CI in children

Implantation in children was initially very controversial, but has now emerged as one of the most exciting areas in the whole field and the one that is expanding most rapidly. The challenge is to use the CI to introduce the child's auditory system to sound, in particular speech sounds, so that he or she can use these stimuli to program the auditory cortex and language areas and thus learn to speak normally. Early opponents declared that it was impossible and, that it was ethically wrong to subject a child to a major operation without its consent with no perceived chance of success. The arguments were vitriolic but have quietened down now that the success of the technique is clear.

The critical period

At birth, the sensory cerebral cortex can be seen as a relatively blank area awaiting input from the new world into which the baby has been delivered (12). The area that will subsequently be used for vision, the visual cortex, needs visual input to program it. If it does not receive this input within a critical period, that part of the cortex will be "taken over" by adjacent areas and cortical blindness will result, even though the eye itself may be functioning normally. Similar mechanisms apply in the auditory system. The part of the brain destined for primary auditory perception (the primary auditory cortex) lies in Heschl's gyri in either hemisphere. It is found on the upper surface of the temporal lobe in the Sylvian fissure. It projects to Wernicke's area for auditory linguistic processing. If the child does not receive the appropriate auditory input in the critical period, these areas

will lose their plasticity and it will be impossible later to reverse the process. Feral children with normal hearing, reintroduced into a human environment when the critical period is over, cannot learn speech and language. It is thus essential that if CI is to have a chance of habilitating congenitally or prelingually deaf children, it must be carried out early. The implant stimulates the spiral ganglion cells, the cochlear nerve is activated, pathways are laid down in the brainstem, and the auditory cortices respond by creating complicated synaptic maps in the same way as in a normally hearing child. Most cochlear implant programmes like to implant these children at the age of two years or less and most of these children will, after four years of implant use, be able to enter mainstream schooling (13). It is clear that, for implantation to be successful, certain prerequisites are essential. There must be a cochlear structure into which one can insert an electrode, there must be a neural structure that the electrode can stimulate (usually the spiral ganglion), and there must be a cochlear nerve to conduct the electrical activity to the brainstem. It is also clear that the brain itself must be capable of dealing with the incoming signals and that cognitive function is sufficient for the individual to ascribe meaning to these signals—so-called central auditory processing.

Deafness in children

Profound hearing loss in children may be congenital or acquired. Of the acquired causes, the commonest is still meningitis, which, in addition to causing deafness, may also have a deleterious effect on central auditory processing. Children who have been through the special care baby unit are at particular risk because there may be more than one contributory factor (e.g., prematurity, low birth weight, hypoxia, hyperbilirubinaemia, renal failure, and ototoxic drugs).

Congenital deafness

About 80% of children with congenital hearing loss have no obvious bony abnormality of the inner ear, and their hearing loss is assumed to be due to abnormalities at a cellular level in the membranous inner ear. The remaining 20% have a bony dysplasia that can be demonstrated on high-quality imaging such as high definition computed tomography (CT) scanning or magnetic resonance (MR) imaging. The inner ear abnormalities, whether dysplastic or nondysplastic, may be isolated or may be part of a multiorgan syndrome. In considering the problems specific to implanting children with genetic deafness, it is valuable to consider the normal development of the inner ear (14).

During the third week after conception, the otic placode appears on the surface ectoderm. This becomes invaginated to form the otic pit and, in turn, the otic vesicle or otocyst by the end of the fourth week. The vesicle divides into a ventral component, which gives rise to the saccule and the cochlear duct, and a dorsal component, which forms the utricle, semicircular canals, and endolymphatic duct. In the sixth week, the saccule forms a tubular outpocketing at its lower pole, the cochlear duct. This penetrates the surrounding mesenchyme and by the end of the eighth week has completed 2½ turns. In the 10th week, vacuolisation in the surrounding mesenchyme around the cochlear duct forms the scala tympani and vestibuli, and following that membranous structures such as the organ of Corti begin to develop in the cochlea. The semicircular canals appear as outpocketings of the utricle about the sixth week. The central portions of these outpocketings eventually become apposed to each other and disappear giving rise to the three semicircular canals. The endolymphatic sac and duct is initially a wide structure, but the proximal portion, the duct narrows about the seventh week. If there is no developmental arrest before the eighth week, a normal cochlea is formed (15).

The statoacoustic ganglion forms from neural crest cells and cells derived from the otic vesicle. It subsequently splits into cochlear and vestibular components, the spiral ganglion and Scarpa's ganglion.

There is increasing interest in the genetic and molecular factors that drive this complicated process. Over 400 syndromes in which deafness is a regular or occasional feature have been described (16), and after more than a decade of molecular biological analysis, around 60 recessive and 48 dominant loci have been identified (3). The subject has been covered in considerable detail elsewhere in this book. Normal expression of the *PAX2 and PAX3* genes is necessary for the normal development of the cochlea and of Nkx5 for the formation of the semicircular canals. The *FGF3* gene seems to be necessary for differentiation within the otic vesicle. The *SLC26A4* (*PDS*) gene mutation results in abnormalities of the endolymphatic system leading to the dilation of the vestibular aqueduct as seen in Pendred syndrome. The *EYA1* gene has an important role in encoding transcription factors. The connexins, of which connexin 26 is the most important, are controlled by at least three connexin genes (*GJB2, GJB3,* and *GJB6*).

Figure 18.1A and B show the normal anatomy of the inner ear and IAM.

CI in dysplastic inner ears

From the point of view of the implanting surgeon, it is important to understand the malformations that may occur when the normal process of development is arrested even if we do not necessarily understand why this has happened. The best review of these developmental anomalies is that given by Sennaroglu and Saatci (15), which really is an update on the valuable original work by Jackler et al. (17), and the following section is based on their classification. It should be emphasised that these abnormalities may occur as isolated phenomena or as components of multiorgan syndromes such as branchio-oto-renal syndrome (18,19) and Waardenburg syndrome (20).

The various types of inner ear malformations may have quite different prognoses for good auditory performance with CI depending on the degree of the dysplasia. It should be emphasised that no single centre has, as yet, assembled a very large series of cochlear implants in dysplastic ears, so a clear picture of the expected outcomes in each group is not possible at this stage.

Michel deformity

Here, there is complete aplasia of all inner ear structures (Fig. 18.2). It may be unilateral or bilateral, or associated with a less severe anomaly on the contralateral side. It may be associated with aplasia of the internal auditory canal. CI is not possible in such cases, but recent thought has embraced the

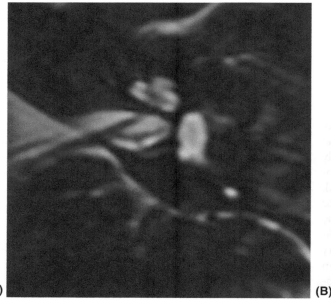

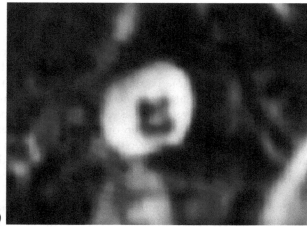

(A)   **(B)**

Figure 18.1 (A) Axial T2 MRI. Normal cochlea and internal meatus. (B) Parasagittal T2 MRI showing four nerves entering the internal auditory meatus. *Abbreviation*: MRI, magnetic resonance imaging.

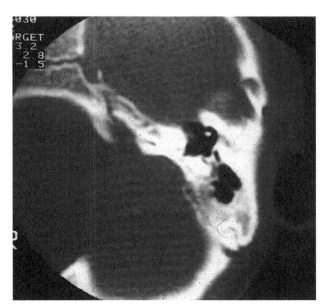

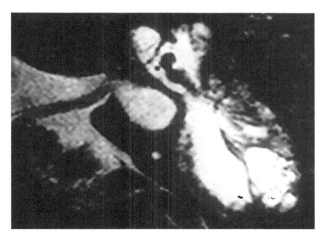

Figure 18.3 T2 magnetic resonance imaging. Common cavity. No separation into cochlear or vestibular components.

Figure 18.2 Michel deformity. There is no recognisable inner structure present.

possibility of brainstem implantation in this situation. This will be discussed later in this chapter.

Cochlear aplasia

Here there is an absent cochlea in the presence of a normal, dilated, or hypoplastic vestibule and semicircular canal system. The internal meatus maybe normal. Because there is no cochlea, CI is not possible in this type of ear, but ABI may be a possibility in the future.

Common cavity

This represents a further stage in the development of the inner ear in which the cochlea and the vestibule are an undifferentiated common cavity and is due to developmental arrest around the fourth week (Fig. 18.3). There may be an internal auditory canal present, but it is often abnormal and there may be connection between the common cavity and the internal auditory canal (IAC) due to lack of the party wall between them. CI has been performed in such cases, but there are problems.

Firstly it is not certain what neural elements may be present in relation to the cavity for the electrode to stimulate and where they might be located. One presumes that they will be in the wall of the cavity. However if the arrest is truly at the fourth week and membranous elements appear later, it is by no means certain that they will exist at all or exist in sufficient quantity to be capable of stimulation. A histological report (21) suggests the presence of ganglion cells in the wall of the cavity but, although the case is reported as a common cavity, it seems to be slightly further along the development pathway. From a surgical point of view, there may be difficulties. The inner ear must be opened through the bony bulge that the cavity produces in the medial wall of the middle ear cleft. If there is continuity with

the IAC, there may be a dramatic flow of cerebrospinal fluid (CSF) into the surgical field, which may require packing or the insertion of a lumbar drain (21). Furthermore, the electrode may pass straight through into the IAC and into the posterior fossa. A preoperative X-ray is essential to check for this occurrence. Conventional electrode design is based on the anatomy of the normal cochlea and may not be appropriate for a common cavity in terms of ease of insertion, positioning within the cavity, and delivery of electrical charge to the place where (we think) it is needed. Beltrame et al. (22) reported the technique of double posterior labyrinthotomy, introducing a custom-made electrode into the common cavity. They described three cases using the technique and found that surgery was technically no more demanding than other standard surgical approaches. They report that the speech processor programs remained stable over time, and auditorily that speech recognition results were similar to those obtained from children with no cochlear abnormalities. Others are not so sanguine! Buchman et al. (23) point out that the level of performance of these recipients is not high. Papsin (24) reported on eight children with a common cavity deformity and found that they had a reduced dynamic range and increased incidence of facial nerve simulation. Despite the fact that no fewer electrodes were inserted, they were judged to be more difficult to program and tended to require greater pulse widths. Mylanus et al. (25) report a single case with a common cavity with some open set speech understanding after one year of use. They also emphasise the risk of a perilymph gusher and the increased likelihood of encountering an aberrant facial nerve.

It is clear that opinion still differs about the possible outcomes from implanting common cavity patients. The discrepancies may be, in part, explained by inaccurate classification and using the term "common cavity" to include anything from a true common cavity to a much more differentiated entity approaching the status of a Mondini deformity.

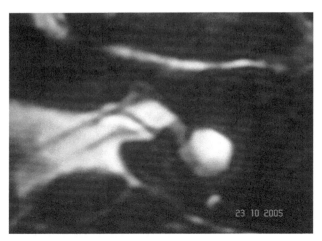

Figure 18.4 T2 magnetic resonance imaging. Incomplete partition type 1. Separation into two cystic components representing undifferentiated cochlea and vestibule.

Incomplete partition type 1: cystic cochleovestibular malformation

This may represent arrest at a later stage than the common cavity, perhaps at about the fifth week (Fig. 18.4). There has been some differentiation from the common cavity with separation into vestibular and cochlear components, giving a cystic dilated vestibule and a cystic dilated cochlea. Again most cases have an abnormal IAC with absence of the lateral wall of the IAC. The vestibular aqueduct is not enlarged in incomplete partition type 1 (IP1). As regards CI in IP1, the issues are really no different from common cavity.

Cochleovestibular hypoplasia

This group of malformations is more differentiated than IP1 with cochlear and vestibular structures clearly seen to be separate from each other. The cochlea is smaller than normal but may have normal internal architecture. Sennaroglu and Saatci (15) feel that it probably represents a failure of development at about the six-week stage.

IP2: Mondini malformation

This is true Mondini dysplasia (Fig. 18.5A and B). The term has been used indiscriminately in the past to include just about any inner ear abnormality, but it is important now that CI is widespread to ensure that the terminology is used accurately. Here the cochlea is of normal size and the internal organisation is much more advanced. The basal turn is normal or perhaps slightly dilated, but there is an interscalar defect between the middle and apical turns giving a cystic appearance. The basal part of the modiolus is present, so there is less likelihood of a defect in the lateral wall of the internal meatus. Ganglion cells are present in the lower part of the cochlea (26), so the prospects for successful implantation are very much better that in IP1. Vestibular anomalies are minimal, but many cases of Mondini malformations are associated with large vestibular aqueducts.

CI in IP2 has been reported by a number of teams, although the numbers are still small. After allowing for inaccuracies in classification, the results are reasonably encouraging. Miyamoto et al. (27) were among the first to describe a case and stated that the dysplastic cochlear anatomy did not preclude successful CI, and that electrical threshold measurements were similar to those recorded in children deafened as a result of other causes.

Munro et al. (28) found no difference in performance between their three patients with Mondini malformations and recipients with normally formed cochleas. Turrini et al. (29) reported a case and, although an unclear relationship existed between the electrode array and the cochlear partition making implant programming difficult, an excellent result was reported.

Arnoldner et al. (30) reported on three cases and stated that results are similar to those in children with normal cochleas.

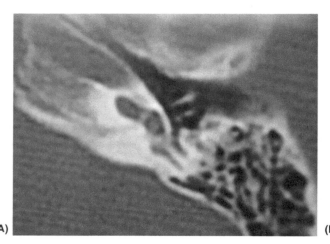

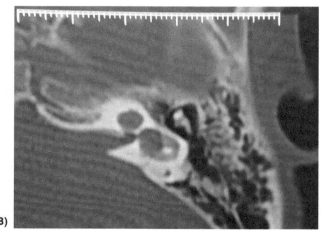

(A)   (B)

Figure 18.5 Computed tomography. Incomplete partition type 2 (Mondini malformation). (A) At the level of the relatively normal basal turn. (B) At the level of the common apical/middle turn.

Large vestibular aqueduct

This occurs as a late developmental anomaly, probably around seven to eight weeks (Fig. 18.6). As stated above, it may be seen as part of the Mondini anomaly but it may also be seen as an isolated entity. It is commonly seen as a feature of Pendred syndrome in which the genetic abnormality has been identified as a mutation of the *SLC26A4* (*PSD*) gene. The gene protein pendrin is involved in the transport of chloride and iodine ions, which explains the thyroid dysfunction and goitre seen in this condition. Patients with a wide vestibular aqueduct experience a progressive but fluctuant hearing loss that may become profound. The fluctuations coincide with relatively minor head injuries. The recovery from the impaired threshold may be delayed and quite dramatic so one should not rush into CI immediately but wait several months before making the decision.

CI in the large vestibular aqueduct syndrome (LVAS) has not been associated with surgical or programming problems, and the results are good (31). Contrary to fears that had been expressed by some, CSF gusher is not a problem when the scala tympani is opened. The endolymphatic compartment is a self-contained entity, and in a pure LVAS, there should be no continuity with the subarachnoid space. Transmitted pulsation in the basilar membrane can be seen through the cochleostomy, but there is no leakage of fluid. The results from a study of 14 adults and 9 children (32) indicated positive outcomes for both children and adults, with auditory and speech recognition performance that did not differ significantly from control subjects. The study by Bichey et al. (33) found an improvement in the quality of life associated with CI in postlingually deafened patients with LVAS similar to that in previous published studies of CI in other types of patients. Their data also indicated a favourable cost-utility when compared with published data about other disease states. Chen et al. (34) compared the characteristics of psychophysical tests of implanted children with LVAS and those with normal inner ears and found that

mapping parameters were not significantly different in the two groups.

In addition to dysplasias of the inner ear it is important to recognise that there may be abnormalities of the internal acoustic meatus that may present problems for the implant team. The normal internal meatus is about 8 to 10 mm in length with a cross section diameter of 4 to 6 mm. It contains four nerves, the cochlear, superior vestibular, inferior vestibular, and facial. The meatus and its contents may be affected by various degrees of developmental failure. Bulbous widening of the internal auditory canal may be associated with profound hearing loss—the large IAM (LIAM). There may be loss of the lateral wall of the IAM and CI may be associated with a CSF gusher (35). This may in fact be a manifestation of the X-linked deafness syndrome in which stapes surgery is also associated with a CSF "gusher" (36).

An important anomaly to recognise is the narrow or very narrow internal meatus, which may be demonstrated on CT or MR imaging. Valvassori (37) drew attention to the fact that a narrow IAC of 2 mm or less is associated with absence of the cochlear nerve. Parasagittal MR is necessary to allow identification of the neural structures in the CP angle and meatus (38). If no cochlear nerve is visible, CI is contraindicated (39,40) (Figs. 18.7, 18.8A and B). Meatal dysplasias may occur in isolation but are commonly seen in association with other developmental anomalies, e.g., microcephaly, syndactyly, tracheoesophageal fistula, duodenal atresia, and imperforate anus in Feingold syndrome (41).

CI in nondysplastic inner ears

Most children's cochleas that are implanted are grossly normal but are deaf as a result of a failure of development at a cellular

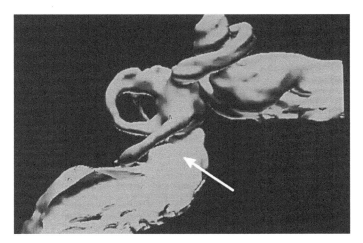

Figure 18.6 Three-dimensional surface rendered T2. Arrow points to large vestibular aqueduct.

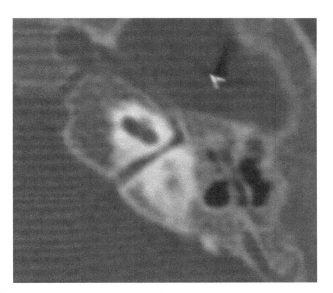

Figure 18.7 Computed tomography of narrow internal auditory canal (Feingold syndrome).

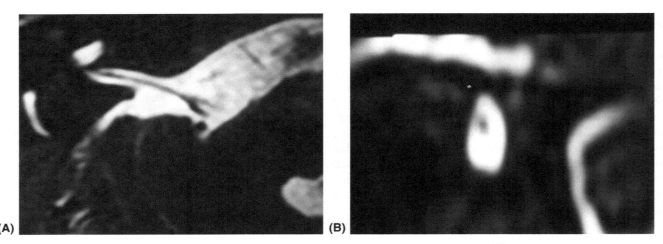

(A)　　　　**(B)**

Figure 18.8 (A) Axial T2 magnetic resonance imaging of narrow internal meatus with only one clearly identifiable nerve. (B) Parasagittal T2 MRI confirming that there is only one nerve entering the internal auditory meatus.

level in the inner ear. In most of these cases the deafness is an isolated phenomenon, but it can be part of a pluri- or multiorgan syndrome. Isolated deafness is commonly a recessively inherited disorder (autosomal recessive nonsyndromic hearing impairment).

Abnormalities of the GJB2 gene

Abnormalities of the *GJB2* gene, which encodes the connexin 26 gap junction protein are found in 50% of such cases. These children present no technical problems for the surgeon, and, assuming that the surgery has been performed early enough and that good rehabilitation, educational, and family support is available, they should make excellent progress with their implant, the majority entering mainstream schooling in due course. There is disagreement in the literature about whether individuals with GJB2-related deafness actually do better than a matched group of implantees with GJB-unrelated deafness. Sinnathuray et al. (42) and Fukushima et al. (43) felt that GFB2-related deafness was a good predictor of outcome, although the numbers in the latter study were very small. Bauer et al. (44) found that children with GJB2 deafness had significantly higher reading and nonverbal cognitive abilities than children without the mutation and suggest that this is because GJB2-related deafness is entirely due to cochlear damage with no effect on the cochlear nerve or the central auditory pathways. By way of contrast, Cullen et al. (45) found that the presence or absence of the *GJB2* mutation did not appear to have an impact on speech recognition. Lustig et al. (46) showed that patients with GJB2-related deafness clearly benefited from CI but outcomes were similar to patients without the *GJB2* mutation.

There are some important syndromes associated with cochlear structure that is grossly normal, but with profound or progressive deafness and comorbidity that may influence surgical decision-making.

The Jervell-Lange-Nielsen or long QT syndrome

This is an association between deafness and cardiac conduction defects. Stress and particularly the stress of general anaesthesia may precipitate irreversible ventricular fibrillation even in children who have a pacemaker fitted.

CHARGE syndrome

CHARGE Syndrome is a nonrandom association characterised by coloboma, heart disease, choanal atresia, retarded growth, and hearing problems. The hearing loss may be associated with a normal cochlea or with a dysplastic inner ear. The importance of the syndrome is the high incidence of heart defects, notably Fallot's spectrum and septal defects, as well as laryngopharyngeal incoordination, which may place the child at increased risk during general anaesthesia for CI (47). Because of the risks of unwelcome cardiac events, every child for cochlear implant surgery should have an electrocardiogram as part of the preoperative work up.

Usher 1 syndrome

Usher 1 syndrome carries the risk of total deafness and blindness. CI should be performed at an early stage so that the child can undergo auditory rehabilitation before the vision is lost.

Neurofibromatosis type 2

This is a dominantly inherited condition characterised by the occurrence of bilateral vestibular schwannomas (acoustic neuromas) (Fig. 18.9). It is caused by mutations in chromosome 22 as a result of which there is loss of the tumour suppressor gene protein, schwannomin or merlin. Deafness occurs as result of damage to the cochlear nerves from the tumours themselves, as a consequence of surgical removal of the tumours, or the effects of stereotactic radiosurgery. Some degree of auditory rehabilitation is possible using the ABI, which is a modification of the cochlear implant that utilises a multichannel surface electrode

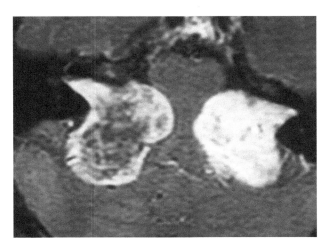

Figure 18.9 T1 magnetic resonance imaging with gadolinium. Neurofibromatosis type 2. Bilateral vestibular schwannomas.

placed on the surface of the cochlear nucleus in the lateral recess of the fourth ventricle. There are some circumstances in which it is possible to carry out CI in neurofibromatosis type 2 (NF2). If a Schwannoma is removed when it is still very small, a functioning auditory nerve may be preserved and a cochlear implant inserted at the same or a subsequent operation (48). This is a preferable option because cochlear implants usually give a much better outcome than ABI and furthermore it avoids the risk, albeit small, of inserting prosthesis into the brainstem.

Auditory brain stem implant

This device is a modification of the cochlear implant, developed to stimulate the cochlear nucleus in individuals who have no neural structure between the cochlea and the brainstem and are thus unsuitable for a CI. The main group of recipients are those described above with NF2, but recent work by has identified a group of nontumour cases who perform outstandingly well with the ABI (49). Of relevance to this chapter is the severe otosclerotic group with intolerable nonauditory stimulation with their CI to the extent that it becomes unusable. The other somewhat controversial group are those children with cochlear nerve aplasia or hypoplasia. Early results indicate that these children do gain access to sound but it is too early to know just what degree of speech understanding and language acquisition they are capable of achieving.

Summary

CI has proved to be highly successful as part of the rehabilitation of many deaf adults and children with severe to profound genetic sensorineural deafness. The success of the procedure is very much dependent on the phenotype. The ease and safety of the surgery to insert the implant is influenced by the presence

and extent of inner ear dysplasia. The less severe the dysplasia, the better the outcome. Outcome is also dependent on the survival of neural structures that can be stimulated electrically. In the most frequently encountered genetic deafness in children, associated with recessively inherited connexin 26 mutation, the outcomes are excellent. Some deafness syndromes are associated with hypoplasia of the auditory nerve, and the ABI may be a possible means of restoring some hearing. More information about outcomes in specific syndromes with deafness is needed.

References

1. Menger DJ, Tange R. The aetiology of otosclerosis: a review of the literature. Clin Otol 2003; 28:112–120.
2. Van den Bogaert K, de Leenheer EM, Chen W, et al. A fifth locus for otosclerosis, OTSC5, maps to chromosome 3q22–24. J Med Genet 2004; 41:450–453.
3. Van Camp G, Smith RJH. Hereditary hearing loss homepage, http://webhost.ua.ac.be./hhh/ (accessed October 2005).
4. Karosi T, Konya J, Szabo LZ, et al. Codetection of measles virus and tumour necrosis factor-alpha mRNA in otosclerotic stapes footplates. Laryngoscope 2005; 115:1291–1297.
5. Niedermeyer HP, Arnold W, Schuster, et al. Persistent measles virus infection and otosclerosis. Ann Otol Rhinol Laryngol 2001; 110:897–903.
6. McKenna MJ, Kristiansen AG, Haines J. Polymerase chain reaction amplification of a measles virus sequence from human temporal bone sections with active otosclerosis. Am J Otol 1996; 17:827–830.
7. Rotteveel LJC, Proops DW, Ramsden RT, et al. Cochlear implantation in 53 patients with otosclerosis: demographics, CT scanning, surgery and complications. Otol Neurotol 2004; 25:943–952.
8. Ramsden RT, Bance M, Giles E, et al. Cochlear Implantation in otosclerosis: a Unique Positioning Problem. J Laryngol Otol 1997; 111:262–265.
9. Li Z, Li R, Chen J, et al. Mutational analysis of the mitochondrial 12S rRNA gene in Chinese pediatric subjects with aminoglycoside-induced and non-syndromic hearing loss. Hum Genet 2005; 117:9–15.
10. Sinnathuray AR, Raut V, Awa A, et al. A review of cochlear implantation in mitochondrial sensorineural hearing loss. Otol Neurotol 2003; 24:418–426.
11. Morrison AW, Mowbray JF, Williamson R, et al. On genetic and environmental factors in Meniere's disease. Am J Otol 1994; 15:35–39.
12. Ryugo DK, Limb CJ, Redd EE. Brain plasticity. The impact of the environment on the brain as it relates to hearing and deafness. In: Niparko J, ed. Cochlear Implants: Principles and Practices. Philadelphia: Lippincott Williams and Wilkins, 2000:33–56.
13. Govaerts PJ, De Beukelaer C, Daemers K, et al. Outcome of cochlear implantation at different ages from 0–6 years. Otol Neurotol 2002; 23:885–890.

14. Sadler TW. Langman's Medical Embryology. 6th ed. Baltimore: Williams and Wilkins, 1990.

15. Sennaroglu L, Saatci I. A new classification for cochleovestibular malformations. Laryngoscope 2002; 112:2230–2241.

16. Gorlin RJ, Toriello HV, Cohen MM, eds. Hereditary Hearing Loss and Its Syndromes. Oxford Monograms on Medical Genetics no. 28. Oxford University Press, 1997.

17. Jackler RK, Luxford WM, House WF. Congenital malformations of the inner ear: a classification based on embryogenesis. Laryngoscope 1987; 97(suppl 40):2–14.

18. Ceruti S, Stinkens C, Cremers CWRJ, et al. Temporal bone anomalies in the branchio-oto-renal syndrome: detailed computed tomographic and magnetic resonance imaging finding. Otol Neurotol 2002; 23:200–2007.

19. Probst EJ, Blaser S, Gordon KA, et al. Temporal bone findings on computed tomography imaging in branchio-oto-renal syndrome. Laryngoscope 2005; 115:1855–1862.

20. Madden C, Halstead MJ, Hopkin RJ, et al. Temporal bone abnormalities associated with hearing loss in Waardenburg syndrome. Laryngoscope 2003; 113:2035–2041.

21. Graham JM, Phelps PD, Michaels L. Congenital malformations of the ear and cochlear implantation in children: review and temporal bone report of common cavity. J Laryngol Otol Supplement. 2000; 25:1–14.

22. Beltrame MA, Frau GN, Shanks M, et al. Double posterior labyrinthotomy technique: results in three Med-El patients with common cavity. Otol Neurotol 2005; 26:177–182.

23. Buchman CA, Copeland BJ, Brown CJ, et al. Cochlear implantation in children with congenital inner ear malformations. Laryngoscope 2004; 114:309–316.

24. Papsin BC. Cochlear implantation in children with anomalous cochleovestibular anatomy. Laryngoscope 2005; 115(suppl 106):1–26.

25. Mylanus EA, Rotteveel LJ, Leeuw RL. Congenital malformation of the inner ear and pediatric cochlear implantation. Otol Neurotol 2004; 25:308–317.

26. Schmidt JM. Cochlear neuronal populations in developmental defects of the inner ear. Implications for cochlear implantation. Acta Otolaryngol 1985; 99:14–20.

27. Miyamoto RT, Robbins AJ, Myres WA, et al. Cochlear implantation in the Mondini inner ear malformation. Am J Otol 1986; 7:258–261.

28. Munro KJ, George CR, Haacke NP. Audiological findings after multichannel cochlear implantation in patients with Mondini dysplasia. Br J Audiol 1996; 30:369–379.

29. Turrini M, Orzan E, Gabana M, et al. Cochlear implantation in a bilateral Mondini dysplasia. Scand Audiol Suppl 1997; 46:78–81.

30. Arnoldner C, Baumgartner WD, Gstoettner W, et al. Audiological performance after cochlear implantation in children with inner ear malformations. Int J Otorhinolaryngol 2004; 68: 457–467.

31. Temple RH, Ramsden RT, Axon PR, et al. The large vestibular aqueduct syndrome: the role of cochlear implant in its management. Clin Otol 1999; 24:301–306.

32. Miyamoto RT, Bichey BG, Wynne MK. Cochlear implantation with large vestibular aqueduct syndrome. Laryngoscope 2002; 112:1178–1182.

33. Bichey BG, Hoversland JM, Wynne MK, et al. Changes in quality of life and the cost-utility associated with cochlear implantation in patients with large vestibular aqueduct syndrome. Otol Neurotol 2002; 23:323–327.

34. Chen X, Han D, Zhao X, et al. Comparing the characteristics of psychophysical tests between cochlear implant children with large vestibular aqueduct syndrome and normal inner ear. Lin Chuang Er Bi Yan Hou Ke Za Zhi 2005; 19:583–584, 587.

35. Birman CS, Gibson WPR. Hearing loss associated with large internal meatus: a report of 5 paediatric cases. J Laryngol Otol 1999; 113:1015–1019.

36. Cremers CW, Hombergen GC, Wentges RT. Perilymphatic gusher and stapes surgery. A predictable complication? Clin Otol 1983; 8:235–240.

37. Valvassori GE. The internal auditory canal revisited. The high definition approach. Otolaryngol Clin North Am 1995; 28(3):431–451.

38. Casselman JE, Offeciers FE, Govaerts PJ, et al. Aplasia and hypoplasia of the vestibulocochlear nerve: diagnosis with MR imaging. Radiol 1997; 202:773–781.

39. Shelton C, Luxford WM, Shelton C. The narrow internal auditory canal in children: a contraindication to cochlear implants. Otolaryngol Head Neck Surg 1989; 100:227–231.

40. Maxwell AP, Mason SP, O'Donoghue GM. Cochlear nerve aplasia and its importance in cochlear implantation. Am J Otol 1999; 20:335–337.

41. Dodds A, Ramsden RT, Kingston H. Feingold syndrome—a cause of profound deafness. J Laryngol Otol 1999; 113:919–921.

42. Sinnathuray AR, Toner JG, Geddis A, et al. Auditory perception and speech discrimination after cochlear implantation in patients with Connexin 26 (GJB2) gene-related deafness. Otol Neurotol 2004; 25:930–934.

43. Fukushima K, Sugata K, Kasai N, et al. Better performance in cochlear implant patients with GJB2–related deafness. Int J Paed Otorhinolaryngol 2002; 62:151–157.

44. Bauer PW, Geers AE, Brenner C, et al. The effect of GJB2 allele variants on performance after cochlear implantation. Laryngoscope 2003; 113:2135–2140.

45. Cullen RD, Buchman MD, Brown CJ, et al. Cochlear implantation for children with GJB2-related deafness. Laryngoscope 2004; 114:1415–1419.

46. Lustig LR, Lin D, Venick H, et al. GJB2 gene mutations in cochlear implant recipients: prevalence and impact. Archs Otolaryngol Head Neck Surg 2004; 130:541–546.

47. Wyse RK, al-Mahdawi S, Burn J, et al. Congenital heart disease in CHARGE association. Paed Cardiol 1993; 14:75–81.

48. Temple RH, Axon PR, Ramsden RT, et al. Auditory rehabilitation in neurofibromatosis type 2: a case for cochlear implantation. J Laryngol Otol 1999; 113:161–163.

49. Colletti V, Carner M, Miorelli V, et al. Auditory brainstem implant (ABI): new frontiers in adults and children. Otolaryngol Head Neck Surg 2005; 133:126–138.

19 Auditory neuropathy caused by the otoferlin gene mutation

Constantino Morera, Laura Cavallé,
Diego Collado, Felipe Moreno

Introduction

Auditory neuropathy

Auditory neuropathy includes different neuropathologies in the auditory pathway from the VIII nerve to the brainstem. This term was introduced by Starr (1) to describe patients who presented with a hearing loss with absent or severely distorted auditory brainstem responses (ABR) and normal otoacoustic emissions (OAEs) and cochlear microphonics. It has been suggested that the hearing loss reflected altered temporal synchrony in the cochlear nerve (1,2). The generalised use of OAEs as a procedure to assess the function of outer hair cells (OHC) of the cochlea facilitates the diagnosis of auditory neuropathy.

Different aetiologies have been described in patients with the condition. These include acquired perinatal aetiologies [hyperbilirubinaemia (HBR) and hypoxia], acquired peri- and postnatal causes (toxic, infectious, immunological and metabolic disorders), nonsyndromal and syndromal causes of genetic origin [Charcot–Marie–Tooth (C–M–T), Friedreich ataxia], and unknown aetiologies (3–6).

In more than 90% of the patients with auditory neuropathy, the hearing impairment is sensorineural, bilateral, and symmetrical (3). Kraus et al. reported that 14% of their patients with absent ABRs correspond to auditory neuropathy (2). Berlin considered that 5 of every 50 or 60 children with profound hearing impairment can be included in this group (7).

The lesion in auditory neuropathy can be located anywhere from the inner hair cells to the brainstem cochlear nucleus (inner hair cells, synapses, spiral ganglion, fibres of the VIII nerve) (8). The most frequent site of the lesion is in the more peripheral regions (9). Harrison reported an experimental model in animals treated with carboplatin, with a loss of the inner hair cells and preservation of the OHC, with preservation of the OAEs and cochlear microphonics while the ABR was affected (10).

Cochlear implantation in auditory neuropathy has been discussed and variable results have been published. Initial studies recommended caution before implanting patients with auditory neuropathy. However, more recent studies report benefits from cochlear implantation (11,12). This could relate to the site of the lesion, which is difficult to identify.

The otoferlin gene

Hearing impairment of genetic origin includes a heterogeneous group of lesions with an approximate incidence of 1 in 1000 newborn babies. Most congenital genetic deafness is nonsyndromal with an autosomal recessive pattern of inheritance (DFNB). Many genes have been described as causing hearing loss. The most frequent is the connexin 26 mutation (13).

Yasunaga et al. reported nonsyndromal congenital deafness with the otoferlin (*OTOF*) gene mutation (Locus DFNB9 in

2P22-P23) (14). Migliosi et al. described the homozygous mutation Q829X as a cause of deafness in the Spanish population. It is the third most frequent cause of genetic prelingual deafness in Spain (13).

The *OTOF* gene encodes otoferlin, which is a cytosolic membrane protein that is expressed mainly in the inner hair cells of the organ of Corti and in type I vestibular hair cells. It is considered that this protein is involved in the synapses of these sensory cells of the inner ear.

Objectives of the present study

Cochlear implant performance in patients with auditory neuropathy is variable. The otoferlin protein encoded by the *OTOF* gene is considered to be implicated in the synapses of the inner hair cells and is common in the Spanish population. In consequence, this study has two objectives:

- To determine the prevalence of the OTOF gene as a cause of auditory neuropathy in Valencia, a Mediterranean area of Spain
- To study the results of cochlear implantation in auditory neuropathy and in the OTOF group, in particular. We hypothesised that the results should be good because the cochlear implant stimulus should bypass such lesions.

Material and methods

The study comprised both prospective and retrospective investigations in relation to cochlear implantation in auditory neuropathy. The prospective group included the patients with audiological and genetic diagnoses prior to implantation. The retrospective group includes patients who had previously been implanted, the diagnosis of auditory neuropathy having been made in a subsequent genetic study.

The study was carried out in a group of 15 patients. This was clinical with a single subject design, with successive audiological tests in the same patients who acted as their own controls. The results have been compared with similar groups of patients implanted without associated pathology.

The study protocol includes the following:

1. Anamnesis, ENT examination and preoperative cochlear implant workup
2. Audiological testing including transient OAEs, ABR, pure tone audiometry (PTA) and speech recognition tests appropriate to the patient's age
3. Radiological exploration
4. Genetic investigation
5. Neurological study
6. Audiological and genetic evaluation of the families

Results

Most of the patients with auditory neuropathy in our series had the Q829X mutation of the *OTOF* gene (66%). The second most common cause was HBR. The other aetiologies were C–M–T polyneuropathy (PN) and a PN of unknown cause (Fig. 19.1).

Ten patients had the homozygous *OTOF* gene mutation (Q829X/Q829X), all with a profound bilateral sensorineural hearing impairment. The median age at diagnosis was of 9.1 years (standard deviation ±5.04). All the parents were heterozygotes for the Q829X mutation and had normal hearing.

The deafness in the *OTOF* gene mutation group was stable over time. The deafness was congenital and, in consequence, prelingual. Three patients had a family history of hearing impairment, one having an affected brother, one a deaf cousin, and the third an affected maternal aunt. No other auditory risk factors were found. The characteristics of these patients are shown in Table 19.1.

Table 19.2 shows the group with diverse aetiologies. Three patients had HBR, one C–M–T PN, and another case had an unknown cause. The age at which hearing loss was first suspected varies from 7 days of life to 11 years. Most frequently, the hearing loss was progressive; in one patient it was stable and in another regressive, with progressive improvement.

The series included 15 patients with auditory neuropathy, including 13 patients who have been implanted. Two patients were not implanted because there were no audiological indications. No malformations were found in the preoperative radiological investigation with computed tomography and magnetic resonance imaging (Fig. 19.2).

The preoperative PTA in implanted cases, showed a bilateral and symmetrical severe-profound hearing impairment (Fig. 19.3). The preoperative sound field audiometry (SFA) threshold with hearing aids is presented in Figure 19.4, and the postoperative improvement in SFA results following implantation in Figure 19.5.

The first tuning was carried out one month after implantation, starting the auditory habilitation/rehabilitation process. Cochlear implant performance was evaluated with

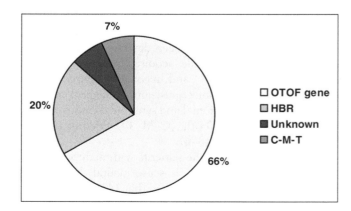

Figure 19.1 Aetiology of auditory neuropathy in our series (15 patients). *Abbreviations*: HBR, hyperbilirubinaemia; *OTOF*, otoferlin; C–M–T, Charcot–Marie–Tooth.

Table 19.1   Auditory neuropathy cases with the *OTOF* gene mutation (10 cases)

Case	Aetiology	HI onset	Type HI	Family history of HI	Other risk factor of HI	General evaluation
1C	Q829X/Q829X	Congenital	Profound	–	–	Normal
2C	Q829X/Q829X	Congenital	Profound	Yes (no OTOF)	–	Normal
3N	Q829X/Q829X	Congenital	Profound	Yes	–	Normal
4R	Q829X/Q829X	Congenital	Profound	–	–	Normal
5F	Q829X/Q829X	Congenital	Profound	–	–	Normal
6F	Q829X/Q829X	Congenital	Profound	–	–	Normal
7R	Q829X/Q829X	Congenital	Profound	Yes?	–	Normal
8I	Q829X/1236delC	Congenital	Profound	–	–	Normal
9C	Q829X/Q829X	Congenital	Profound	–	–	Normal
10C	Q829X/Q829X	Congenital	Profound	–	–	Normal

Abbreviations: HI, hearing impairment; *OTOF*, otoferlin.

Table 19.2   Auditory neuropathy patients without the *OTOF* gene mutation (5 cases)

Case	Aetiology	HI onset	Type HI	Family history of HI	Other risk factor of HI	General evaluation
1M	Unknown	2 yr	Progressive profound	–	–	Normal
2A	C–M–T	8 yr	Progressive profound	–	–	Bilat cataracts PN
3P	HBR	11 yr	Progressive moderate	–	HBR	Normal
4C	HBR	7 days	Stable profound	–	HBR	Normal
5C	HBR	3 mo	Restoration to normal hearing	–	HBR	Normal

Abbreviations: C–M–T, Charcot–Marie–Tooth; HBR, hyperbilirubinaemia; HI, hearing impairment; *OTOF*, otoferlin; PN, polyneuropathy.

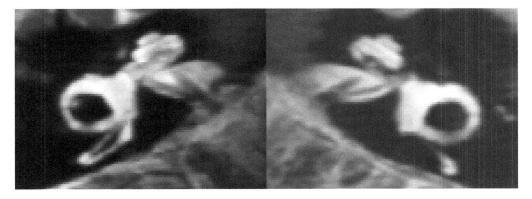

Figure 19.2   Normal magnetic resonance imaging in a patient with *OTOF* gene mutations. *Abbreviation*: *OTOF*, otoferlin.

speech recognition tests appropriate to the age and language development of each patient. These tests were carried out with loudspeakers located 1 m away from the patient's head. The material was presented at 65 dB SPL. In very small children, the Infant Toddler Meaningful Auditory Integration Scale (IT-MAIS) was also carried out.

In the OTOF group, the patients were classified into several groups according to the aetiology of the auditory neuropathy,

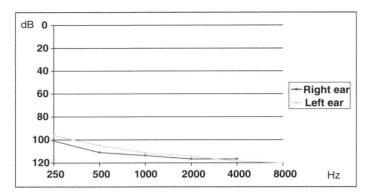

Figure 19.3 Mean preoperative pure tone audiometry in the *OTOF* gene mutation group. *Abbreviation*: *OTOF*, otoferlin.

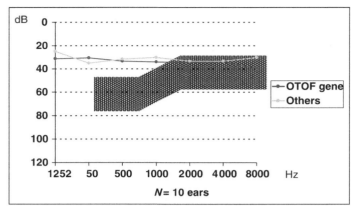

Figure 19.5 Mean postimplantation sound field audiometry postcochlear implantation in the *OTOF* gene mutation group. *Abbreviation*: *OTOF*, otoferlin.

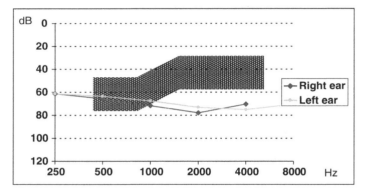

Figure 19.4 Mean preoperative sound field audiometry with hearing aids in the *OTOF* gene mutation group. *Abbreviation*: *OTOF*, otoferlin.

the age of onset of hearing impairment and the experience with their cochlear implant. The first group comprised two children with auditory neuropathy caused by the *OTOF* gene mutation implanted before the age of two years and with one year's

experience with a cochlear implant. A second group is formed by children with auditory neuropathy caused by the *OTOF* gene mutation with more than one year's experience with their cochlear implant. This group was the largest and has been compared with a control group of 37 implanted children with hearing impairments of cochlear origin.

The third group comprised two patients with auditory neuropathy caused by the *OTOF* gene mutation, one implanted at the age of 9 and the other at 24 years. They constitute the group with the worst results. The results of the first, with three years experience with a cochlear implant, are shown in Figure 19.5. The second, the woman implanted at 24 years of age, had very limited benefit with the cochlear implant, similar to what is often found in implanted adults with prelingual hearing impairment.

The preoperative stapedial reflex was absent in all cases. After implantation, we found it to have recovered in all patients. Similarly, good responses were observed with neural

Table 19.3 Cochlear implant results in the auditory neuropathy group with the *OTOF* gene mutation

Case	Age at CI	CI type	CI experience	Post-CI performance
1C	24 yr	MED-EL40+	1 yr	Poor
2F	9 yr	N24M	3 yr	Poor
3F	37 mo	N24M	2 yr	Good
4R	31 mo	N24M	3 yr	Good
5R	28 mo	N24M	3 yr	Very good
6C	24 mo	N24K	1 yr	Good
7C	24 mo	CII	3 yr	Good
8C	24 mo	CII	3 yr	Good
9 N	19 mo	N24C	6 mo	Good
10I	17 mo	N24CA	6 mo	Good

Abbreviation: CI, cochlear implant; *OTOF*, otoferlin.

Table 19.4   Cochlear implant results in the auditory neuropathy group without the *OTOF* gene mutation

Case	Age at suspected HI	Aetiology	Age at CI	CI type	CI experience	Post-CI performance
1M	Postlingual	Unknown	15 yr	MED-EL40 +	8 yr	Very good
2A	Postlingual	PN(C–M–T)	25 yr	N22	2 yr	Moderate
3C	Congenital	HBR	18 mo	CII	6 mo	Good

Abbreviations: CI, cochlear implant; C–M–T, Charcot–Marie–Tooth; HBR, hyperbilirubinaemia; HI, hearing impairment; *OTOF*, otoferlin; PN, polyneuropathy.

response telemetry in those patients in whom we could perform the test.

Tables 19.3 summarise the cochlear implant performance in the group with auditory neuropathy caused by the *OTOF* gene mutation and with auditory neuropathy from other causes. The results of implantation have been classified as good, moderate or poor, according with the results of speech recognition in the adapted tests, relative to the normal range:

- Poor: less than 40% speech recognition
- Moderate: 40% to 70% speech recognition
- Good: 70% to 90% speech recognition
- Very good: more than 90% speech recognition

In the cases of auditory neuropathy caused by the *OTOF* gene mutation, the post–cochlear implantation performance was homogeneous and depended on the age at implantation (Table 19.3).

The implanted performance in patients with auditory neuropathy due to other aetiologies is heterogeneous. For patients with C–M–T, the implanted performance is moderate. The other two patients with HBR and unknown cause had good results.

Discussion

Auditory neuropathy is a clinical entity recently described, and characterised by findings in objective electrophysiological and behavioural tests, compatible with a disorder of the cochlear nerve. The clinical findings are variable (15). The site of the lesion along the auditory pathway is important in order to define and carry out effective treatment (16).

The hearing loss caused by mutation of the *OTOF* gene is the most frequent cause of auditory neuropathy in our series (66%) and it is the third most common cause of genetic deafness of our series after the connexin and mitochondrial mutations, in accord with previous results in Spain (13). The heredity is autosomal recessive, which corresponds to the most common pattern of inheritance in congenital deafness (8). Three patients in the present series had family members who were also affected.

The hearing impairment in the patients with auditory neuropathy caused by the *OTOF* gene mutation is, in all the cases, bilateral, and profound. Hearing impairment in other patients with auditory neuropathy is not homogenous and can be progressive.

All patients with auditory neuropathy caused by the *OTOF* gene mutation showed stapedial reflexes during surgery. They also gave good responses with Neural Response Telemetry, which may be interpreted as a functional recovery of the auditory pathway with the electro-auditory stimulation by the cochlear implant.

The good and homogeneous results obtained with the cochlear implant in the OTOF group are considered to be clinical confirmation of the otoferlin localisation in the synapses of the inner hair cells (14). Cochlear implant performance is similar to that found in other patients with prelingual hearing impairment, and its magnitude is mainly dependent on other variables, particularly the duration of the hearing impairment.

In the non-OTOF auditory neuropathy group, the results were good for two of the cases caused by HBR. The other case was a patient with C–M–T syndrome with poor cochlear implant performance. We conclude that this is because the lesions in these patients were located in rostral sections of the auditory pathway—a view in accord with the opinion of other authors (6,8,9).

Patients with auditory neuropathy have good postnatal Transient OAEs and can pass the neonatal hearing screening using this technique, as in one of our cases. Therefore, although the prevalence of this condition is low, some authors recommend screening programmes based on the use of behavioural testing (17).

Conclusions

1. Cochlear implantation provides an effective treatment for the profound bilateral hearing impairment in most patients with auditory neuropathy.
2. Auditory neuropathy caused by the homozygous Q829X *OTOF* gene mutation shows an autosomal recessive pattern of inheritance and presents clinically as a profound hearing impairment.

3. Cochlear implantation in auditory neuropathy caused by the *OTOF* gene mutation shows good results and we do not observe differences from the control group. This could be regarded as clinical confirmation of site of the lesion as being in the peripheral auditory system with otoferlin deficiency, because this protein is codified by *OTOF* gene and is located in inner hair cell synapses in the organ of Corti.

4. The results of cochlear implantation in patients with auditory neuropathy with non-OTOF causes, are not as good nor as homogeneous as in the *OTOF* gene group.

5. Genetic investigations are very important in auditory neuropathy and in the prognosis of treatment of auditory neuropathy with cochlear implants.

Acknowledgement

This work was honoured with the FIAPAS (Spanish Confederation of Parents and Friends of the Deaf) prize in 2005.

References

1. Starr A, Picton T, Sininger Y, et al. Auditory neuropathy. Brain 1996; 119:741–753.

2. Kraus N, Ozdamar V, Stein L, Reed N. Absent auditory brain stem response: peripheral hearing loss or brain stem dysfunction? Laryngoscope 1984; 94:400–406.

3. Starr A. The Neurology of Auditory Neuropathy: a New Perspective on Hearing Disorders. 1st ed. San Diego, Singular Thomson Learning, 2001:37–50.

4. Rodríguez BM, Del Castillo FJ, Martín Y, et al. Auditory neuropathy in patients carrying mutations in the otoferlin gene. Hum mutation 2003; 22:451–456.

5. Kraus N. Auditory neuropathy: an historical and current perspective. In: Sininger Y, Starr A, eds. Auditory Neuropathy: a New Perspective on Hearing Disorders. 1st ed. San Diego, Singular Thomson Learning, 2001:1–14.

6. Rungby JA, Skibsted R, Johsen T, et al. Hearing loss in hereditary motor and sensory neuropathy: a review. J Audiol Med 1999; 6:131–141.

7. Berlin C. Auditory neuropathy. Curr Opin Otolaryngol Head Neck Surg 1998; 6:325–329.

8. Sininger Y, Oba S. Patients with auditory neuropathy: who are they and what can they hear? In: Sininger Y, Starr A, eds. Auditory Neuropathy: a New Perspective on Hearing Disorders. 1st ed. San Diego, Singular Thomson Learning, 2001:15–36.

9. Hood L. Auditory neuropathy. What is it and what can we do about is? Hear J 1998; 51:8–10.

10. Harrison RV. An animal model of auditory neuropathy Ear Hear 1998; 19:355–356.

11. Miyamoto RT, Kirk KI, Renshaw J, et al. Cochlear implantation in auditory neuropathy. Laryngoscope 1999; 109:181–185.

12. Shallop JK, Peterson A, Facer GW, et al. Cochlear implant in five cases of auditory neuropathy: postoperative findings and progress. Laryngoscope 2001; 111:555–562.

13. Migliosi V, Modamio-Hoybjor S, Moreno-Pelayo MA, et al. Q829X, a novel mutation in the gene encoding otoferlin (OTOF), is frequently found in Spanish patients with prelingual nonsyndromic hearing loss. J Med Genet 2002; 39:502–506.

14. Yasunaga S, Grati M, Cohen-Salmon M, et al. A mutation in OTOF, encoding otoferlin, a fer-1-like protein, causes DFNB9, a nonsyndromic form of deafness. Nature Genet 1999; 21:363–369.

15. Rance G, Beer DE, Cone-Wesson B, et al. Clinical findings for a group of infants and young children with auditory neuropathy. Ear Hear 1999; 20:238–252.

16. Varga R, Kelly PM, Keats BJ, et al. Non-syndromic recessive auditory neuropathy is the results of mutations in the otoferlin (OTOF) gene. J Med Genet 2003; 40:45–50.

17. Joint Committee on Infant Hearing. Year 2000 position statement: principles and guidelines for early hearing detection and intervention programs. Pediatrics 2000; 106:798–871.

Part III
The future

20 Innovative therapeutical strategies to prevent deafness and to treat tinnitus

Jing Wang, Matthieu Guitton, Jérôme Ruel, Rémy Pujol, Jean-Luc Puel

Introduction

Compared to the millions of photoreceptors in the eye or the number of olfactory neurones in the nose, the number of sensory hair cells (15,000) in the cochlea is extremely modest. In addition, as a result of age-related changes, this number continuously diminishes during the course of one's life. Because of the fragility of these hair cells, one can understand the need to protect the cochlea against the dangers of modern life, including certain medicines. In the United States, hearing loss linked to taking drugs affects 2 to 3 patients per 1000. More than 130 drugs are potentially ototoxic, including certain antibiotics (streptomycin, amikacin, neomycin, etc.), anti-inflammatory drugs (duperan, indocid, etc.), diuretics (furosemide), oestrogen, vitamin A (an aggravating factor for otosclerosis), and even quinine, which provokes tinnitus, hyperacusis, and dizziness. Cisplatin, a chemotherapeutic agent used in certain types of cancer, destroys the sensory hair cells, leading to irreversible hearing loss. Among factors having a harmful effect on hearing, noise is the most dangerous. Hearing loss is one of the commonest complaints in the workplace, and industrial noise has a considerable effect on hearing.

More so than hearing loss, tinnitus strongly interferes with the daily lives of millions of people. In industrialised nations, 8% to 20% of the adult population currently experience tinnitus. Unfortunately, few treatments are effective. As tinnitus is the subjective perception of sound in the absence of an external stimulus, animal models are difficult to establish. One possibility for studying tinnitus in animals consists of recording the electrophysiological activity of the neural structures of the auditory pathway. This approach has demonstrated that high doses of salicylate, the active component of aspirin known to induce tinnitus in humans (1), provoked an increase in the spontaneous activity of the cochlear nerve fibres (2–4) and modified the average spectrum of activity recorded from the round window, which is a gross measure of the spontaneous activity of the cochlear nerve (5–7). The characteristics of these changes appear to be similar to those of salicylate-induced tinnitus in animals (5). This suggests that, at least in part, salicylate-induced tinnitus is associated with dysfunction of the cochlear nerve. Nevertheless, the demonstration that abnormal activity at the periphery is responsible for the occurrence of tinnitus requires studies of perception.

This paper summarises the molecular mechanisms of sensory hair cell death and generation of tinnitus. Based on these molecular mechanisms, we propose novel therapeutic strategies to prevent hearing loss and treat tinnitus.

Molecular mechanisms responsible for deafness

Exposure to noise or ototoxic drugs (aminoglycosides antibiotics, cisplatin, etc.) initiates a complex cascade of biochemical processes in the sensory hair cells, which leads to a prominent apoptosis. Apoptosis is an active process of programmed cell death (8) characterised by chromatin condensation, intracellular fragmentation associated with membrane-enclosed cellular fragments called apoptotic bodies, and intranucleosomal DNA fragmentation. These proteolytic processes are largely achieved by activation of caspases (9). A schematic drawing of the cell death pathway that participates in apoptosis is given in Figure 20.1.

In the case of spiral auditory neurons, cell death may be due to an excessive release of glutamate, the neurotransmitter of the inner hair cells (IHCs), an injury called excitotoxicity (10); however, it has also been suggested that degeneration of the neurons occurred secondarily to the loss of the sensory IHCs to which they are connected. Whatever the mechanism triggering neuronal death (lack of presynaptic target or excitotoxicity), recent studies have suggested that an apoptotic process is involved, as in the hair cells (11).

Noise-induced hearing loss

Noise trauma induces hair cell loss at the site maximally stimulated by sound. Fragmented hair cell nuclei are observed in the same region using morphological analyses and specific DNA labelling. Morphological features typical of autolysis (vacuolated cytoplasm, but intact lateral membrane) and of apoptosis (shrinkage of the cell body, increased electron density of the cytoplasm, chromatin compaction with an intact lateral membrane) are observed in the noise-damaged hair cells (Fig. 20.2).

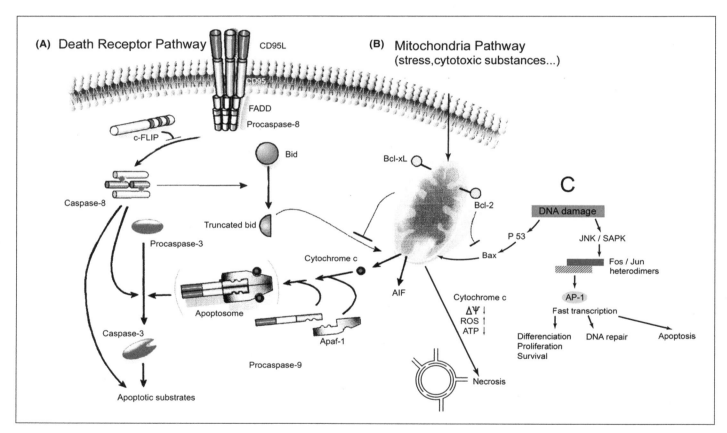

Figure 20.1 A schematic presentation of two major apoptotic pathways thought to be active within damaged mammalian hair cells. (A) The cell death-receptor pathway (left side of fig.) is triggered by members of the cell death-receptor superfamily such as CD95 (Fas). Binding of CD95 ligand (CD95 L) to CD95 induces receptor clustering and formation of a death-inducing signal complex. This complex recruits, via the adaptor molecule FADD, multiple procaspase-8 molecules, resulting in autocatalysis of this procaspase molecule and formation of activated caspase-8. (B) The mitochondrial pathway (right side of fig.) is extensively activated in cells in respond to extracellular signals and internal insults (e.g., DNA damage). These diverse responses converge on mitochondria, often through the activation of proapoptotic members of the Bcl-2 family (e.g., Bax, Bad, and Bik). These proapoptosis cytosolic forms of the Bcl-2 family represent pools of inactive, but potentially lethal proteins. Proapoptotic signals activate and redirect these proteins to the mitochondria, where they interact with antiapoptotic molecules such as Bcl-2 and Bcl-xL at the outer membrane of the mitochondria, where they compete to regulate the formation of pores and the release of cytochrome C from the mitochondria into the cytosol of the affected cell. The cytochrome C associates with Apaf-1, procaspase-9 to form an apoptosome complex. The apoptosome activates procaspase-9, which in turn activates downstream effector caspases (e.g., caspase-3). Cells in which mitochondria have ruptured are at risk of death through a slower nonapoptotic mechanism resembling necrosis because of loss of the electrochemical gradient across the inner membrane ($\Delta\Psi$m), production of high levels of ROS, and a rapid decline in ATP production. The cell death-receptor and mitochondrial cell death pathways converge at the level of procaspase-3 activation. Caspase-8–mediated cleavage of Bid, a proapoptotic Bcl-2 family member, greatly increases its proapoptotic activity and results in its translocation from the cytosol to the outer mitochondria membrane, where it promotes the formation of pores by Bax and the release of cytochrome C. (C) DNA damage and/or oxidative stress can trigger the activation of the JNK signal transduction pathway (right side of fig.). Signal transduction via JNK can induce the phosphorylation of transcription factors such as c-Jun and c-Fos, which are members of the early immediate family of genes. C-Jun and c-Fos, when active as heterodimers, form AP-1, which can trigger rapid transcriptional activity and has been implicated in the regulation of many important biological processes including cell cycle progression, transformation, differentiation, proliferation, DNA repair, and apoptosis. *Abbreviations*: AIF, apoptosis inducing factor; Apaf-1, Fas associated death domain; AP-1, activator protein-1; ATP, adenosine triphosphate; CD 95, Fas receptor; CFLIP, cellular FLICE inhibitory protein; FADD, fas-associated death domain protein; JNK, C-jun N-terminal protein kinase; ROS, reactive oxygen species; SAPK, stress activated protein kinase.

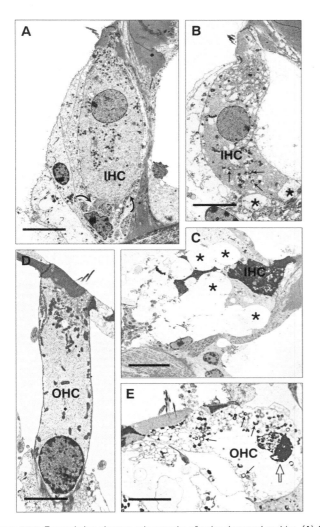

Figure 20.2 Transmission electron micrographs of noise-damaged cochlea. **(A)** An IHC observed in the undamaged region of the organ of Corti six hours after acoustic trauma. Both the IHC and its innervations (*curved arrows*) have a normal appearance. **(B)** Vacuolated IHC undergoing an autolytic process in the noise-damaged region of the organ of Corti, six hours after acoustic trauma. The mitochondria are altered (*arrows*), but the cytoplasmic lateral membrane is preserved. Note the swollen afferent dendrites (*asterisks*) at the basal pole of the IHC. **(C)** Typical apoptotic IHC observed six hours after trauma. This hair cell shows shrinkage of the cell body and increased electron density of the cytoplasm. The cytoplasmic lateral membrane is preserved. All afferent endings are totally disrupted (*asterisks*). **(D)** Normal appearance of an OHC observed 24 hours after noise trauma in the undamaged region of the organ of Corti. **(E)** In the noise-damaged region of the organ of Corti, a degenerating OHC observed 24 hours after noise trauma. Note cellular enlargement, vacuole formation, and organelle disorganisation. Sign of necrosis: distorted mitochondria (*small black arrows*) and the electron dense nucleus due to chromatin compaction (sign of apoptosis; *large white arrow*). Scale bars: (A), (B), (C) = 10 μm; (D) and (E) = 5 μm. *Abbreviations*: IHC, inner hair cell; OHC, outer hair cell. *Source*: From Ref. 12.

Interestingly, individual hair cells sharing both autolytic and apoptotic features are also seen. Moreover, signs of necrosis (cellular debris and disintegrated cytoplasmic membrane) are occasionally seen in the area of the damaged hair cells (Fig. 20.2). The presence of these different phenomena indicates that the

degeneration of the noise-damaged hair cells involves different mechanisms of cell death, including typical apoptosis, autolysis, and, to a lesser extent, necrosis.

In the case of auditory neuronal cell death, however, it is not clear if degeneration of the neurones occurs secondarily to the loss of the sensory IHCs to which they are connected, or if the neuronal death is due to an excessive release of glutamate, the neurotransmitter of the IHCs. Indeed, intracochlear perfusion of glutamate antagonists prevents 50% of the acute threshold elevation by protecting the neuronal endings of the cochlear nerve, but it has no protective effect on the hair cells themselves (13).

Pharmacological strategies have also been used to protect the cochlea against noise trauma. Corticosteroid therapy has been reported to have a significant effect when applied intraperitoneally (i.p.) (14). In these experiments, 20 mg/kg methylprednisolone injected i.p. one hour after trauma resulted in a significant 10 dB functional improvement, although higher doses actually aggravated acoustic trauma. Pirvola et al. (11) used the kinase inhibitor CEP-1347 to block the mitogen-activated protein kinase/c-Jun N terminal kinase (MAPK/JNK) cell death signal pathway. Systemic administration of CEP-1347, a mixed lineage kinase inhibitor, provided partial protection against sound trauma–induced hearing loss.

Recent years have seen increasing interest in the development of local delivery of pharmacological agents to protect the cochlea from noise trauma. Free radical scavengers such as mannitol or deferoxamine are much less potent than glutamate antagonists at preventing acute threshold elevation, but they can reduce hair cell loss by 40% (15). Neurotrophins have also been evaluated as a local protective pharmacological strategy. In these experiments, neurotrophin-3 and glial cell line–derived neurotrophic factor have been shown to rescue 11% of hair cells and to slightly improve auditory thresholds (4). The calpain inhibitor, leupeptin, reduced outer hair cell (OHC) loss following a 105 dB sound pressure level (SPL) exposure by as much as 60% (8). Riluzole, a wide-spectru neuroprotective agent, has also been shown to prevent or attenuate apoptotic and necrotic cell death in rat models of spinal cord (16) and retinal (17) ischaemia. In the light of these findings, Wang et al. (18) have examined the potential protective effect of riluzole against noise-induced hearing loss in the cochlea of the adult guinea pig. Intracochlear perfusion of riluzole protects guinea pig cochleas from damage caused by acoustic trauma, as demonstrated both by functional tests and by morphometric methods. Riluzole-treated animals showed less compound action potential (CAP) threshold elevation and less hair cell loss than noise-exposed controls one month after noise trauma (Fig. 20.3).

The protective effect of riluzole was evident by day 2 and even more pronounced one month after noise trauma. Cytocochleograms prepared one month after noise trauma showed that riluzole treatment (100 μM) protected more than 80% of IHCs and OHCs destined to die. To date, the most efficient way to protect the cochlea against sound is a novel inhibitor peptide D-JNKI-1, a cell permeable peptide that blocks the mitogen-activated protein kinase/c-Jun N terminal kinase (MAPK/JNK) signal pathway (19). When applied directly into the cochlea, D-JNKI-1 peptide also protected the cochlea against permanent hearing loss

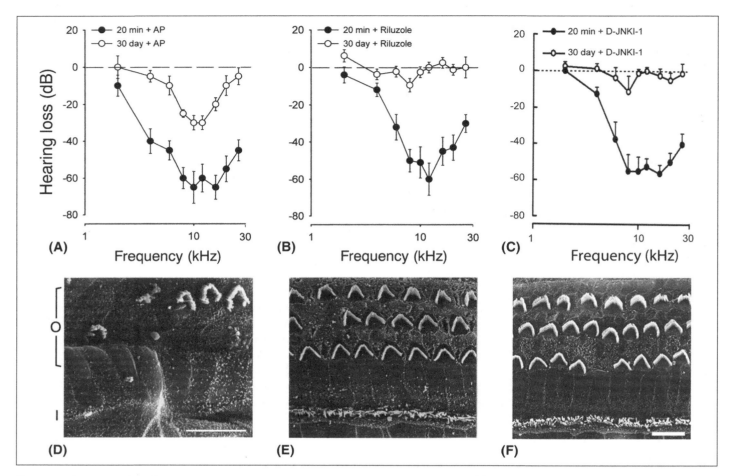

Figure 20.3 Protective effect of riluzole and D-JNKI-1 on noise-induced hearing loss and loss of hair cells. (A) The graphs represent mean audiograms measured 20 minutes (*filled circles*) and 30 days (*empty circles*) after acoustic trauma (6 kHz, 120 dB, 30 minutes) in cochleae perfused with artificial perilymph alone. The average hearing thresholds measured 20 minutes after acoustic trauma were 60 to 70 dB between 12 and 16 kHz (Fig. 2A). There was a partial recovery of CAP thresholds of around 30 dB by 30 days postexposure. This residual impairment represents definitive hearing loss, i.e., PTS. (B) The immediate elevation of CAP thresholds due to noise trauma was not significantly attenuated when the cochlea was perfused with 100 μM riluzole (*filled circles*). In contrast, a clear improvement in the recovery of CAP thresholds, with significantly reduced PTS (*empty circle*), was observed. (C) Protection against a permanent hearing loss was clearly observed for the 10 μM D-JNKI-1–treated cochleae, with a TTS that was similar to the contralateral unperfused cochlea at 20 minutes but with a near-complete recovery of hearing function by 30 days postexposure. (D) and (F) Typical scanning electron micrographs of areas damaged by acoustic trauma from the same cochlea. (D) In the damaged area of the cochleae that received only artificial perilymph, more severe damage was observed in the row of IHCs and in the first row of OHCs than in the second and the third rows of OHCs. (E) Direct delivery of 100 μM of riluzole into the scala tympani of the cochlea prevents noise trauma–induced hair cell loss. (F) Note 10 μM of D-JNKI-1 effectively prevented hair cell loss. Scale bar: (D) and (E) = 25 μm, (F) = 15 μM. *Abbreviations*: CAP, compound action potential; IHC, inner hair cells; JNKI-1, C-Jun N terminal Kinase; OHC, outer hair cells; PTS, permanent threshold shift; TTS, initial hearing loss.

induced by sound trauma and provided near-complete protection of the auditory hair cells (Fig. 20.3). Similar results were obtained when D-JNKI-1 was applied onto the round window membrane via an osmotic minipump. The 50% efficient concentration (EC 50) was calculated as 2.31 μM for intracochlear perfusion of D-JNKI-1 and 2.05 μM for round window application of D-JNKI-1. In addition, D-JNKI-1 protection is still effective for up to 12 hours when applied onto the round window after noise trauma (20).

Cisplatin ototoxicity

Cisplatin [*cis*-diamine-dichloroplatinum II; (CDDP)] is a highly effective and widely used anticancer agent (21). The risk of

ototoxic and nephrotoxic side effects commonly hinders the use of higher doses that could maximise its antineoplastic effects (22). CDDP has been shown to induce auditory sensory cell apoptosis in vitro (23,24) and in vivo (25,26). Recently, Devarajan et al. (27) have reported CDDP-induced apoptosis in an immortalised cochlear cell line. In this model, CDDP toxicity was associated with an increase in caspase-8 activity followed by truncation of Bid, translocation of Bax, release of cytochrome C, and activation of caspase-9. This suggests that both death-receptor and mitochondrial pathways are involved in CDDP-induced apoptosis of hair cells. However, results obtained in vitro may not be directly applicable in vivo. In contrast to the in vitro study showing a transient activation of caspase-8 in an immortalised cell line (27,28) a significant increase in caspase-8 activation was not observed in CDDP-treated guinea pig cochleae. It is worth noting that this immortalised auditory cell line represents OHC precursors, and not adult-like OHCs (27). Thus, the different patterns of caspase-8 activation observed in vitro (27) and in vivo may be due to the differences in these two experimental models. Further functional data reported in our study reveal that local scala tympani perfusion of Z-I-E(OMe)-T-D(OME)-FMK, caspase-8 inhibitor (z-IETD-fmk), a caspase-8 inhibitor, was ineffective in preventing both CDDP-induced hair cell death and hearing loss. This result suggests that in vivo CDDP-induced apoptosis of cochlear cells is caspase-8–independent.

Following its release from the mitochondria, cytochrome C can then trigger either programmed cell death by apoptosis or necrotic cell death processes depending on the level of damage within the affected cell with more severe levels of damage favouring necrosis (29,30). The finding that two pivotal caspases (caspase-9 and caspase-3) are activated during CDDP-induced hair cell death is in agreement with evidence that implicates mitochondria as a primary site of CDDP-damage within auditory hair cells. The evidence is (i) electron microscopy studies show ultrastructural changes in hair cell mitochondria after CDDP exposure (12,31) and (ii) generation of reactive oxygen species (ROS, e.g., H_2O_2) with depletion of intracellular glutathione (GSH) stores, and interference with antioxidant enzymes within the cochleae of CDDP-exposed animals.

Mitochondria are both a target of ROS and a source for the generation of additional ROS. In situ generated ROS can cause cytochrome C release in primary cultures of cerebellar granule neurons (32). Cytochrome C release into the cytosol is required for the formation of the apoptosome and the resultant activation of caspase-9. Numerous studies (24,27,28,33,34) have shown that both an upstream initiator caspase (i.e., caspase-9) and a downstream effector caspase (i.e., caspase-3) were activated in the CDDP-damaged OHCs and some IHCs located in the basal turn of the cochlea. Accordingly, intracochlear perfusion of caspase-3 inhibitor Asp-Glu-Val-Asp-O-methyl-fluoromethylketone, caspase-3 inhibitors (z-DEVD-fmk) and caspase-9 inhibitor Z-Leu-Glu(OMe)-His-Asp(OMe)-FMK, TFA, caspase-9 inhibitor (z-LEHD-fmk) dramatically reduced the ototoxic effects of CDDP, as evidenced by a lack of DNA fragmentation with almost no apoptotic cell death of hair cells or other cell types within the cochlea and almost no loss of hearing in the CDDP-treated animals (28). While z-DEVD-fmk is a potent, cell permeable and irreversible inhibitor of caspase-3, we cannot exclude the possibility that other members of the caspase-3 subfamily are involved in CDDP ototoxicity since caspases-2 and -7 are known to also be inhibited by z-DEVD-fmk (35). Finally, Mandic et al. (36) reported on the possible involvement of calcium-dependent protease calpains in CDDP toxicity in a human melanoma cell line suggesting a role for calpains in CDDP ototoxicity. Although experiments have yet to be done in vivo, the lack of a protective effect of calpain

inhibitors on auditory hair cell and neurones in culture argues against this hypothesis (23). Altogether, these results suggest that CDDP-ototoxicity is mediated through a molecular pathway that involves the mitochondria and the sequential activation of initiator and effector caspases.

A protective role for JNK against DNA damage-induced apoptosis is supported by the results of recent studies on noise trauma (10,19). Wang et al. (28) investigated the involvement of this signal pathway in CDDP-induced apoptosis of cochlear cells in vivo by measuring the levels of activated JNK. CDDP treatment induced a significant increase in activated JNK. Inhibition of this signal pathway by scala tympani perfusion of D-JNKI-1 prevented neither the CDDP treatment initiated activation, subcellular redistribution of Bax, nor mitochondrial release of cytochrome C. Surprisingly, inhibition of this signal cascade by D-JNKI-1 increased the sensitivity of cochlear hair cells to damage by CDDP. This result suggests that the JNK pathway is not involved in the CDDP-induced hair cell death, but may have a role in DNA repair and maintenance of CDDP-damaged sensory cells.

Molecular mechanisms responsible for tinnitus

Guitton et al. (37) developed a behavioural test based on an active avoidance paradigm. Briefly, female adult Long-Evans rats had to perform a motor task (in this case jumping on a climbing pole) on hearing a sound (Fig. 20.4).

The conditioning stimulus (CS) was a 50 dB SPL pure tone with a frequency of 10 kHz and duration of three seconds, and the unconditioned stimulus (US) was a 3.7 mA electric foot shock presented for 30 seconds at most. The time between the CS and the US was one second. Electric shocks were stopped when the animal climbed correctly. Intertrial intervals were one minute. The conditioning paradigm consisted of dispatched sessions with 10 trials per session. Animals were considered to be conditioned when the level of performance (the number of times the rat climbed correctly in response to the sound) was 80% in three consecutive sessions. The behavioural test protocol (nine days) consisted of daily measurement of the correct responses to sound (score) and climbs during intertrial periods (false-positives or responses during silent periods) in the same 10-minute session. The frequency of the CS was selected to match the expected frequency of salicylate-induced tinnitus in rats (38).

Salicylate-treated animals are expected to have tinnitus (37–39). Because they have a sound hallucination (i.e., tinnitus), they are more likely to execute the motor task during the silent periods. If this is true, animals treated with salicylate would show an increase in the number of false-positive responses, i.e., they would behave as if they had heard a sound when no external sound was presented. Our results demonstrate that animals treated with salicylate show a significantly

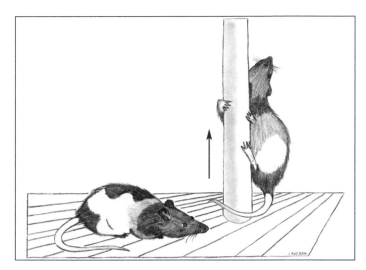

Figure 20.4 The behavioural protocol to quantify tinnitus. The experimental protocol has been described elsewhere (37). Briefly, animals were trained to jump on a climbing pole when hearing a sound. The CS was a 10 kHz pure tone of 50 dB SPL (reference 2.1–5 Pa) and of three-second duration. The US was a 3.7 mA electrical foot shock presented for, at most, 30 seconds (time between CS and US = one second). Once conditioned (correct responses to sound ≥80% in three consecutive sessions), animals were included in the experiments. The behavioural testing protocol consisted of a daily measurement of both the score (correct responses to sound) and false-positive responses. False-positive responses were the number of climbs during the intertrial periods (i.e., responses during silent periods). If animals stayed on the pole more than 10 seconds, they were put down on the floor. Trials were randomised and electrical foot shocks were presented only if the animal did not climb in response to sound. Whatever the score and the false-positive responses, each session included 10 trials and lasted 10 minutes. Both score and false-positive responses were measured in the same session. *Abbreviations*: CS, conditioning stimulus (10 kHz pure tone sound); SPL, sound pressure level; US, unconditioned stimulus (3.7 mA electrical foot shock). *Source*: Courtesy of Jérôme Ruel.

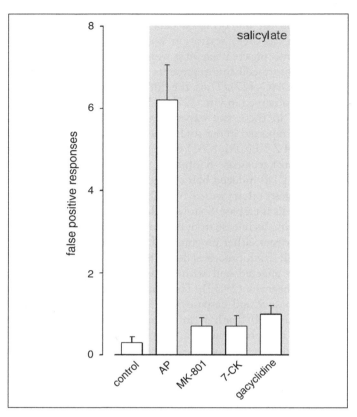

Figure 20.5 Local application of NMDA antagonist abolishes salicylate-induced tinnitus. The measurement of false-positive responses is a behavioural indicator of tinnitus, as animals behave as if they were hearing a sound during a silent period. The number of false-positive responses is shown as a function of the treatment. In the absence of sound, animals will not execute the task during a silent period (control group; $n = 10$). In contrast, salicylate treatment (300 mg/kg/day for four days) leads to a drastic increase in the number of false-positive responses, even in animals receiving intracochlear application of artificial perilymph (AP group; $n = 10$). Local application of the NMDA antagonists, e.g., MK 801 ($n = 10$), 7-chlorokynurenate (7-CK group; $n = 10$), and gacyclidine ($n = 10$), abolishes the increase in the number of false-positive responses. Thus, local application of NMDA antagonists prevents the occurrence of salicylate-induced tinnitus. *Abbreviations*: AP, activated protein; NMDA, *N*-methyl-*D*-aspartate. *Source*: Adapted from Ref. 37.

increased number of false-positive responses (jumping on the climbing pole) during silent periods. One physiological basis of salicylate ototoxicity is likely to originate from altered arachidonic acid metabolism (40–42). Electrophysiological studies (6,43) have demonstrated that arachidonic acid increases the channel-opening probability of the *N*-methyl-*D*-aspartate (NMDA) receptor in various systems, including cerebellar granule cells, dissociated pyramidal cells, cortical neurones, and adult hippocampal slices. We therefore tested the hypothesis that salicylate and mefenamate induce false-positive responses via activation of cochlear NMDA receptors. When applied to the perilymphatic fluids of the cochlea, the NMDA antagonists MK 801 (channel blocker), 7-chlorokynurenate (glycine-site antagonist), and gacyclidine (PCP-site antagonist) strongly reduced the occurrence of false-positive responses induced by salicylates (Fig. 20.5).

Although definite explanations of the molecular mechanisms of the action of salicylate on cochlear NMDA receptors remain to be determined, these results support the implication of cochlear NMDA receptors in the occurrence of salicylate-induced tinnitus.

Local therapy to restore hearing and treat tinnitus

The results presented here were obtained in animal experiments, in which drugs were directly applied into the cochlea. It is clear that systemic application of antiapoptotic molecules or NMDA antagonists will cause side effects. For example, glutamate antagonists have deleterious effects on learning and memory when applied systemically. Similarly, systemic application of antiapoptotic drugs may induce the occurrence of tumours. Therefore, advances in the local pharmacology of humans represent a great hope for the preservation of hearing and the treatment of tinnitus in patients exposed to noise or ototoxic drugs.

Conclusions

Recent advances in molecular pharmacology of the cochlea have led to a much better understanding of the physiology, and especially the pathophysiology of the sensorineural structures of the organ of Corti. Knowledge of the intimate molecular mechanisms of cellular dysfunction is of considerable use in the development of new therapeutic strategies. We have summarised the mechanisms of sensory hair cell death after various injuries. Based on these molecular mechanisms, novel therapeutic strategies to restore hearing have been proposed. In addition to permanent hearing loss, exposure to noise or ototoxic drugs also induces tinnitus. We thus review recent findings obtained from a behavioural model of tinnitus in rats. In addition to providing evidence for the site and mechanism of generation of tinnitus induced by salicylates, these results support the idea that targeting cochlear NMDA receptors may represent a promising therapeutic strategy for treating tinnitus.

References

1. Sée G. Etudes sur l'acide salicylique et les salicylates; traitement du rhumatisme aigu et chronique et de la goutte, et de diverses affections du système nerveux sensitif par les salicylates. Bull Acad Natl Med 1877; 26:689–706.
2. Evans EF, Borerwe TA. Ototoxic effects of salicylates on the responses of single cochlear nerve fibers and on cochlear potentials. Br J Audiol 1982; 16:101–108.
3. Evans EF, Wilson JP, Borerwe TA. Animal models of tinnitus. Ciba Found Symp 1981; 85:108–138.
4. Stypulkowski PH. Mechanisms of salicylate ototoxicity. Hear Res 1990; 46:113–146.
5. Cazals Y, Horner KC, Huang ZW. Alterations in average spectrum of cochleoneural activity by long-term salicylate treatment in the guinea pig: a plausible index of tinnitus. J Neurophysiol 1998; 80:2113–2120.
6. Miller B, Sarantis M, Traynelis SF, Attwell D. Potentiation of NMDA receptor currents by arachidonic acid. Nature 1992; 355:722–725.
7. Schreiner CE, Snyder RL. A physiological animal model of peripheral tinnitus. In: Feldmann H, ed. Proceedings the 3rd International Tinnitus Seminar. Karlsruhe: Harsch Verlag, 1987:100–106.
8. Wang J, Ding D, Shulman A, et al. Leupeptin protects sensory hair cells from acoustic trauma. Neuroreport 1999; 10:811–816.
9. Gorman AM, Orrenius S, Ceccatelli S. Apoptosis in neuronal cells: role of caspases. Neuroreport 1998; 9:49–55.
10. Puel JL, Pujol R, Tribillac F, et al. Excitatory amino acids antagonists protect cochlear auditory neurons from excitotoxicity. J Comp Neurol 1994; 341:241–256.
11. Pirvola U, Qun LX, Virkkala J, et al. Rescue of hearing, auditory hair cells, and neurons by CEP-1347/KT7515, an inhibitor of c-Jun N-terminal kinase activation. J Neurosci 2000; 20:43–50.
12. Wang J, Lloyd Faulconbridge RV, Fetoni A, et al. Local application of sodium thiosulfate prevents cisplatin-induced hearing loss in the guinea pig. Neuropharmacol 2003a; 45: 380–393.
13. Puel J-L, Ruel J, d'Aldin C. Pujol R. Excitotoxicity and repair of cochlear synapses after noise-trauma induced hearing loss. Neuro Report 1998; 9:2109–2114.
14. d'Aldin C, Cherny L, Devriere F, Dancer A. Treatment of acoustic trauma. Ann NY Acad Sci 1999; 884:328–344.
15. Yamasoba T, Schacht J, Shoji F, Miller JM. Attenuation of cochlear damage from noise trauma by an iron chelator, a free radical scavenger and glial cell line-derived neurotrophic factor in vivo. Brain Res 1999; 815:317–325.
16. Lang-Lazdunski L, Heurteaux C, Mignon A, et al. Ischemic spinal cord injury induced by aortic cross-clamping: prevention by riluzole. Eur J Cardiothorac Surg 2000; 18:174–181.
17. Ettaiche M, Fillacier K, Widmann C, et al. Riluzole improves functional recovery after ischemia in the rat retina. Invest Ophthalmol Vis Sci 1999; 40:729–736.
18. Wang J, Dib M, Lenoir M, et al. Riluzole rescues cochlear sensory cells from acoustic trauma in the guinea pig. Neuroscience 2002; 111:635–648.
19. Wang J, Van de Water T, Bonny C, et al. Peptides inhibitor of c-Jun-N-terminal kinase (IB1/JIP-1) protect against both aminoglycoside and acoustic trauma-induced auditory hair cell death and hearing loss. J Neurosci 2003; 23:8596–8607.
20. Wang J, Ruel J, Ladrech S, Bonny C, Van De Water TR, Puel JL. Inhibition of the JNK-mediated mitochondrial cell death pathway restores auditory function in sound exposed animals. Mol Pharmacol 2007; 71:654–666.
21. Trimmer EE, Essigmann JM. Cisplatin. Essays Biochem 1999; 34:191–211.
22. Humes HD. Insights into ototoxicity. Analogies to Nephrotoxicity. Ann NY Acad Sci 1999; 884:15–18.
23. Cheng AG, Huang T, Stracher A, et al. Calpain inhibitors protect auditory sensory cells from hypoxia and neurotrophin-withdrawal induced apoptosis. Brain Res 1999; 850:234–243.
24. Liu W, Staecker H, Stupak H, et al. Caspase inhibitors prevent cisplatin-induced apoptosis of auditory sensory cells. Neuroreport 1998; 9:2609–2614.
25. Alam SA, Ikeda K, Oshima T, et al. Cisplatin-induced apoptotic cell death in Mongolian gerbil cochlea. Hear Res 2000; 141:28–38.
26. Teranishi M, Nakashima T, Wakabayashi T. Effects of alpha-tocopherol on cisplatin-induced ototoxicity in guinea pigs. Hear Res 2001; 151:61–70.
27. Devarajan P, Savoca M, Castaneda MP, et al. Cisplatin-induced apoptosis in auditory cells: role of death receptor and mitochondrial pathways. Hear Res 2002; 174:45–54.
28. Wang J, Ladrech S, Pujol R, et al. Caspase inhibitors, but not c-Jun N-terminal kinase inhibitor treatment prevents cisplatin-induced hearing loss. Cancer Res 2004; 64:9217–9224.
29. Lefebvre PP, Malgrange B, Lallemend F, et al. Mechanisms of cell death in the injured auditory system: otoprotective strategies. Audiol Neurootol 2002; 7:165–170.

30. Liu X, Kim CN, Yang J, et al. Induction of apoptotic program in cell-free extracts: requirement for dATP and cytochrome C. Cell 1996; 86:147–157.

31. Andrews PA, Albright KD. Mitochondrial defects in cis-diamminedichloroplatinum(II)-resistant human ovarian carcinoma cells. Cancer Res 1992; 52:1895–1901.

32. Atlante A, Calissano P, Bobba A, et al. Cytochrome C is released from mitochondria in a reactive oxygen species (ROS)-dependent fashion and can operate as a ROS scavenger and as a respiratory substrate in cerebellar neurons undergoing excitotoxic death. J Biol Chem 2000; 275:37159–37166.

33. Zhang M, Liu W, Ding D, Salvi R. Pifithrin-alpha suppresses p53 and protects cochlear and vestibular hair cells from cisplatin-induced apoptosis. Neurosci 2003; 120:191–205.

34. Watanabe K, Inai S, Jinnouchi K, Baba S, Yagi T. Expression of caspase-activated deoxyribonuclease (CAD) and caspase 3 (CPP32) in the cochlea of cisplatin (CDDP)-treated guinea plus. Auris Nasus Larynx 2003; 30:219–225.

35. Janicke RU, Ng P, Sprengart ML, Porter AG. Caspase-3 is required for alpha-fodrin cleavage but dispensable for cleavage of other death substrates in apoptosis. J Biol Chem 1998; 273:15540–15545.

36. Mandic A, Hansson J, Linder S, Shoshan MC. Cisplatin induces endoplasmic reticulum stress and nucleus-independent apoptotic signaling. J Biol Chem 2003; 278:9100–9106.

37. Guitton MJ, Caston J, Ruel J, et al. Salicylate induces tinnitus through activation of cochlear NMDA receptors. J Neurosci 2003; 23:3944–3952.

38. Jastreboff PJ, Brennan JF, Coleman JK, Sasaki CT. Phantom auditory sensation in rats: an animal model for tinnitus. Behav Neurosci 1988; 102:811–822.

39. Bauer CA, Brozoski TJ, Rojas R, et al. Behavioral model of chronic tinnitus in rats. Otolaryngol Head Neck Surg 1999; 121:457–462.

40. Cazals Y. Auditory sensori-neural alterations induced by salicylate. Prog Neurobiol 2000; 62:583–631.

41. Escoubet B, Amsallen P, Ferrary E, Tran Ba Huy P. Prostaglandin synthesis by the cochlea of the guinea pig. Influence of aspirin, gentamicin, and acoustic stimulation. Prostaglandins 1985; 29:589–599.

42. Jung TT, Rhee CK, Lee CS, et al. Ototoxicity of salicylate, non-steroidal anti-inflammatory drugs, and quinine. Otolaryngol Clin North Am 1993; 26:791–810.

43. Horimoto N, Nabekura J, Ogawa T. Developmental changes in arachidonic acid potentiation of NMDA currents in cortical neurones. Neuroreport 1996; 7:2463–2467.

Stem cells in the inner ear: advancing towards a new therapy for hearing impairment

Marcelo N Rivolta

Introduction: deafness and the potential for cell-based therapy

Deafness is a highly common disability, with substantial social and economic implications. More than 3 million adults in the United Kingdom alone have a bilateral hearing impairment that is moderate to profound (more than 45 dB HL) (1). Almost 90% of these suffer sensorineural loss, which involves loss of sensory hair cells and their associated innervations. These cells are not replaced and hearing loss is irreversible. To compound the problem, congenital deafness affects 1 in 1000 children. There is no cure for deafness although, with a suitable nerve supply, the sensory function of the inner ear can be replaced by a cochlear implant.

The recent developments in stem cell technologies are opening novel therapeutic possibilities for the treatment of deafness. Possible strategies could involve triggering of sensory cell regeneration from existing cells, or, alternatively, replacement of lost cells by transplantation of exogenous in vitro-maintained stem cells. In this chapter I will aim to introduce some general concepts about stem cell biology, to discuss the recent advances of this new discipline in hearing research and to present an outline of its vast therapeutic potential and future challenges.

What is a stem cell?

Stem cells have been defined as "clonal precursors of both more stem cells of the same type and a defined set of differentiated progeny" (2). The enormous potential of therapies employing stem cells has raised great hopes and expectations in almost every area of medicine. The possibilities range from cell replacement to the more ambitious and still futuristic idea of generating whole organs in vitro for transplantation. Stem cells can be classified into different types, depending on the source tissue, the time of derivation, and the potential to produce different lineages.

The primordial, master stem cell is the zygote. The fertilised egg is "totipotent," that is it has the potential to produce any cell type in the body, including extraembryonic tissue such as the trophoblast. "Pluripotent" stem cells have a slightly more restricted potential. They have the ability to generate cell types from all the three germ layers (endoderm, mesoderm, and ectoderm), including all the somatic lineages as well as germ cells but rarely if ever can produce extraembryonic lineages such as those from the placenta. Finally, "multipotent" stem cells have a more limited ability, producing cell types usually restricted to a single organ or germ layer. Pluripotent stem cells have the widest range of potential applications. They can generally be classified as embryonic or adult, depending on their developmental stage of derivation. Some groups are opposed to the use of human embryonic stem cells (hESCs), based on ethical and moral concerns. Our knowledge about the sources and potential of these cells is still very limited and further research is necessary with both stem cell types to understand their possible applications.

Different types of stem cells

Embryonic pluripotent cells

Three different cell types, derived from mammalian embryos, have manifested pluripotency. Embryonal carcinoma (EC) cells were the first to be identified and characterised during the 1960s and 1970s (3). These cells are present in teratocarcinomas, gonadal tumours that can produce cell types from the three embryonic germ (EG) layers (4). It is believed they are derived from primordial germ cells (PGCs), the embryonal precursors of the gametes (5). Human EC cell lines were derived by isolating them from the tumours and growing them on mitotically inactive layers of fibroblasts (feeder layers). Although they had been considered for therapeutic applications, the presence of aneuploidy was a cause for concern (3,6). This limitation led Evans and Kaufman (7) and Martin (8) to isolate cells from normal mouse blastocysts, using culture conditions optimised for EC cells. These embryonic stem cells (ESCs) have a normal karyotype (9) and are maintained in an undifferentiated state by the inclusion of leukaemia inhibitory factor (LIF) in the culture media. Almost two decades later, Thomson et al. (10) succeeded in establishing ESC lines from human blastocysts. A notable difference between human and mouse ESCs is that LIF is not sufficient to maintain human ESCs undifferentiated and it is necessary to grow them on feeder layers or feeder-conditioned medium. ESCs are derived from the inner cell mass of the blastocyst, and they are roughly equivalent to these cells, although in vivo they do not persist for any great length of time. The apparent immortality and the maintenance of undifferentiated features of ESCs are a result of their establishment in vitro. One of the greatest challenges is to control their differentiation predictably to enable selection of specific cell types for therapeutic application (11). Finally, EG cells are derived from PGCs of the postimplantation embryo. They are maintained undifferentiated in the presence of feeder layers and have a similar potential to ESCs (12,13).

Foetal and adult stem cells

There are a few major groups of foetal and adult stem cells, including haematopoietic, mesenchymal, and neural stem cells (NSCs). Given their higher numbers during development, foetal tissue is an ideal source for the initial isolation and setting up of cultures to expand cells in vitro. On the other hand, adult stem cells could be targeted and mobilised by exogenous cues, without the need of transplantation. Pockets of stem cells also exist in specific organs such as the retinal stem cells present in the eye (14). Recently, a population of pluripotent stem cells has been identified in the adult mouse vestibular organ. These cells will be discussed more in detail below.

Haematopoietic stem cells

The ability to produce multiple cell lineages is retained by certain cell types into adult life. Bone marrow haematopoietic stem cells (HSCs) have the capacity to reconstitute the blood cell progenies throughout the life of the individual. Long-term HSCs (LT-HSCs) are named according to their ability to give rise to the lymphoid and myeloerythroid lineages for life after transplantation into lethally irradiated mice. LT-HSCs give rise to short-term HSCs (ST-HSCs), which can only give rise to blood lineages for 8 to 12 weeks when transplanted. ST-HSCs in turn are the source of multipotent progenitors, which progressively lose the potential for self-renewal. An intrinsic advantage of these kinds of stem cells is the possibility of using them for autologous transplants. They can be used to replenish the bone marrow of cancer patients who have undergone chemotherapy. By selecting HSCs based on their surface markers, the possibility of contaminating the transplant with tumour cells and reinducing a spread can be virtually eliminated (15).

The potential applications of HSCs go beyond the fields of oncology and haematology. Lagasse et al. (16) showed that HSCs could repair liver damage by giving rise to new hepatocytes. Furthermore, they were able to treat fumarylacetoacetate hydrolase-deficient mice, a mutation producing a phenotype similar to human fatal hereditary tyrosinemia type I, which leads to severe liver failure. Seven months after transplantation, 30% to 50% of the liver mass in the treated animals was derived from donor cells. The mechanisms underlying this phenomenon are still unclear. Evidence suggests that the new hepatocytes may have been generated by cell fusion rather than by direct differentiation from HSCs (17,18). However, more recent experiments appear to support the idea of differentiation without fusion (19). Regardless of the mechanism, these experiments show that stem cells can be successfully used to treat a genetic condition by replacing a critically targeted cell population.

Mesenchymal stem cells and multipotent adult progenitors cells

Mesenchymal stem cells (MSCs) (also known as stromal cells) are a population located in the bone marrow that can grow as adherent cells in culture and can differentiate into osteoblasts, chondroblasts, and adipocytes in vitro and in vivo. They can be identified by a number of surface markers including CD29, CD44, CD90, and CD106, while they are generally negative for CD34, CD45, or CD14. Human MSC can differentiate in vitro into mesodermal and neuroectodermal-derived tissues (20,21).

A subpopulation of highly plastic MSCs, known as multipotent adult progenitor cells (MAPCs), has created great expectations in the field. They were initially isolated from MSCs and can also grow in vitro as adherent cells (22–25). Human MAPCs do not need LIF for expansion, unlike their murine counterparts. They can proliferate for more than 100 population doublings without undergoing senescence. They lack most of the markers associated with MSCs or HSC such as CD34 or CD44 and express factors characteristic of ESCs such as oct-4 and rex-1. They have the potential to differentiate in vitro not only into mesenchymal progenies, but also into visceral mesodermal, neuroectodermal, and endodermal cell types (24,25). When transplanted into early embryos, they contribute to most, if not all, of the somatic cell types. When grafted into an adult host, they can differentiate into the haematopoietic lineages as well as contributing to the lung, gut, and liver epithelium.

These cells might prove fundamental in treating a broad range of diseases or conditions, regardless of the tissue involved. They could well have the potential to produce inner ear sensory cells if exposed to the right cues and introduced into the appropriate cellular environment. As with HSCs, a critical advantage is that they can be derived from the same patient, enabling autologous transplants that will avoid the complications of tissue rejection. Unfortunately, MAPCs appear to be notoriously difficult to culture and only a few labs worldwide have been able to maintain them.

Neural stem cells

The long-standing dogma that there were no cells in the adult central nervous system with proliferative capacity was shattered by the discovery of proliferating neuronal precursors (26,27). The main sources for derivation of adult NSCs are the subventricular zone, the hippocampus (28), and the olfactory bulb (29). They are normally grown as aggregates in suspension, known as neurospheres, although some labs have grown them as adherent monolayers. The multilineage potential of NSCs appears to stretch beyond the boundaries of neural tissue. Several reports have shown their ability to produce non-neural lineages such as blood (30–32) and even muscle (33). Morshead et al. (34) have explained this non-neural plasticity of NSC as artificially acquired by the passaging in vitro. It is possible that the initial source of derivation would have a substantial effect on the different lineages and neural types produced, since it has been proposed that not all NSCs are equal, and some may be temporally and regionally restricted (35). If this line of thinking proves to be correct, it would indicate the need to derive inner ear-specific NSCs to obtain fully functional, auditory sensory neurons. On the other hand, there is evidence that adult NSCs display a very broad repertoire for differentiation depending upon their cellular environment (36). Injected into the amniotic cavities of stage-4 chick embryos or in clonal culture derived from neurospheres they can form a broad range of phenotypes including neural cells, muscle, mesonephric cells, and epithelial cells of liver and intestine. These results imply that stem cells in different adult tissues may be quite closely related and effective in "non-native" cellular environments.

Adult inner ear stem cells

These cells have been described very recently and a single report has been published so far (37), but given their potentially enormous importance for the treatment of deafness, they are included here as a separate entity. They were isolated from the utricular macular epithelia of three- to four-month old mice by their ability to form floating spheres. When dissociated and plated as adherent cultures, the cells differentiated into hair cell and supporting cell phenotypes. Cells also expressed neuronal markers and, when grafted into chicken embryos, contributed to mesodermal, endodermal, and ectodermal derivatives.

Can stem cells be isolated from the normal cochlea?

Over the past 15 years, it has become clear that supporting cells in mechanosensory epithelia may harbour a limited potential to replace themselves and produce a new hair cell. In 1967, Ruben (38) used tritiated thymidine to detect the last round of mitoses occurring in the mouse organ of Corti. This work showed that hair cells and the surrounding supporting cells are born at around embryonic day 14.5. The synchrony of their terminal mitoses suggested that hair cells and supporting cells probably share a common progenitor. This idea was supported by a study on the effects of retinoic acid (39). Supernumerary hair cells and supporting cells were produced after treating embryonic cochlear explants with exogenous retinoic acid. The additional cells appeared without signs of cell proliferation, implying that retinoic acid had changed the fate of a postmitotic cell population into one with the potential to produce hair cells and supporting cells. This population represents prosensory precursor cells. Laser ablation of hair cells in the developing mouse organ of Corti provided further evidence that new hair cells can be derived from supporting cells (40). A few years later, the lineage relationship between hair cells and supporting cells was demonstrated directly in the chicken basilar papilla, the avian equivalent of the mammalian cochlea (41,42). Replication-defective retroviral vectors were used to label a few progenitor cells around the time of terminal mitoses and the vast majority of clones analysed later contained both hair cells and supporting cells. Hair cells and their immediate supporting cells also share a clonal relationship with the neurons (43). In mammals, there is evidence for low-level regenerative capacity in the utricular macula (44,45). Furthermore, conditionally immortal supporting cell lines derived from the early postnatal mouse utricle have the potential to replace themselves and to produce cells with clear, neonatal hair cell phenotypes (46).

As described before, a population of pluripotent stem cells has been identified in the adult mouse inner ear, although so far these cells have only been isolated from the vestibular organs and not from the cochlea (37). There is no firm evidence for the existence of a real stem cell population in the adult mammalian cochlea, but it is too early to rule out the possibility. Initial attempts to isolate a population of embryonic auditory progenitors have led to the derivation of several mouse and rat immortalised cell lines with different potential (47–51). Malgrange et al. (52) approached this issue by culturing cells from neonatal rat cochleae in the presence of epidermal growth factor (EGF) and fibroblast growth factor 2 (FGF2). They used nestin as a marker for potential stem cells. Suspensions of nestin-positive cells formed "otospheres," reminiscent of the neurospheres formed from NSCs, and from these cells it was possible to differentiate a variety of cell phenotypes, including hair cells. In a similar study, but working with E13.5 math1-green fluorescent protein (GFP) transgenic mice, Doetzlhofer et al. (53) were able to culture a population of progenitors that differentiate in vitro into cells displaying hair and supporting cell markers. These cells were only capable of producing math1-GFP cells for up to three weeks in vitro. The in vitro–generated hair cells needed EGF and the support of periotic mesenchyme for their survival. The frequency of math1-GFP cells dropped substantially when the cells were isolated from postnatal day 2 cochleae.

Pirvola et al. (54) demonstrated with great elegance that FGF receptor 1 is required for proliferation of the prosensory cell population in the developing mouse organ of Corti. It is not clear how the prosensory cells are specified or how FGF signalling is related to the expression of the cyclin-dependent kinase inhibitor p27. However, FGF signalling appears to regulate a population of "transit amplifying cells" in a manner that may shed light on the regulation of an endogenous stem cell population. The prosensory cells express the transcription factor SOX2 (55). This gene has been associated with multipotency and with the proliferation and maintenance of stem cells from diverse origins. In the ear, however, it has been proposed as having an instructive role, helping on the specification of the prosensory field by acting upstream of math1.

A population of nestin-positive cells is normally located in the most basal, supporting cell layer of the sensory epithelia and in the inner spiral sulcus, remaining in the inner spiral sulcus of the rat cochlea up to two weeks of age (56). Using a GFP-nestin transgenic mouse, Lopez et al. (57) have described a small population of Deiters cells, located underneath the outer hair cells, which remained positive for GFP-nestin as late as postnatal day 60. This work provides a preliminary indication that cochlear stem cells might exist in postnatal life. However, nestin alone cannot be considered an exclusive marker for stem cells.

Attempts to isolate populations from the adult cochlea have produced very limited results. A population of neural precursors has been isolated from adult guinea pig and human spiral ganglions, although with very limited proliferative capacity and restricted lineage potential (58). Zhao (59) attempted to derive stem cells from young adult guinea pigs. Cells from six to eight organs of Corti were cultured in a keratinocyte medium supplemented with EGF, bovine pituitary extract, and 10% foetal bovine serum. Epithelial clones were derived, which appeared to have the potential to differentiate hair cells. Further experimental evidence is needed to identify the proliferative capacity and potency of these cells, but the results should serve to encourage more studies of this kind.

Studies in the mammalian retina illustrate the kind of evidence that may be required (14). There is no evidence for natural regeneration in the mammalian retina, either in the sensory neural epithelium or in the retinal pigmented epithelium. Nevertheless, pigmented cells from the ciliary margin

(PCM cells) of two- to three-month old mice can form self-renewing colonies that can differentiate into retinal epithelial cells, including photoreceptors. These cells are distinct from the retinal progenitors that are produced during development and which have a limited lifespan. The fact that PCM cells are clustered in a discrete "niche" is an important issue because they must inhabit an environment that maintains their identity (11). It is not clear if the nestin-positive cells identified by Malgrange et al. (52) form such a niche, although they do lie in a region within which ectopic hair cells can be induced by transfection with math1 (60). Evidence for a true adult stem cell population should ideally come from a defined group of cells in adults with direct evidence that they can proliferate and are multipotent. Interestingly, PCM cells proliferate without exogenous growth factors but they do not normally produce a regenerative response. The suggestion is that, like the spinal cord (61), the cellular environment is inhibitory and that if the inhibition is removed then the endogenous stem cells might effect repair.

Efforts to drive stem cells into ear phenotypes and cell transplantation

Given their immense capacity to proliferate and expand in vitro, ESCs are an ideal source to generate different cell types. Li et al. (62) demonstrated that it is possible to direct stepwise differentiation of murine ESCs into inner ear phenotypes. Initially, cells were allowed to aggregate into embryoid bodies in the presence of EGF and insulin-like growth factor 1 (IGF) and then the ear progenitors expanded by adding bFGF. A detailed experimental protocol can be found in Ref. (63). These manipulations induce the coordinated expression of hair cell transcription factors brn3c and math1 in a single cell. Transplantation into developing chicken otocysts was followed by further differentiation of hair cell characteristics. Given that progenitors are generated after the first stage of induction, it is surprising that a vast majority of hair cell phenotypes were observed, with relatively few grafted cells that did not express hair cell markers. It is not yet clear if this is a peculiarity of the system or if other instructive signals are needed to support the differentiation of these progenitors into the remaining cell types, i.e., supporting cells and neurons. In a different study, murine ESCs were transplanted into mouse ears after having been treated with stromal cell–derived inducing activity. This activity, obtained by growing the ESC on PA6 feeder cells promotes neural differentiation (64). Cells survived for four weeks and expressed the neuronal marker βIII-tubulin, but no hair cell ones. Differentiation was not complete, since cells were still proliferating and expressing stage-specific embryonic antigen 3 (SSEA3), a marker of the undifferentiated state (65). An independent study transplanted untreated ESCs into the vestibulocochlear nerve and detected cells migrating centrally into the brain stem (66).

In very preliminary attempts to explore therapeutic applications of NSCs, NSCs derived from adult rat hippocampus were transplanted into newborn rat cochleae in the hope that they might be incorporated into the sensory epithelia (67). The experimental evidence in this study is limited but there was some indication of survival and integration after two to four weeks. In a similar work, the survival of adult NSCs was slightly improved by damaging the sensory epithelia with neomycin. NSCs that were transduced with the neurogenic gene *ngn2* showed better differentiation as neurons, but no cells were found that displayed hair cell markers (68).

Preliminary transplantation studies of naïve, untreated bone marrow MSC into adult chinchilla cochleae showed that although some cells had grafted, the proportion that presented neuronal differentiation was low (about 0.4%) (69). Differentiation of MSC could improve greatly by in vitro manipulations. In a more recent study, differentiation of glutamatergic sensory neurons was induced from MSC after exposure in culture to sonic hedgehog and retinoic acid. It is unclear if the initial population isolated from the bone marrow included MAPCs, since no characterisation of the surface markers was performed (70).

Some attempts have been performed using allograft and xenograft implants of foetal dorsal root ganglion into adult rat and guinea pig cochleas (71–73). This tissue survived in the host for a few weeks, and cells were retained mainly in the scala tympani and along the auditory nerve fibres of the modiolus, but no evidence has yet been produced of the formation of synaptic connections with the host hair cells. These are not stem cells or progenitors, and hence they do not offer an expandable, renewable source. This type of experiment, however, could offer insights into the feasibility of integration and survival of donor tissue and help to ascertain different surgical approaches.

Stem cell–based therapy holds promise, but many challenges lie ahead

The application of stem cells to the development of therapies for deafness is creating hopes and expectations. They have a potential that goes beyond other technologies. Gene therapy for instance aims to replace or correct a single defective gene. Unlike most metabolic disorders where the defect lies in an enzymatic gene, many forms of hereditary deafness are produced by mutations in genes encoding cytoskeletal, structural, or channel proteins, whose lack of function leads to a direct or secondary degeneration of several cell types (74–77). Although exciting results including restoration of auditory function have been obtained by replacing the *math1* gene into acutely deafened guinea pigs (78), this kind of approach alone may not work in many chronic conditions where the general cytoarchitecture of the inner ear has been disrupted. A cell-based therapy could contribute not only to restoring the critical hair cells and neurons, but also to rebuilding the entire cytological frame. Other important cell types, like those in the stria vascularis, could also be targeted in this kind of therapy.

Endogenous stem cells or transplantation?

As mentioned before, there are two ways of exploiting our knowledge of stem cells in the inner ear. The first is to transplant stem cells into the region of the damaged tissue. The second is to awaken any dormant, endogenous stem cells and encourage them, possibly by removing inhibitory signals, to regenerate lost tissue. Assuming that endogenous stem cells exist in the adult cochlea, it will be necessary to goad them into action with the appropriate signals. Latent neural progenitors in the adult hippocampus can be stimulated by EGF and FGF2 to repair ischaemic damage to CA1 pyramidal neurons (79). The response is subtle. If the growth factors are applied simultaneously with the ischaemia, they do not protect the CA1 neurons from subsequent degeneration and apoptotic death. However, they stimulate upregulation of cell-specific transcription factors within the first day. Proliferation of replacement neurons occurs within four days of treatment, preceding neuronal loss. By 28 days, there are clear signs of both structural and functional recovery. This work suggests that stimulation with the appropriate growth factors at the appropriate time can activate an effective endogenous response. It will be of interest to know whether this can also be done following long-term damage.

By drawing information from other systems and the limited studies in the ear so far, it could be suggested that a more successful approach would be obtained when stem cells, regardless of their origin, are exposed in vitro to specific signals that would trigger the initial programs of differentiation. Transplanted "naïve" stem cells, although homing and surviving into the different regions of the cochlea, may not produce the diversity of fully differentiated cell types needed. It is likely that the necessary signals and cues to drive a particular lineage are no longer in place in the adult cochlea and the cells would need to be "jump-started" into a given lineage a priori. The "priming" of cells pretransplantation would be particularly important with ESCs and other pluripotent cells types, when highly undifferentiated cells could pose a tumourigenic risk.

Transplantation experiments depend largely upon trial and error because there are so many unknown variables in the in vivo environment. The main targets for transplantation have been Parkinson's disease, Huntington's disease, epilepsy, and stroke (80). In these cases, clinical trials have been based mainly upon the use of primary foetal neural tissue, a rather ill defined and controversial source. Successful experiments with retinal tissue have been discussed earlier. However, functional replacement of hair cells by transplantation is probably harder than replacement of brain cells, retinal cells, or pancreatic cells.

This is because hair cells are highly structurally specialised and need to be placed with micron accuracy to be coupled to the sound stimulus. Replacement of surrogate hair cells may be beneficial if they secrete the appropriate growth factors and thus help to retain the innervations. This kind of intervention would be most constructive in conjunction with cochlear implants. In the same context, it may be easier to replace or regenerate spiral ganglion neurons.

How to deliver them?

The delivery of stem cells will very likely require improvement and sophistication of current surgical techniques. A potential way of access could involve the round window, a route increasingly used for drug administration (81), or a cochleostomy in its proximity, as normally performed to place the array of electrodes in a cochlear implant (82). Experiments performed so far have delivered the cells into the modiolus (69,83) or into the perilymphatic space by drilling a small hole either into the scala tympani at the basal cochlear turn (73) or into the lateral semicircular canal (84). These ways of delivery should be appropriate for neurons, but for the replacement of the sensory epithelium, cells would ideally have to be injected directly into the scala media. Iguchi et al. (84) have experimented by

drilling through the stria vascularis of the second turn. A considerable number of transplanted cells were located in the scala media, but as expected, a substantial elevation of the ABR thresholds was produced.

Xenotransplantation

To transfer this technology to a clinical application, sources for stem cells will need to be scrutinised, not only in terms of tissue of origin, but also in terms of species. The use of animal tissue as donors for transplantation into humans, or xenotransplantation, is certainly a possibility. Pig cells, for instance, have been used to treat certain conditions such as diabetes (85) and Parkinson's disease (86). This approach, although attractive for the relatively availability of the source, is saddled with several limitations. Xenotransplants elicit a significant immune rejection both from the acquired and from the innate systems. This is a formidable obstacle to overcome, requiring substantial immmunosuppression, even considering that the inner ear may be an immunoprivileged organ. Moreover, the possibility of pathogens crossing across species is a certain risk. Porcine endogenous retrovirus, for instance, has been shown to infect human cells (87), and more control experiments and closely monitored trials are required (88). Besides (or perhaps because

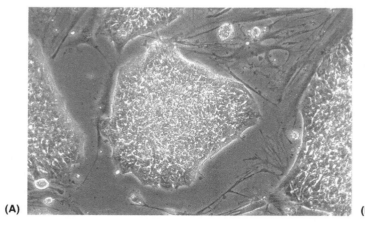

(A)

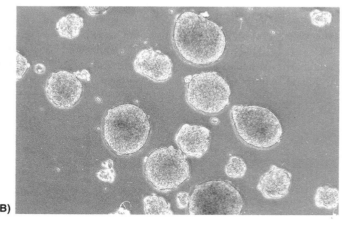

(B)

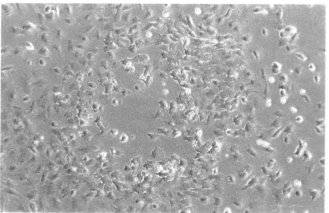

(C)

Figure 21.1 Human embryonic stem cells in culture. (A) Colonies of undifferentiated cells growing on mouse feeder layers. (B) Differentiation is induced by detaching the colonies and allowing the cells to aggregate into embryoid bodies. (C) Embryoid bodies are later dissociated and grown as a monolayer.

of) all these limitations, an increased resistance is building up among patients to receive cell-based therapies from other species. Even in potentially life-threatening conditions such as diabetes type 1, more than 70% of the patients interviewed rejected the idea of pig islet xenotransplants (89).

The problems presented by xenotransplantation could be minimised by the use of human stem cells. Our laboratory is developing ways to direct hESCs cells into auditory phenotypes (Fig. 21.1), as well as establishing human auditory stem cells from other sources (90). hESCs also appear to offer the peculiar advantage of possessing immunoprivileged properties, not eliciting an immune response (91).

The therapeutic application is not the only reason to develop a human-based system. Basic differences in the biology of human stem cells are becoming more apparent when compared to other species. For instance, the surface antigens SSEA-3 and SSEA-4 are expressed by human but not mouse ESCs, while SSEA-1 is expressed by mouse but not human ESCs (92). More important is the dependence of undifferentiated mouse ESCs on LIF. Human ESCs do not require LIF but need to grow on feeder layers (10). Comparison of the transcriptome of human and mouse ESCs by gene expression arrays (93,94) as well as by massively parallel signature sequencing (95) has shown substantial differences in the profile of transcripts expressed as well as in the use of signalling cascades. Human stem cells could therefore provide species-specific answers to fundamental biological questions.

Conclusions

Although the field of auditory stem cell research is still in its infancy, important advances are already taking place. The discovery of a population of pluripotent stem cells in the adult vestibular epithelia has opened the possibility of devising strategies to recruit these cells to repair injury. An equivalent cell type found in the adult cochlea would be a phenomenal therapeutic target, but all the attempts so far to prove if that population indeed exists have failed. Using alternative stem cell sources that can be coerced into inner ear cell types is then a sensible complementary strategy and a few labs worldwide are working on finding ways to instruct these stem cells into the path of auditory fate. Improving the surgical techniques available will facilitate their delivery. Finally, the identification and isolation of human auditory stem cells will take these technologies closer to a realistic clinical application.

References

1. Davis A. The prevalence of hearing impairment. In: Graham JMM, ed. Ballantyne's Deafness. 6th ed. London: Whurr, 2001.
2. Weissman IL, Anderson DJ, Gage F. Stem and progenitor cells: origins, phenotypes, lineage commitments, and transdifferentiations. Annu Rev Cell Dev Biol 2001; 17:387–403.
3. Andrews PW. From teratocarcinomas to embryonic stem cells. Phil Trans R Soc Lond B Biol Sci 2002; 357:405–417.
4. Martin GR, Evans MJ. The morphology and growth of a pluripotent teratocarcinoma cell line and its derivatives in tissue culture. Cell 1974; 2:163–172.
5. Donovan PJ, Gearhart J. The end of the beginning for pluripotent stem cells. Nature 2001; 414:92–97.
6. Andrews PW. Teratocarcinomas and human embryology: pluripotent human EC cell lines. Review article. Apmis 1998; 106:158–167; discussion 167–168.
7. Evans MJ, Kaufman MH. Establishment in culture of pluripotential cells from mouse embryos. Nature 1981; 292:154–156.
8. Martin GR. Isolation of a pluripotent cell line from early mouse embryos cultured in medium conditioned by teratocarcinoma stem cells. Proc Natl Acad Sci U S A 1981; 78:7634–7638.
9. Bradley A, Evans M, Kaufman MH, Robertson E. Formation of germ-line chimaeras from embryo-derived teratocarcinoma cell lines. Nature 1984; 309:255–256.
10. Thomson JA, Itskovitz-Eldor J, Shapiro SS, et al. Embryonic stem cell lines derived from human blastocysts. Science 1998; 282:1145–1147.
11. Lovell-Badge R. The future for stem cell research. Nature 2001; 414:88–91.
12. Matsui Y, Zsebo K, Hogan BL. Derivation of pluripotential embryonic stem cells from murine primordial germ cells in culture. Cell 1992; 70:841–847.
13. Resnick JL, Bixler LS, Cheng L, Donovan PJ. Long-term proliferation of mouse primordial germ cells in culture. Nature 1992; 359:550–551.
14. Tropepe V, Coles BL, Chiasson BJ, et al. Retinal stem cells in the adult mammalian eye. Science 2000; 287:2032–2036.
15. Weissman IL. Translating stem and progenitor cell biology to the clinic: barriers and opportunities. Science 2000; 287:1442–1446.
16. Lagasse E, Connors H, Al-Dhalimy M, et al. Purified hematopoietic stem cells can differentiate into hepatocytes in vivo. Nat Med 2000; 6:1229–1234.
17. Vassilopoulos G, Wang PR, Russell DW. Transplanted bone marrow regenerates liver by cell fusion. Nature 2003; 422: 901–904.
18. Wang X, Willenbring H, Akkari Y, et al. Cell fusion is the principal source of bone-marrow-derived hepatocytes. Nature 2003; 422:897–901.
19. Jang YY, Collector MI, Baylin SB, Diehl AM, Sharkis SJ. Hematopoietic stem cells convert into liver cells within days without fusion. Nat Cell Biol 2004; 6:532–539.
20. Pittenger MF, Mackay AM, Beck SC, et al. Multilineage potential of adult human mesenchymal stem cells. Science 1999; 284:143–147.
21. Woodbury D, Reynolds K, Black IB. Adult bone marrow stromal stem cells express germline, ectodermal, endodermal, and mesodermal genes prior to neurogenesis. J Neurosci Res 2002; 69:908–917.
22. Reyes M, Lund T, Lenvik T, Aguiar D, Koodie L, Verfaillie CM. Purification and ex vivo expansion of postnatal human marrow mesodermal progenitor cells. Blood 2001; 98:2615–2625.

23. Reyes M, Dudek A, Jahagirdar B, Koodie L, Marker PH, Verfaillie CM. Origin of endothelial progenitors in human postnatal bone marrow. J Clin Invest 2002; 109:337–346.

24. Jiang Y, Jahagirdar BN, Reinhardt RL, et al. Pluripotency of mesenchymal stem cells derived from adult marrow. Nature 2002; 418:41–49.

25. Jiang Y, Henderson D, Blackstad M, Chen A, Miller RF, Verfaillie CM. Neuroectodermal differentiation from mouse multipotent adult progenitor cells. Proc Natl Acad Sci U S A 2003; 100 Suppl 1:11854–11860.

26. Reynolds BA, Weiss S. Generation of neurons and astrocytes from isolated cells of the adult mammalian central nervous system. Science 1992; 255:1707–1710.

27. Lois C, Alvarez-Buylla A. Proliferating subventricular zone cells in the adult mammalian forebrain can differentiate into neurons and glia. Proc Natl Acad Sci U S A 1993; 90:2074–2077.

28. Gage FH. Mammalian neural stem cells. Science 2000; 287:1433–1438.

29. Pagano SF, Impagnatiello F, Girelli M, et al. Isolation and characterization of neural stem cells from the adult human olfactory bulb. Stem Cells 2000; 18:295–300.

30. Bjornson CR, Rietze RL, Reynolds BA, Magli MC, Vescovi AL. Turning brain into blood: a hematopoietic fate adopted by adult neural stem cells in vivo. Science 1999; 283:534–537.

31. Shih CC, Weng Y, Mamelak A, LeBon T, Hu MC, Forman SJ. Identification of a candidate human neurohematopoietic stem-cell population. Blood 2001; 98:2412–2422.

32. Vescovi AL, Rietze R, Magli MC, Bjornson C. Hematopoietic potential of neural stem cells. Nat Med 2002; 8:535; author reply 536–537.

33. Galli R, Borello U, Gritti A, et al. Skeletal myogenic potential of human and mouse neural stem cells. Nat Neurosci 2000; 3:986–991.

34. Morshead CM, Benveniste P, Iscove NN, van der Kooy D. Hematopoietic competence is a rare property of neural stem cells that may depend on genetic and epigenetic alterations. Nat Med 2002; 8:268–273.

35. Temple S. The development of neural stem cells. Nature 2001; 414:112–117.

36. Clarke DL, Johansson CB, Wilbertz J, et al. Generalized potential of adult neural stem cells. Science 2000; 288:1660–1663.

37. Li H, Liu H, Heller S. Pluripotent stem cells from the adult mouse inner ear. Nat Med 2003; 9:1293–1299.

38. Ruben RJ. Development of the inner ear of the mouse: a radioautographic study of terminal mitoses. Acta Otolaryngol 1967; (suppl 220):1–44.

39. Kelley MW, Xu XM, Wagner MA, Warchol ME, Corwin JT. The developing organ of Corti contains retinoic acid and forms supernumerary hair cells in response to exogenous retinoic acid in culture. Development 1993; 119:1041–1053.

40. Kelley MW, Talreja DR, Corwin JT. Replacement of hair cells after laser microbeam irradiation in cultured organs of Corti from embryonic and neonatal mice. J Neurosci 1995; 15:3013–3026.

41. Fekete DM, Muthukumar S, Karagogeos D. Hair cells and supporting cells share a common progenitor in the avian inner ear. J Neurosci 1998; 18:7811–7821.

42. Lang H, Fekete DM. Lineage analysis in the chicken inner ear shows differences in clonal dispersion for epithelial, neuronal, and mesenchymal cells. Dev Biol 2001; 234:120–137.

43. Satoh T, Fekete DM. Clonal analysis of the relationships between mechanosensory cells and the neurons that innervate them in the chicken ear. Development 2005; 132:1687–1697.

44. Warchol ME, Lambert PR, Goldstein BJ, Forge A, Corwin JT. Regenerative proliferation in inner ear sensory epithelia from adult guinea pigs and humans. Science 1993; 259:1619–1622.

45. Forge A, Li L, Corwin JT, Nevill G. Ultrastructural evidence for hair cell regeneration in the mammalian inner ear. Science 1993; 259:1616–1619.

46. Lawlor P, Marcotti W, Rivolta MN, Kros CJ, Holley MC. Differentiation of mammalian vestibular hair cells from conditionally immortal, postnatal supporting cells. J Neurosci 1999; 19:9445–9458.

47. Rivolta MN, Grix N, Lawlor P, Ashmore JF, Jagger DJ, Holley MC. Auditory hair cell precursors immortalized from the mammalian inner ear. Proc Biol Sci 1998; 265:1595–1603.

48. Germiller JA, Smiley EC, Ellis AD, et al. Molecular characterization of conditionally immortalized cell lines derived from mouse early embryonic inner ear. Dev Dyn 2004; 231:815–827.

49. Lawoko-Kerali G, Milo M, Davies D, et al. Ventral otic cell lines as developmental models of auditory epithelial and neural precursors. Dev Dyn 2004; 231:801–814.

50. Ozeki M, Duan L, Hamajima Y, Obritch W, Edson-Herzovi D, Lin J. Establishment and characterization of rat progenitor hair cell lines. Hear Res 2003; 179:43–52.

51. Rivolta MN, Holley MC. Cell lines in inner ear research. J Neurobiol 2002; 53:306–318.

52. Malgrange B, Belachew S, Thiry M, et al. Proliferative generation of mammalian auditory hair cells in culture. Mech Dev 2002; 112:79–88.

53. Doetzlhofer A, White PM, Johnson JE, Segil N, Groves AK. In vitro growth and differentiation of mammalian sensory hair cell progenitors: a requirement for EGF and periotic mesenchyme. Dev Biol 2004; 272:432–447.

54. Pirvola U, Ylikoski J, Trokovic R, Hebert JM, McConnell SK, Partanen J. FGFR1 is required for the development of the auditory sensory epithelium. Neuron 2002; 35:671–680.

55. Kiernan AE, Pelling AL, Leung KK, et al. Sox2 is required for sensory organ development in the mammalian inner ear. Nature 2005; 434:1031–1035.

56. Kojima K, Takebayashi S, Nakagawa T, Iwai K, Ito J. Nestin expression in the developing rat cochlea sensory epithelia. Acta Otolaryngol Suppl 2004; 551:14–17.

57. Lopez IA, Zhao PM, Yamaguchi M, de Vellis J, Espinosa-Jeffrey A. Stem/progenitor cells in the postnatal inner ear of the GFP-nestin transgenic mouse. Int J Dev Neurosci 2004; 22:205–213.

58. Rask-Andersen H, Bostrom M, Gerdin B, et al. Regeneration of human auditory nerve. In vitro/in video demonstration of neural progenitor cells in adult human and guinea pig spiral ganglion. Hear Res 2005; 203:180–191.

59. Zhao HB. Long-term natural culture of cochlear sensory epithelia of guinea pigs. Neurosci Lett 2001; 315:73–76.

60. Zheng JL, Gao WQ. Overexpression of math1 induces robust production of extra hair cells in postnatal rat inner ears. Nat Neurosci 2000; 3:580–586.

61. Schwab ME. Repairing the injured spinal cord. Science 2002; 295:1029–1031.

62. Li H, Roblin G, Liu H, Heller S. Generation of hair cells by stepwise differentiation of embryonic stem cells. Proc Natl Acad Sci U S A 2003; 100:13495–13500.

63. Rivolta MN, Li H, Heller S. Generation of inner ear cell types from embryonic stem cells. In: Turksen K, ed. Embryonic Stem Cells: Methods and Protocols. 2nd ed. Totowa, New Jersey: Humana Press, 2005.

64. Kawasaki H, Mizuseki K, Nishikawa S, et al. Induction of midbrain dopaminergic neurons from ES cells by stromal cell-derived inducing activity. Neuron 2000; 28:31–40.

65. Sakamoto T, Nakagawa T, Endo T, et al. Fates of mouse embryonic stem cells transplanted into the inner ears of adult mice and embryonic chickens. Acta Otolaryngol Suppl 2004; 551: 48–52.

66. Regala C, Duan M, Zou J, Salminen M, Olivius P. Xenografted fetal dorsal root ganglion, embryonic stem cell and adult neural stem cell survival following implantation into the adult vestibulocochlear nerve. Exp Neurol 2005; 193:326–333.

67. Ito J, Kojima K, Kawaguchi S. Survival of neural stem cells in the cochlea. Acta Otolaryngol 2001; 121:140–142.

68. Hu Z, Wei D, Johansson CB, et al. Survival and neural differentiation of adult neural stem cells transplanted into the mature inner ear. Exp Cell Res 2005; 302:40–47.

69. Naito Y, Nakamura T, Nakagawa T, et al. Transplantation of bone marrow stromal cells into the cochlea of chinchillas. Neuroreport 2004; 15:1–4.

70. Kondo T, Johnson SA, Yoder MC, Romand R, Hashino E. Sonic hedgehog and retinoic acid synergistically promote sensory fate specification from bone marrow-derived pluripotent stem cells. Proc Natl Acad Sci U S A 2005; 102:4789–4794.

71. Olivius P, Alexandrov L, Miller J, et al. Allografted fetal dorsal root ganglion neuronal survival in the guinea pig cochlea. Brain Res 2003; 979:1–6.

72. Olivius P, Alexandrov L, Miller JM, Ulfendahl M, Bagger-Sjoback D, Kozlova EN. A model for implanting neuronal tissue into the cochlea. Brain Res Brain Res Protoc 2004; 12:152–156.

73. Hu Z, Ulfendahl M, Olivius NP. Survival of neuronal tissue following xenograft implantation into the adult rat inner ear. Exp Neurol 2004; 185:7–14.

74. Steel KP, Kros CJ. A genetic approach to understanding auditory function. Nat Genet 2001; 27:143–149.

75. Rozengurt N, Lopez I, Chiu CS, Kofuji P, Lester HA, Neusch C. Time course of inner ear degeneration and deafness in mice lacking the Kir4.1 potassium channel subunit. Hear Res 2003; 177:71–80.

76. Kudo T, Kure S, Ikeda K, et al. Transgenic expression of a dominant-negative connexin 26 causes degeneration of the organ of Corti and non-syndromic deafness. Hum Mol Genet 2003; 12:995–1004.

77. Kurima K, Peters LM, Yang Y, et al. Dominant and recessive deafness caused by mutations of a novel gene, TMC1, required for cochlear hair-cell function. Nat Genet 2002; 30:277–284.

78. Izumikawa M, Minoda R, Kawamoto K, et al. Auditory hair cell replacement and hearing improvement by Atoh1 gene therapy in deaf mammals. Nat Med 2005; 11:271–276.

79. Nakatomi H, Kuriu T, Okabe S, et al. Regeneration of hippocampal pyramidal neurons after ischemic brain injury by recruitment of endogenous neural progenitors. Cell 2002; 110:429–441.

80. Bjorklund A, Lindvall O. Cell replacement therapies for central nervous system disorders. Nat Neurosci 2000; 3:537–544.

81. Banerjee A, Parnes LS. The biology of intratympanic drug administration and pharmacodynamics of round window drug absorption. Otolaryngol Clin North Am 2004; 37:1035–1051.

82. Copeland BJ, Pillsbury HC 3rd. Cochlear implantation for the treatment of deafness. Annu Rev Med 2004; 55:157–167.

83. Tamura T, Nakagawa T, Iguchi F, et al. Transplantation of neural stem cells into the modiolus of mouse cochleae injured by cisplatin. Acta Otolaryngol Suppl 2004; 551:65–68.

84. Iguchi F, Nakagawa T, Tateya I, et al. Surgical techniques for cell transplantation into the mouse cochlea. Acta Otolaryngol Suppl 2004; 551:43–47.

85. Groth CG, Korsgren O, Tibell A, et al. Transplantation of porcine fetal pancreas to diabetic patients. Lancet 1994; 344:1402–1404.

86. Deacon T, Schumacher J, Dinsmore J, et al. Histological evidence of fetal pig neural cell survival after transplantation into a patient with Parkinson's disease. Nat Med 1997; 3:350–353.

87. Patience C, Takeuchi Y, Weiss RA. Infection of human cells by an endogenous retrovirus of pigs. Nat Med 1997; 3:282–286.

88. Magre S, Takeuchi Y, Bartosch B. Xenotransplantation and pig endogenous retroviruses. Rev Med Virol 2003; 13:311–329.

89. Deschamps JY, Roux FA, Gouin E, Sai P. Reluctance of French patients with type 1 diabetes to undergo pig pancreatic islet xenotransplantation. Xenotransplantation 2005; 12: 175–180.

90. Chen W, Moore H, Andrews PW, Rivolta MN. Isolation and characterization of human auditory stem cells and multipotent progenitors. 3rd Annual Meeting of the International Society for Stem Cell Research, 2005. San Francisco, CA, 2005.

91. Li L, Baroja ML, Majumdar A, et al. Human embryonic stem cells possess immune-privileged properties. Stem Cells 2004; 22:448–456.

92. Henderson JK, Draper JS, Baillie HS, et al. Preimplantation human embryos and embryonic stem cells show comparable expression of stage-specific embryonic antigens. Stem Cells 2002; 20:329–337.

93. Ginis I, Luo Y, Miura T, Thies S, et al. Differences between human and mouse embryonic stem cells. Dev Biol 2004; 269:360–380.

94. Sato N, Sanjuan IM, Heke M, Uchida M, Naef F, Brivanlou AH. Molecular signature of human embryonic stem cells and its comparison with the mouse. Dev Biol 2003; 260:404–413.

95. Wei CL, Miura T, Robson P, et al. Transcriptome profiling of human and murine ESCs identifies divergent paths required to maintain the stem cell state. Stem Cells 2005; 23:166–185.

22 Tissue transplantation into the inner ear

Mats Ulfendahl

Introduction

For hearing impaired individuals, rehabilitative measures have traditionally been based on technical solutions. These include primarily hearing aids, which essentially only amplify and filter the incoming sound signals and present them to the ear using the natural pathways (auditory canal–middle ear–inner ear) without interfering with the integrity of the auditory system. Cochlear prostheses (cochlear implants) represent a much more invasive approach to regain auditory function. By implanting an electrode (or rather, an array of electrodes) into the fluid-filled scala tympani, the damaged sensory cells are by-passed and the neural pathways leading to more central auditory nuclei are stimulated directly (Fig. 22.1). This elicits a sensation of hearing despite missing sensory receptors. The efficacy of the cochlear prosthesis depends very much on the number and functional state of the remaining spiral ganglion neurons (1,2). Another key factor for stimulation is the quantity and quality of the contacts between the neural elements (nerve cells and neural processes) and the electrode. To establish optimal stimulation conditions, the electrode surfaces should be as close as possible to the spiral ganglion neurons. Ideally, spiral ganglion cells should be in direct physical contact with the electrode plates on the cochlear implant. The necessity for a significant cell population and/or close electrode-cell contacts has instigated attempts to increase the number of spiral ganglion cells within the cochlea and to find ways of bridging the distance between the stimulating electrode and the target cells. For replacing cells within the injured mammalian cochlea, several possible approaches could be proposed. Generation of new sensory cells or neurons by activating cochlear stem cells or rather progenitor cells (3,4) (Wei D et al., unpublished work), or by conversion of supporting cells (5) seems no longer unrealistic but is for the foreseeable future not clinically feasible. An interesting and more immediate alternative could be a cell replacement therapy based on tissue or cell transplantation.

Tissue transplantation approaches have been applied to several other biological systems in order to treat incapacitating disorders. In addition to whole organ transplantation, e.g., heart, kidney, and liver, there has been an increasing interest in the therapeutic potential of cell transplantation. Significant work has been performed, both experimentally and clinically, to study beneficial effects of cell-based therapies on Parkinson's disease (6–8). The loss of dopaminergic neurons in the substantia nigra causes severe motor deficits, some of which can be reduced by drugs such as dopamine and levodopa. For a more permanent treatment effect, replacing the dopaminergic neurons by neural transplantation has been tested. The results were initially very promising and provided proof of the principle that transplanting foetal dopaminergic neurons could give significant and prolonged functional effects. Recent double-blind studies have presented less-convincing results and have drawn attention to issues that remain to be resolved in order to make cell therapy a reliable clinical tool in the treatment of Parkinson's disease (9,10). Neural tissue as well as embryonic and adult stem cells has been tested in the treatment of several nervous system disorders, e.g., Huntington's disease, Alzheimer's disease, and spinal cord injuries (11–18). In the olfactory system, it has been shown that the adult neural stem cells can generate olfactory bulb neurons following injury (19). However, among the sensory systems, most interest has been focused on the eye and the possibility of retinal repair. Experimental observations have shown that the embryonic retina transplanted to the rat brain can establish projections to the superior colliculus (20) and can even drive a pupillary reflex in the eye of the host animal (21). This work clearly demonstrates that sensory tissue can integrate both structurally and functionally. Transplantation of retinal tissue and retinal pigment epithelium directly to the retina, the subretinal space, and the vitreous has shown promising results in terms of survival and differentiation (22). Retinal cells have been transplanted to visually impaired patients, e.g., individuals having macular degeneration or retinitis pigmentosa, but so far the visual benefits have been less promising (23). The present focus has shifted towards using stem cells, which have been reported to migrate, integrate structurally, and even differentiate when

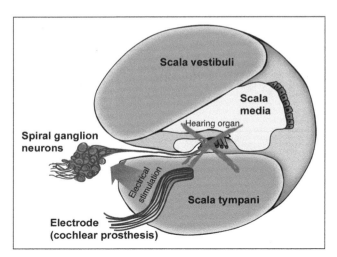

Figure 22.1 Schematic illustration of the fluid-filled scalae of the cochlea. The main site for inner ear cell transplantation is scala tympani, which is adjacent to the spiral ganglion inside Rosenthal's canal. Scala tympani is also the location of the cochlear prosthesis electrode, which, in patients with severe degeneration of the hearing organ, is used for stimulating the spiral ganglion neurons.

transplanted to the degenerating retina. However, as brain-derived progenitor cells do not seem to readily differentiate into the proper retinal neurons (22), other approaches are being explored. Differentiation along a retinal lineage could possibly be facilitated by using the more adaptable embryonic stem cells or modifying the brain-derived stem cells prior to transplantation. An alternate approach would be to isolate progenitor cells from the retina itself and use these cells for transplantation purposes. Indeed, it has been shown that when transplanted to the diseased adult retina, these progenitor cells express both an integrative plasticity and the capacity to differentiate into retinal neurons and photoreceptors (22).

Although far from conclusive in terms of clinical applicability, the very promising results from experiments on neurodegenerative or sensory disorders such as Parkinson's disease and visual impairment have prompted similar studies focusing on the auditory system. This chapter will outline the rationale underlying recent efforts to make use of cell and tissue transplantation for treating the injured inner ear. It should be noted already here that inner ear transplantation is still at an early experimental level and thus very far from being a clinical tool. Irrespective of whether tissue transplantation will be implemented in clinical practice, the efforts are revealing valuable fundamental principles. Recent observations, primarily from our own laboratory (24), illustrating the approaches used so far will be discussed, as well as the future steps that need to be taken to fully prove the concept.

Transplantation rationale

The aim of tissue transplantation into the inner ear, as defined here, is to create a cell-based therapy for the injured or

degenerating inner ear. Before discussing how this can be realised, it is essential to define the objectives, i.e., the reasons for transplanting cells as well as what cells to target. The overall reason, of course, is to regain auditory function following severe inner ear trauma or degeneration, suggesting that clinically, tissue transplantation would be considered primarily in adult individuals. This adds a significant constraint, as the mature inner ear most likely is less "receptive" to foreign tissue. Not only will structural integration be more challenging in a system already formed, but also the immune response is expected to be more efficient thus causing the graft to be rejected.

At the cochlear level, transplanting tissue or cells into the inner ear can have different purposes. The most obvious reason for transplantation is to "replace" missing or injured cells with exogenous cells. This goal imposes, however, considerable requirements for the transplantation to be successful. The new cells must not only survive at the proper site in the host inner ear but also completely integrate both structurally and functionally, and, if transplanting immature cells, differentiate to the specific cell type they are to replace. Inner ear pathologies primarily affect the sensory inner and outer hair cells within the hearing organ and, as a secondary effect of hair cell loss, the spiral ganglion neurons. The mammalian hearing organ has an exquisite three-dimensional organisation where each cellular element needs to be precisely positioned and connected in order to maintain normal auditory function. For the hair cells, this is especially true. Realistically, it is hard to imagine exogenous cells to functionally replace inner or outer hair cells. A more probable cell target would be the spiral ganglion neurons, which are less-strictly organised. In addition to replacing the neurons per se, implanted exogenous cells could function as an intermediate cellular "building block," bridging the distance between a cochlear prosthesis electrode and the spiral ganglion neurons (Fig. 22.1).

It should be noted that the purpose of transplanting cells need not necessarily be to replace old cells but can equally well be to supply exogenous factors to "support" or "maintain" the host cells, and thus halt or slow down an ongoing degenerative process. There is ample evidence that exogenously administered substances such as neurotrophic factors and antioxidants can prevent inner ear injuries and stop the progress of degenerative processes (25). The idea would be to introduce cells into the cochlea that could release, for example, neurotrophic factors needed to maintain viable spiral ganglion neurons or hair cells. The requirements for the final location of the implanted cells within the cochlea would be much less precise and there would be no need for the cells to form functional contacts with the host tissue. Moreover, by genetically modifying the cells, theoretically any biological substance could be released. Although the focus of present research, as well as of this chapter, is on replacement therapies, efforts to augment auditory function will most likely increase in the near future. Not only is there a clinical urgency to find cures against progressive hearing loss, e.g., presbycusis, but also it will undoubtedly be much easier to rescue cells that are already present and integrated than to introduce new cells and expect them to become fully interconnected and functional.

If a cell replacement therapy aiming at introducing exogenous cells to replace missing spiral ganglion cells should ever be considered clinically feasible, there are a number of important issues to address. What cell types could be used and from which donors? What are the possible transplantation sites in the inner ear? Will exogenous cells survive at all in the inner ear—and for how long? Will immature cell types differentiate into functionally appropriate cochlear cells? Will implanted cells migrate to functionally relevant regions and can they integrate with the host tissue, e.g., to establish contacts that may convey auditory information to the nervous system? And finally, can exogenous cells play a functional role in their new environment?

Donor tissue

There are several cell types that could be used for transplantation into the inner ear. Among the candidates that are being explored are embryonic and adult stem cells, embryonic neural tissue, and auditory progenitor cells, but there are likely several other cell types that will prove interesting. Moreover, modern molecular tools make it feasible to further design the donor cells. In addition to the particular cell type, the species of the donor must be considered. As with all transplantations, there is a potential risk of an adverse immune response against the grafted tissue—a host-versus-graft reaction—leading to transplant rejection. Most advantageous would be the use of cells from the individual (the recipient or host) itself, so-called autografting (Fig. 22.2). An autologous approach, which essentially eliminates the host reaction, is used in, e.g., cancer treatment in order to protect the patient's bone marrow (the cells of which are

collected before onset of treatment and then retransplanted). This approach, also using bone marrow cells, has been applied to the inner ear with positive results (26). An alternative is to use tissue from another individual of the same species, allografting. This is currently the most common situation for clinical tissue transplantation. When using tissues from another individual, it is important to find donors as close to the recipient as possible to have optimal human leukocyte antigen (HLA) matching. HLA antigens are formed by the major histocompatibility complex (MHC), which assists the immune system in discriminating self from nonself, i.e., identifying foreign bodies in the organism. It is, however, very unlikely for unrelated people to be MHC-identical. The need for close HLA matching depends on the transplantation site. In bone marrow transplantation, HLA matching is essential whereas in, e.g., corneal transplantation, it is less significant. The eye and some other tissues such as the brain are considered to be immunologically privileged sites where the immune system activity is very much reduced. The inner ear, however, is not an immune-privileged site as once thought (27). For clinical applications where human tissue is not readily available, e.g., for ethical reasons, the use of tissues from other species, i.e., xenografting must be considered. With the possible exception of autografting, transplantation often requires some kind of immmunosuppression to avoid adverse tissue reactions.

Stem cells

A stem cell is characterised by its capacity to self-renew and give rise to a wide range of different cell types. The stem cell needs to maintain full phenotypic plasticity, multipotentiality, for several generations until the occurrence of so-called asymmetric cell division when one daughter cell remains multipotent while the other differentiates into a mature cell. There has been a massive focus on stem cells due to their potential to replace degenerated cells, both for endogenous cell regeneration and for therapeutic purposes (28–30). Two principally different types of stem cells are considered for transplantation into the inner ear, embryonic stem cells, and adult stem cells. However, within each group, there are numerous types of stem cells, each with its specific origin and lineage commitment, survival capability, etc. It is thus very difficult to compare the outcome of different experiments.

Embryonic stem cells are obtained from a very early stage of embryological development, from the inner cell mass of the blastocyst. These cells are especially interesting as transplantation candidates as they are both very proliferative and totipotent, i.e., capable of generating all tissues of the mammalian body (28–30). The cells can replicate indefinitely in vitro and it is thus feasible to culture them on a large scale. Their capacity to give rise to new cell types can be demonstrated by injecting embryonic stem cells into immunodeficient mice, resulting in the formation of benign teratomas containing cells of all three germ layers. If embryonic stem cells can be made to differentiate

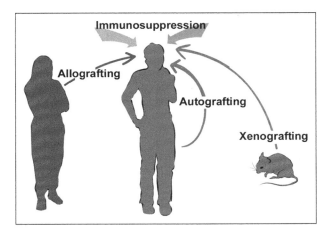

Figure 22.2 Possible donors for cell and tissue transplantation. Allografting is defined as transplanting tissue from individuals of the same species while xenografting involves a donor from another species, e.g., mouse-to-human. In both cases, immmunosuppression is often required to limit host-versus-graft reactions. Tissue can also be obtained from and transplanted to the same individual, autografting.

into true spiral ganglion cells, it would create a nearly unlimited source of transplantable cells for inner ear treatment.

There are several human embryonic stem cell lines available today. These cells are potentially very interesting in that they are expected to elicit less immune response in a clinical context as compared to cells from other species and would thus be a practical source for transplantation (allografting). However, as human embryonic stem cells primarily originate from discarded embryos produced for in vitro fertilisation, there are significant ethical and political issues that need to be addressed as well.

Stem cells are not restricted to foetal development but exist also in several tissues of the adult body. Multipotent adult stem cells thus normally produce new differentiated cells necessary for maintaining functional tissues and restoring degenerated cells. However, the differentiation potential of adult stem cells is much more restricted than that of embryonic stem cells. An important observation is that adult stem cells seem to be able to transdifferentiate, i.e., differentiate into cell types other than that of the original tissue (31). It would thus be possible to employ an autologous approach by which stem cells from a patient would be isolated, transdifferentiated into the proper progenitor cell, and transplanted back (autografting) to the impaired tissue of the same individual. This should not only reduce or eliminate an adverse immune response to the graft but also circumvent the ethical problems related to human embryonic stem cells. However, adult stem cells are relatively rare in mature tissues, and as methods for expanding their numbers in cell culture have not been fully worked out (in contrast to embryonic stem cells), it may be difficult to obtain the large numbers of cells that are needed for stem cell replacement therapies.

The multipotentiality of stem cells offers great possibilities for a stem cell chosen for transplantation purposes to differentiate into the desired cell type. However, what cell type a certain stem cell eventually will produce is impossible to predict. It may thus be more practical to use progenitor cells, i.e., more specialised cells that will develop into mature, differentiated cells of a specific type. Using progenitor cells may also reduce the risk of uncontrolled proliferation following transplantation, as undifferentiated stem cells by definition are tumourigenic.

Neural tissue

Stem cells, by definition, do not have a definite lineage commitment. Thus, to overcome the uncertainty as to what will be the resulting cell type when transplanting undifferentiated stem cells, more specialised or mature cells could be used, e.g., neurons. Transplantation of foetal or adult neural tissue has been tested with relatively positive results in both animal models and patients with Parkinson's disease (32,33). For inner ear treatment, the obvious choice would be to transplant spiral ganglion neurons since these are the cells to be replaced. Fetal and adult spiral ganglion cells can be obtained quite easily in experimental models. Also adult human spiral ganglion cells have been isolated (34), but the numbers are most likely too few for transplantation. It is thus of interest to test also other, nonauditory cell types such as cranial nerve or sensory ganglion cells. For example, cells from dorsal root ganglia have been used for grafting in the peripheral nervous system (14). As immature tissue generally has a greater capacity for regeneration than that of the adult, embryonic or foetal neural tissue should preferably be used for transplantation.

Auditory progenitor cells

The observations of pluripotent stem cells in a wide range of tissues in the mature individual, including the adult brain, suggest that also the inner ear contains stem cells. Auditory stem cells would certainly constitute the ideal candidate for a cell replacement therapy, but it is questionable whether the number of stem cells present in the adult inner ear is sufficient. It is probably more feasible to imagine that progenitor cells could be isolated for transplantation purposes. While these cells should have lost their multipotentiality, they would, compared to embryonic or nonauditory adult stem cells, already have adopted the proper lineage and be "set" to become cochlear cells. Recent findings of inner ear progenitor-like cells (3,4) (Wei et al., unpublished work) are very promising and offer exciting possibilities. The number of progenitor cells that can be obtained is very low and a cell line based on these cells would need to be established in order to more readily provide cells for implantation.

Transplantation sites

The site of transplantation should ideally be the same as the location of the cells that are to be replaced. In the cochlea this is however not feasible. The spiral ganglion cells are to be found in Rosenthal's canal, located within the bony tissue well inside of the cochlear scalae. To directly place cells here would significantly risk destroying the integrity of the cochlea and further injuring remaining functional elements. Moreover, the spiral ganglion is not contained at a single restricted location but "spirals" along the length of the cochlea and is thus not so easily targeted. Fortunately, transplanted cells, and especially stem cells (35), seem to readily migrate from the transplantation site to the target. It is thus feasible to transplant cells into the fluid-filled scalae and expect the cells to reach relevant locations further away. Surgically, the scala tympani in the basal cochlear turn is easily reached and by either penetrating the round window or making a small cochleostomy, cells can be introduced into the cochlea. Once inside the scala tympani and within the perilymphatic compartment, the cells can theoretically reach throughout the cochlea. The transplantation site is adjacent to, but separated from, both the hearing organ and the spiral ganglion, but the physical barriers between the compartments are not absolute. There are plenty of microscopic fenestrations [canaliculae perforantes (36,37)] within the bone separating the scala tympani from Rosenthal's canal, thus providing a possible path for the implanted cells to reach the spiral ganglion neurons. Implanted cells can then, by following the nerve fibres, reach also the hearing organ. There are fenestrations also connecting Rosenthal's canal to the scala vestibuli, but this site is somewhat further away from the spiral ganglion and also less accessible. The perilymphatic compartment can also be accessed via the vestibular part of the inner ear, e.g., the lateral semicircular canal (38). Another alternative is to transplant cells into the scala media, an approach that has been used, e.g., for viral vector administration aimed at the cells within the hearing organ (5). This would, however, position the cells within the endolymphatic compartment and they would not be expected to reach the spiral ganglion.

Transplantation outcome

Inner ear tissue transplantation is as yet at a very early stage and the measures for evaluating its outcome must thus be defined accordingly. At this time the emphasis should be on proving the concept, demonstrating that transplanting exogenous cells to the inner ear could be of potential use for treating hearing impairment. A key issue is whether exogenous cells will survive at all in the inner ear. The primary transplantation site, the scala tympani, is fluid-filled and essentially lacks a structural matrix that may be critical for cell growth. It is also important to explore whether implanted cells will migrate to functionally relevant regions. In the case of immature cells, it must be demonstrated that they can differentiate into appropriate cell types. The exogenous cells need to interact with the local milieu and a critical assessment will be whether the cells integrate with the host tissue. Finally, the most important question is to what extent transplanted cells can play a functional role. A few recent observations illustrating these aspects of cell and tissue transplantation to the inner ear will be reviewed here.

Survival of transplanted cells in the host inner ear

All different cell types transplanted into the inner ear up to now seem to survive. For example, when embryonic (embryonic days 13–14) dorsal root ganglion cells were transplanted to the adult inner ear, surviving donor cells were found in more than half of the recipient animals (39–42). A somewhat surprising observation was that there was no apparent difference between allografting (transplanting guinea pig cells into guinea pigs) and xenografts (mouse to rat). For time periods of up to 10 weeks,

surviving cells could be found in the cochlea but there was a clear tendency for decreasing survival rates with time. Simultaneous application of growth factors (e.g., nerve growth factor or a combination of brain-derived neurotrophic factors and ciliary neurotrophic factor) enhanced cell survival (39–43). There was no obvious difference between cell survival in normal and deafened animals. This is contrary to when transplanting adult neural stem cells (44), where cell survival was greater following transplantation into the damaged inner ear. The results suggest that injured inner ear tissue may release factors promoting, e.g., cell survival, similar to what has been described in other systems (35,45), but that the impact of these factors depends on the characteristics of the transplanted tissue.

The survival of transplanted adult neural stem cells was noticeably lower than for dorsal root ganglion cells. In about half of the implanted animals, surviving cells were found at two weeks after transplantation. However, at four weeks, no surviving cells could be found (44). The survival rate of neural stem cells was undoubtedly low but is in line with results presented by Iguchi et al. (46). A slight improvement was observed after transfecting the cells with neurogenin 2 in an attempt to increase cell survival by promoting differentiation into a neural fate (44). Still, it was estimated that less than 0.1% of the implanted adult stem cells actually survived within the cochlea. Using embryonic stem cells expected to proliferate extensively and even to form teratomas at the transplantation site, the results were equally discouraging (47). However, cell survival was greatly enhanced when the stem cells were implanted together with embryonic neural tissue (cografting) (47) suggesting that an essential component for the survival of implanted cells is missing in the normal adult cochlea.

When tissue is transplanted into the scala tympani, the cells are placed in a fluid-filled compartment without much structural support and possibly lacking tropic factors. In a non-permissive local environment, low survival rates are only to be expected. Cells thus need to migrate to more accommodating locations, e.g., the spiral ganglion region. The tropic support is most likely better among the host neurons but it should be noted that the spiral ganglion is tightly enclosed in Rosenthal's canal, a bony canal leaving little room for cell proliferation, at least in the normal inner ear. The physical properties of the cochlea may actually constitute an environment that is unfavourable for the survival and proliferation of exogenous cells and it is thus crucial to identify permissive factors for developing a cell substitution therapy. The positive results on cell survival when embryonic stem cells were cografted with dorsal root ganglion tissue support this notion.

Localisation to functional relevant sites in the inner ear

While in the scala tympani, the implanted cells are at a distance from and physically separated from their main target, the spiral ganglion region in Rosenthal's canal. Ideally, the cells should migrate to more functionally relevant locations. It is, however, interesting to observe where the exogenous cells localise also within the scala tympani. A consistent observation was that surviving cells were found close to the spiral ganglion region, along the bony wall separating the scala tympani from Rosenthal's canal, suggesting the release of tropic factors at the location. This was true for both embryonic dorsal root ganglion cells and stem cells. Cells were also found inside Rosenthal's canal, among the spiral ganglion cells. The experimental procedures were quite different and it is difficult to make direct comparisons but it appeared as if the number of surviving dorsal root ganglion cells found within Rosenthal's canal was greater than for stem cells. Implanted cells, both dorsal root ganglion neurons and stem cells, were also seen at locations along the nerve fibres projecting to the organ of Corti (Fig. 22.3). Transplanted stem cells were often found in the scala vestibuli of the same turn, demonstrating that cells placed into the scala tympani have the potential to reach functionally relevant regions also well outside of the actual transplantation site. This observation is in agreement with results reported by other groups (26,46).

For a cell therapy approach aiming at restoring impaired function, implanted cells need to be able to convey auditory information from the periphery to more centrally located nuclei. Although strictly speaking not an inner ear transplantation approach, interesting results have been obtained from experiments where cells have been transplanted directly to the auditory nerve, i.e., centrally of the cochlea and the inner ear. It was thus shown that dorsal root ganglion cells or embryonic stem cells transplanted to the transected auditory nerve migrated along the nerve fibres in the internal auditory meatus and in some cases even reached close to the cochlear nucleus in the brain stem (42). Interestingly, Ito et al. reported that embryonic brain tissue transplanted to the acutely transected ventral cochlear tract resulted in not only regeneration but also functional recovery (48). The results indicate that a target of

inner ear tissue transplantation could very well be also within the central auditory nervous system.

Differentiation to neural cells

Whereas cells of the dorsal root ganglion have a predetermined, definite neural fate, the end result is much more uncertain when transplanting stem cells. It is thus important to clarify to what extent cells with much less clear lineage commitment will differentiate into relevant cell types in the inner ear. A clearly disappointing finding was that adult neural stem cells transplanted into the normal inner ear expressed no neural differentiation at all. There was only sporadic differentiation into glial cells (44). On the other hand, lack of cell differentiation is maybe not so remarkable from a functional perspective. In the normal, unperturbed inner ear one would not expect the necessary cues for initiating stem cell proliferation or differentiation to be present, rather the opposite. Thus it was attempted to induce a functional "need" for neural differentiation by chemically deafening the inner ear using neomycin, creating extensive hair cell loss and a progressive degeneration of spiral ganglion neuron. Indeed, when adult neural stem cells were transplanted into the injured inner ear not only was the survival rate greater but the cells were also observed to differentiate into cells staining positive for a neuronal marker (βIII-tubulin) (44). Similar results have been reported by Tateya et al. (49). This clearly indicates that the injured inner ear may release factors that are beneficial for implanted cells. Identifying these factors is not only of great scientific interest but also is imperative for furthering the cell therapy approach. Transplanted embryonic stem cells were observed to differentiate into neuronal cell types [βIII-tubulin positive (47)] also in the normal inner ear. The ratio was, however, still discouragingly low and, contrary to what was observed using adult stem cells, no improvement was seen when implanting cells in the injured inner ear (47).

A methodologically very interesting approach to enhance cell differentiation is to genetically modify the cells prior to transplantation. For example, transducing adult neural stem cells with neurogenin 2 has been shown to significantly increase neural differentiation (50). Transplantation of similarly transduced cells to the inner ear gave encouraging results but the survival rate was still low (44). However, the results would most likely improve by delivering other genes, more suited for the differentiation into sensory cells [e.g., neurogenin 1 (51)].

It is evident that the specific characteristics of the host local environment will affect survival and differentiation of the exogenous cells and thus determine the transplantation outcome. This is illustrated by an experiment, in which small tissue pieces of embryonic (E13–14) dorsal root ganglia were transplanted into the scala tympani at the same time as embryonic stem cells (47). The hypothesis that the embryonic neural tissue would release factors beneficial to the implanted cells was clearly supported by the findings that the presence of a cograft

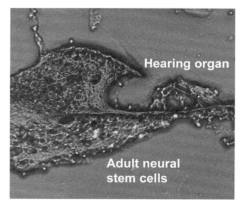

Figure 22.3 Adult neural stem cells (expressing green fluorescent protein) localised along the nerve fibres projecting to the hearing organ two weeks following transplantation into scala tympani (xenograft: mouse-to-guinea pig). *Source*: Modified from Ref. 44.

not only enhanced cell survival but also promoted neuronal differentiation of transplanted, undifferentiated embryonic stem cells. However, more work is undoubtedly required to clarify the environmental requirements for cell differentiation.

Structural integration of exogenous cells in the host inner ear

The encouraging observations of surviving transplanted exogenous cells adjacent to and even within the spiral ganglion as well as along the nerve tracts lead to the important issue of integration—will the cells actually establish contacts? Although present results are not entirely conclusive they clearly suggest this to be possible. For example, implanted embryonic dorsal root ganglion cells, supported by exogenously applied nerve growth factor (41) were observed to form extensive neurite-like projections reaching towards the host spiral ganglion cells (Fig. 22.4). On the other hand, no contact formation was observed in experiments where adult neural stem cells were transplanted (44) and for embryonic stem cells, neurite-like projections were only seen in the presence of an embryonic neural cograft (47). Again, differences in the experimental conditions could explain these discrepancies but it could also be that the more differentiated neural tissue is more capable of interacting with the host tissue. It should be noted that neurite and contact formation could just as well be initiated by the host cells. For example, it has been demonstrated using in vitro coculture systems that spiral ganglion cells form processes contacting adult neural stem cells (Wei et al., unpublished work).

Cellular integration leading to altered auditory function

Interesting as it may be, cell survival, differentiation, and even structural integration have no clinical relevance unless it can

be demonstrated that also auditory function is affected. In conditions where replacing auditory spiral ganglion neurons would be considered, the sensory receptors, the hair cells, will most certainly also be missing. Consequently, cell therapy would not be expected to offer any functional relief unless it was combined with, for example, a cochlear prosthesis (cochlear implant). When there is significant loss of sensory cells, cochlear prostheses can be used to electrically excite the remaining spiral ganglion neurons and afferent fibres (Fig. 22.1). A key issue is the electrode-cell interface, not only the number of remaining spiral ganglion neurons (1,2,52,53) but also the distance between the electrode and the neurons. It has been hypothesised that if the spiral ganglion cell population was to be supplemented with exogenous cells, preferably in close relation to the electrode, the efficiency of the cochlear prosthesis would improve. Experiments demonstrating a functional effect of cell implantation are however lacking. A major problem at this point is the very low survival rate of implanted cells. The resulting population of exogenous cells in the cochlea is probably not large enough to change the efficacy of electrical stimulation.

Conclusions and future directions to prove the concept

It has been demonstrated that exogenous cells transplanted into the adult cochlea can survive for prolonged time periods and even tend to migrate to functionally relevant locations. Transplanted cells can extend processes that seem to contact spiral ganglion neurons, suggesting the capacity of donor tissue to interact with the host nervous system. Immature cells can differentiate into neural-like cells, at least in the presence of tissue specific factors (e.g., from injured tissue or from exogenous embryonic material). The survival rate is very low, indicating that the cochlear environment may not be permissive for exogenous cell survival. The results are encouraging but it must be concluded that the true potential of an inner ear transplantation therapy still needs to be demonstrated.

In order to prove the concept of inner ear cell therapy, there are a number of issues that should be addressed. To create a functionally significant population of appropriate exogenous cells, the intrinsic problems with cell survival and differentiation need to be solved. In addition to identifying suitable donor tissue, this will most certainly involve genetic engineering to provide the donor cells with genes appropriate for the targeted tissue type. Genetic engineering could also solve problems with tissue incompatibility and host-versus-graft reactions and thus make it feasible to use tissues from other individuals or species more freely. Another approach would be to manipulate the local environment in the recipient by providing humoral signalling compounds and/ or a physical matrix supporting cell proliferation and differentiation.

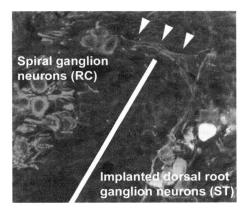

Figure 22.4 Three weeks following transplantation, extensive neurite-like connections (*arrow heads*) were observed between surviving mouse dorsal root ganglion neurons within scala tympani and the host (rat) spiral ganglion neurons inside Rosenthal's canal. The white line indicates the thin bone separating Rosenthal's canal and scala tympani. *Abbreviations*: RC, Rosenthal's canal; ST, scala tympani. *Source*: Modified from Ref. 47.

References

1. Blamey P. Are spiral ganglion cell numbers important for speech perception with a cochlear implant? Am J Otolaryngol 1997; 18:S11–S12.

2. Nadol JB Jr. Patterns of neural degeneration in the human cochlea and auditory nerve: applications for cochlear implantation. Otolaryngol Head Neck Surg 1997; 117:220–228.

3. Li H, Liu H, Heller S. Pluripotent stem cells from the adult mouse inner ear. Nat Med 2003; 9:1293–1299.

4. Li H, Robling G, Liu H, Heller S. Generation of hair cells by stepwise differentiation of embryonic stem cells. Proc Natl Acad Sci U S A 2003; 100:13495–13500.

5. Izumikawa M, Minoda R, Kawamoto K, et al. Auditory hair cell replacement and hearing improvement by *Atoh1* gene therapy in deaf mammals. Nat Med 2005; 11:271–276.

6. Björklund LM, Sanchez-Pernaute R, Chung S, et al. Embryonic stem cells develop into functional dopaminergic neurons after transplantation in a Parkinson rat model. Proc Natl Acad Sci U S A 2002; 99:2344–2349.

7. Björklund A, Dunnett SB, Brundin P, et al. Neural transplantation for the treatment of Parkinson's disease. Lancet Neurol 2003; 2:437–445.

8. Kim JH, Auerbach JM, Rodriguez-Gomez JA, et al. Dopamine neurons derived from embryonic stem cells function in an animal model of Parkinson's disease. Nature 2002; 418:50–56.

9. Harrower TP, Barker RA. Is there a future for neural transplantation? Biodrugs 2004; 18:141–153.

10. Winkler C, Kirik D, Björklund A. Cell transplantation in Parkinson's disease: how can we make it work? Trends Neurosci 2005; 28:86–92.

11. Sugaya K, Brannen CL. Stem cell strategies for neuroreplacement therapy in Alzheimer's disease, Med Hypotheses 2001; 57:697–700.

12. Blesch A, Lu P, Tuszynski MH. Neurotrophic factors, gene therapy, and neural stem cells for spinal cord repair. Brain Res Bull 2002; 57:833–838.

13. Armstrong RJ, Watts C, Svendsen CN, et al. Survival, neuronal differentiation, and fiber outgrowth of propagated human neural precursor grafts in an animal model of Huntington's disease, Cell Transplant 2000; 9:55–64.

14. Rosario CM, Dubovy P, Sidman RL, Aldskogius H. Peripheral target reinnervation following orthotopic grafting of fetal allogeneic and xenogeneic dorsal root ganglia. Exp Neurol 1995; 132:251–261.

15. Rosser AE, Dunnett SB. Neural transplantation in patients with Huntington's disease. CNS Drugs 2003; 17:853–867.

16. McDonald JW, Liu XZ, Qu Y, et al. Transplanted embryonic stem cells survive, differentiate and promote recovery in injured rat spinal cord. Nat Med 1999; 5:1410–1412.

17. Kozlova EN, Seiger Å, Aldskogius H. Human dorsal root ganglion neurons from embryonic donors extend axons into the host rat spinal cord along laminin-rich peripheral surroundings of the dorsal root transitional zone. J Neurocytol 1997; 26:811–822.

18. Levinsson A, Holmberg H, Schouenborg J, et al. Functional connections are established in the deafferented rat spinal cord by peripherally transplanted human embryonic sensory neurons. Eur J Neurosci 2000; 12:3589–3595.

19. Storch A, Schwarz J. Neural stem cells and neurodegeneration. Curr Opin Investig Drugs 2002; 3:774–781.

20. McLoon LK, Lund RD, McLoon SC. Transplantation of reaggregates of embryonic neural retinae to neonatal brain: differentiation and formation of connections. J Comp Neurol 1982; 205:179–189.

21. Klassen H, Lund RD. Retinal transplants can drive a pupillary reflex in host rat brains. Proc Natl Acad Sci U S A 1987; 84:6958–6960.

22. Klassen H, Sakaguchi DS, Young MJ. Stem cells and retinal repair. Prog Retinal Eye Res 2004; 23:149–181.

23. Berson EL, Jakobiec FA. Neural retinal cell transplantation: ideal versus reality. Ophthalmology 1999; 106:445–446.

24. Ulfendahl M, Hu Z, Olivius P, et al. A cell therapy approach to substitute neural elements in the inner ear. Physiol Behav 2007 In press.

25. Duan ML, Ulfendahl M, Laurell G, et al. Protection and treatment of sensorineural hearing disorders caused by exogenous factors: experimental findings and potential clinical application. Hearing Res 2002; 169:169–178.

26. Naito Y, Nakamura T, Nakagawa T, et al. Transplantation of bone marrow stromal cells into the cochlea of chinchillas. Neuroreport 2004; 15:1–4.

27. Ryan AF, Keithley EM, Harris JP. Autoimmune inner ear disorders. Curr Opin Neurol 2001; 14:35–40.

28. Levy YS, Stroomza M, Melamed E, Offen D. Embryonic and adult stem cells as a source for cell therapy in Parkinson's disease. J Mol Neurosci 2004; 24:353–386.

29. Wobus AM, Boheler KR. Embryonic stem cells: prospects for developmental biology and cell therapy. Physiol Rev 2005; 85:635–678.

30. Gepstein L. Derivation and potential applications of human embryonic stem cells. Circ Res 2002; 91:866–876.

31. Passier R, Mummery C. Origin and use of embryonic and adult stem cells in differentiation and tissue repair. Cardiovasc Res 2003; 58:324–335.

32. Lindvall O, Björklund A. Cell therapy in Parkinson's disease. Neurorx 2004; 1:382–393.

33. Nakao N, Shintani-Mizushima A, Kakishita K, Itakura T. The ability of grafted human sympathetic neurons to synthesize and store dopamine: a potential mechanism for the clinical effect of sympathetic neuron autografts in patients with Parkinson's disease. Exp Neurol 2004; 188:65–73.

34. Rask-Andersen H, Boström M, Gerdin B, et al. Regeneration of human auditory nerve. In vitro/in video demonstration of neural progenitor cells in adult human and guinea pig spiral ganglion. Hear Res 2005; 203:180–191.

35. Kulbatski I, Mothe AJ, Nomura H, Tator CH. Endogenous and exogenous CNS derived stem/progenitor cell approaches for neurotrauma. Curr Drug Targets 2005; 6:111–126.

36. Küçük B, Abe K, Ushiki T, et al. Microstructures of the bony modiolus in the human cochlea: a scanning electron microscopic study. J Electron Microsc (Tokyo) 1991; 40:193–197.

37. Glueckert R, Pfaller K, Kinnefors A, et al. The human spiral ganglion: new insights into ultrastructure, survival rate and implications for cochlear implants. Audiol Neurootol 2005; 10:258–273.

38. Iguchi F, Nakagawa T, Tateya I, et al. Surgical techniques for cell transplantation into the mouse cochlea. Acta Otolaryngol 2004; (suppl 551):43–47.

39. Olivius NP, Alexandrov LI, Miller JM, et al. Allografted fetal dorsal root ganglion neuronal survival in the guinea pig cochlea. Brain Res 2003; 979:1–6.

40. Hu Z, Ulfendahl M, Olivius NP. Survival of neuronal tissue following xenograft implantation into the adult rat inner ear. Exp Neurobiol 2004; 185:7–14.

41. Hu Z, Ulfendahl M, Olivius NP. NGF stimulates extensive neurite outgrowth from implanted dorsal root ganglion neurons following transplantation into the adult rat inner ear. Neurobiol Disease 2005; 18:184–192.

42. Hu Z, Ulfendahl M, Olivius NP. Central migration of neuronal tissue and embryonic stem cells following transplantation along the adult auditory nerve. Brain Res 2004; 1026:68–73.

43. Olivius NP, Alexandrov LI, Miller JM, et al. A model of implanting neuronal tissue into the cochlea. Brain Res Prot 2004; 12:152–156.

44. Hu Z; Wei D, Johansson CB, et al. Survival and neural differentiation of adult neural stem cells transplanted into the mature inner ear. Exp Cell Res 2005; 302:40–47.

45. Picard-Riera N, Nait-Oumesmar B, Baron-Van Evercooren A. Endogenous adult stem cells: limits and potential to repair the injured central nervous system. J Neurosci Res 2004; 76:223–231.

46. Iguchi F, Nakagawa T, Tateya I, et al. Trophic support of mouse inner ear by neural stem cell transplantation. Neuroreport 2003; 14:77–80.

47. Hu Z, Andäng M, Ni D, Ulfendahl M. Neural co-graft stimulates the survival and differentiation of embryonic stem cells in the adult mammalian auditory system. Brain Res 2005; 1051:137–144.

48. Ito J, Murata M, Kawaguchi S. Regeneration and recovery of the hearing function of the central auditory pathway by transplants of embryonic brain tissue in adult rats. Exp Neurol 2001; 169:30–35.

49. Tateya I, Nakagawa T, Iguchi F, et al. Fate of neural stem cells grafted into injured inner ears of mice. Neuroreport 2003; 13:1677–1681.

50. Falk A, Holmström N, Carlén M, et al. Gene delivery to adult neural stem cells. Exp Cell Res 2002; 279:34–39.

51. Ma Q, Chen Z, del Barco Barrantes I, et al. Neurogenin1 is essential for the determination of neuronal precursors for proximal cranial sensory ganglia. Neuron 1998; 20:469–482.

52. Incesulu A, Nadol JB Jr. Correlation of acoustic threshold measures and spiral ganglion cell survival in severe to profound sensorineural hearing loss: implications for cochlear implantation. Ann Otol Rhinol Laryngol 1998; 107:906–911.

53. Shinohara T, Bredberg G, Ulfendahl M, et al. Neurotrophic factor intervention restores auditory function in deafened animals. Proc Natl Acad Sci U S A 2002; 99:1657–1660.

23 Gene therapy of the inner ear

M Pfister, A K Lalwani

Introduction

Epidemiology of hearing loss

Hearing loss is the most frequently occurring sensory deficiency and the second most common chronic illness in humans after arthritis (1). According to epidemiological studies by the British MRC Institute of Hearing Research, the total number of persons with hearing loss of at least 25 dB in 2005 was over 560 million, worldwide. Around 190 million hearing-impaired people are reckoned to live in the industrialised countries: 80 million in Europe and over 30 million in the United States and Canada (2). These figures will continue to rise. It is estimated that in 2015, there will be over 700 million people with a significant loss of hearing, worldwide (2). Exposure to noise in the workplace together with the noise trauma associated with stationary recreational activities will lead to hearing damage amongst the younger population (3,4). According to statistical studies in Sweden, more than 50% of people with a hearing impairment today are under 65 years and, thus, of working age (5). The imminent demographic crisis of an aging population in industrial societies will aggravate this problem since more than a third of the population in these is over 65 years (1).

Consequences of hearing loss

The ability to hear and thus communicate has profound effects on the quality of life in nearly all professional and social areas and makes hearing loss one of the main problems of health care in a society dependent on communication (6). The economic costs incurred due to loss of productivity caused by untreated hearing loss are currently estimated at €75 billion a year in Europe alone. This is expected to increase to €87 billion in 2005. These costs could be compared to those incurred in building a motorway five times all the way around the German border (7).

Causes and current treatment for hearing loss

Around 80% of those affected by hearing loss suffer from a sensory deficit of the inner ear. Causal treatment options for this are not available in current clinical practice. Loss of hearing in the inner ear is often caused by the irreversible loss of sensory cells located in the inner ear. Sensory cells convert physical acoustic signals into electrical and chemical signals, which are transferred to the central nervous system. A loss of sensory cells results in an irreversible loss of hearing, also known as sensorineural hearing loss or perception hearing loss. This form of deafness can currently only be alleviated by providing prosthetic hearing aids. This solution is, however, often unsatisfactory for those concerned due to a lack of speech discrimination, and it means that hearing aids are actually used by only a relatively small proportion of those with a hearing impairment. Furthermore, there is a negative attitude to hearing devices amongst those concerned due to social stigmatism and cosmetic considerations. There are additional limitations for specific jobs.

The objective of approaches concerning gene therapy is therefore to throw light upon the cellular and molecular causes of deafness directly. Understanding these mechanisms forms the knowledge basis for a causal treatment of loss of hearing based on gene therapy.

Routes for application of gene therapy to the inner ear

Various forms of application for the inner ear are currently being investigated in experimental studies and some have even begun clinical trials. The main routes for administering substances are via

1. Diffusion through the membranous round window of the middle ear using carrier substances such as Gelfoam (8).
2. Injection through the round window directly into the perilymphatic space of the inner ear (9–12).
3. Injection after opening the bony wall of the labyrinth directly into the perilymphatic space of the inner ear via a cochleostomy or a canalostomy (13,14–18).
4. Injection into the endolympatic space of the inner ear via an endolymphatic sac (19).

All these methods result in a detectable expression (with vector systems) in the inner ear, with varying intensity and duration. It is important to consider not only the location of administration but also the quantity applied, in particular. With excessive quantities, there is a risk of membrane rupture in the inner ear, with the possibility of a consequential loss of hearing.

Cochleostomy to introduce a viral vector via infusion with a miniosmotic pump was characterised by an evidence of trauma at the basal turn adjacent to the cochleostomy, with an inflammatory response and connective-tissue deposition. After miniosmotic pump infusion via a cocheostomy, Carvalho et al. (13) demonstrated a preservation of preoperative auditory brainstem response (ABR) thresholds in the lower frequencies (1–2 kHz), mild postoperative elevation of thresholds (<10 dB) in the mid-frequencies (4–8 kHz), and a marked rise (>30 dB) in ABR thresholds at higher frequencies (>16 kHz). However, in general, cochleostomy has been shown to cause histopathological alterations (including localised surgical trauma and inflammation) and may lead to hearing loss (13).

Several studies have documented that direct microinjection through the round window membrane (RWM) can be accomplished without causing permanent hearing loss or tissue destruction seen with cochleostomy (20). Histologically, cochleae microinjected through the round window demonstrated intact cochlear cytoarchitecture and an absence of inflammatory response two weeks after microinjection via the round window. Further, microinjection through the RWM did not cause permanent hearing dysfunction (20). To avoid potential hearing loss associated with the direct manipulation of the cochlea, gene-transfer vectors have also been delivered through the vestibular apparatus via canalostomy (21). This delivery modality yielded transgene expression mainly in the perilymphatic space, with the preservation of cochlear function.

The potential for surgical trauma, inflammation, and hearing loss associated with these infusion or microinjection techniques has led to the investigation of a less-invasive delivery method. Diffusion across the RWM has been shown to be an effective, atraumatic, but vector-dependent method of delivery for gene-transfer vectors. Jero et al. (8) investigated the potential to deliver a variety of vectors across an intact RWM by loading vectors onto a Gelfoam patch that was placed in the round window niche. Adenovirus and liposome vectors, but not the adeno-associated virus (AAV) vector, effectively infected inner ear tissues as evidenced by detection of reporter genes.

Gene-transfer systems

The possibility of transfecting exogenous DNA into specific cells means that it is possible to develop new molecular-based therapeutic strategies on the sensory organ of the inner ear. In the meantime, new application methods using both viral and nonviral vectors (Fig. 23.1) have enabled successful transfection in the animal model, without any functional damage occurring to the sense organ. Further developments now aim to improve the efficiency of transfection, improve pharmacokinetics, and increase cellular specificity. In addition to the therapeutic approach, the ability to introduce exogenous genes into the inner ear can also, according to experiments, contribute to the further clarification of the function and the control of inner ear–specific genes and proteins. The combination of new data from application research and molecular genetic research will ultimately make causal therapy possible. However, gene-therapy techniques are currently restricted to the animal model.

Viral vector systems

The first successful transfection of the inner ear in vivo was described in 1996 (10,16). As transfer systems, viral vectors (adeno-associated viruses or adenoviruses) were used with a β-galactosidase reporter gene in both studies and applied via a pump system (Alzet™ pump) or by injection through the round window (Fig. 23. 2). The expression of the reporter gene could be detected in various cell types of the inner ear. In particular, expression was detected in receptors, hair cells of the cortical organ and neurons, spiral ganglion cells as well as spiral ligamentum. Apart from the successful transfection of the ipsilaterally treated inner ear, expression of the reporter gene was also detected in the contralateral, nontreated inner ear and in the cerebellum (23). This nonspecific transfection was, however, only observed when using viral vectors. In addition to adeno-associated viruses and adenoviruses, a successful transfection in vivo in the inner ear could also be detected for herpes and lentiviruses (18). However, common to all viral vectors is the possibility that immunological reactions could occur and that an insertional mutagenesis could arise if the vector integrates into the host genome. Furthermore, vector/DNA production is more expensive and more time-consuming than nonviral transfer systems. However, the benefits of viral vectors are better transfection efficiency and higher expression in the target tissue.

Nonviral vector systems

The risks of the viral transfer systems can be avoided by the use of nonviral vectors. Nonviral vector systems are a heterogenous group and can be subdivided into at least six subgroups based on their composition: DNA per se, RNA per se, cationic liposomes, lipopolylysines, polycationic constructs, and viral hybrids. The advantage of nonviral systems is that DNA is not formed in the genome and, therefore, insertional mutagenesis is practically ruled out. According to histological and immunohistochemical studies, immunological reactions are also more rare. Furthermore, plasmid DNA of nearly any size can be combined with nonviral vectors and applied both quickly and easily. Using cationic liposomes, a successful transfection of the inner ear could also be detected (15). Expression and specificity, on the other hand, are significantly reduced in comparison to viral vectors. Reduced duration of transfection is a disadvantage with nonviral systems in the inner ear, but it may not be crucial. Expression was

GENE TRANSFER VECTORS								
Vector	Genome	Insert Size	Site	Efficiency	Cell Division	Expression	Advantages	Disadvantages
AAV	ssDNA	4.5 kB	Genome	variable	Not required	permanent	No human disease	Difficult to produce
Retrovirus	RNA	6-7kB	Genome	low	required	permanent	Suited for neoplastic cells	Insertional mutagenesis
Adenovirus	dsDNA	7.5 kB	Episome	Moderate	Not required	Transient	Ease of production	Inflammatory response
Herpes Virus	dsDNA	10-100kB	Episome	Modderate	Not required	Transient	Neural tropism	Human disease
Plasmid	RNA/DNA	Unlimited	Episome	Very low	Not required	Transient	Safe, easy production	Low transfection
Liposome		Unlimited	Episome	Very low	Not required	Transient	Safe, easy production	Low transfection

Figure 23.1 Gene-tranfer vectors. *Abbreviation*: AAV, adno-associated virus. *Source*: From Ref. 22.

detected six or nine weeks after application of liposomes, and, if necessary, the problem can be solved by multiple applications.

Therapeutic approaches

The general strategies of gene therapy for the sensory system of the ear are based on:

1. Gene amplification for loss of hearing caused by recessive genes or correction of a mutation for loss of hearing caused by dominant genes.
2. Specific gene amplification in otoprotection.
3. Specific influence of gene expression in regeneration.

Correcting genetic hearing loss

A number of new hearing-loss genes and pathogenic mutations have been identified in the past few years when investigating hearing loss. In many cases, the physiological and epidemiological significance of these genes in the hearing process is still unclear. However, one such gene, *Connexin 26*, was found to play a significant role in profoundly deaf patients. Of the profoundly deaf people in Germany, 10% to 15% could be traced back to a mutation in this gene. For this reason, an early therapeutic approach appears worthwhile for this type of hearing loss

(DFNB1). The development of new strategies is, however, currently restricted by the lack of animal models for this gene. A mouse model with a different gene defect (*Shaker 2*) was, however, successfully used to prove that inserting the *myo15* gene in *Shaker 2* zygotes led to normal inner ear morphology in hearing mice (24). This strategy is thus potentially useable.

Otoprotection

Various models for studying otoprotection are available. These include animal models for which loss of hearing is due to

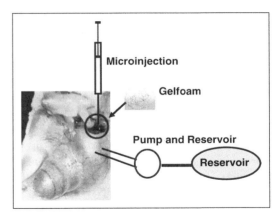

Figure 23.2 Delivery methods for viral vector systems. See text for details.

noise exposure or administering ototoxic substances (e.g., aminoglycoside antibiotics). Neuroprotective factors are currently being introduced to the inner ear of animal models by different methods and vector systems in order to prevent or at least reduce apoptotic cell death of sensory cells and neurons (11). In the auditory system, glial cell-line derived neurotrophic factor (GDNF), brain-derived neurotrophic factor (BDNF), and neurotropin-3 (NT-3), in particular, are described as active neurotrophic factors that contribute to the development of the neuritogenesis of auditory projections and the survival of neurons (25–27). These factors can prevent ototoxic damage in in vivo experiments (28–30). In preclinical application studies, Staecker et al. (31) used a herpes simplex virus-1 (HSV-1) vector to deliver BDNF to the inner ear and assessed its protective effect against neomycin. The gene-therapy group demonstrated a 94.7% salvage rate for spiral ganglion neurons (SGNs) in contrast to a 64.3% loss of SGNs in control animals without the BDNF transgene. Interestingly, while BDNF expression was ubiquitous in inner ear tissues, this was not the case for the reporter gene, β-galactosidase. This reporter gene was detected in only 50% of the cells, thus identifying the cells specifically transduced by the HSV-1 vector. This transduction rate was sufficient to affect cochlea-wide BDNF distribution and ensure 95% SGN survival. The authors speculate that SGNs must require only a small number of BDNF-producing cells to ensure the survival of the entire ganglion.

Lalwani et al. (32) used both in vitro and in vivo models to test the protective effect of AAV-mediated BDNF expression. They found a significant survival, relative to controls, of SGN in cochlear explants transduced with AAV–BDNF and challenged with aminoglycoside. Although direct expression of transgenic BDNF could not be recorded, the vector's ability to salvage SGNs was tested against a gradient of known BDNF concentrations applied directly to the cochlear explants. They found that the vector system was able to achieve the same protective effects as 0.1 ng/mL of BDNF. This is subtherapeutic because the most efficient dose was determined to be 50 ng/mL, a concentration of BDNF that results in almost total SGN protection. In the in vivo experiment, animals infused with AAV–BDNF with an osmotic minipump displayed enhanced SGN survival. The protection from AAV–BDNF therapy was region specific; there was protection at the basal turn of the cochlea but not at the middle or the apical turn. The authors propose that this regional selectivity is a pharmacokinetic phenomenon.

NT-3–mediated protection against cisplatin-induced ototoxicity has been documented using an HSV-1–derived viral vector (33,34). Chen et al. (34) established the efficacy of the vector in an in vitro study, where HSV-1–mediated transfer of NT-3 (demonstrated by production of NT-3 mRNA and protein and by reporter-gene expression) conferred increased survival to cochlear explants after cisplatin exposure. Bowers et al. (33) confirmed these effects in an in vivo model, where HSV-1–mediated transfer of NT-3 to SGNs suppressed cisplatin-induced apoptosis and necrosis. The authors suggest that these findings may not only be useful to prevent cisplatin-related

injury but it may also provide preventative treatment for hearing degeneration due to normal aging.

Several studies have established the ability of an adenovirus vector carrying the GDNF gene (Ad.GDNF) to protect against a variety of ototoxic insults. When administered prior to aminoglycoside challenge, Ad.GDNF significantly protects cochlear (35) and vestibular (36) hair cells from cell death. Pretreatment with Ad.GDNF also provides significant protection against noise-induced trauma (37). Finally, Ad.GDNF enhances SGN survival when administered four to seven days after ototoxic deafening with aminoglycosides (38).

The studies described above have assessed the therapeutic efficacy of gene transfer against chemically or physically induced ototoxicity in animal models. The results of these studies are promising as preventative countermeasures.

Regeneration

Regeneration represents another significant therapeutic approach. Unlike in other vertebrates, in humans and in other mammals, hair cells are not replaced once they have been lost. Their loss and the restriction of function connected with this are permanent and irreversible. The only causal approach to treatment is replacing lost hair cells through the biological process of hair-cell regeneration.

The aim of regeneration biology for hearing is to throw light upon cellular and molecular mechanisms that permit a regeneration of hearing by creating sensory cells de novo in the inner ear. Unlike the situation with humans and mammals, other vertebrates and warm-blooded birds, in particular, are able to regenerate hair cells spontaneously. In these cases, hair-cell regeneration involves forming new hair cells from cell division in neighbouring support cells. Traditional thinking has, up until now, rated the chances of such regeneration in mammals as very low. Acoustic organ cells were not considered capable of entering the cell cycle and thus regeneration based on cell renewal was inconceivable. However, this biological dogma was contradicted by the identification of a relevant cell-cycle regulator, cyclin-dependent kinase inhibitor p27^{Kip1}. The influence of this regulator could be used to show on a molecular level that cell division is also possible in the adult sensory acoustic organ (39). From a therapeutic point of view, suppressing expression of this gene could be thought of as an induction of the hair-cell regeneration process. With reference to these therapeutic implications, it is worth mentioning that when using antisense oligonucleotides that target the mRNA of p27^{Kip1}, a p27^{Kip1}-mediated cell-cycle arrest could be overcome in cell cultures in vitro (40). A prerequisite for a regenerative effect in the inner ear would be that newly divided cells are also differentiated from hair cells.

On the level of differentiation, another gene has also been independently discovered, which is necessary for the differentiation of hair cells during development of precursor cells. After terminal mitosis, i.e., the last cell division to take place during development in the sensory epithelium, cell-specific differentiation is started. At this time, expression of the *Math1* gene is found in the cortical organ and in the prosensory cells that later differentiate into hair cells. This gene encodes a basic helix-loop-helix transcription factor and is a key regulator of hair-cell development. When *Math1* is deleted, differentiation of hair cells takes place entirely in the sensory epithelium (41). Overexpression of *Math1* (induced exogenously by plasmid transfection in postnatal explants), on the other hand, leads to the production of ectopic hair cells in transfected support cells in the inner sulcus. With the exogenously induced expression of *Math1*, it is clear that at this time, these cells can still change their fate and be differentiated into hair cells (42). In March 2005, Raphael and his group reported that *Atoh1* (another name for *Math1*) induces regeneration of hair cells and substantially improves hearing thresholds in the mature deaf inner ear after delivery to nonsensory cells through adenovectors (43). This is the first demonstration of cellular and functional repair in the organ of Corti of a mature deaf mammal. These data suggest a new therapeutic approach based on expressing crucial developmental genes for cellular and functional restoration in the damaged auditory epithelium and other sensory systems.

The recent discovery of stem cells in the adult inner ear that are capable of differentiating into hair cells, as well as the finding that embryonic stem cells can be converted into hair cells, open an additional exciting possibility for the future development of a stem cell–based regeneration of the inner ear (44). However, many obstacles have to be overcome before these treatment options can be used in humans.

Risks and limitations

Major risk factors associated with the introduction of the gene-transfer vector into the inner ear are twofold: damage to the cochlear structure and function as a consequence of delivery modality and the relative safety of the gene-transfer vector. Delivery modalities that prevent damage to the cochlear structure/function have been described above. The safety of the gene-transfer agent is determined by assessing its immunogenicity and toxicity. Unwanted dissemination of the therapeutic agent outside of the target region also represents a potential risk factor.

Utilising AAV as the gene-therapy vector, Lalwani et al. (23) observed transgene expression within the contralateral cochlea of the AAV-perfused animal, albeit much weaker than within the directly perfused cochlea. Subsequently, Stover et al. (45) demonstrated transgene expression in the contralateral cochlea using an adenovirus. Expression of the transgene away from the intended target site, i.e., within the contralateral cochlea, raises concern about the risks associated with dissemination of the virus from the target tissue. The appearance of the virus distant from the site of infection may be due to its hematogenous dissemination to near and distant tissues. However, this is unlikely (23,46). Other possible explanations include migration of AAV via the

bone-marrow space of the temporal bone (23) or via the cerebrospinal fluid (CSF) space to the contralateral ear (23,46). The perilymphatic space into which the virus is perfused is directly connected to the CSF via the cochlear aqueduct; transgene expression within the contralateral cochlear aqueduct has been demonstrated following introduction of the viral vector in the ipsilateral cochlea. Collectively, these results suggest potential routes for AAV dissemination from the infused cochlea via the cochlear aqueduct or by extension through the temporal bone-marrow spaces. Subsequent investigations have shown that dissemination outside the target cochlea can largely be eliminated by utilising microinjection or round window application of vector and avoiding the infusion technique (8,18,47).

The future

Demonstrating the possibility of successfully introducing genes into the peripheral auditory system using various routes and viral and nonviral transfer systems (vectors) is the first significant step towards a possible molecular-genetic therapeutic strategy for diseases of the inner ear. The chosen application is the microinjection or positioning of the transfer system at the round window. The current transfer systems (vectors), however, require further development as regards higher specificity and lower risks for other organ systems. Exciting new research data on regeneration in the inner ear, based on stem cells or genes, will trigger research to overcome current obstacles and to develop, at the end, a molecular-based therapy for this most common sensory deficit in humans.

References

1. The National Health Interview Survey. National Institute of Health Statistics http://www.ntis.gov (1994).
2. Davis A. Public health implications of hearing impairment in Europe. In: MRC Institute of Hearing Research WoH, Brussels, ed. World of Hearing. Nottingham: UK, 1999.
3. Smith P, Davis A. Social noise and hearing loss. Lancet 1999; 353:1185.
4. Zenner HP, Struwe V, Schuschke G, et al. Hearing loss caused by leisure noise. Hno 1999; 47:236–248.
5. Hearing Research Foundation HR, www.hrf.se, Sweden 1998.
6. NCOA Research. The National Council on the Aging 409 Third St. S, Suite 200 Washington, DC 20024 USA Seniors Research Group. The Consequences of Untreated Hearing Loss in Older Persons 1999.
7. Better Hearing Institute, Washington, DC 20013 USA. http://www.betterhearing.org, 1999.
8. Jero J, Mhatre AN, Tseng CJ, et al. Cochlear gene delivery through an intact round window membrane in mouse. Hum Gene Ther 2001; 12:539–548.
9. Derby ML, Sena-Esteves M, Breakefield XO, et al. Gene transfer into the mammalian inner ear using HSV-1 and vaccinia virus vectors. Hear Res 1999; 134:1–8.

10. Raphael Y, Frisancho JC, Roessler BJ. Adenoviral-mediated gene transfer into guinea pig cochlear cells in vivo. Neurosci Lett 1996; 207:137–141.

11. Yagi M, Magal E, Sheng Z, et al. Hair cell protection from aminoglycoside ototoxicity by adenovirus-mediated overexpression of glial cell line-derived neurotrophic factor. Hum Gene Ther 1999; 10:813–823.

12. Komeda M, Roessler BJ, Raphael Y. The influence of interleukin-1 receptor antagonist transgene on spiral ganglion neurons. Hear Res 1999; 131:1–10.

13. Carvalho GJ, Lalwani AK. The effect of cochleostomy and intra-cochlear infusion on auditory brain stem response threshold in the guinea pig. Am J Otol 1999; 20:87–90.

14. Stover T, Yagi M, Raphael Y. Cochlear gene transfer: round window versus cochleostomy inoculation. Hear Res 1999; 136: 124–130.

15. Wareing M, Mhatre AN, Pettis R, et al. Cationic liposome mediated transgene expression in the guinea pig cochlea. Hear Res 1999; 128:61–69.

16. Lalwani AK, Walsh BJ, Reilly PG, et al. Development of in vivo gene therapy for hearing disorders: introduction of adeno-associated virus into the cochlea of the guinea pig. Gene Ther 1996; 3:588–592.

17. Jero J, Tseng CJ, Mhatre AN, et al. A surgical approach appropriate for targeted cochlear gene therapy in the mouse. Hear Res 2001; 151:106–114.

18. Han JJ, Mhatre AN, Wareing M, et al. Transgene expression in the guinea pig cochlea mediated by a lentivirus-derived gene transfer vector. Hum Gene Ther 1999; 10:1867–1873.

19. Yamasoba T, Yagi M, Roessler BJ, et al. Inner ear transgene expression after adenoviral vector inoculation in the endolymphatic sac. Hum Gene Ther 1999; 10:769–774.

20. Kho ST, Pettis RM, Mhatre AN, et al. Cochlear microinjection and its effects upon auditory function in the guinea pig. Eur Arch Otorhinolaryngol 2000; 257:469–472.

21. Kawamoto K, Oh SH, Kanzaki S, et al. The functional and structural outcome of inner ear gene transfer via the vestibular and cochlear fluids in mice. Mol Ther 2001; 4:575–585.

22. Mathre, Lalwani. Molecular genetics of neurotology. Neurotology 2005.

23. Kho ST, Pettis RM, Mhatre AN, et al. Safety of adeno-associated virus as cochlear gene transfer vector: analysis of distant spread beyond injected cochleae. Mol Ther 2000; 2:368–373.

24. Probst FJ, Fridell RA, Raphael Y, et al. Correction of deafness in shaker-2 mice by an unconventional myosin in a BAC transgene. Science 1998; 280:1444–1447.

25. Ylikoski J, Pirvola U, Moshnyakov M, et al. Expression patterns of neurotrophin and their receptor mRNAs in the rat inner ear. Hear Res 1993; 65:69–78.

26. Pirvola U, Arumae U, Moshnyakov M, et al. Coordinated expression and function of neurotrophins and their receptors in the rat inner ear during target innervation. Hear Res 1994; 75:131–144.

27. Wheeler EF, Bothwell M, Schecterson LC, et al. Expression of BDNF and NT-3 mRNA in hair cells of the organ of Corti: quantitative analysis in developing rats. Hear Res 1994; 73:46–56.

28. Ernfors P, Van De Water T, Loring J, et al. Complementary roles of BDNF and NT-3 in vestibular and auditory development. Neuron 1995; 14:1153–1164.

29. Zheng JL, Stewart RR, Gao WQ. Neurotrophin-4/5 enhances survival of cultured spiral ganglion neurons and protects them from cisplatin neurotoxicity. J Neurosci 1995; 15:5079–5087.

30. Magal E, Kuang R, Hever G, et al. Cochlear hair cells are protected by GDNF against ototoxins. 34th Workshop on Inner Ear Biology, 1997: O26,8.

31. Staecker H, Kopke R, Malgrange B, et al. NT-3 and/or BDNF therapy prevents loss of auditory neurons following loss of hair cells. Neuroreport 1996; 7:889–894.

32. Lalwani AK, Jero J, Mhatre AN. Current issues in cochlear gene transfer. Audiol Neurootol 2002; 7:146–151.

33. Bowers WJ, Chen X, Guo H, et al. Neurotrophin-3 transduction attenuates cisplatin spiral ganglion neuron ototoxicity in the cochlea. Mol Ther 2002; 6:12–18.

34. Chen X, Frisina RD, Bowers WJ, et al. HSV amplicon-mediated neurotrophin-3 expression protects murine spiral ganglion neurons from cisplatin-induced damage. Mol Ther 2001; 3:958–963.

35. Yagi M, Kanzaki S, Kawamoto K, et al. Spiral ganglion neurons are protected from degeneration by GDNF gene therapy. J Assoc Res Otolaryngol 2000; 1:315–325.

36. Takumida M, Anniko M. Nitric oxide in guinea pig vestibular sensory cells following gentamicin exposure in vitro. Acta Otolaryngol 2001; 121:346–350.

37. Kanzaki S, Kawamoto K, Oh SH, et al. From gene identification to gene therapy. Audiol Neurootol 2002; 7:161–164.

38. Yamane H, Nakai Y, Takayama M, et al. Appearance of free radicals in the guinea pig inner ear after noise-induced acoustic trauma. Eur Arch Otorhinolaryngol 1995; 252:504–508.

39. Lowenheim H, Furness DN, Kil J, et al. Gene disruption of p27(Kip1) allows cell proliferation in the postnatal and adult organ of corti. Proc Natl Acad Sci U S A 1999; 96:4084–4088.

40. Coats S, Flanagan WM, Nourse J, et al. Requirement of p27Kip1 for restriction point control of the fibroblast cell cycle. Science 1996; 272:877–880.

41. Bermingham NA, Hassan BA, Price SD, et al. Math1: an essential gene for the generation of inner ear hair cells. Science 1999; 284:1837–1841.

42. Zheng JL, Gao WQ. Overexpression of Math1 induces robust production of extra hair cells in postnatal rat inner ears. Nat Neurosci 2000; 3:580–586.

43. Izumikawa M, Minoda R, Kawamoto K, et al. Auditory hair cell replacement and hearing improvement by Atoh1 gene therapy in deaf mammals. Nature Med 2005; 11:271–276.

44. Li H, Corrales CE, Edge A, et al. Stem cells as therapy for hearing loss. Trends Mol Med 2004; 10:309–315.

45. Stover T, Yagi M, Raphael Y. Transduction of the contralateral ear after adenovirus-mediated cochlear gene transfer. Gene Ther 2000; 7:377–383.

46. Suzuki M, Yagi M, Brown JN, et al. Effect of transgenic GDNF expression on gentamicin-induced cochlear and vestibular toxicity. Gene Ther 2000; 7:1046–1054.

47. Wheling M. Specific, nongenomic actions of steroid hormones. Annu Rev Physiol 1997; 59:365.

24 Mechanisms for hair cell protection and regeneration in the mammalian organ of Corti

Sara Euteneuer and Allen F Ryan

Introduction

In normal hearing, sound pressure variations entering the human inner ear are sensed in the organ of Corti by the hair cell's stereociliary bundle on the apical membrane, then converted within the cell to transmitter release at the basal membrane. The latter generates an action potential in the fibres of the spiral ganglion neurones (Fig. 24.1). Two types of hair cells—inner and outer—work together to accomplish this highly efficient mechanism of sound processing: Outer hair cells frequency specifically amplify the mechanical signal, while inner hair cells convert the mechanical signal into neuronal impulses.

The average number of cochlear hair cells, 15,000 per human inner ear, is quite small and there is little (if any) redundancy in these highly specific cells. Thus, hair cell loss is associated with compromised hearing in the cell's specific frequency range, since hair cells are organized in the organ of Corti in a tonotopical order. In contrast to many avian and other non mammalian species, hair cell regeneration does not occur in mammals in vivo. Therefore, once a mammalian hair cell is lost, hearing in the specific cell's frequency is lost as well.

From the pathophysiologist's point of view, the hearing impairment at a specific frequency is not the only matter of concern: the loss of a hair cell also puts the remaining hair cells at risk. Considering that the apical surface of the organ of Corti is immersed in K^+ rich endolymph, a fluid toxic to the basal parts of the cells, even a brief open connection in one spot might endanger the entire organ. Therefore a highly complex

and regulated mechanism of cell death and scar formation in the organ of Corti is needed. Understanding this mechanism is necessary not only to identify possible ototoxic agents in advance, but also to develop treatment concepts for prevention of hair cell damage and/or rescue of injured hair cells.

Mechanisms of hair cell death: apoptosis and necrosis

At least two different modes of cell death can be distinguished: apoptosis and necrosis. The later form of cell death results from nonspecific, severe, acute cell injury. Morphologically the cells show degradation of cytoskeletal proteins, energy depletion, cell swelling and finally cell rupture. The released cytoplasmatic proteins then trigger a pronounced inflammatory response in the surrounding tissue.

As opposed to necrosis, the term "apoptosis" was coined by Kerr et al. as early as 1972, describing a programmed, energy-dependent process of cell deconstruction (1). This process includes cellular and nuclear shrinkage, disassembly of intracellular structures, DNA fragmentation and division of the cell into apoptotic bodies; however, the integrity of the plasma membrane is preserved. Finally the degradated cell fragments are "safely" removed by phagocytosis without release of cytoplasmatic proinflammatory mediators into the surrounding tissue.

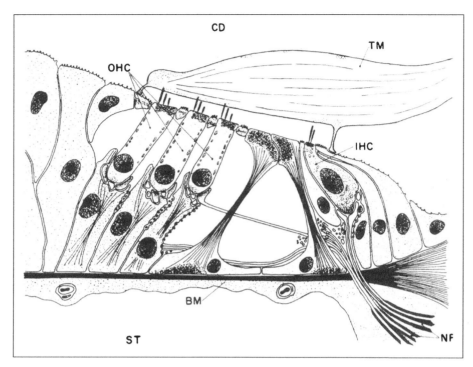

Figure 24.1   Structure of the organ of Corti. *Abbreviations*: BM, basilar membrane; CD, cochlea duct; IHC, inner hair cells; OHC, outer hair cells; ST, scala tympani; TM, tectorial membrane. *Source*: From Robinette MS, Glattke TJ. Otoacoustic Emissions Clinical Applications. New York: Thieme Medical Publishers Inc., 1997:22.

Even if the mechanisms involved in necrosis and apoptosis blend into each other, apoptosis seems to be important in the cochlea for the sake of sealing the gap in the sensory epithelium in an orderly manner, before it even arises (2,3). Supporting cells rapidly expand their apical domains, constricting the hair cell beneath their membranes, therefore sealing the reticular lamina prior to any endolymph leak (3).

Many different factors and conditions can serve as initial signals for active cell death. This includes absence of trophic factors, diffusible molecules that bind to specific cell-surface receptors ("death receptors," DR) and different kinds of cellular stress (Fig. 24.2). Generalizing, there are two major biochemical routes that lead to activation of caspases, the cystein proteases that specifically cleave a variety of substrates leading to fragmentation of nuclear DNA and disassembly of the cell (Fig. 24.2) (4).

The "extrinsic" pathway is triggered by ligation of ligands to DRs such as Fas, the TNF-family receptors, DR-3, DR-4, DR-5 and others. Death ligand binding leads to recruitment of downstream signalling partners, which ultimately results in activation of the "initiator" caspase 8. Subsequently, activation of the "effector" caspases such as caspase 3 and finally cell death, by protein and DNA cleavage, occurs. The "intrinsic" pathway involves increases in mitochondrial membrane permeability with release of mitochondria-specific proteins, like cytochrome C or endonuclease G, into the cytoplasm (5). Once in the cytoplasm, the proteins bind the scaffolding protein apoptotic protease-activating factor-1 (Apaf-1), which recruits the "initiator" caspase 9 to a high-molecular mass complex, the

so called apoptosome. Caspase 9 is activated and subsequently activates the "effector" caspases-3, -6 and -7 proteolytically. The effector caspases then execute cell death by protein and DNA degradation.

Various intracellular signalling pathways can lead to impairment of mitochondrial function and mitochondrial membrane integrity. These pathways often lead to changes in protein function of the B-cell CLL/lymphoma 2 (Bcl-2) family proteins, which are key players in regulation of mitochondrial membrane integrity (5). Bcl-2 itself is an integral membrane protein in the cytoplasmatic face of the outer mitochondrial membrane. It carries out its pro-survival function by inhibiting the translocation of the multi-Bcl-2 Homology (BH)-protein Bax to the mitochondrial membrane, as well as by inhibiting its colocalisation with the multi-BH-protein Bak in the mitochondrial membrane. The Bax-Bak homo-oligomers otherwise coalesce into larger complexes and permeabilize the mitochondrial membrane, allowing release of cytochrome C into the cytoplasm. The BH3-only proteins, such as Bim, Bid, Bad and others, also promote apoptosis, by targeting Bcl-2 and ablating its inhibition of Bax (Fig. 24.2) (5). The BH3-only protein Bid can also activate Bax-Bak oligomerization directly. In some cells, so called "type II" cells, Bid can be activated by DRs, thereby linking the extrinsic to the intrinsic pathway in these cells. Type I cells, in which the extrinsic pathway operates via caspase 8 only, are primarily leukocytes. If DRs are involved in cochlear cell death, it seems likely that they would respond like type II cells, not only via caspase 8 activation but via Bid and caspase 9 as well.

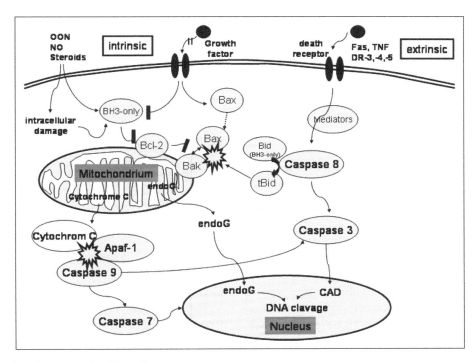

Figure 24.2 Schematic overview of apoptotic signalling pathways.

Mechanisms for hair cell damage in humans

Ototoxic drugs

Clinically important ototoxic drugs are the chemotherapeutic drug cisplatin and aminoglycoside antibiotics.

Cisplatin, cis-diamminedichloroplatinum(II), is a widely used chemotherapeutic agent. However its use is limited by serious side effects including neuro-, nephro- and ototoxicity. The most vulnerable cells for cisplatin cytotoxicity in the inner ear are outer hair cells, followed by inner hair cells. Supporting cells and the stria vascularis are the least damaged. Functionally, hearing loss first appears in the high frequencies and then progresses to lower frequencies.

Binding of nuclear DNA and formation of DNA complexes with consecutive disturbance of transcription and DNA replication is believed to be the main biological cytotoxic effect of cisplatin, and is responsible for its anticancer properties (6). However, before reaching the nucleus, cisplatin also interacts with the cell membrane and various proteins in the cytoplasm. Binding to phospholipids in the cell membrane leads to ceramide synthesis. The latter can initiate apoptosis via activation of the MAP kinase JNK, which inhibits Bcl-2 (7). Nevertheless, inhibition of the JNK pathway fails to protect hair cells from cisplatin-induced apoptosis, suggesting that other classes of MAP kinases such as p38 MAPK might be involved as well (8).

In the cytoplasm, cisplatin also exhibits strong reactivity against nucleophiles, like thiol-containing proteins, especially glutathione. The latter is one of the most important antioxidants of the cytoplasm. Therefore cisplatin raises intracellular levels of radical oxygen species (ROS) by depleting antioxidants. ROS are pro-apoptotic by oxidation of mitochondrial membrane proteins, and therefore destabilizing their membrane, as well as by activating intracellular stress pathways. Hair cells seem to be the most vulnerable cell type in the inner ear for antioxidant depletion. Especially the outer hair cells have relatively lower glutathione levels, and therefore antioxidant capacity, than other cell types in the cochlea. There is also a gradient of outer hair cell glutathione levels in the cochlea, rising towards the apex (9). This may help to explain the vulnerability of the basal cochlea to hair cell damage.

Aminoglycoside antibiotics, such as gentamicin, are primarily administered during infections with gram negative bacteria to irreversibly inhibit their protein biosynthesis. In the cochlea, aminoglycosides destroy outer hair cells in a systematic manner first, then inner hair cells as well as supporting cells. As with cisplatin, damage starts with the outer hair cells in the basal turn progressing to the apex, resulting initially in high frequency hearing loss (10). The formation of ROS is believed to be an early step in aminoglycoside ototoxicity. Aminoglycosides can form complexes with iron, which subsequently reacts with unsaturated fatty acids of membrane lipids to form lipid oxides and free ROS. Lipid oxides in the cell membrane can trigger the intrinsic apoptotic pathway. The overproduction of ROS puts oxidative stress on the cell's antioxidant systems, finally depleting them and initiating apoptosis. Beside ROS activation, aminoglycosides seem to activate various cell signalling networks involved in apoptosis as well as cell survival. A death pathway leading from kRas to cdc42 and JNK plays a critical role (11,12). Survival pathways that oppose hair cell death are also activated, including an hRas-Mek-Erk pathway (11) and a PI3K/Akt/PKC pathway (13). It is the balance of activity in these damage and survival pathways that determine the fate of the cell. Blocking these damage mechanisms or stimulating survival pathways can protect hair cells.

Noise-induced hearing loss (NIHL)

Exposure to sound of sufficient intensity produces a threshold shift in hearing level. Hearing function can recover completely or residual or permanent threshold shift might occur. With repeated exposure, a permanent threshold shift can accumulate, leading to increasingly debilitating hearing loss. Common histological findings affect the spiral limbus, the ligament with the organ of Corti, as well as the stria vascularis.

Genetic studies in various animal models suggest the involvement of genes similar to those involved in ototoxic hair cell damage. Stress-signal induced factors, first of all ROS, as well as iron and intracellular calcium levels seem to be important (for a review see Ref. 14). As in ototoxicity, cell signalling networks involving cell death as well as cell survival pathways appear to be centrally involved in NIHL. Signalling proteins identified to link noise exposure to hair cell death are Src protein tyrosine kinase, activated by mechanical alterations of cell-cell and cell-extracellularmatrix interactions (15), the JNK pathway (16) and proteins induced by transcription factor NFkB (17) have all been implicated.

Age-related hearing loss (ARHL)

As early as in the 1960s, Schucknecht and Gacek proposed a framework for age-related hearing loss (ARHL). They emphasized the occurrence of relatively isolated degeneration in either the organ of Corti, afferent neurones or the stria vascularis (18). These separate mechanisms have been seen in various animal models such as mice, cats and guinea pigs (14). The intracellular mechanisms which mediate ARHL are still vague, but studies with transgenic mice shed some light upon the possible players. Until now, three so-called ahl (aging induced hearing loss) genes, ahl1, ahl2 and ahl3, have been identified in mice (14,19). Ahl1 codes for cadherin 23 (Cdh 23), which is a constituent of hair cell sterocilia (19). Mutations in Cdh23 have been shown to cause late-onset hearing loss and deafness in mice and humans (20). Products for the ahl2 and ahl3 genes have not yet been identified.

It seems likely that some of the same damage processes that operate in other forms of SNHL also occur in ARHL. Genes that modulate the amount of intracellular ROS, as well as the melatonin metabolism, appear to be involved (for a review see Ref. 14). Decline in protective pathways may also be relevant. The recent work of Rüttiger et al. (21) suggests that a reduced amount of neurotrophic factors, like BDNF, in the spiral ganglion dendrites may play a role.

Genetic hearing loss

In the last decade many genes associated with hearing loss have been identified in humans, as well as in animal models (20). These are detailed in other chapters of this volume. Many of the mutations that result in hearing loss are characterized by loss of hair cells. Relatively little is known about the intracellular mechanisms that lead to cell damage. However, it is possible that some of the same cell damage pathways that act in noise and ototoxic injury are involved.

Protecting hair cells: Prevention of hair cell damage and recovery of injured hair cells

Considering the different mechanisms described in the previous sections, hair cell protection by prevention of hair cell damage seems highly desirable. Prevention of damage requires knowledge that danger is ahead to counteract the toxic event before it occurs. Damage by noise exposure cannot always be predicted in advance. Since ototoxic drugs are administered by intention, their effect is predictable, as is ageing. In late-onset forms of genetic deafness, hearing loss can also be predicted well in advance.

ROS are major players in inducing apoptosis not only in aminoglycoside and cisplatin ototoxicity, and also in noise-induced hearing loss. ROS act upstream in damage and apoptotic pathways so that their elimination suppresses the toxic mechanism near the very onset. Many agents blocking either the formation of ROS or scavenging ROS once they are formed (antioxidants) have been studied intensively in vitro as well as in vivo in different animal models (for a detailed summary see Ref. 22). Iron chelators, like deferoxamine, 2,2'-dipyridyl, salicylate, D-methionine and 2,3 dihydroxybenzoate, which inhibit aminoglycoside binding to free iron and consecutive ROS formation, have demonstrated protection against aminoglycoside toxicity in mice and in guinea pigs in vitro and in vivo. Salicylates and D-methionine act as antioxidants as well. Both have proved protection against aminoglycoside and cisplatin toxicity in vitro and in vivo in different animal models. Recently Sha et al. (24) demonstrated in a randomised, double-blind study that high dose salicylate treatment (3 gr aspirin per day) reduced gentamicin-induced hearing loss in humans.

Stress activated protein kinase pathways, especially the c-Jun N-terminal Kinase (JNK)-cascade, appear to be another important target in prevention of aminoglycoside and noise-induced hair cell loss. Besides the activation of pro-apoptotic transcription factors, JNK activates pro-apoptotic members of the Bcl-2 family and inactivates Bcl-2 itself by phosphorylation in the cytosol (Fig. 24.2). Simultaneous inhibition of JNK signalling with neomycin administration and noise exposure respectively has been shown to diminish hair cell damage in vitro and in vivo in mice as well as in guinea pigs (16). In contrast, cisplatin ototoxicity does not appear to be mediated by JNK, but rather by the alternative stress MAPK, p38 (8).

Downstream in the apoptotic pathways, various caspase inhibitors have proven to attenuate hair cell loss from noise, cisplation and aminoglycoside damage (4,8). However, effector caspases are activated late and typically after mitochondrial damage. Therefore, inhibition of effector caspases may only delay hair cell loss but not rescue hair cells, since the apoptotic signal may be diverted upstream due to metabolic enzymes and other effectors take over for caspases.

In addition to damaged pathways, cellular stress may lead to enhanced cell damage by interruption of pro-survival pathways like Erk/MAPK, as well as PI3K/Akt/PKC signalling (4,11,13). Indeed, FGF-2, glial cell line derived neurotrophic factor, BDNF, NT-3 among others have shown to prevent hair cell loss from various damage (25–28) possibly by activation of survival signalling.

Finally, insertion of a bacterial resistance gene into the mammalian genome has been shown to protect hair cells from aminoglycosides (29), and would presumably protect other tissues such as kidney, without influencing the bacteriocidal effect of the antibiotic.

Understanding the embryonic development of the organ of corti— key knowledge for cell replacement

The inner ear evolves from the otic placode, on the lateral side of the embryo, which invaginates and forms the early otocyst in the first trimester of development in humans. The otocyst develops outgrowths, which extend to form the vestibular and cochlear divisions of the membranous labyrinth. Undifferentiated sensory epithelia form on the walls of the developing labyrinth. Just after the time at which cell division ceases in the epithelia, the hair cells differentiate from the surrounding cells, which become supporting cells.

The signalling events that lead to the specification of individual cell types in the inner ear and their exit from the cell cycle are still largely unknown. However, a variety of cellular interactions that play roles during the highly complex development and morphogenesis of the inner ear, especially in hair cell development, have been identified (for recent review see Ref. 30). The pair-box transcription factor Pax2, Sox2 and the cell cycle modulator $p27^{KIP1}$ are expressed in early proliferating progenitors of hair cells (31) and then down regulated with further differentiation. Notch-ligand Jagged-1 (32), the cell cycle modulator $p27^{KIP1}$ (33) and the signalling proteins BMP4 and BMP7 (34) play an important role in the switch from the proliferative sensory progenitors to the differentiating sensory epithelium. Atoh1 (also known as Math1/Hath1 in mouse and human) and Brn-3.1 (POU4F3) are essential for the terminal differentiation

of hair cells (35,36). Hair cells are generated to survive—without renewal—for a whole lifetime. They lose their capability for renewal when they exit the cell-cycle before birth.

Replacing hair cells: hair cell regeneration by trans-differentiation of supporting cells

Non-mammalian vertebrates, especially birds and amphibians, regenerate hair cells constantly throughout their lives (37). New hair cells can form from progenitor cells that remain present in both the vestibular as well as the auditory part of the adult avian inner ear. Alternatively, they may derive from supporting cells, either by asymmetrical cell division or straightforward transdifferentiation (37). Supporting cells of the mammalian inner ear are post mitotic in vivo, and therefore unable to go through cell division and therefore regeneration. However, several studies showed that over-expression of the gene Atoh1, necessary for final hair cell differentiation during development, could induce transdifferentiation of supporting cells into hair cell phenotypes in the adult mammalian ear in vitro and in vivo (38–40).

Raphael and colleagues (39,40) demonstrated that in vivo inoculation of adenovirus with the Atoh1 gene into the cochlear endolymph of mature guinea pigs led to the expression of the gene in supporting cells of the organ of Corti as well as adjacent cells. Thirty to sixty days after transgene inoculation, the transfected cells had developed a hair cell-like morphology and expressed the hair cell marker myosin VII. In addition, some spiral ganglion dendrites extended towards the new myosin VII positive cells (39). In their later publication they confirmed these results in previously deafened adult guinea pigs, 8 weeks after transgene inoculation. In addition they observed normal surface morphology and orientation of new hair cells within the organ of Corti, leading to a partial recovery of hearing function in these animals with a threshold as low as 65 db (40). Surprisingly they detected an increase in the number of nuclei in the supporting cell area of the organ of Corti after Atoh1 treatment. They hypothesised the existence of unidentified supporting cell precursors capable of replicating.

Recently White et al. (41) demonstrated this potential for cell mitosis and replication in the mammalian inner ear. They showed that post mitotic supporting cells isolated from the neonatal mouse organ of Corti retained the ability to both divide and transdifferentiate into hair cells in vitro upon co-culture with periotic mesenchymal cells. First, the supporting cells down-regulated the cell cycle inhibitor $p27^{KIP1}$ and proliferated in culture. Later, in culture these cells expressed the hair cell marker myosin VII. The observed capacity to down-regulate $p27^{KIP1}$ upon stimulation and therefore to regenerate seemed to fade with ageing of the animal. In cultures from postnatal day 14 (P14) inner ears, only 2% of cells down-regulated p27^{KIP1} and re-entered the cell cycle. Nevertheless the capacity for transdifferentiation, as identified by the yield of hair cells generated by the P14 supporting cells, was comparable to what was observed in the neonatal cultures.

Replacing hair cells: hair cell regeneration from stem cells

Because the capacity for transdifferentiation of supporting cells into hair cells is limited, especially because of the limited number of supporting cells, the idea of replacing hair cells with proliferating stem cells is particularly exciting. In general, there are four principal resources for stem cells to regenerate organ-specific cell types: 1) embryonic stem cells (ESC) either derived from the inner cell mass of the blastocyst; or 2) designed by cloning of a differentiated cell's nucleus of into a blastocyst's cell body; 3) adult stem cells (ASC) from the organ to be regenerated itself; or 4) adult stem cells from other organs like the brain or the haematopoetic system stimulated to express the target organ's genes.

Hair cells from embryonic stem cells (ESC)

Even if considered highly controversial in humans, ESC have the greatest capacity for differentiation into multiple cell types because they are the precursors of all adult cells. They also have the capacity for self renewal (symmetrical division) and therefore can expand into large numbers. In addition ESC have the capacity for asymmetrical cell division, i.e., one of the two daughter cells is still a stem cell while the other daughter cell can differentiate into a specific adult cell type. Directing ESC differentiation into a specific cell types in vitro has been successful among other things in producing dopaminergic neurones for the potential treatment of Parkinson's disease (42), insulin-secreting cells for diabetes (43) and motor neurones for spinal cord injuries (44).

Recently, similar results were achieved in the inner ear: mammalian ESC were differentiated into inner-ear progenitors in vitro by applying growth factors that are involved in normal embryonic development (45). The application of epidermal growth factor (EGF), insulin-like growth factor-1 (IGF-1) and basic fibroblast growth factor (bFGF)—all physiological cues leading to the demarcation of the otic placode early in development—to murine ESC in vitro led to the development of cells expressing physiological markers for the otic placode and otic vesicle (Pax2, BMP7, Jagged-1). Withdrawal of growth factors, the mitogenic stimuli, led to further differentiation of the generated cells. Markers of the maturing organ of Corti like Atoh1, Brn3.1, p27^{KIP1}, as well as markers of fully differentiated hair cells (myosinVIIa and epsin) and supporting cells (p27^{KIP1}, Jagged-1) could be detected.

Still, the in vivo situation for application of ESC is much more challenging because stem cells need a highly controlled environment. One set of conditions is required to remain undifferentiated and multipotent. Different cues are needed for initiation, completion and stabilization of differentiation. This potential niche for ESC in the inner ear still needs to be identified. Last, but definitely not least, before the therapeutic administration of human ESC, the problem of incompatibility between the major histocompatibility complex of the recipient and the grafted ESC with necessity for immunosuppression needs to be addressed.

Hair cells from adult stem cells (ASC)

Because of the ethical objections against ESC and the potential for immune rejection by the recipient, the concept of using ASC from the same individual for regeneration of the inner ear's sensory epithelium has drawn increasing attention in the last few years. This is particularly true after the discovery of quiescent ASC in the adult mouse and human inner ear (46,47). Li et al. (46) isolated pluripotent stem cells from the utricular macula of adult mice and found that these ASC could differentiate not only into a hair cell phenotype but also into supporting cell types and even neuronal marker expressing cell types as well as muscle marker-expressing cells. These findings suggest that these cells may be the source for the previously described regenerative capability of the mammalian utricular sensory epithelium (48). Rask-Andersen et al. (47) isolated neuronal stem cells from adult human and guinea pig spiral ganglia and stimulated these cells to differentiation in to mature neurones and glial cells.

In addition to these two studies, the work of Malgrange et al. (49) and Oshima et al. (50) suggests the presence of stem cells in the mammalian organ of Corti, at least neonatally. Malgrange et al. (49) isolated sphere-forming cells from the organ of Corti of newborn rats and induced their differentiation into hair cell marker (myosin VIIa) expressing cells in vitro. Oshima et al. (50) confirmed these results in early postnatal animals and also isolated substantially lower numbers of sphere-forming cells from more mature tissue. The latter data suggest a postnatal loss of stem cells in the mammalian organ of Corti, and increase interest in other possible sources for ASC that could be differentiated into hair cells.

Haematopoetic stem cells seem particularly interesting from the clinical standpoint since they are more readily accessible. Recently Jeon et al. (51) reported the differentiation of mesenchymal bone marrow stem cells into neuroectoderm progenitors, based on the progenitors expression profile of nestin, BMP4, BMP7 and Atoh1. Even neuronal stem cells could be differentiated towards Brn-3c and myosin VII expression (52).

Clinical applications: Where are we? Where can we go?

In the last decade, substantial progress has been made in understanding key positions in cochlear development as well as in cell death mechanisms in the cochlea.

Nevertheless, most studies investigating cell death mechanisms in the cochlea have been performed in vitro with ototoxic drugs, or in animals in vivo with ototoxic drugs or noise exposure. It remains to be seen if any of the anti-apoptotic agents or factors in these recent studies can also rescue hair cells from death due to genetic disease or ageing. In addition, nearly all studies cited in this chapter have been carried out on animal models that have suffered relatively acute hearing loss before treatment and it remains to be seen how long-term hearing loss, the more likely situation in humans, reacts to the same treatments. Most likely there will be no single drug or treatment to prevent the complex and interactive process of hair cell death. Further studies focusing on the combination of treatments in vitro and in vivo in the established animal models are necessary. Recent success in studies intending to replace hair cells by gene manipulation, of Atoh1 and p27^{KIP1} (40,41), as well as stem cell therapy raise different challenges regarding safe delivery to the cochlea without causing damage to residual hearing. The development of safe and reliable strategies for long term local delivery into the cochlea will be crucial for the translation of experimental achievements into patient therapy.

Before translation of the promising results achieved in basic stem cell research is possible, the obstacles to appropriate integration into the cochlea need to be overcome. Finally, more studies like that of Izumikawa et al. (40), showing partial restoration of hearing after hair cell recovery, are needed to determine the functional consequences of hair cell recovery or restoration.

In summary, substantial progress in basic research into cell death and restoration mechanisms in the cochlea has been made. Initial results regarding the functional consequences of cochlear therapy have been obtained. Inner ear research therefore seems poised to tackle the obstacles of translation of basic science knowledge into clinical application. The years to come will be exciting for those participating in this area.

References

1. Kerr JF, Wyllie AH, Currie AR. Apoptosis: a basic biological phenomenon with wide-ranging implications in tissue kinetics. Br J Cancer 1972; 26:239–257.

2. Rosenblatt J, Raff MC, Cramer LP. An epithelial cell destined for apoptosis signals its neighbors to extrude it by an actin- and myosin-dependent mechanism. Current Biol 2001; 11:1847–1857.

3. Raphael Y. Cochlear pathology, sensory cell death and regeneration. Br Med Bull 2002; 63:25–38.

4. Lamelland F, Lefebvre P, Hans G, Moonen G, Malgrange B. Molecular pathways involved in apoptotic cell death in the injured cochlea: cues to novel therapeutic strategies. Curr Pharm Des 2005; 11:2257–2275.

5. Adams JM. Ways of dying: multiple pathways to apoptosis. Genes Develop 2003; 17:2481–2495.

6. Fuertes MA, Castilla J, Alonso C, Perez JM. Cisplatin biochemical mechanism of action: from cytotoxicity to induction of cell death through interconnections between apoptotic and necrotic pathways. Current Med Chem 2003; 10:257–266.

7. Ruvolo PR. Ceramid regulates cellular homeostasis via diverse stress signalling pathways. Leukemia 2001; 15:1153–1160.

8. Wang J, Van DE, Water TR, et al. A peptide inhibitor of c-Jun N-terminal kinaxe protects against both aminoglycoside and acoustic trauma-induced auditory hair cell death and hearing loss. J Neurosci 2003; 23:8596–8607.

9. Sha SH, Taylor R, Forge A, Schacht J. Differential vulnerability of basal and apical hair cells is based on intrinsic susceptibility to free radicals. Hear Res 2001; 155:1–8.

10. Forge A, Schacht J. Aminoglycoside antibiotics. Audiol Neurootol 2000; 5:3–22.

11. Battaglia A, Pak K, Brors D, Bodmer D, Frangos JA, Ryan AF. Involvment of ras activation in toxic hair cell damage of the mammalian cochlea. Neurosci 2003; 122:1025–1035.

12. Bodmer D, Brors D, Pak K, Gloddek B, Ryan AF. Rescue of auditory hair cells from aminoglycoside toxicity by clostridium difficile toxin B, an inhibitor of the small GTPase Rho/Rac/Cdc 42. Hear Res 2002; 172:81–86.

13. Chung W-H, Pak K, Lin B, Webster N, Ryan AF. A P13K pathway mediates hair cell survival and opposes gentamicin toxicity in neonatal rat organ of Corti. J Assoc Res Otolaryngol 2006; 7(4) 373–382.

14. Ohlemiller KK. Contribution of mouse models to understanding of age and noise-related hearing loss. Brain Res 2006; 1091:89–102.

15. Harris KC, Hu B, Hangauer D, Henderson D. Prevention of noise-induced hearing loss with Src-PTK inhibitors. Hear Res 2005; 208:14–25.

16. Wang J, Ladrech S, Pujol R, Brabet P, van De Water, Puel JL. Caspase inhibitors, but not c-Jun NH2-terminal inhibitor treatment prevent cisplatin-induced hearing loss. Cancer Res 2004; 64:9217–9224.

17. Masuda M, Nagashima R, Kanzaki S, Fujioka M, Ogita K, Ogawa K. Nuclear factor-kappa B nuclear translocation in the cochlea of mice following acoustic overstimulation. Brain Res 2006; 237–247.

18. Schuknecht HF, Gacek MR. Cochlear pathology in presbyacusis. Ann Otol Rhinol Laryngol 1993; 102:1–16.

19. Johnson KR, Zheng QY, Erway LC. A major gene affecting age-related hearing loss is common to at least ten inbred strains of mice. Genomics 2000; 80:171–180.

20. Petit C, Levilliers J, Hardelin JP. Molecular genetics of hearing loss. Ann Rev Genet 2001; 35:589–646.

21. Rüttiger L, Panford-Walsh R, Schimmang T, et al. BDNF mRNA expression and protein localization are changed in age-related hearing loss. Neurobiol Aging 2007; 28(4):586–601.

22. Rybak LP, Whitworth CA. Ototoxicity: therapeutic opportunities. Drug Discovery Today 2005; 10:1313–1321.

23. Lautermann J, Dehna N, Schacht J, Jahnke K. Aminoglycoside- and cisplatin-ototoxicity: from basic science to clinics. Laryngo-Rhinol-Otol 2004; 83:317–323.

24. Sha SH, Qui JH, Schacht J. Aspirin to prevent gentamicin-induced hearing loss. N Engl J Med 2006; 354:1856–1857.

25. Low W, Dazert S, Baird A, Ryan AF. Basic fibroblast growth factor (FGF-2) protects rat cochlear hair cells in organotypical

culture from aminoglycoside injury. J Cell Physiol 1996; 167:443–450.

26. Ylikoski J, Privola U, Virkkala J, et al. Guinea pig auditory neurons are protected by glial cell line-derived growth factor from degeneration after noise trauma. Hear Res 1998; 124:17–26.

27. Ruan DS, Leong SK, Mark I, Yeoh KH. Effects of BDNF and NT-3 on hair cell survival in guinea pig cochlea damaged by kanamycin treatment. Neuroreport 1999; 10:2067–2071.

28. Shoji F, Miller AL, Mitchell A, Yamasoba T, Altschuler A, Miller JM. Differental protective effects of neurotrophins in the attenuation of noise-induced hair cell loss. Hear Res 2000; 146:134–142.

29. Dulon D, Ryan AF. The bacterial *neo* gene confers neomycin resistance to mammalian cochlear hair cells. Neuro Rep 1999; 10:1189–1193.

30. Bryant J, Goodyear RJ, Richardson GP. Sensory organ development in the inner ear: molecular and cellular mechanisms. Br Med Bull 2002; 63:39–57.

31. Lawoko-Kerali G, Rivolta MN, Holley M. Expression of the transcription factors GATA3 and Pax2 during development of the mammalian inner ear. J Comp Neurol 2002; 442:387–391.

32. Lanford PJ, Lan Y, Jiang R, et al. Notch signalling pathway mediates hair cell development in mammalian cochlea. Nature Genet 1999; 21:289–292.

33. Chen P, Segil N. p27^{Kip1} links cell proliferation to morphogenesis in the developing organ of Corti. Develop 1999; 126:1581–1590.

34. Li H, Corrales CE, Wnag Z, et al. BMP4 signalling is involved in the regeneration of inner ear sensory epithelia. BMC Dev Biol 2005; 17:5–16.

35. Bermingham NA, Hassan BA, Price SD, et al. Math1: an essential gene for the generation of inner ear hair cells. Science 1999, 284:1837.

36. Erkman L, McEvilly RJ, Luo L, et al. Role of transcription factors Brn.-3.1 and Brn3.2 in auditory and visual systems development. Nature 1996; 381:603–606.

37. Stone JS, Rubel EW. Cellular studies of auditory hair cell regeneration in birds. PNAS 2000; 97:11714–11721.

38. Shou J, Zheng JL, Gao WQ. Robust generation of new hair cells in the mature mammalian inner ear by adenoviral expression of Hath1. Mol Cell Neurosci 2003; 23:169–179.

39. Kawamoto K, Ishimoto SI, Minoda R, Brough DE, Raphael Y. Math1 gene transfer generates new cochlear hair cells in mature guinea pigs in vivo. J Neurosci 2003; 23:4395–4400.

40. Izumikawa M, Minoda R, Kawamoto K, et al. Auditory hair cell replacement and hearing improvement by Atho1 gene therapy in deaf mammals. Nature Med 2005; 11:271–276.

41. White PM, Doetzelhofer A, Lee YS, Groves A, Segil N. Mammalian cochlear supporting cells can divide and trans-differentiate into hair cells. Nature 2006; 441:984–987.

42. Kim JH, Auerbach JM, Rodriguez-Gomez JA, et al. Dopamine neurons derived from embryonic stem cells function in an animal model of Parkinson's disease. Nature 2002; 418:50–56.

43. Lumelsky N, Blondel O, Laeng P, Velasco I, Ravin R, McKay R. Differentiation of embryonic stem cells to insulin-secreting structures similar to pancreatic islets. Science 2001; 292:1389–1394.

44. Wichterle H, Lieberam I, Porter JA, Jessell TM. Directed differentiaion of embryonic stem cells into motor neurons. Cell 2002; 110:385–397.

45. Li H, Roblin G, Liu H, Heller S. Generation of hair cells by stepwise differentiation of embryonic stem cells. PNAS 2003; 100:13495–13500.

46. Li H, Liu H, Heller S. Pluripotent stem cells from the adult mouse inner ear. Nature Med 2003; 9:1293–1299.

47. Rask-Andersen H, Boström M, Gerdin B, et al. Regeneration of human auditory nerve. In vitro/in vivo demonstration of neural progenitor cells in adult human and guinea pig spiral ganglion. Hear Res 2005; 203:180–191.

48. Warchol ME, Lamert PR, Goldstein BJ, Forge A, Corwin JT. Regenerative proliferation in the inner ear sensory epithelia from adult guinea pigs and humans. Science 1993; 259:1619–1622.

49. Malgrange B, Belachew S, Thiry M, et al. Proliferative generation of mammalian auditory hair cells in culture. Mech Dev 2002; 112:79–88.

50. Oshima K, Senn P, Corrales E, Grimm C, Holt JR, Heller S. Cochlear stem cells exist but their number substantially decreases during postnatal cochlear maturation. ARO Abstracts, 2006, 29, p 286, Abstract 849.

51. Jeon S, Heler S, Edge A. Expression of hair cell markers in cells differentiated from bone marrow stem cells. ARO Abstracts, 2006, 29: 284, Abstract 843.

52. Kojima K, Tamura S, Nishida AT, Ito J. Generation of inner hair cell immunophenotypes from neurospheres obtained from fetal rat central nervous system in vitro. Acta Otolaryngol Suppl 2004; 551:26–30.

Index

A

ABR. *See* auditory brainstem response
acoustic reflex thresholds (ARTs)
adaptation
    pathological, 27
Affymetrix platform, 216
age-related hearing impairment, 69–90, 133,
        189, 193, 308
age and NIHL, 98
allele,15
aminoglycoside deafness, 254, 307
        (*See also* ototoxicity)
anotia, 23, 239
APEX arrayed primer extension, 216
apoptosis, 221, 305
ARHI. *See* age-related
        hearing impairment
ascorbic acid, 225
aspirin 308
association, 40
atresia auris. *See* congenital
        atresia auris
audiometric configuration, 24–26,
        185–204
audiometric profiles. *See* audiometric
        configuration
Audioscan, 23
ABI (auditory brainstem implant), 261
auditory brainstem response (ABR),
        31, 32, 206, 207
auditory neuropathy, 70, 81,
        207, 263–268
auditory plasticity, 174–177, 255
auditory steady state response, 33
automated brainstem audiometry.
        See auditory brainstem
        response (ABR)
autosome,15
autosomal inheritance
    dominant, 15
    recessive, 15

B

BAHA bone anchored hearing aid, 241–242,
        247–248
Balance, 56–57
Base,15
    Pair,15
BDNF, 220, 302, 308
Békésy audiometry, 21–23
BOA behavioural observation audiometry,
        206
British Sign Language (BSL), 163

C

calpain, 228
carrier, 15
caspase, 222, 306
CDNA, 15
cerebral plasticity, 175
CHARGE, 41–42, 45, 260
cholesteatoma (in aural atresia), 245
chromatin,15
chromosome, 3,4
cisplatin, 307
cleft palate, 44
coactivator,15
cochlear aplasia, 257
cochlear blood flow, 220–221
cochlear nerve, 21
cochleovestibular hypoplasia, 258
cochleovestibular malformation, 258
codon, 15
common cavity, 257
communication disorders, 173–178, 205
communicative skills, 146–147
congenital atresia auris, 239–251
consanguineous, 15
COR conditioned orientation reflex, 206
Corepressor, 15

cortisone. *See* corticosteroids
corticosteroids, 230–232
CT (computed tomography), 240–241

D

dead regions (cochlear), 28
deaf community, 163–170
deafblindness, 55
    acquired, 55
    congenital, 55
deformation, 40
deformity, Michel, 256
deletion
    of chromosome 1p36, 42
    of chromosome 4qter, 43
    of chromome 2q22-q23, 45
dexametazone. *See* corticosteroids
DFN2,188, 193, 194
DFN3, 69, 188, 194
DFN4, 188
DFN6, 191
DFNA,186
DFNA1, 68, 193
DFNA2, 6, 86, 189, 194
DFNA3, 6, 188, 189
DFNA4, 67, 191
DFNA5, 36, 69, 86, 190, 194
DFNA6, 70, 193
DFNA7, 190
DFNA8, 69, 190, 193
DFNA9, 36, 68, 86, 100, 190, 194
DFNA10, 36, 69, 192, 194
DFNA11, 26, 67, 192
DFNA12, 69, 190, 193
DFNA13, 68, 192, 193
DFNA14, 70, 193
DFNA15, 69, 190, 194
DFNA16, 190, 194
DFNA17, 67, 86, 190, 194
DFNA18, 192

DFNA20, 68, 100, 190, 194
DFNA21, 192
DFNA22, 67, 186
DFNA23, 188, 190
DFNA24, 188, 190
DFNA25, 192
DFNA26, 68, 100, 190, 194
DFNA28, 69, 192
DFNA30, 190
DFNA31, 192
DFNA36, 70, 86, 190, 194
DFNA38, 193
DFNA41, 192, 194
DFNA42, 190
DFNA43, 192, 194
DFNA44, 193
DFNA47, 190
DFNA48, 67, 190
DFNA49, 193
DFNA50, 192
DFNA54, 193
DFNB, 186, 190
DFNB1, 26, 186, 190, 192, 215
DFNB2, 67
DFNB3, 67
DFNB4, 26, 186, 209
DFNB5, 86–87
DFNB6, 70
DFNB7, 70
DFNB8, 70, 186, 190
DFNB9, 70
DFNB1, 70, 186, 190
DFNB11, 70
DFNB13, 186
DFNB16, 68, 190
DFNB18, 67
DFNB21, 69, 193
DFNB22, 68
DFNB23, 66
DFNB30, 67, 190
DFNB31, 67
DFNB36, 68
DFNB37, 27, 67
disruption, 39
D-methionine
DNA, 3, 11
DNA chips See DNA microarrays
DNA microarrays, 16, 72, 209
dominant negative effect, 15
DPOAE, 30, 80, 81, 96, 223
dyslexia, 173
dysplasia, 39

E

ear
    external, 20
    inner, 21, 80
    middle, 20

middle ear admittance, 28
early-detection and
            hearingintervention(EDHI), 206
electrocochleography, 30–31, 207
environmental risk factors, 83, 134
epidemiology of HI, 79–80
    NIHL, 92
eugenetics, 166–167
eukaryote, 15
EVA enlarged vestibular aqueduct, 208, 259
Exons, 8,15
Expressed Sequence Tag(EST), 15

F

family history of hearing problems, 147–156
fetal alcohol syndrome, 174
function
    gain of, 14
    loss of, 14

G

GDNF, 224, 229
gene, 3
    ACTG1, 67
    ALMS1, 58
    Atoh1 (Math1), 219, 311
    CDH23 (Cadherin), 57, 71, 84
    CDH23, 26, 66
    Claudin 14 (CLDN14), 65
    COCH (cochlin), 68, 86, 216
    COL11A1, 26
    COL11A2, 68
    COL1A1, 113
    COL1A2, 113
    connexins. See GJB
    DIAPH1, 68
    EDN3, 50
    EDNRB, 50
    ESPN, 68
    expression, 10
    EYA1, 51, 215, 256
    EYA4, 69
    FGFR2, 48
    FOXP2, 178
    genetic testing, 14
    GJA1, 216
    GJB2 (Cx26), 64, 187, 207, 215, 216,
            256, 260
    GJB3 (Cx31), 65, 216, 256
    GJB6 (Cx30), 64, 215, 216, 256
    harmonin, 57
    HDIA1, 216
    identifying, 11
    KCNQ4, 58, 86
    mapping, 11, 12
    MITF, 50

modifier, 71
MTO1, 71
MYH14, 67, 216
MYH9, 67, 86
MYO15A, 67, 216
MYO6, 67, 216
MYO7A, 26, 57, 67, 216
NDP, 58
OTOA (otoancorin), 68
OTOF (otoferlin), 69, 216, 263–268
PAX2, 256
PAX3, 26, 49, 215, 256
PCDH15, 26
PCDH15, 57, 66
PDS, 48, 208
Pendrin. See SLC26A4; PDS
POU, 69, 216, 308
PRES (prestin), 68
SANS, 57
SLC26A4, 26, 66, 215, 216, 256
SLC26A5, 216
SOX10, 50
STRC (stereocillin), 68
TECTA (alfa-Tectorin), 69, 216
TFB1M, 71
TFCP2L3, 69
TMC1 (transmembrane channel 1), 70, 86
TMIE (transmembrane inner ear), 70
TMPRSS3, 70
Usherin, 57
WFS1 (wolframin), 59, 70, 215
WFS2, 59
Whirlin. See WHRN
WHRN, 67
WLGR1, 57
ZFHX1B, 45
gene therapy, 299–304
genetic marker, 15
genetic testing, 164–166, 168–170, 213–217
genotype, 15
genotype-phenotype relationship,
        26, 208
gentamicin See aminoglycoside deafness
        (See also ototoxicity)
glutamate, 221, 228
glutathione, 225

H

haplo insufficiency, 16
haplotype, 16
hearing conservation programs, 102–103
hearing impairment
    progressive, 23
heterozygous, 16
homozygous, 16
hybridisation, 16
hydrocortisone. See corticosteroids

I

inheritance patterns, 4 (*See also* autosomal
        inheritance)
    maternal, 124
introns, 8, 16
isoforms, 16

L

language disorders, 178–181, 205
language development, 174–179
language processing, 177
latanoprost, 232–233
Leber hereditary optic neuropathy
        (LHON), 125
locus, 16
locus heterogeneity, 16
lod score, 16
Lyonisation, 16

M

malformation, 39
    Mondini, 208, 258
MAPK/JNK, 222–224, 273–274, 307
mapping. *See gene* mapping
marker, 16
medical risk factors, 83, 134
meiosis, 16
melatonine, 225
mendelian, 16
microarray. *See* DNA microarrays
microsatellites, 12, 16
microtia, 239
mitochondria, 121
    ageing, 130–131, 133–136
    ARHI, 129,
    heteroplasmy, 125
    mitochondrial deletions, 85
    mitochondrial gene, 101–102, 216
    mitochondrial mutations, 6, 70–71
    mitochondrial oxidative phosphorilation
        (OXPHOS), 121–126
    mitochondrial syndromes, 125–128,
        254–255
    mt DNA, 122–124
mitosis, 16
Mondini malformation. *See* malformation
mosaicism, 6, 16
    germinal, 16
mutations
    35delG. *See* GJB2
    235delC. *See* GJB2
    effect of, 13
    mechanics of, 13

N

N-acetylcysteine, 225
nanoparticle NP, 233–234
necrosis, 221, 305–306
neurofibromatosis 2, 157–158, 260
newborn hearing screening program, 170,
        206
NFG gene, 224
NGF, 229
NIHL. *See* noise-related hearing impairment
nitric oxide NO, 228
NMDA receptors, 229
noise, 93
    trauma, 230
noise-related hearing impairment, 91–109,
        220–221, 272–274, 308
nonpenetrance, 16
nucleotide, 16

O

OAE (otoacustic emissions), 26, 29, 96, 206,
        207
obligate carrier, 16
open reading frame, 16
ossicula malformations, 242–246
otoprotection, 301–302 (*See also* BDNG,
        NGF)
otosclerosis, 111–119, 156–157, 254
    aetiology, 112
    epidemiology, 113
    genetics, 115
    histopathology, 112
    loci, 113, 192
ototoxicity, 129–130, 274–275, 307
OTSC loci. *See* otosclerosis

P

pedigree, 5
penetrance, 16
    in otosclerosis, 115
perchlorate test, 48
phenocopy, 16
phenotype, 16
poly (A) tail, 6
polymerase chain reaction (PCR), 6
positional cloning, 2
prednisone. *See* corticosteroids
presbyacusis. *See* age-related HL
prenatal genetic testing (PND). *See* genetic
        testing
primary transcript, 16
probe, 16
promoter, 17

prostaglandins, 232–233
pseudogene, 17
pure-tone hearing threshold, 19

Q

quality of life, 146–147

R

recessive, 17
recruitment, 27
regeneration (inner ear), 302–303, 310
retinitis pigmentosa, 56–59
RNA, 6, 11
ROM reactive oxygen metabolites), 221
ROS (reactive oxygen species), 84, 219, 225,
        275, 307–308

S

sequence, 40
sibs (siblings), 17
SNPs (single nucleotide polymorphisms),
        12, 17, 85
specific language impairment (SLI), 177–180
specific reading isability (SRD), 180
speech audiometry, 33–35
    SRT (speech reception threshold), 34
stapedial reflexometry, 28
stapes, 111, 243
stem cells, 279–287, 289, 291–293, 310
syndrome, 40
    Alstrom, 58
    Angelman, 179
    Antley-Bixler, 47–48
    BOR, 52, 69
    DIDMOAD, 59
    Down, 179
    Duane, 52
    EVA, 66
    Jervell Lange Nielsen, 260
    Kearns-Sayre, 125, 127
    Keipert, 47
    Klinefelter, 179
    Marshall, 26
    MELAS, 127, 128
    MERF, 127
    Mohr-Tranebjaerg, 58
    Mowat-Wilson, 46–47
    Norrie, 58
    Otofaciocervical, 52
    Pendred, 48, 208
    Prader-Willi, 179

Refsum, 59
Stickler, 26, 68
Usher, 56–58, 209, 260
    USH1, 26, 56–57, 66–67,
    USH2 57
    USH3, 58
Waardwnburg, 26, 49–52, 209
Waardenburg-Shah, 50
Wolfram, 59, 70

T

TEN test, 28
TEOAE. *See* OAE
TFAM transcription factor A of
    mitochondria, 124

tinnitus, 149, 150, 154–156, 232, 275–276
TNF tumor necrosis factors,
    222, 226–227, 306
    antagonists, 226–227
tocopherols, 225
translation, 9
transcription, 7
transcription factor, 17
transplantation, 284, 289–297
tympanogram, 28–29

U

universal neonatal hearing screening
    (UNHS). *See* newborn hearing
    screening program

V

VEGF vascular endothelial growth factor,
    224–225
viral vectors, 300–301, 303
vision, 56–57
VRA visual reinforced audiometry,
    206–207

X

Xenotransplantation,
    284–285
X-inactivation, 17
X-linked inheritance, 17

T - #0255 - 071024 - C0 - 279/216/18 - PB - 9780367388997 - Gloss Lamination